# Clinical Neurology
## A Cure for Neurophobia[1]

## 2nd Edition

**Affiliate Professor Peter Gates** OAM MBBS FRACP FAAN

**Deakin University Geelong Victoria, Australia**

**Associate Professor Melbourne University Parkville, Victoria Australia**

**Visiting Neurologist St Vincents Hospital, Fitzroy, Victoria, Australia**

1  Two reviewers of the 1st edition stated it was a cure for neurophobia.

# Copyright

Author: Peter Gates

Title: Clinical Neurology: A Cure for Neurophobia / Peter Gates

prof.petergates@gmail.com
www.understanding neurology.com

BISG Codes:
MED005000 Medical / Anatomy
MED056000 Medical / Neurology
MED024000 Medical/Education and Training

Dewy Number: 616.8

---

**1st edition** © 2010 Elsevier Australia
ISBN: 9780729539357
Copyright was terminated April 6 2021

---

**2nd edition** published 2023 © 2021 Peter Gates
ISBN: 978-0-6455156-0-2

# Contents

# Foreword

There have been many attempts over the years to distil the knowledge needed for medical students and young doctors to begin to engage in neurological diagnosis and treatment.

This book by Professor Peter Gates is one of the best books developed to date. Peter Gates is an outstanding clinical neurologist and teacher who has been acknowledged in his own university as one of the leading teachers of undergraduates and registrars in recent times. He takes a classical approach to neurological diagnosis stressing the need for anatomical diagnosis and to learn as much as possible from the history in developing an understanding of likely pathophysiologies and aetiologies. In this book he sets out the lessons of a lifetime spent in clinical neurology and distils some of the principles that have led him to become a master diagnostician.

The first chapter is devoted to neuroanatomy from a clinical viewpoint. The concept of developing diagnosis through an understanding of the vertical and horizontal meridians of the nervous system is developed and intriguingly labelled under latitude and longitude. All the key issues around major anatomical diagnosis are distilled in a very understandable way for the novice. This chapter (and subsequent chapters) is widely illustrated with case studies and the illustrations are excellent. Key points are emphasised and important clinical questions stressed. A great deal of thought has gone into the clinical anecdotes chosen to illustrate major diagnostic issues. These reflect the learnings of a lifetime spent in neurological practice.

Subsequent chapters take the reader through the neurological examination and major neurological presentations and neurological disorders. Key aspects are illustrated with great clarity. This is a book that can be consulted from the index to get points about various disorders and their treatments but, more importantly, should be read from cover to cover by young doctors interested in coming to terms in a more major way with the diagnosis and treatment of neurological disorders. It also contains a lot of material that will be of interest to more experienced practitioners. The book has a clinical orientation and the references are comprehensive in listing most of the relevant key papers that the reader who wishes to pursue the basis of clinical neurology further may wish to consult. The final chapter is an excellent overview of how one can approach information gathering and keeping up-to-date using the complex information streams available to the medical student and young doctor today.

This book is clearly aimed at medical students and young doctors who have a special interest in developing further understanding of the workings of the nervous system, its disorders and their treatments. I would recommend it to senior medical students, to young doctors at all stages and also to those beginning their neurological training. It also has some information that may be of interest to the more senior neurologist in terms of developing their own approach to teaching young colleagues. It is the best introduction to the diagnosis and treatment of nervous system disorders that I have seen for many years and contains a font of wisdom about a speciality often perceived as difficult by the non-expert.

The second edition of this neurological classic builds on the first with an updated treatment guide and extension of Peter Gates diagnostic approach which has been widely taken up in the rule of four of the brain stem with new formulations for simplifying the approach to the neurology of the upper and lower limbs. In addition, some thoughts are developed that further understanding of a number of neurological disorders. This edition builds on the approach developed in the first edition of demystification of the examination and disorders of the nervous system guided by a master clinician who shares the learnings of a lifetime as a busy consultant neurologist.

It is of great potential value to both medical students interested in learning more of well thought out and more easily mastered approach to neurological disorders and more advanced trainee who has begun to  train for a life in neurological practise. As with the first edition, I commend it strongly to health professionals interested in learning more of neurological diagnosis from a well credentialed master in the field.

**Edward Byrne AC**

# Preface

The purpose of the first edition was to elucidate fundamental principles of clinical neurology that will remain relevant well into the future. Those basic principles remain in the second edition. The emphasis is on the clinical skills of history taking and the neurological examination. This book is the culmination of more than 40 years of clinical practice and teaching in neurology and is an attempt to make neurology more understandable, enjoyable, and logical. The aim is to provide an approach to the more common neurological problems starting from the symptoms that are encountered in everyday clinical practice. It describes how best to retrieve the most relevant information from the history, the neurological examination, investigations, colleagues, textbooks, and the Internet. This book in no way attempts to be a comprehensive textbook of neurology and as such is not intended for the practising neurologist. Investigations and treatments in the text will very quickly be out of date but the basic principles of clinical neurology developed more than 100 years ago are still relevant now and will be for many years to come.

The first edition sold out. One reviewer suggested the book was a cure for neurophobia, [1] a second reviewer suggested it could be the birth of a classic textbook. [2] Despite these and other wonderful and very kind reviews, Elsevier was unwilling to publish a second edition. I have received several requests for copies of the book. Thus, I obtained the copyright from Elsevier and have elected to self-publish a second edition. I have altered the title to Clinical Neurology, a primer, second edition. A cure for neurophobia.

The book contains my rule of 4 of the brainstem, downloaded more than 100,000 times from Internal Medicine Journal [3] and published on request in Practical Neurology [4] and Notfall Rettungsmed. [5] Since the first edition, I have created two new rules. The first is the 5*3*5 rule for examining the upper limbs [6] and the 2*2*4 rule for examining the lower limbs (unpublished). These rules enable the diagnosis of every nerve and nerve root problem causing weakness in the limbs without the need for detailed knowledge of neuroanatomy. All that is required is to ascertain the exact muscles that are weak and consult the tables.

The appendices and text dealing with investigation and management have been updated to reflect current guidelines at the time of writing. I have added four new appendices. The treatment of Parkinson's. Two are my published hypotheses regarding the aetiology of Meniere's disease [7] and essential hypertension. [8] My theory regarding the possible role of temporary lumbar drainage in the management of Idiopathic Intracranial Hypertension (IIH).

I have also added text boxes labelled contrarian thoughts where I express my views that are at odds to current opinion. It is important to note that these are my views only. They are in text boxes to indicate that they may change and are not proven.

This book takes a very different approach to most neurology texts and contains many simple concepts that are intended to assist medical students, nurses, allied health students, chiropractors, osteopaths, neurology residents and registrars, general practitioners (family doctors) and general physicians in understanding neurology and improving their ability to diagnose the common neurological problems they will encounter in their everyday practice. It contains concepts that other neurologists might wish to incorporate into their teaching.

# References

1.  Wijeratne, T., *Book Review:A cure for neurophobia.* MJA, 2011. 194(4): p. 193.

2.  Scalding, N., *Book Review: Clinical neurology: a primer.* Pract Neurol, 2011. 11: p. 178-179.

3.  Gates, P., *The rule of 4 of the brainstem: a simplified method for understanding brainstem anatomy and brainstem vascular syndromes for the non-neurologist.* Intern Med J, 2005. 35(4): p. 263-6.

4.  Gates, P., *Work out where the problem is in the brainstem using 'the rule of 4'.* Pract Neurol, 2011. 11(3): p. 167-72.

5.  Gates, P., *Recognising brainstem problems in the emergency department using the rule of 4 of the brainstem.* Notfall + Rettungsmedizin, 2015. 18(5): p. 364-369.

6.  Gates, P., *5.3.5 Rule for examining the muscles of the upper limb.* Postgrad Med J, 2019. 95(1127): p. 465-468.

7.  Gates, P., *Hypothesis: could Meniere's disease be a channelopathy?* Intern Med J, 2005. 35(8): p. 488-9.

8.  Gates, P.C., *Arteriosclerosis is the cause not the consequence of Essential Hypertension.* Medical Hypotheses, 2020. 144(110236).

# Acknowledgements

I would like to thank my colleagues the late John Balla, Ross Carne, Richard Gerraty and Richard McDonnell for reviewing sections of the manuscript. The 1st edition was published by Elsevier, and I would like to acknowledge and thank Sophie Kaliniecki for accepting my book proposal, Sabrina Chew, Eleanor Cant and Linda Littlemore for all the support and encouragement they provided during the writing of the manuscript, and also to Greg Gaul for the illustrations. I would particularly like to thank Stephen Due, Joan Deane, Helen Skoglund and Serena Griffin at the Geelong Hospital library who have been a tremendous support over many years, especially but not only during the writing of this book. Also, I thank the radiologists and radiographers at Barwon Medical Imaging for providing most of the medical images. My thanks also to the many patients and friends who generously consented to have pictures or video taken to incorporate in this book. Kevin Sturges from GGI Media Geelong (https://ggi-media.com/), a friend and technological whiz, helped me with all the images and video production. Sandra Coventry of Nitty Gritty Graphics (http://nittygrittygraphics.com.au/) for her wonderful illustrations and last but not least my son Jeremy Gates who maintains my website (www.understandingneurology.com)

Thank you also to the students and colleagues who anonymously reviewed the manuscript for their many wonderful suggestions and words of encouragement.

I have indeed been fortunate to have been taught by many outstanding teachers during my training and, although to name them individually runs the risk of omission and causing offence, there are a few that I would like to acknowledge: Robert Newnham, rheumatologist at the Repatriation General Hospital in Heidelberg who, in 1975, first taught the symptom-oriented approach while I was a final-year medical student; at St Vincent's Hospital in Melbourne the late John Billings, neurologist, who introduced me to the excitement of neurology and John Niall, nephrologist, for challenging me to justify a particular treatment with evidence from the literature; the late Arthur Schweiger, the late John Balla, the late Les Sedal, Rob Helme, Russell Rollinson and Henryk Kranz (neurologists) for the opportunity to enter neurology training at Prince Henry's Hospital Melbourne where John Balla encouraged me to write my first paper; the late Lord John Walton, neurologist, for the opportunity to work and study in Newcastle upon Tyne; Peter Fawcett, neurophysiologist, for the opportunity to study neurophysiology; Dr Mike Barnes, neurologist in rehabilitation, who helped in 1983 at the Newcastle General Hospital to make the video of John Walton taking a history.

I also wish to thank the late Henry Barnett, neurologist, in London, Ontario, for the opportunity to work on the EC-IC bypass study; and Dave Sackett, Wayne Taylor and Brian Haynes in the department of epidemiology at McMaster University for opening my eyes to clinical epidemiology and evidence-based medicine. And last but not least my long standing friend Ed Byrne, for his friendship and wise council over many years.

This book is dedicated to my children, Bernard, Amelia and Jeremy, and my wife Rosie, for without their support over the many years this project would not have been possible.

x

# Changes in the 2nd edition

The 5*3*5 rule for examining the upper limbs enables diagnosis of every nerve and nerve root problem causing weakness in the arm without the need for detailed neuro-anatomy.[1] and

The 2*2*4 rule for examining the lower limbs (unpublished) enables diagnosis of every nerve and nerve root problem causing weakness in the leg without the need for detailed neuro-anatomy

My Hypothesis that Meniere's disease is a sodium dependent channelopathy. [2]

My hypothesis that essential hypertension is the consequence not the cause of arteriosclerosis with secondary atherosclerosis. [3]

A discussion on a possible role for a temporary lumbar drain in the management of idiopathic intracranial hypertension.[4-6]

Contrarian thought boxes where I question current dogma.

Updated treatments contained in the text boxes and in the appendices included an additional appendix discussing the treatment of Parkinson's disease.

The text has been modified in several places where what had been written was not as clear as one would desire.

## Corrections:

The caption to figure 8.1.

Figure 11.8 was duplicated in the 1st edition, figure 11.9 now contains the correct image

1.  Gates, P., *5.3.5 Rule for examining the muscles of the upper limb.* Postgrad Med J, 2019. 95(1127): p. 465-468.
2.  Gates, P., *Hypothesis: could Meniere's disease be a channelopathy?* Intern Med J, 2005. 35(8): p. 488-9.
3.  Gates, P.C., *Arteriosclerosis is the cause not the consequence of Essential Hypertension.* Medical Hypotheses, 2020. 144(110236).
4.  Lee, S.W., et al., *Idiopathic intracranial hypertension; immediate resolution of venous sinus "obstruction" after reducing cerebrospinal fluid pressure to<10cmH(2)O.* J Clin Neurosci, 2009. 16(12): p. 1690-2.
5.  Gates, P. and P. McNeill, *A Possible Role for Temporary Lumbar Drainage in the Management of Idiopathic Intracranial Hypertension.* Neuroophthalmology, 2016. 40(6): p. 277-280.
6.  Gates, P., P. McNeill, and N. Shuey, *Indication to use a non-pencil-point lumbar puncture needle.* Pract Neurol, 2019. 19(2): p. 176-177.

The videos that accompany this book can be found at:

http://www.understandingneurology.com/textbook-videos/

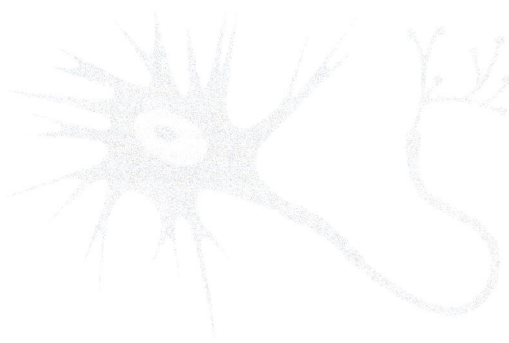

# Clinically Oriented Neuroanatomy

## 'Meridians of Longitude and Parallels of Latitude'

| Key Terms | |
|---|---|
| **Meridians of Longitude:** | The descending motor pathway and the two ascending sensory pathways. |
| **Parallels of Latitude:** | The dermatomes, myotomes and reflexes in the limbs, the dermatomes on the trunk, the cranial nerves in the brainstem, the cerebellum and the cortical symptoms and signs in the cerebral hemispheres. |
| **Central nervous system:** | The spinal cord (excluding the anterior horn cells and dorsal sensory nerve roots), brainstem, cerebellum, and cerebral hemispheres. |
| **Peripheral nervous system:** | The anterior horn cells, anterior motor nerve roots and dorsal sensory nerve roots in the spinal cord, the brachial and lumbosacral plexuses, the peripheral nerves, neuromuscular junction, and muscle. |
| **Upper motor neuron (UMN):** | Strictly speaking, this refers to motor signs, but is often used with symptoms and signs from problems within the central nervous system. |
| **Lower motor neuron(LMN):** | Once again, strictly speaking this refers to motor signs but is used with symptoms and signs from problems within the peripheral nervous system. |
| **Dermatomes:** | The nerve roots that supply sensation to particular parts of the skin on the limbs and trunk. |
| **Myotomes:** | The nerve roots that innervate the individual muscles. |
| ⚷ | Key Point(s) |

Although most textbooks on clinical neurology begin with a chapter on history taking, there is an excellent reason for neuroanatomy being the initial chapter. It is because *clinical neurologists use their detailed knowledge of neuroanatomy when examining a patient and when obtaining a neurological history* to determine the site of the problem within the nervous system. This chapter describes a unique approach to neuroanatomy, likening the nervous system to a map grid with

1

meridians of longitude and parallels of latitude. The site of the problem is where the meridians of longitude meet the parallel(s) of latitude. Examples will be given to explain this concept. It explains upper vs lower motor neuron signs. There is a brief discussion of the anatomy of the central and peripheral nervous systems.

---

The underlying principle of clinical neurology is to evaluate every symptom in terms of its nature (i.e., weakness, altered sensation, visual problems etc.) and its distribution(i.e. what is the exact area of the body affected by those symptoms) to determine the site of the lesion in the nervous system.

Although the nature and distribution of the symptoms and signs (if present) indicate the site of the problem within the nervous system, they DO NOT indicate the underlying pathology.

---

In clinical neurology, it is essential to understand the difference between upper and lower motor neuron signs. The terms are more often (and not unreasonably) used to refer to the central and peripheral nervous systems, CNS and PNS, respectively. More specifically, upper motor neuron refers to motor signs that result from disorders affecting the motor pathway above the level of the anterior horn cell, i.e., within the brain or spinal cord of the CNS. In contrast, lower motor neurons refer to motor symptoms and signs related to PNS disorders, the anterior horn cell, motor nerve root, brachial or lumbosacral plexus or peripheral nerve (see Table 1.1). The pattern of weakness, tone, reflexes, and plantar responses (scratching the lateral aspect of the sole to see which way the big toe points) are different in upper and lower motor neuron problems.

---

The pathology is always at the level of the lower motor neuron signs and above the upper motor neuron signs.

---

The 'student of neurology' cannot be expected to remember detailed neuroanatomy. However, understanding the basic concepts presented in these first few chapters, combined with the correct technique when taking the neurological history (Chapter 2) and performing the neurological examination (Chapter 3–5), together with the illustrations in this chapter will enable the 'non-neurologist to localise the site of the problem in most patients almost as well as a neurologist. This book and in particular this chapter is intended to serve as a resource and be kept on the desk or next to the examination couch. Three rules also eliminate the necessity for detailed knowledge of neuroanatomy. These are the 'rule of 4 of the brainstem', the '5*3*5' rule of the upper limb and the '2*2*4 rule' of the lower limb. Using these rules and consulting the anatomy illustrations in this book will enable any non-neurologist to localise the site of the problem accurately.

---

**Contrarian Thought**

It has never made sense to me why handgrip is in the neurological observation charts. It will be one of the last muscles to become weak with an UMN problem.

---

| Table 1.1 Upper and Lower Motor Neuron Signs | | |
|---|---|---|
| | **Upper Motor Neuron** | **Lower Motor Neuron.** |
| Weakness | The UMN pattern** | Either in the distribution of a peripheral nerve(s) or nerve root(s) |
| Tone | Increased | Decreased |
| Reflexes | Increased | Decreased or absent |
| Plantar Response | Upgoing | Down-going |
| Pain and temperature | Sensory level if present | Either in the distribution of a nerve(s) or nerve root(s). |
| Vibration and proprioception | Reduced or absent below the site of the pathology | Reduced or absent in extremities with neuropathy. |

**The UMN pattern of weakness in the arms is initially weakness of wrist and finger extension. If the weakness is more severe, shoulder abduction followed by elbow extension weakness occur. In the legs, as the weakness increases, hip flexion is followed by weakness of dorsiflexion of the feet and then weakness of knee flexion. When the arm or leg is totally paralysed, all muscles are weak. Thus, the first muscle group to be affected in the arms is extension of the fingers and wrist, whilst it is hip flexion in the legs. If the strength in these two muscle groups is normal in patients with suspected central nervous system problems, there is no need to test any more muscles.

Case 1.1 illustrates how these concepts work

**CASE 1.1** A patient presents with difficulty walking

A 65-year-old man presents with weakness in his legs. His doctor requests a computerised tomography (CT) scan of the lumbosacral spine, which is normal. A CT scan of the lumbosacral spine will only detect problems affecting the peripheral nervous system (including the cauda equina) as it only scans between the 3rd lumbar nerve root (L3) and the first sacral (S1) nerve root.

The patient is referred for a specialist opinion. When examined, there are signs of a UMN problem with weakness of hip flexion and dorsiflexion of the feet, increased tone and reflexes indicating the involvement of the motor pathway (meridian of longitude) in the central and *not* the peripheral nervous system.

The lesion *has to be above the 1st lumbar vertebrae*, the level at which the spinal cord ends. Imaging has been performed below this level and thus missed the problem. The appropriate investigation is to look at the spinal cord above this level.

# Meridians of Longitude and Parallels of Latitude

The nervous system can be likened to a map grid (see Figure 1.1). Establishing the 'meridians of longitude' and 'parallels of latitude' from the history and examination will localise the pathological process.

# The Meridians of Longitude

The three meridians of longitude are:
1. The descending motor pathway from the motor cortex to the muscle
2. The ascending sensory pathway for pain and temperature[1] from the peripheral sensory organs to the cortex
3. The ascending sensory pathway for vibration and proprioception from the peripheral sensory organs to the cortex

# The Parallels of Latitude

## Central Nervous System

In the central nervous system (brain and spinal cord) the cerebral cortex and the cranial nerves of the brainstem are the parallels of latitude.

## Peripheral Nervous System

In the peripheral nervous system, the nerve roots and peripheral nerves are the parallels of latitude.

Using these pathways, we need to appreciate that:
- If the patient has weakness, the pathological process must affect the motor pathway between the cortex and the muscle.
- The pathology must be somewhere between the sensory nerves in the periphery and the cortical sensory structures if there are sensory symptoms.
- The presence of motor and sensory symptoms or signs together immediately rules out conditions confined to muscle, the neuromuscular junction, the motor nerve root, and the anterior horn cell because there are no nerves related to sensation at these sites.

Figure 1.1 shows the meridians of longitude and parallels of latitude.

The following examples combine weakness with various parallels of latitude to help explain this concept. The parallels of latitude follow the + sign.
- Weakness + marked wasting = the peripheral nervous system, as marked wasting does not occur with central nervous system problems
- Weakness + cranial nerve involvement = brainstem
- Weakness + visual field disturbance (not diplopia) or speech disturbance (i.e., dysphasia) = cortex
- Weakness in both legs + loss of pain and temperature sensation on the torso = spinal cord
- Weakness in a limb + sensory loss in a single nerve (mononeuritis) or nerve root (radiculopathy) distribution = peripheral nervous system

---

1  The ascending sensory pathway for pain and temperature may not according to some anatomy textbooks extend all the way to the subcortical region but not to the cortex.

MERIDIANS OF LONGITUDE

MOTOR PATHWAY

SENSORY PATHWAYS
Vibration & proprioception
Pain & temperature

PARALLELS OF LATITUDE

BRAIN

Cortex

Internal capsule

Brainstem

Foramen magnum

Motor and sensory nerve roots
- Myotomes

- Dermatomes

- Reflexes

Anterior horn cell

SPINAL CORD

Brachial and lumbosacral plexuses

Peripheral nerves

Neuromuscular junction

Muscle

PERIPHERAL NERVOUS SYSTEM

Peripheral sensory receptors

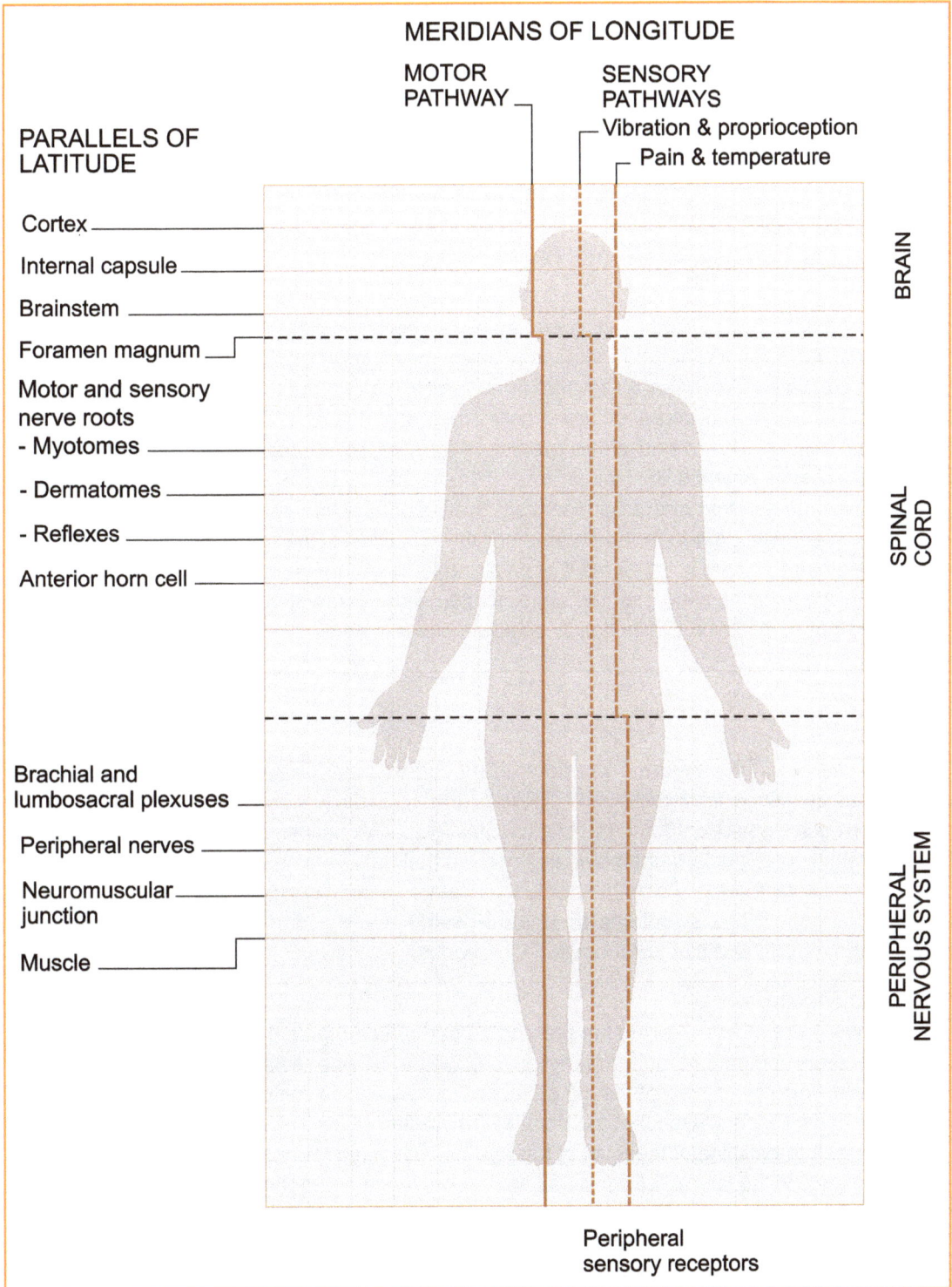

Figure 1.1 Meridians of Longitude and parallels of latitude. *Note:* The descending motor pathway and the Ascending sensory pathway for vibration and proprioception both cross at the level of the foramen magnum. The Ascending sensory pathway for pain and temperature sensation (the spinothalamic tract) crosses immediately it enters the spinal cord.

It is the pattern of weakness and sensory symptoms and/or signs affecting these ascending and descending pathways together with the parallels of latitude that are used to determine the site of the pathology.

# The Meridians of Longitude
# Localising the pathways affected

The descending motor pathway (also referred to as the corticospinal tract) and the ascending sensory pathways represent the meridians of longitude. The dermatomes, myotomes, reflexes, brainstem cranial nerves, basal ganglia and the cortical signs represent the parallels of latitude. The motor pathways and dorsal columns both cross at the level of the foramen magnum, the junction between the lower end of the brainstem and the spinal cord. The spinothalamic tract crosses soon after entering the spinal cord. If there are left-sided upper motor neuron signs or impairment of vibration and proprioception, the lesion is either on the left side of the spinal cord below the level of the foramen magnum or the right side of the brain above the level of the foramen magnum. If there is impairment of pain and temperature sensation affecting the left side of the body, the lesion is always on the opposite side either in the spinal cord or brain. If the face is also weak or numb the problem has to be above the mid pons.

# The Motor Pathway

The motor pathway (see Figure 1.2) refers to the corticospinal tract within the central nervous system that descends from the motor cortex to the contralateral lower motor neurons in the ventral horn of the spinal cord and the corticobulbar tract that descends from the motor cortex to several cranial nerve nuclei in the pons and medulla that innervate muscles plus the motor nerve roots, plexuses, peripheral nerves, neuromuscular junction, and muscle in the peripheral nervous system. If a patient has symptoms or signs of weakness, the problem must be somewhere between the muscle and the motor cortex in the contralateral frontal lobe (see Figure 1.2).

The motor pathway:
- arises in the motor cortex in the pre-central gyrus (see Figure 1.5) of the frontal lobe
- descends in the cerebral hemispheres through the corona radiata and internal capsule
- passes into the brainstem via the crus cerebri (level of the midbrain) and descends in the ventral and medial aspect of the pons and medulla
- Crosses the midline at the level of the foramen magnum (decussation of pyramids)
- descends in the lateral column of the spinal cord to the anterior horn cell where it synapses with the lower motor neuron
- leaves the spinal cord through the anterior (motor) nerve root
- passes through the brachial plexus to the arm and the lumbosacral plexus to the leg and via the peripheral nerves to the neuromuscular junction and muscle.

Cases 1.2 and 1.3 illustrate how to use the meridians of longitude.

---

**CASE 1.2** A patient with upper motor neuron signs

A patient has weakness affecting the right arm and leg, associated with increased tone and reflexes (upper motor neuron signs).

This indicates a problem along the motor pathway in the CNS, either in the upper cervical spinal cord on the same side above the level of C5 or on the left side of the brain above the level of the foramen magnum (where the motor pathway crosses).

If the right side of the face is also affected, the lesion cannot be in the spinal cord and must be in the upper pons or higher on the left side because the facial nerve nucleus is at the level of the mid pons. In the absence of any other symptoms or signs, this is as close as we can localise the problem. It could be in the midbrain, internal capsule, corona radiata or cortex.

If present, the parallels of latitude would be a left 3rd nerve indicating a left midbrain lesion (this is known as Weber's syndrome). Dysphasia (speech disturbance) or cortical sensory signs (see Chapter 5) indicating a cortical lesion.

---

**CASE 1.3** A patient with weakness in the right hand without sensory symptoms or signs

A patient has weakness in the right hand in the absence of any sensory symptoms or signs. In addition to the weakness, the patient has noticed marked wasting of the muscle between the thumb and index finger.

Weakness indicates involvement of the motor system and the lesion has to be somewhere along the 'pathway' between the muscles of the hand and the contralateral motor cortex. The absence of sensory symptoms suggests the problem may be in a muscle, neuromuscular junction, motor nerve root or anterior horn cell, the more common sites that cause weakness in the absence of sensory symptoms or signs. Motor weakness without sensory symptoms can also occur with peripheral nerve lesions.

Wasting is a lower motor neuron sign, a parallel of latitude, and indicates that the problem is in the PNS (marked wasting does not occur with problems in the neuromuscular junction or with disorders of muscle; it usually points to a problem in the anterior horn cell, motor nerve root, brachial plexus, or peripheral nerve). Plexus or peripheral nerve lesions are usually, but not always, associated with sensory symptoms or signs.

The examination demonstrates weakness of all the interosseous muscles, the abductor digiti minimi muscle and flexor digitorum profundus muscle with weakness flexing the distal phalanx of the 2nd, 3rd, 4th and 5th digits, which are referred to as the long flexors. All these muscles are innervated by the C8–T1 nerve roots, but the long flexors of the 2nd and 3rd digits are innervated by the median nerve while the long flexors of the 4th and 5th digits are innervated by the ulnar nerve (see the 5*3*5 rule in chapter 3). The parallel of latitude is the wasting and weakness in the distribution of the C8–T1 nerve roots.

---

# The Sensory Pathways

There are two sensory pathways: one conveys vibration and proprioception and the other pain and temperature sensation; both convey light touch sensation.

## Proprioception and Vibration

The pathway (see Figure 1.3):
- arises in the peripheral sensory receptors in the joint capsules and surrounding ligaments and tendons (proprioception) or the Pacinian corpuscles in the subcutaneous tissue (vibration) [1]
- ascends up the limb in the peripheral nerves
- traverses the brachial or lumbosacral plexus
- enters the spinal cord through the dorsal (sensory) nerve root

- ascends in the *ipsilateral* dorsal column of the spinal cord with the sacral fibres pushed medially by neurons entering the cord higher up with the cervical fibres most lateral
- The dorsal columns <u>cross the midline at the level of the foramen magnum</u>, where the spinal cord meets the brainstem
- ascends in the medial lemniscus in the medial aspect of the brainstem and via the thalamus to the sensory cortex in the parietal lobe.
- Abnormalities of vibration and proprioception may occur with peripheral neuropathies but rarely are they affected with isolated nerve or nerve root lesions. Pain and Temperature Sensation

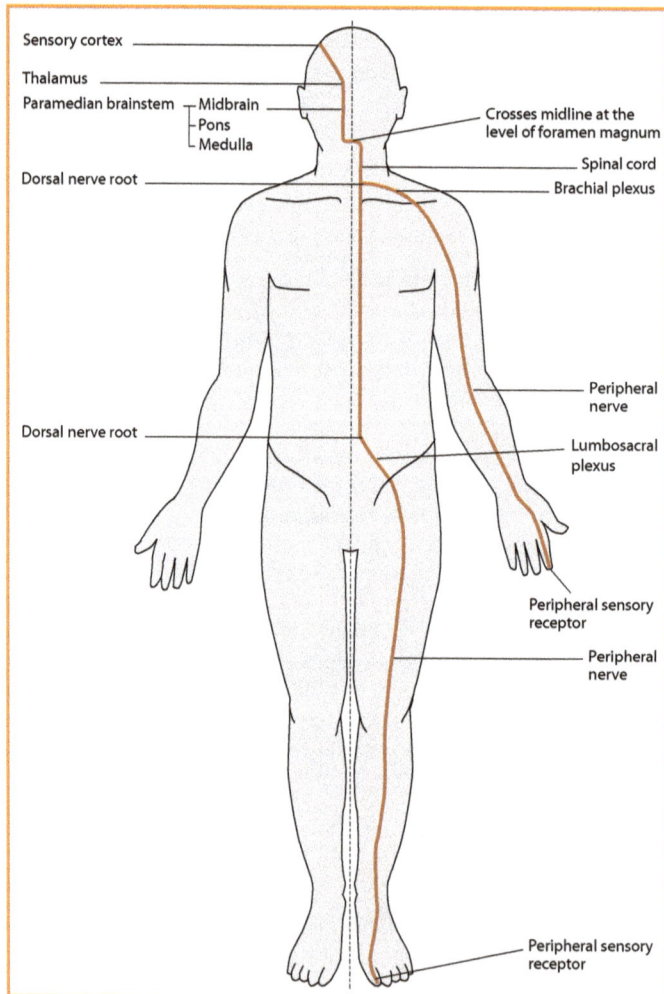

**Figure 1.2:** The motor pathway. Note that the pathway crosses at the level of the foramen magnum where the spinal cord meets the lower end of the medulla.

The spinothalamic pathway (see Figure 1.4):
- includes the nerves conveying pain and temperature that arise in the peripheral sensory receptors in the skin and deeper structures [1]
- coalesces to form the peripheral nerves in the limbs or the nerve root nerves of the trunk
- from the limbs, traverses the brachial or lumbosacral plexus
- enters the spinal cord through the dorsal (sensory) nerve root

- <u>crosses the midline close to the point of entry into the spinal cord</u>
- ascends in the spinothalamic tract located in the anterolateral aspect of the spinal cord, with nerves from higher in the body pushing those from lower laterally in the spinal cord
- ascends in the lateral aspect of the brainstem to the thalamus.

---

The spinothalamic tracts cross the midline almost immediately after entering the spinal cord.

If a patient has impairment of pain and temperature sensation, the lesion must either be in the ipsilateral peripheral nerve or the sensory nerve root or contralateral in the CNS between the level of entry into the spinal cord and the cerebral hemisphere (see Figure 1.4).

---

- Although there is some debate about whether the spinothalamic tract projects to the cortex, abnormal pain and temperature sensation can occur with deep white matter hemisphere lesions and in this setting often affect the trunk to the midline.
- If the history and/or examination detects unilateral impairment of the sensory modalities affecting the face, arm, and leg, this can only localise the problem to above the 5th cranial nerve nucleus in the mid pons of the brainstem on the contralateral side to the symptoms and signs, i.e., there is no 'parallel of latitude' to help localise the problem more accurately than that. The presence of a hemianopia and/or cortical sensory signs would be the parallels of latitude that would indicate that the pathology is in the cerebral hemispheres affecting the parietal lobe and cortex.
- Case 1.4 illustrates a patient with both motor and sensory pathways affected.

---

**CASE 1.4** A 70-year-old woman with difficulty walking

A 70-year-old woman presents with difficulty walking due to weakness and stiffness in both legs. There is no weakness in her upper limbs. She has been instable in the dark and has a sensation of tight stockings around her legs. The examination reveals bilateral weakness of hip flexion associated with increased tone and reflexes and upgoing plantar responses.

There is impairment of vibration and proprioception in the legs and there is decreased pain sensation in both legs and on both sides of the abdomen up to the level of the umbilicus on the front of the abdomen and several centimeters higher than this on the back.

The weakness in both legs indicates that the motor pathway is affected.

The increased tone and reflexes are upper motor neuron signs and, therefore, the problem must be in the CNS not the PNS, either the spinal cord or brain.

The fact that the signs are bilateral indicates that the motor pathways on both sides of the nervous system are affected and the most likely place for this to occur is in the spinal cord, although it can also occur in the brainstem and the medial aspect of the cerebral hemispheres. (For more information on the cortical representation of the legs, not illustrated in this book, look up the term 'cortical homunculus' which is a physical representation of the primary motor cortex.)

The alteration of vibration and proprioception also indicates that the relevant sensory pathway is involved.

The impairment of pain sensation is the 3rd meridian of longitude and indicates that the spinothalamic tract is involved.

The upper motor neuron pattern of weakness and involvement of the pathway conveying vibration and proprioception in the legs simply indicate that the problem is above the level of L1. The sensory level on the trunk at the level of the umbilicus is the parallel of latitude and localises the lesion to the 10th thoracic spinal cord level (see Figures 1.12 and 1.13).

This is not an uncommon presentation. It is said that a thoracic cord lesion in a middle-aged or elderly female is due to a meningioma until proven otherwise.

Sensory cortex

Thalamus

Paramedian brainstem — Midbrain
— Pons
— Medulla

Crosses midline at the
level of foramen magnum

Spinal cord

Dorsal nerve root

Brachial plexus

Peripheral
nerve

Dorsal nerve root

Lumbosacral
plexus

Peripheral sensory
receptor

Peripheral
nerve

Peripheral sensory
receptor

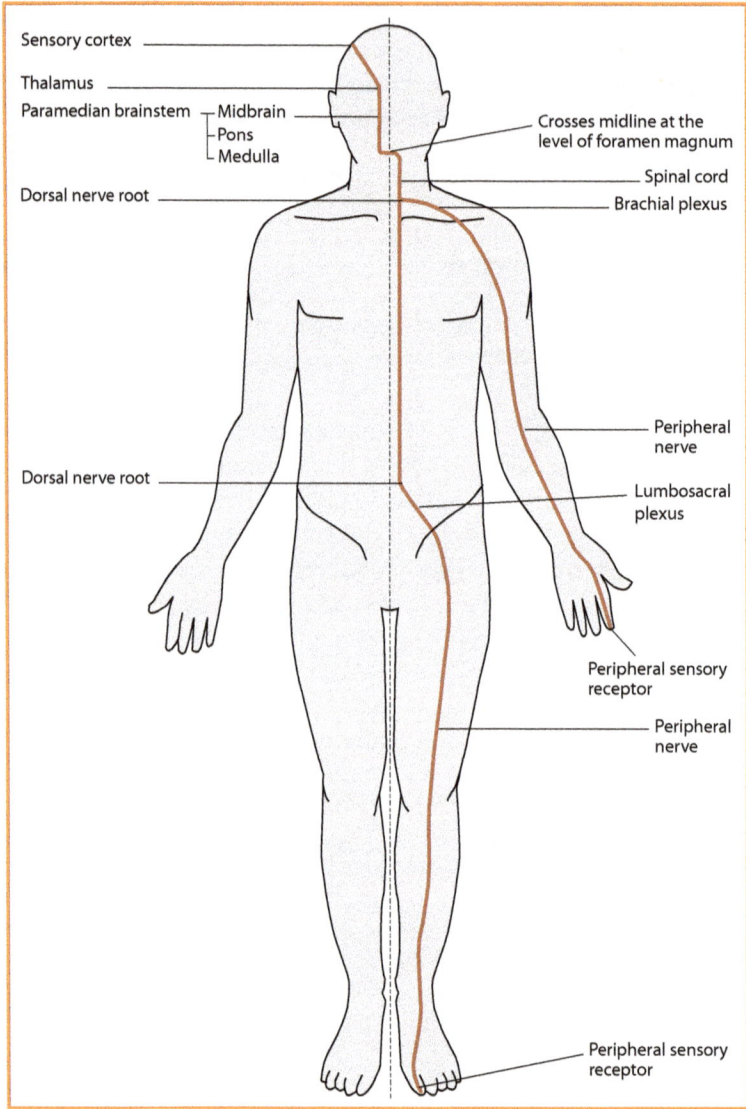

**Figure 1.3** Pathway conveying Proprioception and Vibration.

# The Parallels of Latitude:
## Finding the Site of Pathology

The parallels of latitude refer to the structures within the CNS and PNS that indicate the site of the pathology. For example, if the patient has a right hemiparesis and a non-fluent dysphasia, it is the dysphasia that indicates that the weakness must be related to a problem in the dominant left frontal cortex.

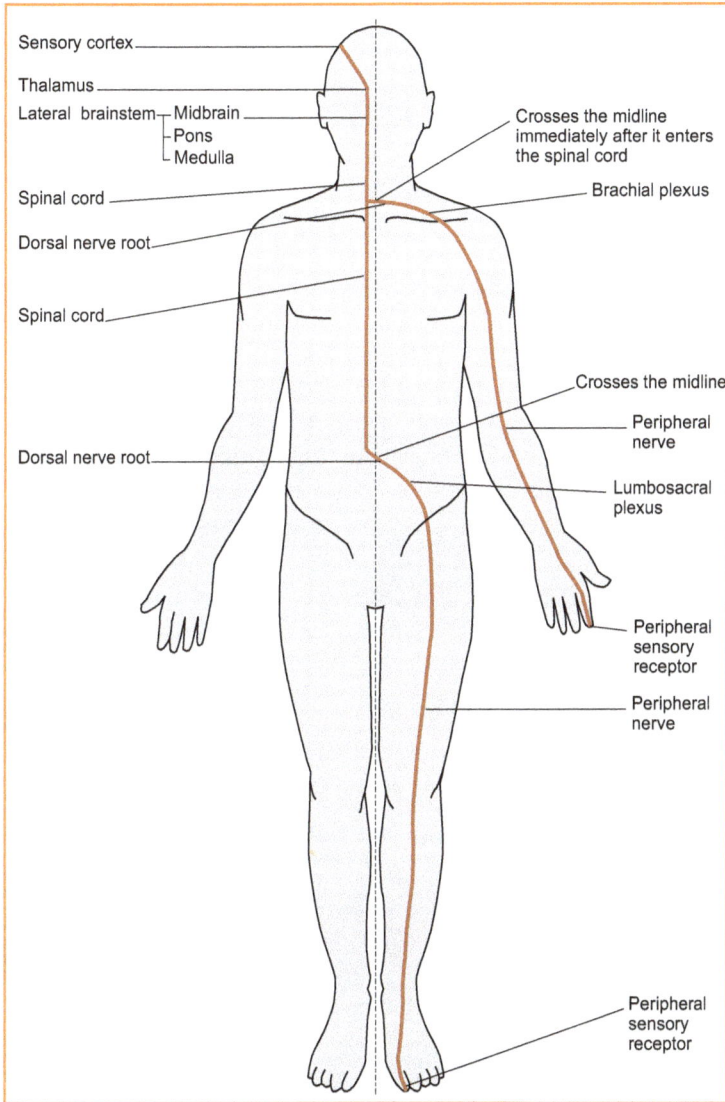

**Figure 1.4** The Spinothalamic Pathway

**In the CNS, the parallels of latitude consist of:**
- **the cortex** — vision, memory, personality, speech, and specific cortical sensory and visual phenomena such as visual and sensory inattention, graphaesthesia etc. (see Chapter 5).
- **the cranial nerves** of the brainstem (see Chapter 4) — each cranial nerve is at a different level in the brainstem and thus represents a parallel of latitude. For example, if the patient has a LMN 7th nerve palsy the problem either has to be in the 7th nerve or the brainstem at the level of the pons.

**In the PNS the parallels of latitude consist of:**
- **The motor and sensory nerves** when affected will result in a very focal pattern of weakness and or sensory loss that indicates that the problem is in the peripheral nerve (Chapter 11 and Chapter 12).

11

- **The nerve roots include:**
- **myotomes** — motor nerve roots supplying muscles produce a classic pattern of the weakness affecting several muscles supplied by that nerve root; specific nerve roots are part of the reflex arc and if, for example, the patient has an absent biceps reflex the lesion is at the level of C5–6.
  - **dermatomes** — areas of abnormal sensation from the involvement of sensory nerve roots (Figures 1.12, 1.13 and 1.22).

# Parallels of Latitude in the Central Nervous System

If a patient has a problem within the CNS, involvement of either the cortex or the brainstem will produce symptoms and signs that will enable accurate localisation. For example, the patient who presents with weakness involving the right face, arm and leg has a problem affecting the motor pathway (the meridian of longitude) on the left side of the brain above the mid pons. The presence of a left 3rd nerve palsy (the parallel of latitude) would indicate the lesion is on the left side of the mid-brain while the presence of a non-fluent dysphasia (another parallel of latitude) would localise the problem to the left frontal cortex. Case 1.5 illustrates how to use the parallels of latitude in the CNS.

---

**CASE 1.5** A man with right facial and arm weakness, vision, and speech impairment

A 65-year-old man presents with weakness of his face and arm on the right side together with an inability to see to the right and a disturbance of his speech. He knows what he wants to say but is having difficulty expressing the words. The examination detects impairment of vibration and proprioception sensation in the right hand.

The weakness of his face and arm indicates a lesion affecting the motor pathway or meridian of longitude on the left side of the brain above the mid pons.

The difficulty expressing his words indicates the presence of a non-fluent dysphasia (the parallel of latitude), accurately localising the problem to the left frontal cortex.

The inability to see to the right is another parallel of latitude and it reflects the involvement of the visual pathways between the optic chiasm and the left occipital lobe, resulting in right homonymous hemianopia (Chapter 5).

The impairment of vibration and proprioception in the right hand indicates that the meridian of longitude conveying this sensation is affected. Since the other symptoms and signs point to a left-hemisphere lesion, the abnormality of vibration and proprioception indicates involvement of the parietal lobe, and this also would indicate that the visual disturbance is almost certainly in the left parietal lobe and not the occipital lobe. This sort of presentation is very typical of a cerebral infarct affecting the middle cerebral artery territory (see Chapter 10).

---

## The Hemispheres

Figure 1.5 is a simplified diagram showing the main lobes of the brain and the cortical function associated with those areas. If the patient has cortical hemisphere symptoms and signs this establishes the site of the pathology in the cortex of a particular region of the brain.

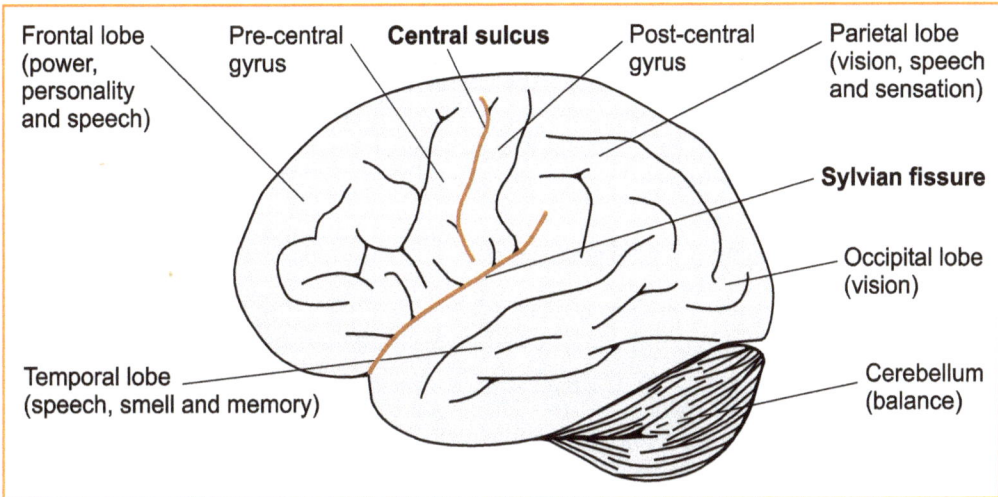

**Figure 1.5** The left lateral aspect of the cerebral hemisphere. *Note*: The central sulcus separates the frontal lobe from the parietal lobe (see Chapter 5, 'The cerebral hemispheres and cerebellum').

## The Brainstem

Figure 1.6 shows the site of the cranial nerves in the brainstem with the numbers added: the 9th, 10th, 11th and 12th cranial nerves at the level of the medulla; the 5th, 6th, 7th and 8th at the level of the pons; and the 3rd and 4th at the level of the midbrain (see Chapter 4 for a detailed discussion of the brainstem and cranial nerves). Also note that the 3rd, 6th and 12th cranial nerves exit the brainstem close to the midline while the other cranial nerves exit the lateral aspect of the brainstem. The importance of this will become apparent when we discuss the rule of 4 of the brainstem in chapter 4.

# Parallels of Latitude in the Peripheral Nervous System

## Cranial Nerves

The presence of cranial nerves signs means the pathology must be at the level of that cranial nerve, either in the nerve itself or in the brainstem.

The exception to this rule is the 6th nerve palsy that is a false localising sign with raised intracranial pressure and the 3rd for nerve palsy which can occur with transtentorial herniation (where a mass lesion in the hemisphere causes raised intracranial pressure resulting and coning that is downward herniation of the brain through the tentorium.

In Figure 1.7 the important points to note are:
*   The 1st division of the trigeminal nerve extends over the scalp to somewhere between the vertex and two-thirds of the way back towards the occipital region where it meets the greater occipital nerve supplied by the 2nd cervical nerve root. In a trigeminal nerve lesion, the sensory loss will not extend to the occipital region, whereas it will with a spinothalamic/quintothalamic tract problem.

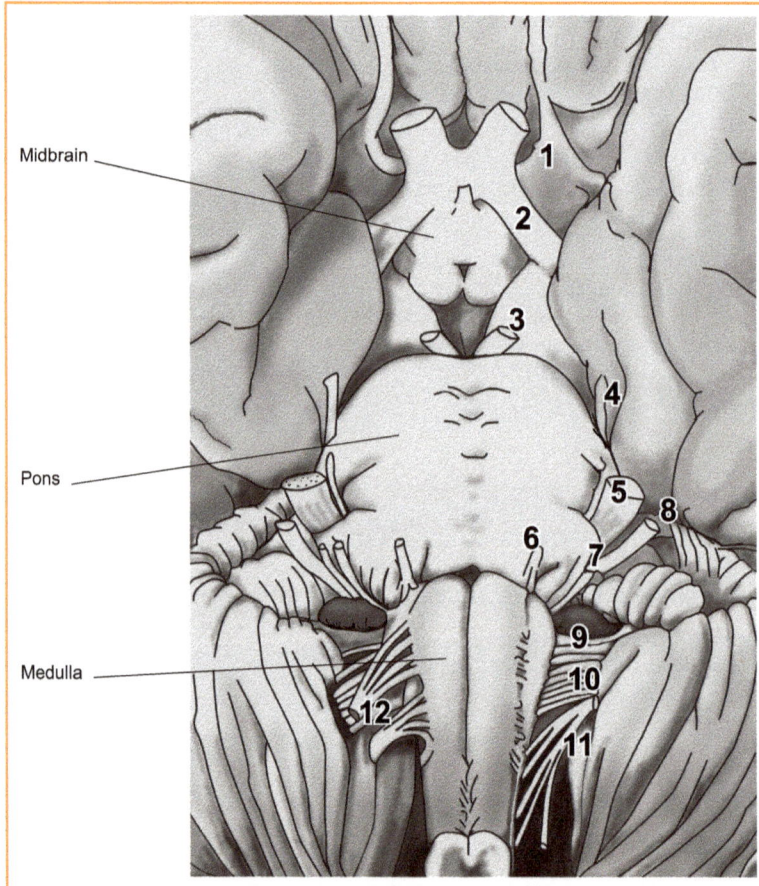

**Figure 1.6** The ventral aspect of the brainstem showing the cranial nerves. Reproduced and modified from *Gray's Anatomy*, 37th edn, edited by PL Williams et al, 1989, Churchill Livingstone, Figure 7.81 [2]. This view is looking up from underneath the hemispheres. The cerebellum can be seen on either side of the medulla and pons, the olfactory nerves (labelled 1) lie beneath the frontal lobes, and the undersurface of the temporal lobes can be seen lateral to the 3rd and 4th cranial nerves.

*   The 2nd and 3rd (predominantly the 3rd cervical sensory nerve root supply the angle of the jaw helping to differentiate isolated trigeminal nerve sensory loss from the involvement of the spinothalamic/quintothalamic tract. The angle of the jaw and neck are affected by lesions of the quinto/spinothalamic tract. Sensory loss on the face without affecting the angle of the jaw indicates the lesion is involving the 5th cranial nerve.
*   The upper lip is supplied by the 2nd division and the lower lip by the 3rd division of the trigeminal nerve.
*   The trigeminal nerve ends in front of the ear lobe.

- The corneal reflex afferent arc is the 1st division of the trigeminal nerve; the nasal tickle reflex is the 1st or 2nd division (Chapter 4).
- The anatomy of the muscles to the eye, the visual pathway and the vestibular pathway are discussed in Chapter 4.

The illustrations in the remainder of this chapter are to serve as a reference point for future use, and it is not anticipated that the reader will remember them all. With this textbook at the bedside or on their desk, the clinician can quickly refer to the illustrations to work out the anatomical basis of the pattern of weakness or sensory loss they elicit with the neurological history and examination. Later in the book, I discuss two new rules that I have developed since the 1st edition that help the non-neurologist work out which nerve or nerve root is affected. These are the 5*3*5 rule for the upper limb and the 2*2*4 rule for the lower limb.

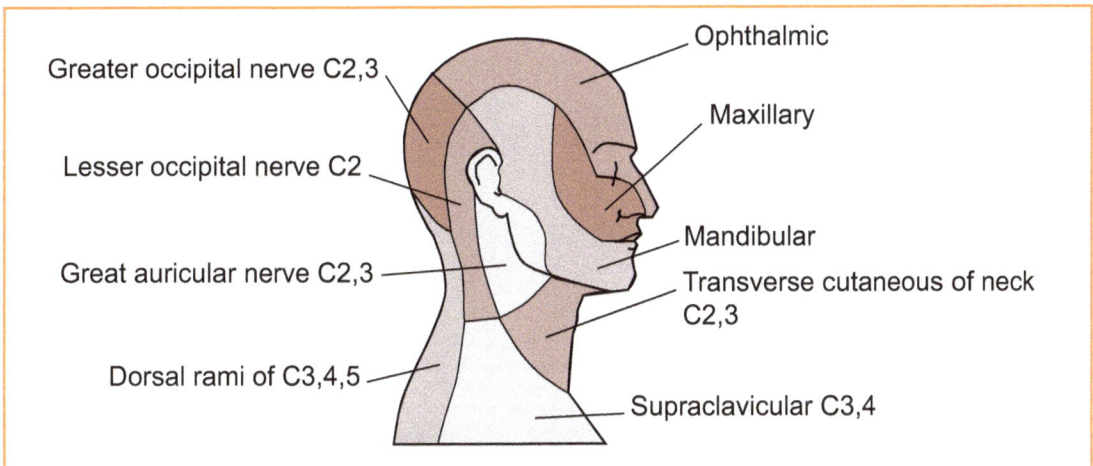

**Figure 1.7** Dermatomes and nerves of the head and neck Reproduced from *Gray's Anatomy*, 37th edn, edited by PL Williams et al, 1989, Churchill Livingstone, Figure 7.242 [2] Note: The ophthalmic, maxillary, and mandibular nerves are the three components of the 5th cranial nerve, the trigeminal nerve.

## Nerves and Nerve roots

In the peripheral nervous system, the weakness or sensory loss will reflect the pattern of weakness or sensory loss seen with either a single nerve, a single nerve root or multiple nerves or nerve roots. The rest of this chapter discusses the individual nerves and nerve roots.

# Upper Limbs
## Brachial Plexus

The most important aspects to note in Figure 1.8 are:
- The suprascapular nerve and the long thoracic nerve arise from the nerve roots (C5, C6 and C7) proximal to the junction of C5 and C6, helping to differentiate between a brachial plexus lesion at the level of C5–C6 and a nerve root lesion. In a brachial plexus lesion the supraspinatus, infraspinatus and serratus anterior will be spared.
- The radial nerve arises from C5, C6 and C7.

- The median nerve arises from C5, C6, C7, C8 and T1.
- The ulnar nerve arises from the C8 and T1. The clinical features of an ulnar nerve lesion and a C8–T1 nerve root problem are very similar. A detailed examination is required to differentiate between these two entities (see chapter 3).

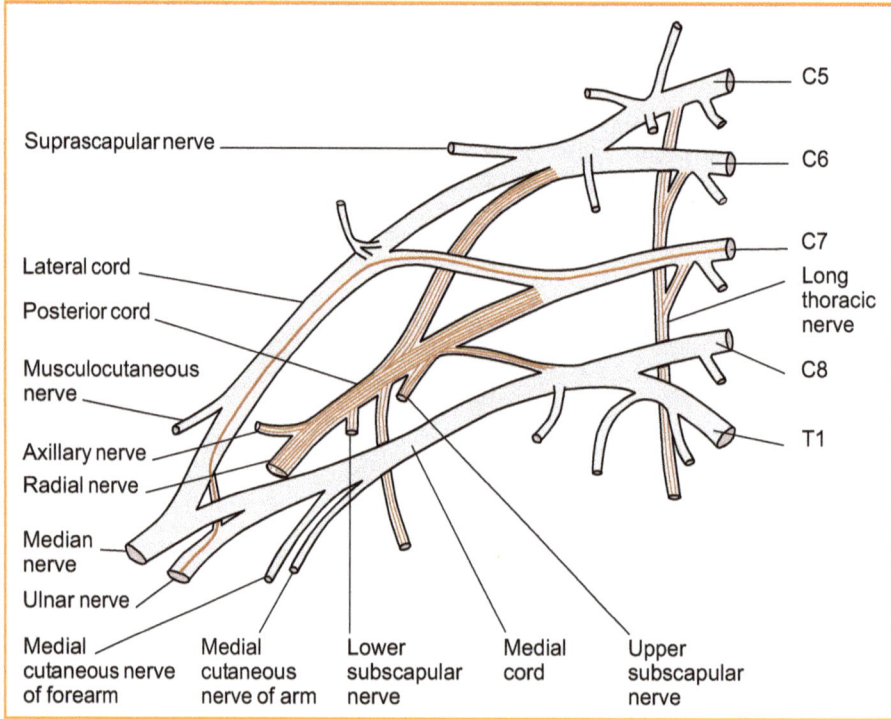

**Figure 1.8** Brachial plexus Reproduced and modified from *Gray's Anatomy,* 37th edn, edited by PL Williams et al, 1989, Churchill Livingstone, Figure 7.243 [2] *Note*: For simplification, the names of several nerves have been removed as they are rarely examined in clinical practice.

# Motor Nerves and Muscles of the Upper Limb
## Axillary and Radial Nerves

Figure 1.9 shows the muscles innervated by the axillary and radial nerves. The important points to note are:

- The axillary only supplies the deltoid muscle, not the other muscles (supraspinatus, infraspinatus, and subscapularis) around the shoulder that collectively form the rotator cuff. Weakness isolated to the deltoid will indicate an axillary nerve lesion (occasionally seen with a dislocated shoulder).
- The branches of the radial nerve to the triceps muscle arise from above the spiral groove of the humerus. The spiral groove is a common site for compression and thus the triceps is not affected.
- The branches to the brachioradialis, extensor carpi radialis longus and extensor carpi radialis brevis arise proximal to the posterior interosseous nerve, these will be affected by a radial nerve palsy but spared if the problem is confined to the posterior interosseous nerve.

# Median Nerve

Figure 1.10 shows the muscles supplied by the median nerve. The points to note are:

- The branches to the flexor carpi radialis (flexes the wrist) and flexor digitorum superficialis (flexes the medial four fingers at the proximal interphalangeal joint) arise near the elbow, proximal to the anterior interosseous nerve.
- The anterior interosseous nerve supplies the flexor pollicis longus (flexes the distal phalanx of the thumb), the pronator quadratus (turns the wrist over so that the palm is facing downwards) and the lateral aspect of the flexor digitorum profundus (flexes the distal phalanges of the 2nd and 3rd digits).
- The nerve to abductor pollicis brevis, the muscle that elevates the thumb when the hand is fully supinated (palm facing the ceiling), arises at or just distal to the wrist in the region of the carpal tunnel.

AXILLARY NERVE

Deltoid

Triceps, long head

Triceps, lateral head

Teres minor

Triceps, medial head

RADIAL NERVE

Brachioradialis

Extensor carpi radialis longus

Extensor carpi radialis brevis

Supinator
Extensor carpi ulnaris
Extensor digitorum
Extensor digiti minimi
Abductor pollicis longus
Extensor pollicis longus
Extensor pollicis brevis
Extensor indicis

POSTERIOR
INTEROSSEOUS NERVE

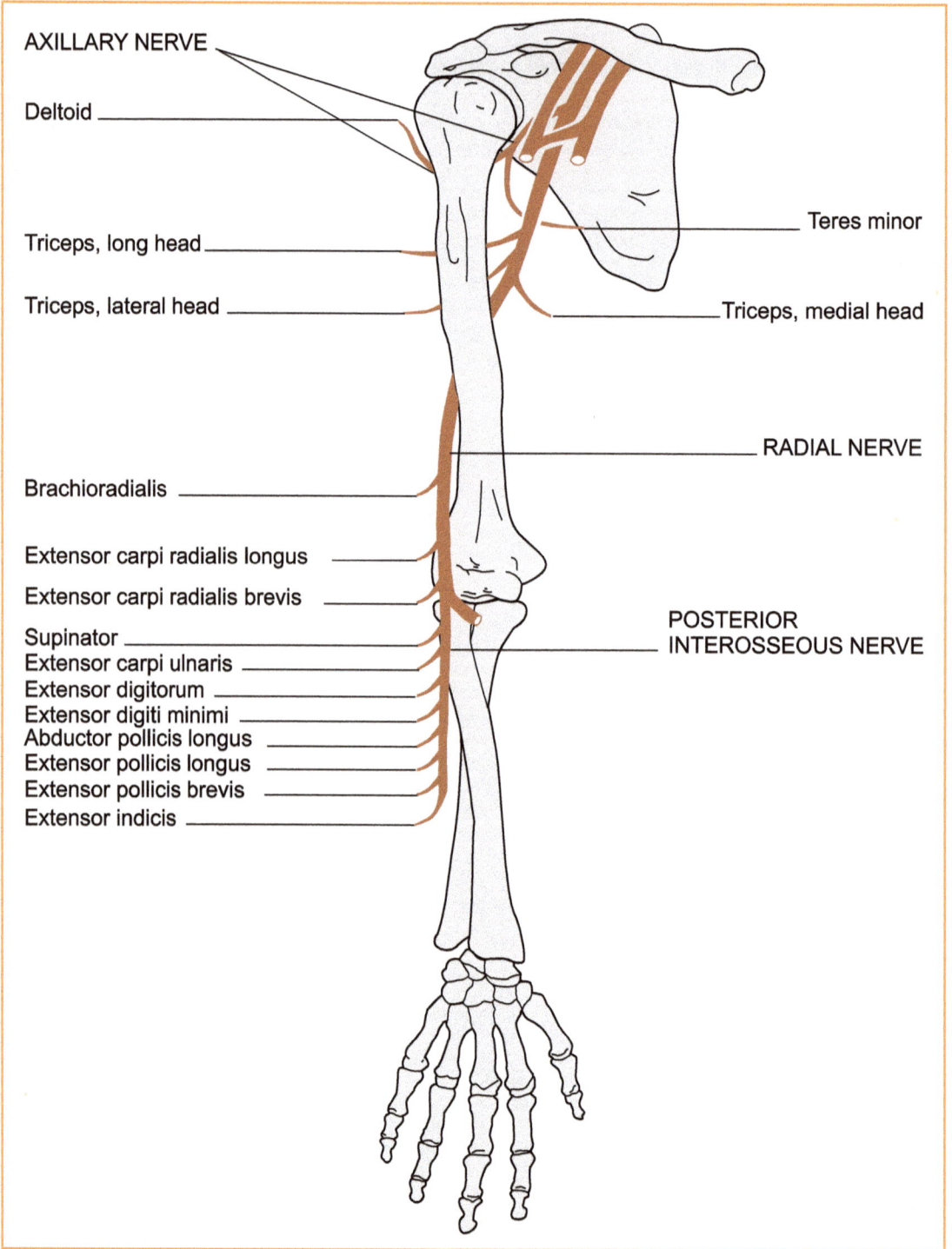

**Figure 1.9** The axillary nerve and radial nerve Reproduced from *Aids to the Examination of the Peripheral Nervous System,* 4th edn, Brain, 2000, Saunders, Figure 15, p 12 [3]

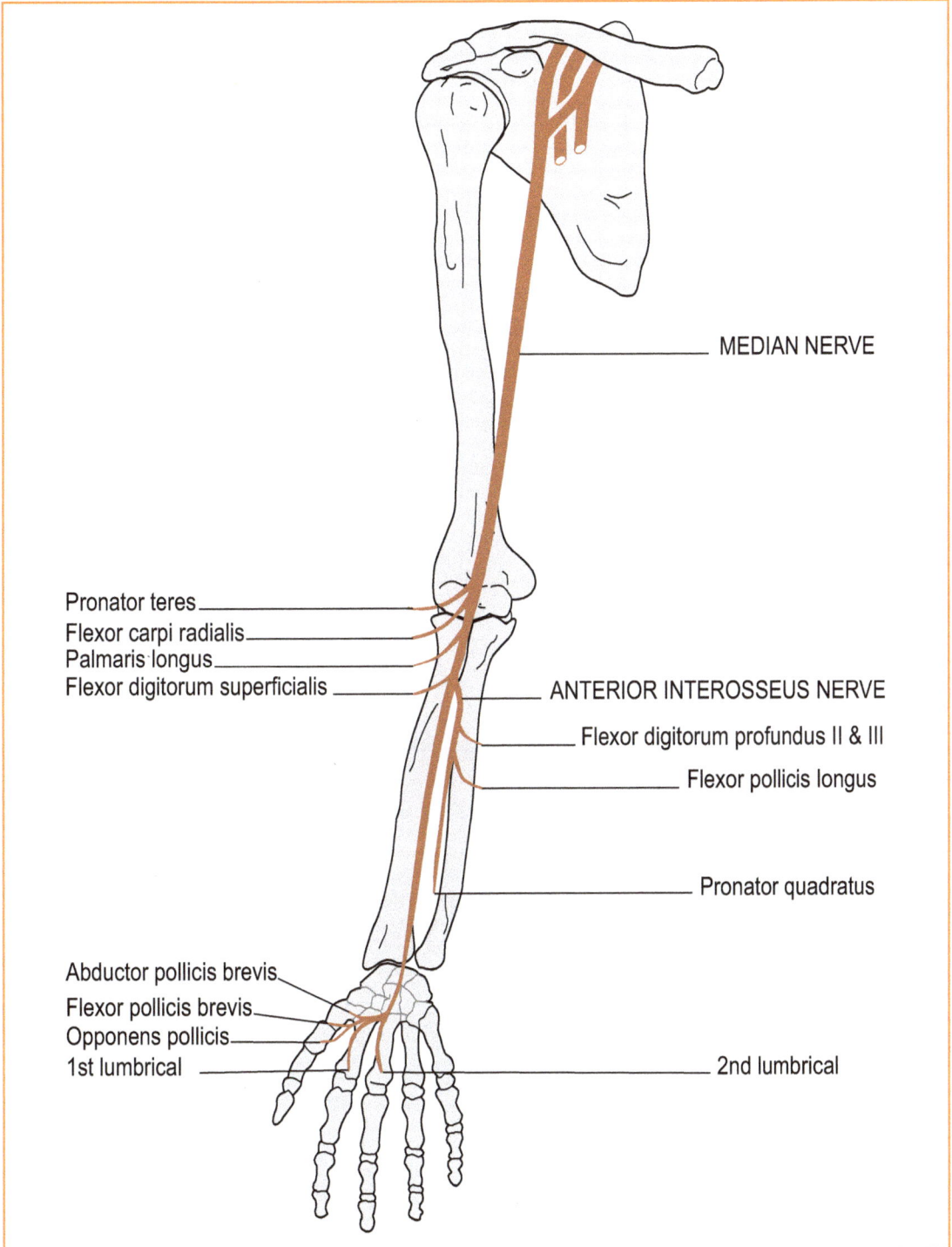

MEDIAN NERVE

Pronator teres

Flexor carpi radialis

Palmaris longus

Flexor digitorum superficialis

ANTERIOR INTEROSSEUS NERVE

Flexor digitorum profundus II & III

Flexor pollicis longus

Pronator quadratus

Abductor pollicis brevis

Flexor pollicis brevis

Opponens pollicis

1st lumbrical

2nd lumbrical

**Figure 1.10** The Median nerve Reproduced from *Aids to the Examination of the Peripheral Nervous System*, 4th edn, Brain, 2000, Saunders, Figure 27, p 20 [3]

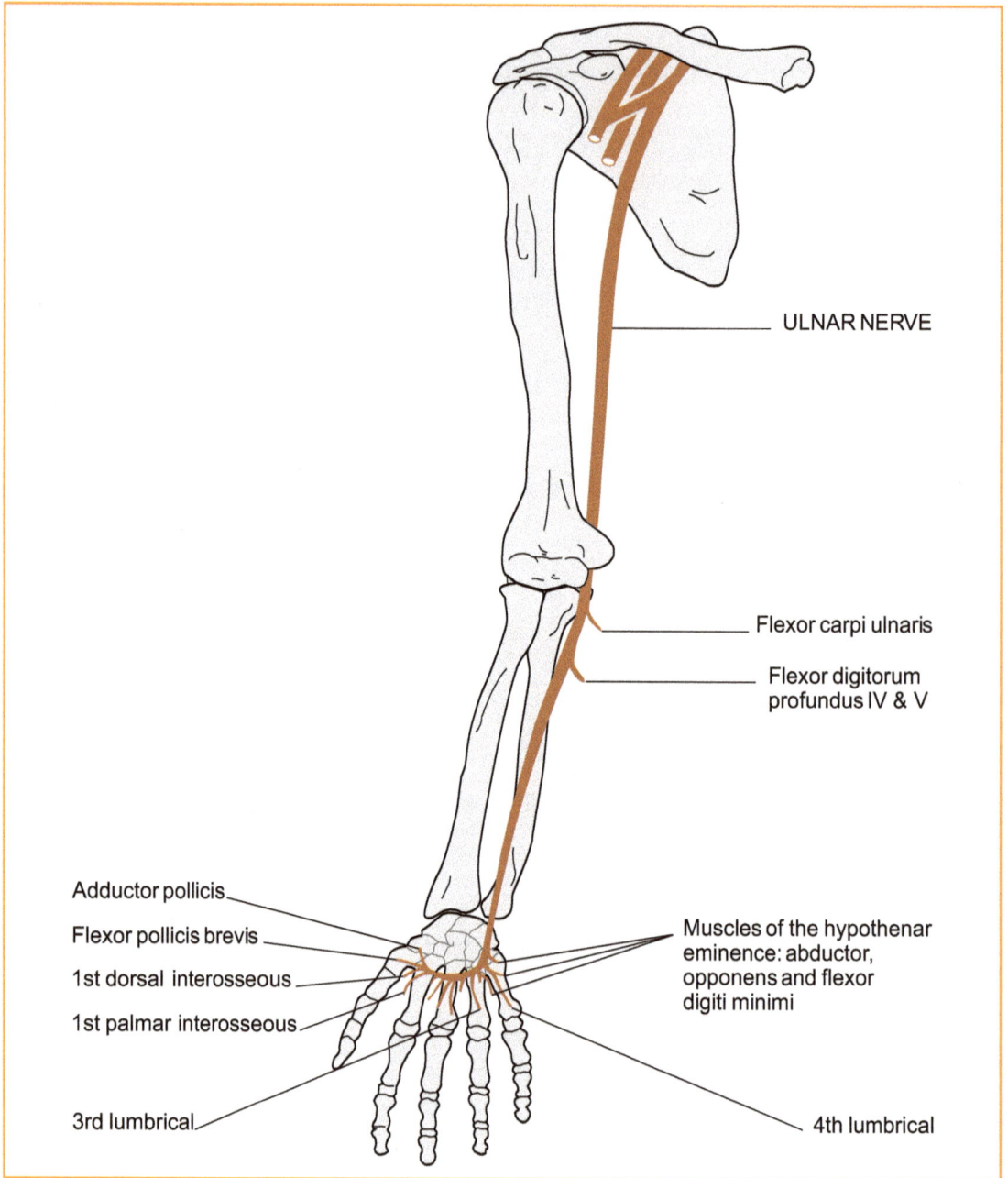

**Figure 1.11** The Ulnar nerve Reproduced from *Aids to the Examination of the Peripheral Nervous System,* 4th edn, Brain, 2000, Saunders, Figure 36, p 26 [3]

The remaining illustrations in this section show the areas supplied by the various sensory nerves that detect light touch, pain, and temperature. Neurologists remember these but 'students of neurology' do not need to remember them, although by remembering a few landmarks it is not hard to fill in the gaps. They are included in this chapter to provide a reference source for the clinician.

## Ulnar Nerve

Figure 1.11 shows the muscles innervated by the ulnar nerve. The points to note are:

- The branches to the flexor carpi ulnaris (flexes the wrist) and medial aspect of the flexor digitorum profundus (flexes the distal phalanges of the 4th and 5th digits) arise just distal to the medial epicondyle and will be affected by lesions at the elbow, a common sight of compression of the ulnar nerve. The lateral aspect of the flexor digitorum profundus is innervated by the median nerve and, thus, flexion of the 2nd and 3rd distal phalanges will be normal with an ulnar nerve lesion at the elbow whilst they will be affected by C8–T1 nerve root or lower cord brachial plexus lesions.
- All other branches arise in the hand.

## Case 1.6 illustrates a problem with the ulnar nerve.

| CASE 1.6 A 35-year-old man with weakness in his right hand |
|---|

A 35-year-old man presents with long-standing weakness confined to his right hand. He has noticed thinning of the muscle between his thumb and index finger. He has also noticed pins and needles affecting his little finger, the medial half of his 4th finger and the medial aspect of his palm and the back of the hand to the wrist. The examination reveals reduced pain sensation in the distribution of the symptoms and weakness of abduction of the medial four digits and also bending the fingertips of the 4th and 5th but not the 2nd or 3rd fingers. The thumb is not affected.

- The presence of weakness indicates that the motor pathway (meridian of longitude) is affected and the altered sensation to pain indicates that either a peripheral nerve, nerve root or the spinothalamic pathway to that part of the hand is affected.
- The presence of wasting is the parallel of latitude and indicates that the problem is in the PNS.
- The pattern of weakness is another parallel of latitude as it involves the muscles innervated by the ulnar nerve at the elbow (Figure 1.11).
- The sensory loss affecting the medial 1½ digits and the medial aspect of both the palm and the dorsal aspect of the hand up to the wrist is another parallel of latitude as the sensory loss is within the distribution of a peripheral nerve, the ulnar nerve (see Figures 1.14 and 1.15).

# The Cutaneous Sensation of the Upper Limbs and Trunk

Below each illustration are the one or two important features that are most useful at the bedside.

---

🗝️

The dermatomes are higher on the back than they are on the front of the trunk. If the sensory loss is at the same horizontal level on both the anterior and posterior aspects of the trunk it is <u>not</u> related to organic pathology and is more likely to be of functional origin.

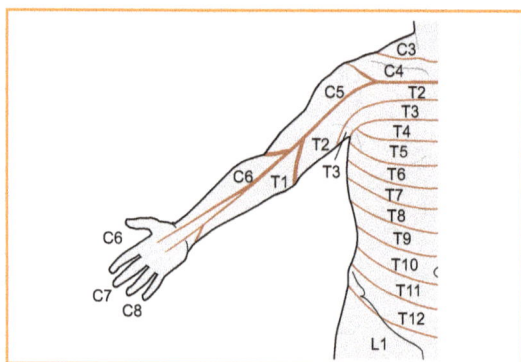

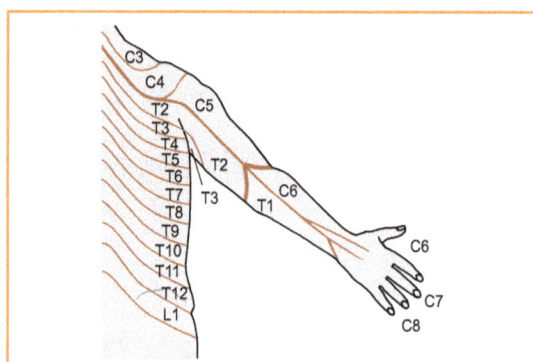

---

**Figure 1.12** (Left) Dermatomes of the trunk and upper limb (anterior aspect) Reproduced from *Aids to the Examination of the Peripheral Nervous System,* 4th edn, Brain, 2000, Saunders, Figure 87, p 56 [3]

**Figure 1.13** (Right) Dermatomes of the trunk and upper limb (posterior aspect) Reproduced from *Aids to the Examination of the Peripheral Nervous System,* 4th edn, Brain, 2000, Saunders, Figure 88, p 57) [3]

Figure 1.13 shows why it is important to roll the patient over or sit them up to examine any sensory loss on the trunk. *The dermatomes are higher on the back than they are on the front of the trunk.* The sensory loss that is at the same horizontal level on both the anterior and posterior aspects of the trunk is not related to organic pathology and is more likely to be of functional origin.

The areas of sensation in the upper limb and trunk supplied by the sensory nerve roots, the dermatomes, are shown in Figures 1.12 and 1.13. A simple method of remembering the dermatomes is:

- The arm—C7 affects the 3rd finger, C6 is lateral to this and C8 is medial to this.
- The trunk—T2 is at the level of the clavicle and meets C4; T8 is at the level of the xiphisternum (the lower end of the sternum), T10 is at the level of the umbilicus and T12 is at the level of the groin.

If you remember these landmarks, you can work out the areas in between supplied by the other dermatomes.

Figures 1.14 and 1.15 show the areas supplied by the individual nerves in the upper limbs.

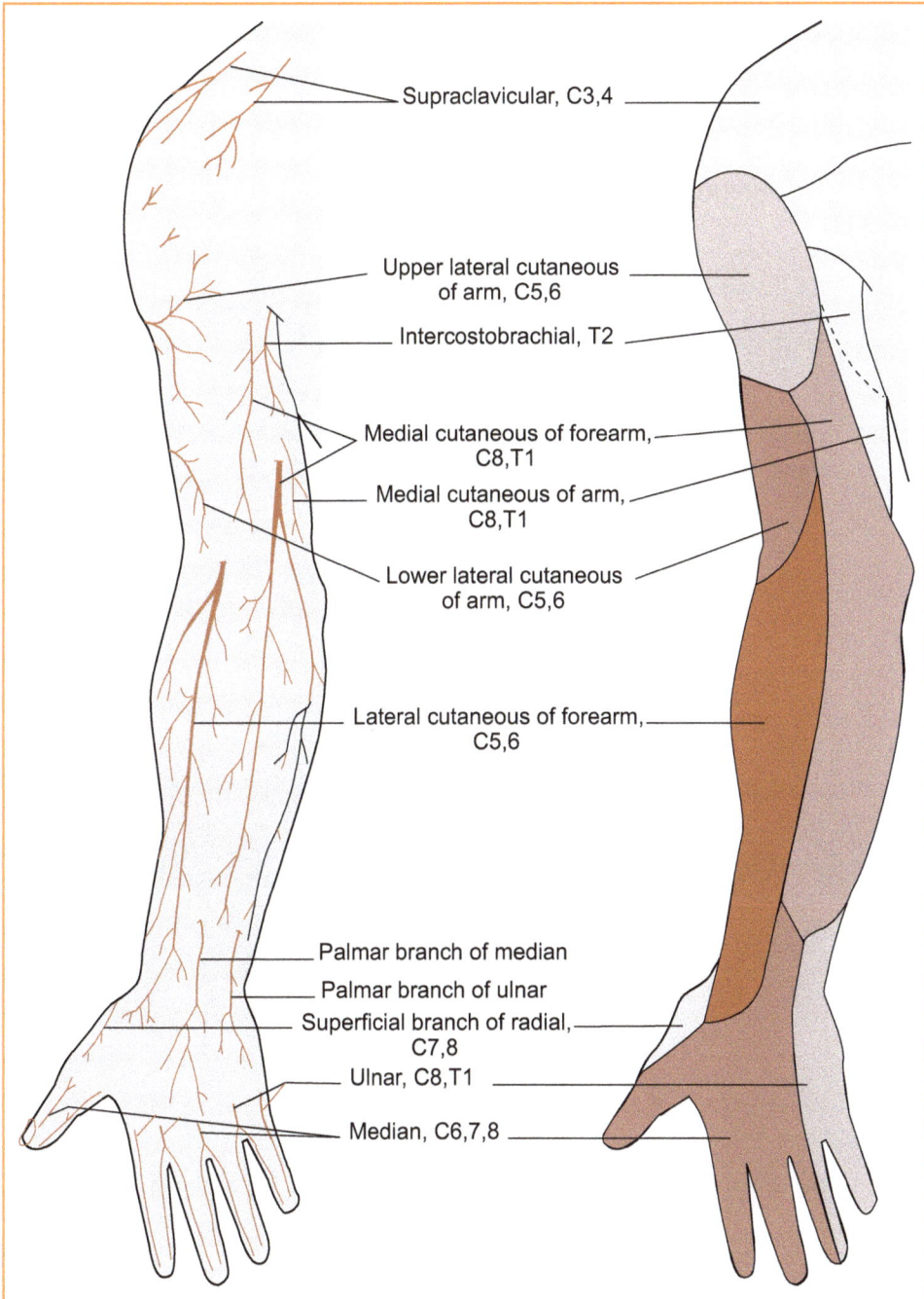

**Figure 1.14** Sensory nerves of the upper limbs (anterior aspect) Reproduced from *Gray's Anatomy*, 37th edn, edited by PL Williams et al, 1989, Churchill Livingstone, Figure 7.244 [2] *Note*: The nerve root origin of the nerves is also shown. Note that the median nerve supplies the lateral 3 ½ digits while the ulnar nerve supplies the medial 1½ digits.

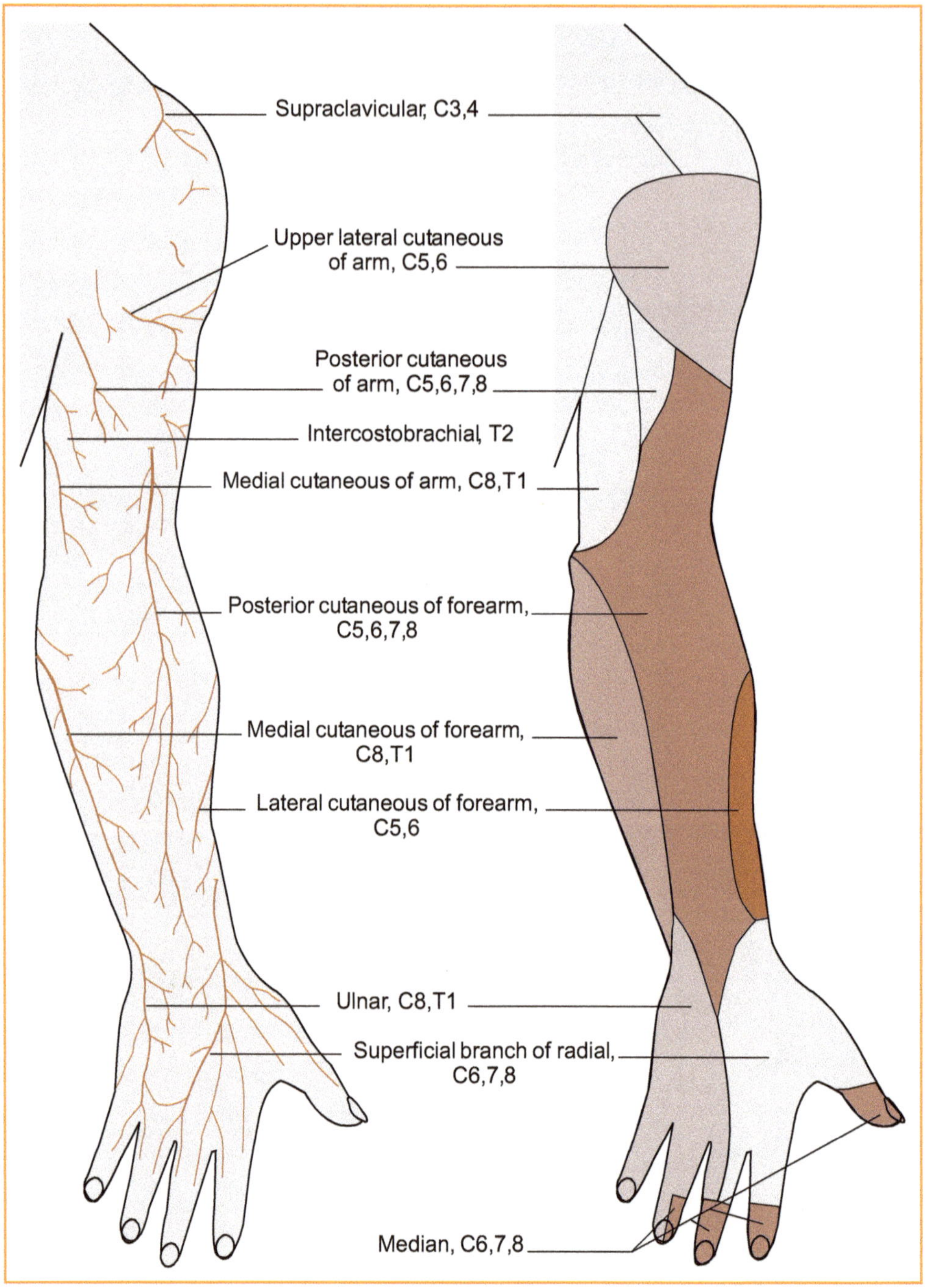

Supraclavicular, C3,4
Upper lateral cutaneous of arm, C5,6
Posterior cutaneous of arm, C5,6,7,8
Intercostobrachial, T2
Medial cutaneous of arm, C8,T1
Posterior cutaneous of forearm, C5,6,7,8
Medial cutaneous of forearm, C8,T1
Lateral cutaneous of forearm, C5,6
Ulnar, C8,T1
Superficial branch of radial, C6,7,8
Median, C6,7,8


**Figure 1.15** Sensory nerves of the upper limbs (posterior aspect) Reproduced from *Gray's Anatomy*, 37th edn, edited by PL Williams et al, 1989, Churchill Livingstone, Figure 7.245) [2] *Note*: The nerve root origin of the nerves is also shown.

# The Lower Limbs

## Lumbosacral Plexus

Unlike the brachial plexus, there is little in the lumbosacral plexus (Figure 1.16 A and B) that helps localise whether the problem is in the lumbosacral plexus or the nerve roots. It is important to note that the sciatic nerve arises from predominantly the 5th lumbar and the 1st and 2nd sacral nerve roots. The point to note (Figure 1.17) is that the common peroneal nerve arises from the sciatic nerve above the popliteal fossa and above the level of the neck of the fibula, a common site for compression and that there are no branches between where it arises and the neck of the fibula.

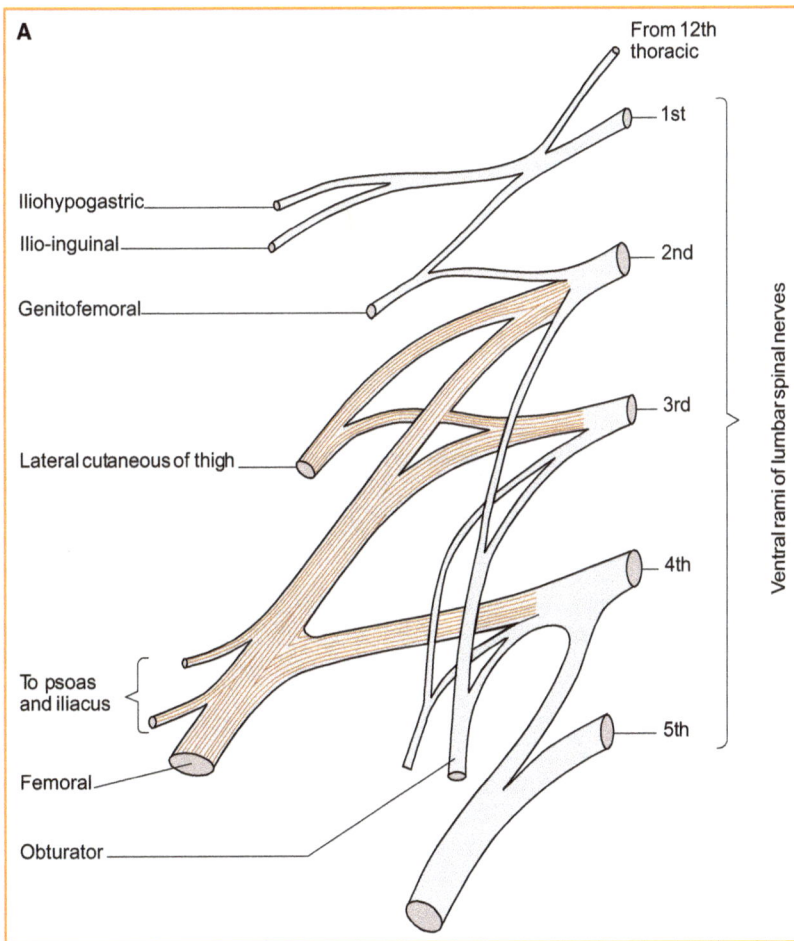

**Figure 1.16 A** Lumbar Plexus *Note*: The main nerve to arise from the lumbar plexus is the femoral nerve. It is formed from the 2nd, 3rd and 4th lumbrical nerve roots. Reproduced from *Gray's Anatomy*, 37th edn, edited by PL Williams et al, 1989, Churchill Livingstone, Figures 7.252 [2]

# The Motor Nerves of the Lower Limb

## Femoral Nerve

The femoral nerve arises from the 2nd to 4th lumbar nerve roots. The obturator nerve arises from the nerve roots proximal to the plexus and would be affected with a radiculopathy but not a plexus lesion.

## Sciatic Nerve

The point to note is that the tibialis posterior muscle is supplied by the posterior tibial nerve while the tibialis anterior muscle is supplied by the common peroneal nerve (see Figure 1.18). Examining these muscles individually in patients with a foot drop helps to differentiate between a common peroneal nerve palsy and an L5 nerve root lesion. Inversion is stronger in a common peroneal nerve lesion while eversion is stronger with an L5 nerve root lesion. (See Chapter 12, 'Back pain and common leg problems with or without difficulty walking')

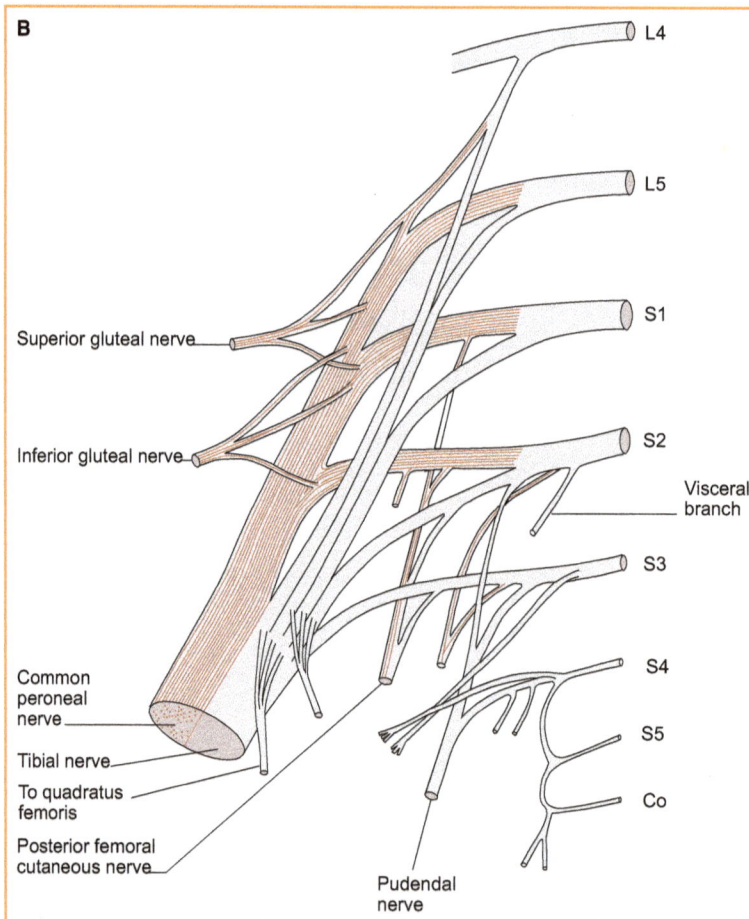

**Figure 1.16** B Sacral Plexus Reproduced from *Gray's Anatomy*, 37th edn, edited by PL Williams et al, 1989, Churchill Livingstone, Figures 7.256. [2]

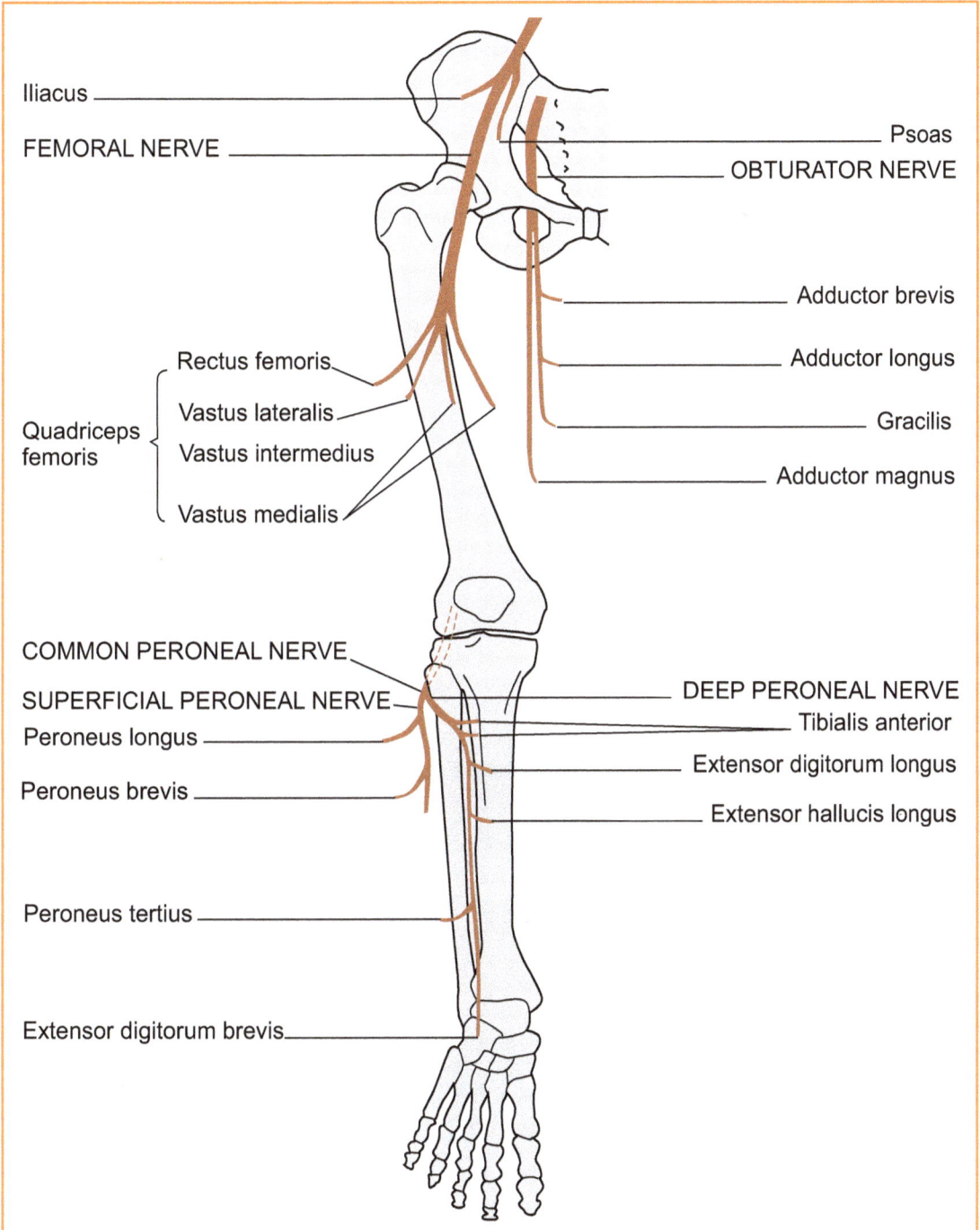

**Figure 1.17** The Femoral nerve, Obturator nerve and Common peroneal nerve of the right lower limb Reproduced from *Aids to the Examination of the Peripheral Nervous System,* 4th edn, Brain, 2000, Saunders, Figure 46, p 32 [3]

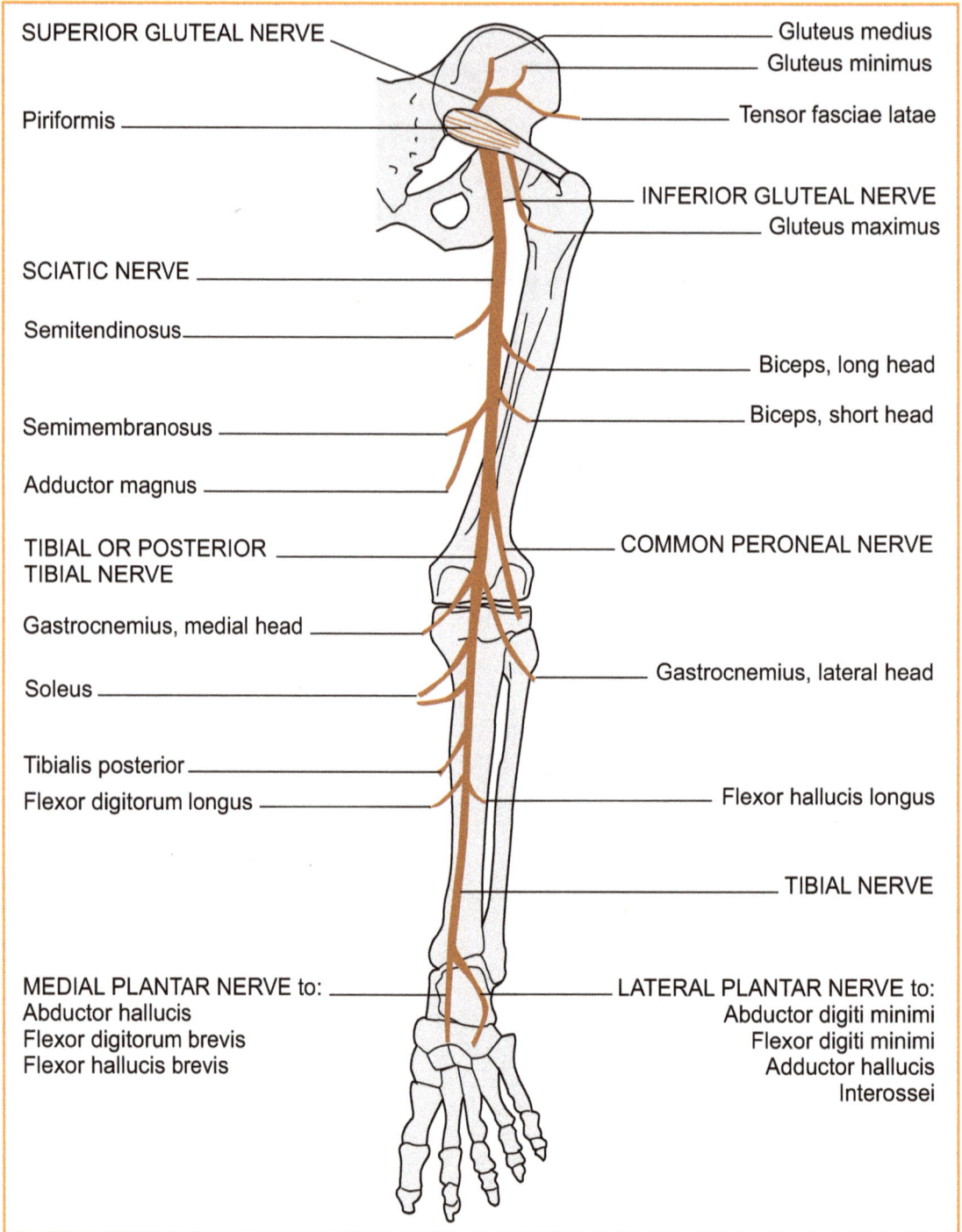

SUPERIOR GLUTEAL NERVE

Gluteus medius

Gluteus minimus

Piriformis

Tensor fasciae latae

INFERIOR GLUTEAL NERVE

Gluteus maximus

SCIATIC NERVE

Semitendinosus

Biceps, long head

Biceps, short head

Semimembranosus

Adductor magnus

TIBIAL OR POSTERIOR TIBIAL NERVE

COMMON PERONEAL NERVE

Gastrocnemius, medial head

Gastrocnemius, lateral head

Soleus

Tibialis posterior

Flexor digitorum longus

Flexor hallucis longus

TIBIAL NERVE

MEDIAL PLANTAR NERVE to:
Abductor hallucis
Flexor digitorum brevis
Flexor hallucis brevis

LATERAL PLANTAR NERVE to:
Abductor digiti minimi
Flexor digiti minimi
Adductor hallucis
Interossei

**Figure 1.18** The Sciatic nerve and posterior tibial nerve Reproduced from *Aids to the Examination of the Peripheral Nervous System,* 4th edn, Brain, 2000, Saunders, Figure 47, p 33 [3]

# The Cutaneous Sensation of the Lower Limbs

As discussed regarding the upper limbs and trunk, Figures 1.19–1.22 are supplied as a reference source along with some important clinical clues.

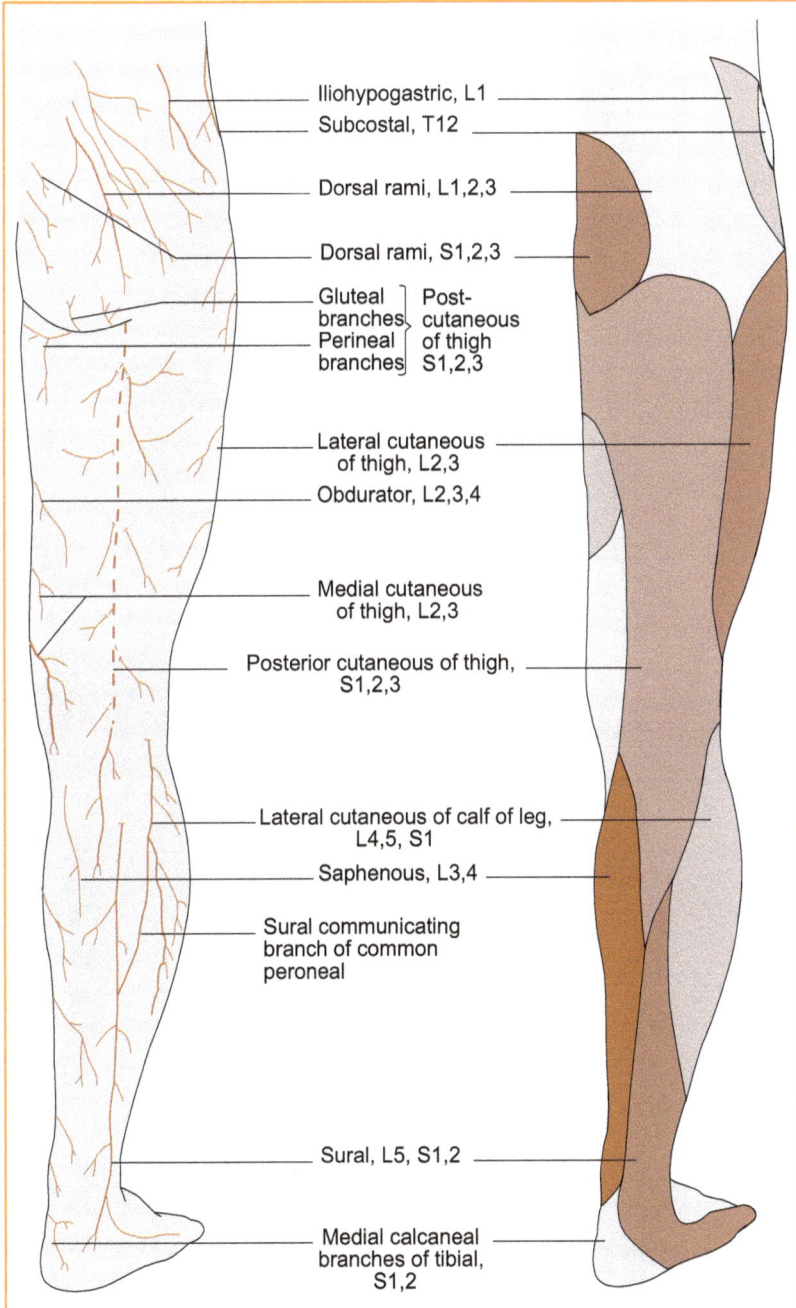

Iliohypogastric, L1

Subcostal, T12

Dorsal rami, L1,2,3

Dorsal rami, S1,2,3

Gluteal branches / Perineal branches } Post-cutaneous of thigh S1,2,3

Lateral cutaneous of thigh, L2,3

Obdurator, L2,3,4

Medial cutaneous of thigh, L2,3

Posterior cutaneous of thigh, S1,2,3

Lateral cutaneous of calf of leg, L4,5, S1

Saphenous, L3,4

Sural communicating branch of common peroneal

Sural, L5, S1,2

Medial calcaneal branches of tibial, S1,2

**Figure 1.19** The Sensory nerves of the lower limbs (posterior aspect) Reproduced from *Gray's Anatomy*, 37th edn, edited by PL Williams et al, 1989, Churchill Livingstone, Figure 7.258) [2] *Note*: The nerve root origin of the nerves is also shown.

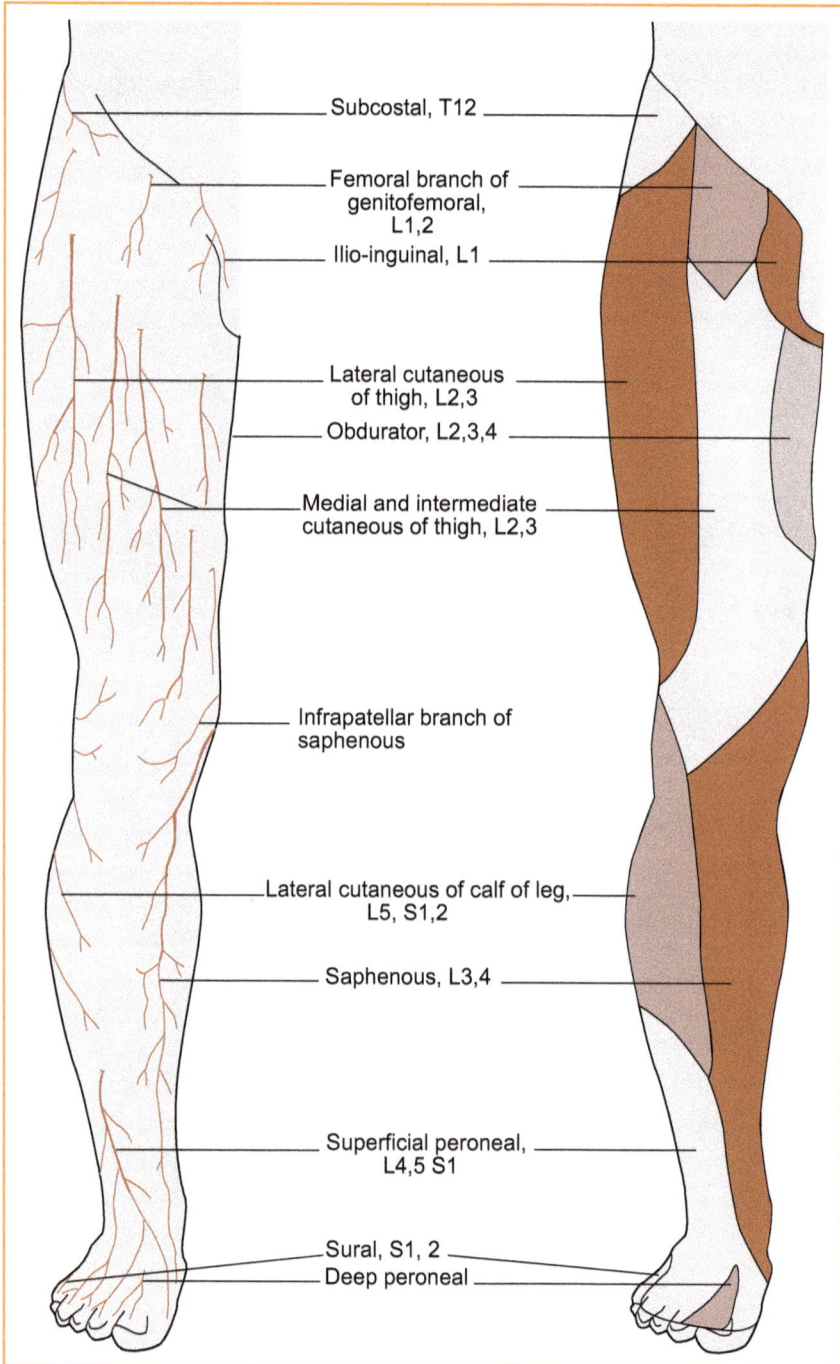

Subcostal, T12

Femoral branch of
genitofemoral,
L1,2

Ilio-inguinal, L1

Lateral cutaneous
of thigh, L2,3

Obdurator, L2,3,4

Medial and intermediate
cutaneous of thigh, L2,3

Infrapatellar branch of
saphenous

Lateral cutaneous of calf of leg,
L5, S1,2

Saphenous, L3,4

Superficial peroneal,
L4,5 S1

Sural, S1, 2
Deep peroneal

**Figure 1.20** The Sensory nerves of lower limbs (anterior aspect) Reproduced from *Gray's Anatomy,* 37th edn, edited by PL Williams et al, 1989, Churchill Livingstone, Figure 7.254 [2] *Note*: The nerve root origin of the nerves is shown.

Tibial, S1,2

Lateral
plantar

Medial plantar

Sural, L5, S1,2

Saphenous, L3,4

Deep
branch

Lateral plantar,
S1,2

Medial plantar,
L4,5

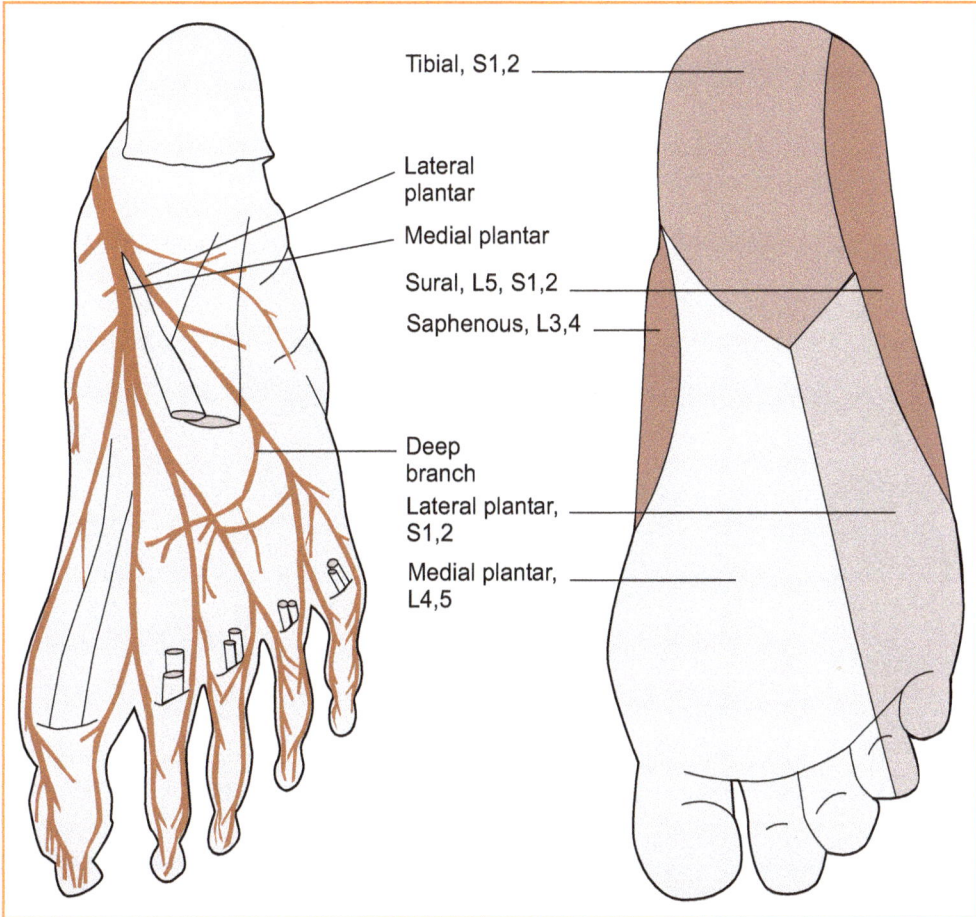

**Figure 1.21** The Sensory nerves of the soles of the feet Reproduced from *Gray's Anatomy,* 37th edn, edited by PL Williams et al, 1989, Churchill Livingstone, Figure X, p Y [2]

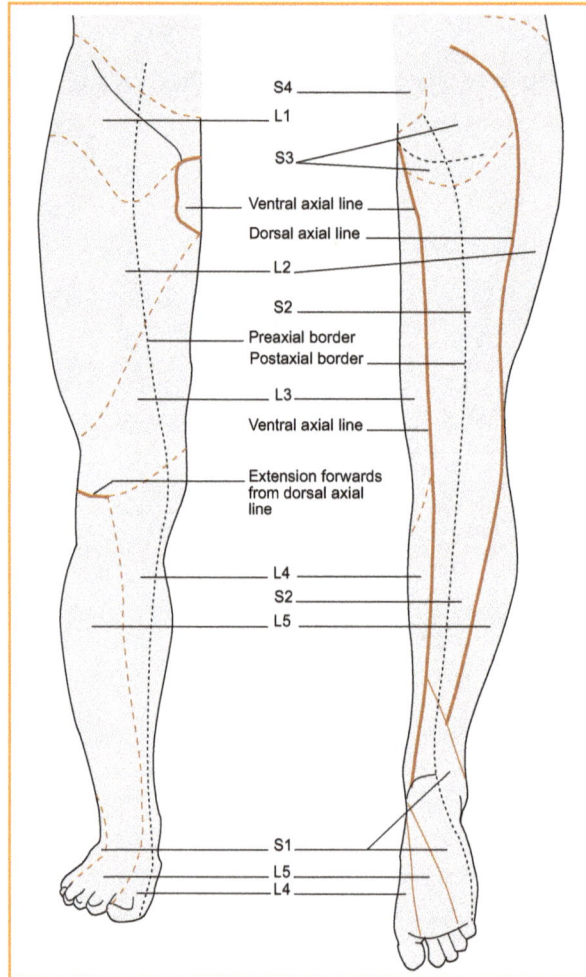

**Figure 1.22** The Dermatomes of the lower limbs Reproduced from *Aids to the Examination of the Peripheral Nervous System,* 4th edn, Brain, 2000, Saunders, Figure 89, p 58 [3] *Note*: T12 meets L1 at the groin, L3 crosses the knee and L5 affects the outside of the shin and the dorsal aspect of the foot. If you remember these landmarks, you can work out the area in between supplied by the other dermatomes.

**Useful Landmarks for Remembering Cutaneous Sensation**

Rather than trying to remember all the dermatomes, the following landmarks can be used.
- T12 is at the level of the groin (see Figure 1.12).
- L3 crosses the knee (see Figure 1.22).
- S1 supplies the outside of the foot (see Figure 1.22).

Then put the intervening dermatomes in between these landmarks.

# References

1    Brodal A. *Neurological anatomy*. 2nd edn London: Oxford University Press; 1969, 807.
2    Gray's anatomy PL, editor. *Williams*. 37th edn London: Churchill Livingstone; 1989.

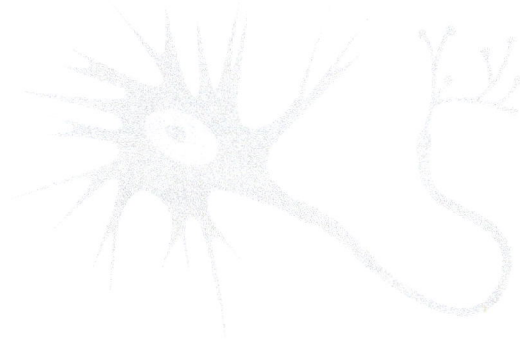

# The Neurological History

| Key Terms | |
|---|---|
| **Meridians of Longitude:** | A term used to describe long pathways where symptoms can arise from any part of that pathway. In addition to the descending motor pathway and the two ascending sensory pathways discussed in the previous chapter, the visual pathway from the eye to the occipital lobe and the vestibular pathway from the inner ear via the brainstem to the cerebellum and vestibular cortex in the temporal and parietal lobes can also be viewed as meridians of longitude. If someone has visual disturbance or vertigo it must be somewhere along these two pathways. |
| **Parallels of Latitude:** | A term used to indicate the exact site of the problem is along the meridian of longitude. The parallels of latitude are the dermatomes, myotomes and reflexes in the limbs, the dermatomes on the trunk, the cranial nerves in the brainstem, the cerebellum and the cortical symptoms and signs in the cerebral hemispheres. |
| **Circumstantial Evidence** | Circumstantial evidence refers to information in the past, family and social history that only increases the likelihood of a particular illness. It does not indicate the presence of that diagnosis. |
| **The Likely Pathology** | The likely pathology is established by eliciting the exact mode of onset and progression of symptoms. |
| **Likely Site of the Problem** | The likely site of the problem in the nervous system is established by eliciting the exact nature and distribution of symptoms. |

This chapter provides a basic understanding of the principles of history taking to make taking a history more rewarding, than just asking a list of questions. Neurologists have been taught to ask two questions; where is the lesion? and what is the underlying pathology?

**Where is the lesion?** Is it in the cerebral hemispheres, brainstem, cerebellum, spinal cord, nerve roots, brachial or lumbosacral plexus, peripheral nerve, neuromuscular junction, or muscle? Determining the site of the problem in the nervous system is best answered by obtaining the nature of the symptoms (i.e., weakness, sensory symptoms, visual or speech disturbance) and their exact distribution in terms of which parts of the body are affected. Whist taking the history, neurologists are thinking about the underlying neuroanatomy that each symptom represents. Their knowledge of the underlying neuroanatomy enables them to localise the problem within the nervous system. Non-neurologists can use the illustrations in this book to work out the site of the problem in the nervous system if they take the history as suggested.

**What is the pathology?** Eliciting the illness's mode of onset and progression will point to the likely pathological process causing the symptoms.

Almost invariably, *the difference between making the correct diagnosis and not* is a direct consequence of the time spent taking a very detailed history. The most common mistake that inexperienced clinicians make when taking a history is that they elicit the nature of the symptoms but do not clarify their exact distribution or how the symptoms evolved. Migraine, subarachnoid haemorrhage, meningitis and a hangover present with headaches, nausea, vomiting and photophobia. It is not the symptoms that indicate the likely diagnosis but rather how those symptoms have evolved.

Using the history-taking techniques described in this chapter, there is no reason why an inexperienced student or hospital medical officer cannot obtain the same history as an experienced clinician. There is always an experienced clinician on the other end of a telephone who can be more helpful if given a good history.

Consider Cases 2.1 and 2.2. In both of these, the referring physician has used the nature of the symptoms, the age of the patient and the past and family history to make an incorrect diagnosis. In the first case, the clinician has assumed that patients of this age with multiple risk factors on prior probability are most likely to suffer from a stroke. However, the patient's symptoms evolved over several weeks and were related to a malignant brain tumour.

| CASE 2.1 A 65-year-old woman with right-sided weakness |
| --- |
| Dear Dr,<br>Thank you for admitting this 65-year-old woman with a stroke. She presents with left-sided weakness. There is has a history of hypertension, diabetes and hypercholesterolaemia. She is a heavy smoker, and both her father and older brother died of a stroke.<br>Yours sincerely, |

In the second case, the past and family history were used to make an incorrect diagnosis of migraine. However, his symptoms were of instantaneous onset and related to a ruptured berry aneurysm causing subarachnoid haemorrhage (bleeding into the subarachnoid space – the space beneath the outer lining of the brain, referred to as the dura mater and the surface of the brain).

| CASE 2.2 A 25-year-old man with a "migraine." |
| --- |
| Dear Dr,<br>Thank you for seeing this 25-year-old man with a migraine. He has headache, nausea, vomiting and photophobia. He suffered from migraine in childhood. His mother and sister both suffer from migraine.<br>Yours sincerely, |

A history of prior medical problems <u>does not preclude the patient from suffering from an unrelated illness.</u> Using the past medical history to influence the diagnosis of the current problem often leads to a delay in diagnosing new issues in patients with chronic diseases.

| |
|---|
| A past history of an illness or risk factors for an illness only increases the patient's likelihood of having a particular problem. Only a detailed analysis of the current symptoms should be used to make a diagnosis. |

| |
|---|
| The nature and distribution of the symptoms can only localise the problem within the nervous system and cannot infer a particular pathological diagnosis. |

In most instances, prior probability is correct. This lulls clinicians into thinking that they are clever when in fact it is difficult for them to be wrong. For example, an older person with hemiparesis in the setting of multiple risk factor is most likely to have had a stroke. Another example is the general practitioner (GP), who diagnoses most patients as having a tension-type headache and is correct the vast majority of the time, simply because most patients attending a GP with headaches do suffer from tension-type headaches.

The age of the patient, the past, family and social history simply increase the likelihood of a particular illness being present. This information should be regarded as **circumstantial evidence**. As in law, where many innocent people have been found guilty based on circumstantial evidence, in medicine, many incorrect diagnoses are made using the age of the patient and the past, family, social and medication history to make a diagnosis.

Spencer [1] stated that it is impossible to learn how to take a good history from a textbook. The clinical environment is the only setting where history taking, physical examination, clinical reasoning, decision making, empathy and professionalism can be taught and learnt as an integrated whole. Although this is mainly correct, one could use the analogy of learning to play golf. You can either hack away for years or have lessons at the start that will make the practice more effective. This chapter aims to outline the basic skills of history taking that can be taken to the wards when seeing patients.

Traditionally, students have been taught to ask a long list of neurological questions about headache, dizziness, weakness, numbness etc. in the forlorn hope that, after this 'fishing expedition' (also referred to as 'looking for the pony'[1]) [2], a diagnosis will be apparent. In other words, in the hope of finding the diagnosis ('the pony'), one collects an extensive list of answers to numerous questions that essentially only relate to the nature of the symptoms with little understanding about what the answers represent. It has been suggested that students should be taught to take a history this way and then taught not to take it that way. I disagree. I recommend that students be taught how to take a history in a meaningful way rather than just collecting useless information they do not know how to use.

---

1   "Looking for the pony" comes from a Christmas tale of two brothers, one of whom was an incurable pessimist and the other, an incurable optimist. On Christmas Day, the pessimist was given a room full of new toys and the optimists, a roomful of horse manure. The optimist threw himself into the muck and began burrowing about in it. When his horrified parents extricated him from the excrement and asked why on earth, he was thrashing about in it, he joyfully cried, "with all this horse manure, there's got to be a pony in here somewhere!"

# Principles of Neurological History Taking

When obtaining the history from a patient with a neurological problem it is important to establish whether the problem is:

- a monophasic illness or
- recurrent episodes of intermittent symptoms

An alternative method of obtaining the history is recommended in patients presenting with or recurrent episodes of intermittent disturbances of neurological function, e.g., epilepsy or headache. In essence, it is better to obtain a blow-by-blow description of several individual episodes with intermittent disturbances. This alternative approach is described in Chapter 7 and Chapter 8.

Having established that the problem is a monophasic illness, the three basic principles of history taking are simple:

- *Define the likely underlying pathological basis by **eliciting the mode of onset, progression, and duration of each and every symptom*** (i.e., the time course of the illness).
- *Establish the site of the disorder within the nervous system by **determining the nature and more importantly the distribution of symptoms.***
- ***Elicit other facts that may*** *either support or refute your initial thoughts regarding the cause for the problem or, more importantly, **influence subsequent management of the patient***. This includes the family history, past history, coexistent medical problems, prescribed drugs, and natural remedies the patient is taking, social factors and the patient's concerns.

Difficulties making a diagnosis are almost invariably the result of failure to establish the mode of onset, progression, and duration of symptoms.

Some patients are not capable of giving an accurate history. This is often (but not always) due to the presence of an inability to speak the language, dementia, confusion, or amnesia. In these circumstances, it is necessary to question a relative or an eyewitness. If that is not possible, one has no choice but to use circumstantial evidence (the past and family history) and prior probability (certain conditions affect particular people of a certain sex and age) to come to a possible diagnosis, keeping in mind that the suspected diagnosis may be incorrect.

# The Underlying Pathological Process

## Mode of Onset, Duration and Progression of Symptoms

Different pathological processes evolve over variable periods. It is this variability that can be used to determine the most **likely pathology**. Three modes of onset can be loosely defined: sudden onset within seconds to minutes, gradual onset over hours to days and a very gradual onset over months to years (see Figure 2.1). The expression 'mode of onset' refers to the time for all symptoms to fully develop. Symptoms can worsen by either increasing in intensity or spreading to affect a larger area of the body.

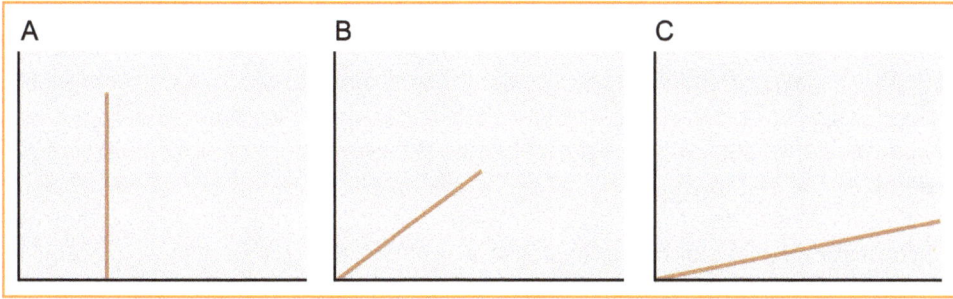

**Figure 2.1** The three 'modes of onset' of an illness: A acute, seconds to minutes; B subacute, hours to days; C chronic, months to years

The pathological processes that reflect these modes of onset are:

**A. Instantaneous – seconds, rarely minutes**
- Electrical: an epileptic seizure or an arrhythmia such as a tachyarrhythmia (fast heartbeat), bradyarrhythmia (slow heartbeat) or complete heart block (no impulse between the right atrium and ventricles, the Stokes–Adams attack)
- Vascular: subarachnoid haemorrhage, cerebral embolus
- Mechanical: trauma, a slipped intervertebral disc or positional vertigo

**B. Subacute – hours to days**
- Infective: meningitis, encephalitis
- Inflammatory: multiple sclerosis, acute inflammatory neuropathies
- Metabolic disorders: hyponatraemia, diabetic coma

**C. Chronic – months to years**
- Neoplastic: benign and occasionally malignant tumours
- Degenerative: cervical spondylitic myelopathy and the various genetic disorders
- Chronic endocrine problems: hypothyroidism, Cushing's disease, pituitary disorders
- Chronic inflammatory/infective processes: polymyositis, chronic inflammatory demyelinating peripheral neuropathies, cryptococcal or tuberculous meningitis

Although the majority of diseases that clinicians encounter fit into one of these three basic patterns, it is important to remember that *they are only a guide* and there are always exceptions to the rule.

**Some exceptions to the rule include:**
- Symptoms such as diplopia (double vision) and vertigo will, as a result of their very nature, always begin abruptly and need not necessarily indicate a pathological process with a vascular or mechanical basis (see the section 'The nature and distribution of symptoms').
- At times, neoplastic disorders can present with a rapid evolution of symptoms as a result of a seizure and the rapid onset of a focal neurological deficit after the seizure; tumours can also appear to evolve more rapidly when there is a superimposed mechanical shift due to the mass effect.
- Vascular disorders can have a slower onset: for example, the stroke-in-evolution that may or may not be stepwise; the intracerebral haemorrhage that evolves over many minutes; the subdural that develops over hours to days (although here the bleeding results in a mass lesion); or the giant aneurysm that behaves as a tumour with symptoms due to the mass.

In older patients with a chronic disease, the deterioration is so slow that it is assumed that their increasing disability is simply related to old age until there is a crisis, such as a fall where they are unable to get up. Patients present under these circumstances with an apparent illness of sudden onset, whereas in reality, it is simply the 'straw that broke the camel's back' phenomenon. The true nature is only clarified when a careful and detailed history of slowly evolving disability is obtained.

In this situation, it *is imperative to elicit whether the symptoms progressed after they were first noticed*. Progression can either be more intense symptoms, the spread of the symptoms to other parts of the body or the appearance of additional symptoms.

There are two circumstances where it is not possible to establish the exact time of onset of the initial symptom(s):

If the symptoms are present on awakening, even if the patient awoke at an unusual hour unless you can determine that the symptoms awoke the patient (this is very unlikely). The best estimate for the onset is the time between falling asleep and waking.

If the symptoms are only noticeable with an external stimulus (e.g., the patient becomes aware of altered temperature sensation when they sit on a cold surface.

# The Nature and Distribution of Symptoms

Neurologists use the nature of the symptoms and their distribution over the body to determine what part of the nervous system is involved by the disease process. In doing this, it is essential to remember that many patients use terms differently from the medical profession. Therefore, it is important to clarify what the patient means.

# Symptom clarification

Symptom clarification involves having the patient explain exactly what they mean when they describe their symptoms. The term *collapse* in the toilet can be anything from a severe bout of diarrhoea to sudden death. The complaint of weakness or numbness does not necessarily imply a loss of strength or sensation, respectively. It is not unusual for patients with facial nerve palsy (Bell's palsy) to describe their face as numb when in fact it is weak. The term *weakness* is used by some patients to describe a loss of function regardless of the cause, and actual weakness can be described as a feeling of heaviness, numbness or even a loss of feeling. When some patients say they have double vision what they mean is that their vision is blurred, not that they see two objects! Dizziness is another very vague term that means different things to different patients.

When clarifying the nature of symptoms, the following sample questions may be helpful:
- By weakness, do you mean an actual loss of strength?
- You said you had double vision – do you mean you saw two objects and, if you did, were they side-by-side or one above the other?
- When you say you are dizzy, what do you mean? Do you have a feeling of light-headedness or is it a sensation that the room or your head is spinning?
- When you say your speech is slurred, do you mean it sounds as if you are intoxicated (this would be the description of dysarthria) or do you mean that either you have difficulty

finding the words that you want to say or, even though you can think of what you want to say, you are unable to say those words (this is the description of dysphasia)?

# The Nature of Symptoms

Some symptoms can point to the involvement of a specific part of the nervous system, whilst others only indicate involvement of a particular pathway or system within the nervous system. Some symptoms are so non-specific that they have no value in localising the problem.

Symptoms that Localise to a Particular Part of The Nervous System
- Unilateral visual loss indicates that either the ipsilateral eye or optic nerve is affected.[2]
- Visual loss affecting both temporal fields (lateral vision): optic chiasm.[3]
- Hemianopia (loss of vision to one side): the optic radiation or occipital cortex.
- Vertical diplopia: brainstem, specifically the midbrain, 3rd, or 4th cranial nerve (very rarely due to local muscle; superior and inferior recti or superior and inferior oblique muscle problems in the orbit).
- Horizontal diplopia: brainstem, specifically the pons, 6th cranial nerve or medial longitudinal fasciculus (very rarely due to local muscle; medial or lateral rectus problems within the orbit).
- The 'pill-rolling' tremor at rest of Parkinson's: basal ganglia – specifically the subthalamic nucleus.
- Variability of weakness with exercise suggests the neuromuscular junction and myasthenia gravis or Lambert–Eaton syndrome.[4] Increased weakness with exercise indicates possible myasthenia gravis, while increased strength (and increased reflexes if examined before and after exercise) with exercise the Lambert–Eaton syndrome.
- A loss of speech is referred to as aphasia, while impairment of speech is referred to as dysphasia affecting the production and/or comprehension of written or spoken language. This almost invariably indicates a dominant hemisphere problem, usually cortical. Very rarely, a subcortical or even a thalamic problem can cause dysphasia.

# Symptoms that only Indicate Involvement of a Pathway

Vertigo (room or head-spinning): vestibular system, anywhere from the inner ear through the vestibular nerve to the brainstem and the central vestibular cortex in the temporal lobe
- Weakness: motor pathway between the cerebral cortex and the muscle
- Altered sensation: sensory pathways between the peripheral nerves and the cerebral cortex
- Marked wasting or fasciculations (visible twitching) of muscles: the lower motor neuron from the anterior horn cells in the spinal cord through the anterior nerve roots, brachial or lumbosacral plexus and peripheral nerves. Wasting does not occur in diseases of the neuromuscular junction or muscle, although occasionally long-standing muscle diseases can have wasting.

---

2  A note of caution: patients can confuse a visual loss in one side of their vision (hemianopia) with a monocular or unilateral visual loss, for example when the patient has Visual phenomena on the right, they sometimes assume it is in the right eye. It may, however, be in the right visual field. It is important to clarify whether the patient could see all or only one half of an object, it would be helpful if they had covered each eye, but most patients do not do this.

3  Optic chiasm lesions are extremely rare, and most patients are not aware of the bilateral visual disturbance

4  Fatigue and exercise-induced worsening of symptoms are very common in many chronic neurological disorders and does not imply problems at the neuromuscular junction.

# Non-Specific Symptoms

- Dysarthria: has no localising value (other than it indicates the problem is above the level of the foramen magnum). It can result from non-dominant hemisphere lesions, deep dominant hemisphere lesions, brainstem pathology and problems affecting the 9th, 10th and 12th cranial nerves, the neuromuscular junction and even disorders of muscle. Neurologists can often differentiate between the different causes of dysarthria, but this is difficult for non-neurologists.
- Anosmia: is the loss of the sense of smell; if it is of neurological origin it points to the involvement of the olfactory pathway, but in most patients', it does not relate to any disorder of the nervous system but is rather due to local nasal pathology.
- Exacerbation of symptoms from heat and exercise: transient worsening of symptoms with heat or exercise that is not relieved by immediate rest is very common with many neurological disorders. One of the most common conditions in which this is a feature is multiple sclerosis.
- Ataxia (or unsteadiness on the legs): is a very non-specific symptom. Although it suggests a cerebellar problem, it can also be present in patients with arthritis in the joints of the legs, weakness, or a proprioceptive disturbance in the legs and in patients with vertigo that is vestibular and not cerebellar in origin. A useful question to ask is whether the instability relates to a feeling in the head, indicating probable involvement of the vestibular system, hypotension, or a cerebellar problem, or to a sense of unsteadiness on the legs in the absence of any altered sensation in the head, suggesting a problem of weakness or sensory disturbance in the legs.
- Pain: is most often related to non-neurological disorders. If it is of neurological origin, it is almost invariably an indication of involvement of the peripheral nervous system as central pain syndromes are exceedingly rare. It will be in the distribution of a nerve root most likely or a peripheral nerve. Central pain syndromes develop after thalamic infarction in which there is pain in the distribution of the contralateral hemi-sensory loss.
- Urinary or bowel sphincter disturbance: sphincter disturbance is a prominent symptom of intrinsic spinal cord problems (as opposed to extrinsic cord compression in which sphincter disturbance develops late), sacral nerve root lesions or autonomic nervous system involvement. However, in females, urinary incontinence is more often of gynaecological origin and not related to a neurological problem. In men, prostatic hypertrophy or malignancy can cause incontinence.
- Dysphagia: (or difficulty swallowing) can occur with brainstem (medulla) or hemisphere problems and is therefore in itself a poor localising symptom.

Weakness with sensory symptoms immediately indicates that the problem CANNOT be related to diseases of muscle, the neuromuscular junction or anterior horn cell within the spinal cord, as these sites result in pure motor syndromes.

# The Distribution of Symptoms

As discussed in Chapter 1, always think about the underlying neuroanatomy that the nature and distribution of symptoms represent. In most instances, the history can assist in establishing whether the pathology is affecting the brain, spinal cord (in the central nervous system) or peripheral nervous system.

As you take the history, think of the nervous system as a map grid with the **meridians of longitude and parallels of latitude.** Although the neurological examination is far more critical when it comes to accurate localisation, many patients present with transient neurological symptoms, without any neurological signs. For example, the history elicits that the patient has weakness affecting the entire left side of the body, including the face. This points to a problem in the central nervous system and on the contralateral side above the mid pons, the site of the facial nerve nucleus.

---

By defining the meridians of longitude and the parallels of latitude that the symptoms (and subsequent signs, if present) represent, it is possible in most instances to accurately localise the site of the problem in the nervous system.

---

# Patterns of Weakness

If the symptom is weakness, ask questions to define the exact pattern of weakness. If the weakness is confined to one limb, ascertain if it is the whole limb or only part of the limb. If the whole limb is weak, this is more suggestive of a central nervous system problem.

Suppose only part of the limb is weak. In that case, it is more likely (but not always) related to the involvement of the peripheral nervous system, either a nerve root, an individual nerve, the brachial plexus in the arm or lumbosacral plexus in the leg. Establish what part of the limb is weak. Muscle wasting and or fasciculations (involuntary twitching of parts of muscles) are both occasionally observed by patients and localise the problem to the lower motor or peripheral nervous system.

An example of how the pattern of weakness can help localise the problem while taking a history is shown in Case 2.3.

---

**Case 2.3** A 55-year-old man presents with 'right-sided weakness'

When the weakness involves the whole leg, it most likely reflects an upper motor neuron or central nervous system problem above the level of L2 in the lumbar spinal cord.

If the ipsilateral arm is also affected, this places the pathology above the level of C5 in the cervical spinal cord or contralateral brain. If the ipsilateral face is also affected, the lesion is above the facial nerve nucleus in the contralateral mid pons of the brainstem.

In the absence of any additional symptoms, this is as far as we can go to localise the problem.

On the other hand, if the patient has impaired speech in the form of dysphasia, this indicates involvement of the speech area in the left hemisphere cortex.

The right-sided weakness is the meridian of longitude, indicating the involvement of the motor pathway. Dysphasia is the parallel of latitude indicating the involvement of the cortical structures in the cortex of the left frontal lobe.

---

The patterns of weakness that indicate involvement of a particular part of the nervous system include:

- Weakness confined to one limb: weakness affecting the entire arm or the entire leg, particularly when it begins suddenly, is most likely to be due to a central rather than a peripheral nervous system problem. The history is not particularly useful when there is a focal weakness in a limb. Focal weakness in a limb can be either of central or peripheral nervous system origin, and a neurological examination is needed to sort out the various causes. On the other hand, establishing precisely what part of the limb is weak can narrow down the possibilities if the problem is in the PNS.

- Weakness of the hand or forearm: C7, C8, T1 nerve root, median, ulnar, or radial nerve (Case 2.4 discusses weakness in the right arm accompanied by some sensory loss.)
- Weakness of the upper arm or shoulder: C5—C6 nerve root, axillary, musculocutaneous or suprascapular nerve problems
- Weakness of the upper leg: L2, L3, L4 nerve root or femoral nerve
- Weakness in the lower part of the leg: L5—S1 nerve root, sciatic, common peroneal or posterior tibial nerve problem.
- Hemiparesis: weakness of the arm and leg with or without facial involvement is almost certainly a central nervous (upper motor neuron) system problem. It is often related to a problem in the contralateral hemisphere, less likely the contralateral brainstem and very rarely in the ipsilateral spinal cord above the level of C5.
- Paraparesis: weakness confined to both legs is most often related to a spinal cord problem or a lower motor neuron problem such as peripheral neuropathy.
- Quadriparesis: four-limb weakness indicates a cervical spinal cord problem above the C5 level, less often a peripheral neuropathy or muscle disease.

Once a patient has symptoms affecting the cranial nerves, vision, speech, hearing, vertigo, memory or cognition, the problem CANNOT be in the spinal cord.

# Patterns of Sensory Symptoms

When a patient complains of numbness in the hand, we can ascertain that the problem must be between the peripheral nerve and the contralateral cerebral sensory cortex. On the other hand, if we ask the patient to clarify the exact area of altered sensation, we can determine whether it is in the distribution of a single nerve, nerve root, or one of the sensory pathways.

For example, a patient complains of numbness affecting the medial 1½ fingers on both the palmar and dorsal aspects of the fingers and the medial aspect of the hand up to the wrist. This pattern of sensory loss is the area supplied by the ulnar nerve. (See Figures 1.14 and 1.15) A second example is a patient who complains of numbness in the leg. A careful history establishes that the numbness is confined to the lateral aspect of the thigh below the groin and above the knee. This is the area supplied by the lateral cutaneous nerve of the thigh, and the diagnosis is meralgia paraesthetica. (See Figure 1.20). Cases 2.4 and 2.5 illustrates numbness originating from a peripheral and a central nervous system problem, respectively.

---

**Case 2.4** A young man with weakness in the right arm and focal sensory loss

A 20-year-old man has fallen asleep in a chair after a heavy night of drinking. He awakens the next morning and notices a severe weakness in his right arm. He is unable to extend his wrist and fingers, and his handgrip is very weak. He is not aware of any pain, but there is a small area of sensory loss between his thumb and index finger on the back of his hand. He is right-handed, and his speech is normal.

The patient has noticed his symptoms on waking, and therefore the exact mode of onset cannot be determined except to say that they arose sometime between when he fell asleep and when he woke. Therefore, the onset could have been very sudden, or it could have come on gradually over minutes or hours.

The patient has a focal weakness in the right arm with an inability to extend the wrist and fingers. This occurs with a stroke, a radial nerve palsy or with C7 radiculopathy. The weakness is usually mild with C7 radiculopathy and in general associated with severe pain down the arm to the middle 3 fingers. Severe weakness in the right hand in a right-handed person due to a central nervous system problem in the left frontal lobe will almost invariably be associated with a severe speech disturbance. A wrist drop is unusual for a stroke. However, it is the very focal sensory loss between the first and second fingers combined with weakness confined to muscles innervated by the radial nerve that enables the correct diagnosis of a radial nerve problem or "Saturday night palsy as it is known".

As shown in Figure 1.15, the area of skin between the first and second digits is supplied by the superficial radial nerve. C7 radiculopathy would produce sensory loss affecting the middle three digits of the hand.

---

Sensory symptoms affecting the ipsilateral leg, arm and face indicate a lesion above the contralateral 5th nerve nucleus in the brainstem.

Patients are often referred with suspected tarsal tunnel syndrome due to compression of the medial or lateral plantar nerves at the level of the medial malleolus when they have symptoms affecting the top and the sole. The problem is beyond the distribution of the medial or lateral plantar nerves, which only supply the sole. Therefore, the problem cannot be tarsal tunnel syndrome.

---

**Case 2.5** A 25-year-old woman with numbness and tingling in her legs and lower body

A 25-year-old woman presents with the gradual onset of numbness and tingling commencing in the toes and spreading over three days to affect her body from the breasts down. She has also noticed difficulty urinating and has been constipated.

The distribution of the sensory symptoms indicates involvement of the sensory pathways because they affect both the legs and the trunk and cannot represent problems associated with individual nerves or nerve roots.

Sensory symptoms do not occur on the entire trunk in problems affecting the peripheral nervous system, but sensory disturbance on either side of the midline can be seen in, for example, diabetic truncal neuropathy. A truncal neuropathy results in a band of sensory loss extending a few centimetres on either side of the midline rather than sensory loss affecting the whole trunk.

The sensory symptoms extended up to the level of the breasts, which is consistent with a lesion at the level of T4 in the thoracic spinal cord. The disturbance of sphincter function also indicates that the problem is in the spinal cord. The mode of onset is gradual over several days and this suggests an inflammatory or infective process, most likely transverse myelitis, or a manifestation of multiple sclerosis.

---

# Pain

In most instances, pain is unrelated to a neurological problem. Pain in the region of a joint made worse by moving that joint reflects local joint pathology. Pain with localised tenderness is related to a process at the site of tenderness, e.g., acute gout in a joint or the tenderness just below the lateral epicondyle in "tennis elbow" with pain radiating down the back of the forearm.

When pain does reflect a neurological problem, when taking the history, don't just ascertain that the patient has limb pain. Ask them for the exact distribution of the pain. In doing so, one can have a much better idea of whether it is a nerve root or peripheral nerve problem. Central pain is infrequent. It can occur after a stroke affecting the contralateral thalamus, with pain down the opposite side of the body to the midline. Pain due to compression or irritation of a nerve root radiating into the arm or leg is referred pain as the site of the pain is not at the site of the pathological process. Where the pain radiates to in the limb will depend on which nerve root is involved. For example, if the pain radiates down the arm from the neck to the thumb, this is in keeping with a C6 nerve root problem.

If the patient has pain confined to the lateral 3½ fingers of the hand, this indicates a median nerve problem. Pain limited to one or more branches of the trigeminal nerve on the face suggests "probable" involvement of that nerve. It is essential to understand that dental pain is also restricted to the distribution of the 2nd or 3rd divisions of the trigeminal nerve. Pain beyond the trigeminal nerve distribution excludes trigeminal neuralgia. (See Chapter 9) Case 2.6 and 2.7 illustrate how the distribution of pain and altered sensation can aid in diagnosis.

---

**Case 2.6** A 70-year-old man with severe pain radiating from his right buttock to the ankle

A 70-year-old man experiences the sudden onset of severe pain radiating from his right buttock down his right leg to the ankle while bending over in the garden. He retires to bed and, when he stands the following morning, he has difficulty walking because he cannot lift his right foot. When he touches his right leg, he notices reduced sensation affecting the top of his foot and the lateral aspect of his shin.

- The onset of his pain is sudden and occurred whilst bending over, suggesting a mechanical problem. The weakness of dorsiflexion of the right foot is in keeping with either L5 radiculopathy or a common peroneal nerve lesion. The presence and distribution of the pain is more in keeping with radiculopathy. Of course, the pattern of sensory symptoms is clearly in the distribution of the L5 nerve root (see Figure 1.22), not in the peroneal nerve distribution.

- This is a classical presentation of sciatica. Exactly why the weakness and sensory disturbance develops some hours later when the disc compresses the nerve root at the time of the original injury is unclear, but possibly represents an inflammatory response to the nerve root compression.

---

**Case 2.7** A 40-year-old man with pain over his left thigh

A 40-year-old-man developed pain down the lateral aspect of his left thigh that was made worse with standing and was not present lying flat. He had degenerative changes in his left hip and a left L4-5 disc protrusion. He underwent a total left hip joint replacement without benefit and subsequently developed altered sensation down the lateral aspect of the thigh in the same distribution as the pain. An L4-5 discectomy did not relieve his pain.

His pain was not influenced by moving his hip; thus, it is not surprising that hip surgery didn't relieve the pain. The distribution of the sensory loss was not that of an L5 nerve root lesion, so it is not surprising that the discectomy did not relieve his pain. His pain and sensory loss involved the distribution of the lateral cutaneous nerve of the thigh. The diagnostic test was to compress his lateral cutaneous nerve beneath the inguinal ligament just medial to the anterior superior iliac spine. His pain resolved with a corticosteroid injection combined with local anaesthetic into the region where the nerve is compressed beneath the inguinal ligament. In this case, neither the orthopaedic surgeon nor the neurosurgeon elucidated the exact nature and distribution of his symptoms.

# Past History, Family History and Social History

The family history, previous medical problems and social history should not be used to diagnose the present problem. The exception to this is when one cannot obtain a reliable account. These aspects of the history support the diagnosis made from analysing the presenting symptoms as outlined above.

Another reason why we should ignore the past and family history is that the diagnosis may have been incorrect. It is crucial that there was proof of the diagnosis or that the symptoms were consistent with that diagnosis. This is particularly so with a past or family history of an illness such as migraine, for which there is no test to confirm the diagnosis. In many instances, on detailed questioning, the prior headaches do not fulfil the criteria for migraine as defined by the International Headache Society [3]. Other examples include where relatives are told that the cause of death was a heart attack when patients suffer sudden death or succumb during sleep without any pathological confirmation of the diagnosis.

In many patients with chronic neurological diseases, there is a tendency for both the patient and the inexperienced practitioner to assume that all new symptoms are related to that chronic neurological illness. However, a diagnosis of Parkinson's disease does not exclude the patient from suffering a stroke, spinal cord compression or some other neurological problem. In a patient with a chronic, slowly progressive neurological problem, *the vital clue that there may be an additional illness is a sudden change in the rate of progression of the disability.* Two examples of this seen by the author are one patient with slowly progressive difficulty walking over years related to Parkinson's disease who developed a rapid decline in function from walking to being bedridden within six months. This rapid deterioration was due to dermatomyositis. A second patient with slowly progressive Parkinson's disease developed rapidly worsening difficulty walking, was found to have leg weakness, not a feature of Parkinson's, and had spinal cord compression.

Many incorrect diagnoses are sustained by simply accepting the patient's statement that they or a relative had a particular illness in the past.

In patients with chronic neurological disorders, beware of new symptoms or an alteration in the rate at which the illness is worsening. This often indicates the presence of a second problem.

# The Process of Taking the History

Patients often come to the consultation with a preconceived idea about what they intend to say. Some have many, many pages of notes, much of which is not relevant. I have developed the trick of asking the patient to give me the notes to read them and decide what is relevant. After the initial introductions, *it is essential to allow the patient time to describe the symptoms without interruption*, recording brief comments that you can explore later.

If you interrupt the patient at this early stage, a vital piece of information may be missed. Other patients may feel 'cheated' and complain that the doctor did not listen to what they had to say! This usually takes a few minutes. In many cases, one has very few clues after the patient's initial comments and, frequently, there is a lot of information that does not help determine the nature of the problem. At some stage, it is necessary to take charge of the history-taking process and clarify (where possible):

- The mode of onset and progression of every symptom
- The exact nature and distribution of every symptom
- The past, family, social and medication history that may influence subsequent management.

This is best achieved by using the approach illustrated in Figure 2.2.

There is a link[5] to my website that contains a lecture explaining the principles in this chapter. There is also a video of Lord John Walton, Professor of Neurology at Newcastle upon Tyne (UK). He is taking a history from a patient. He asks repeated questions to establish precisely when the patient first noticed their symptoms. In this instance, the patient only became aware of a problem when she sat on a cold surface. Therefore, exactly when the initial symptoms commenced cannot be established.

Further questioning elicits that the symptoms progressed by spreading to other body parts after they were first noticed. In this manner, John Walton is identifying the possible pathological process. He clarifies the exact nature and distribution of every symptom, thus defining the site of the problem within the nervous system. Finally, he asks about symptoms in the past that would indicate any previous neurological illness that may relate to the current illness.

---

5  Professor Peter Gates website: http://www.understandingneurology.com/

When were you last well?

↓

What was the first symptom you noticed?
Exactly what part of the body did it involve?

↓

Did it improve or worsen either in intensity
or extent (spread to another part of the
body) after it was first noticed? If so,
over what period of time?

↓

What was the next symptom you noticed?
did it get worse after you first noticed it?
If so, how quickly?
(Repeat this question until all
symptoms are descibed)

↓

How long did it last?
(Repeat this question until all
symptoms are descibed)

↓

Is there any family history of a
similar problem?

↓

What medical problems have you had
in the past?

↓

What medications are you taking?

↓

Do you live alone or is there someone
either at home or who lives nearby
who can help you?

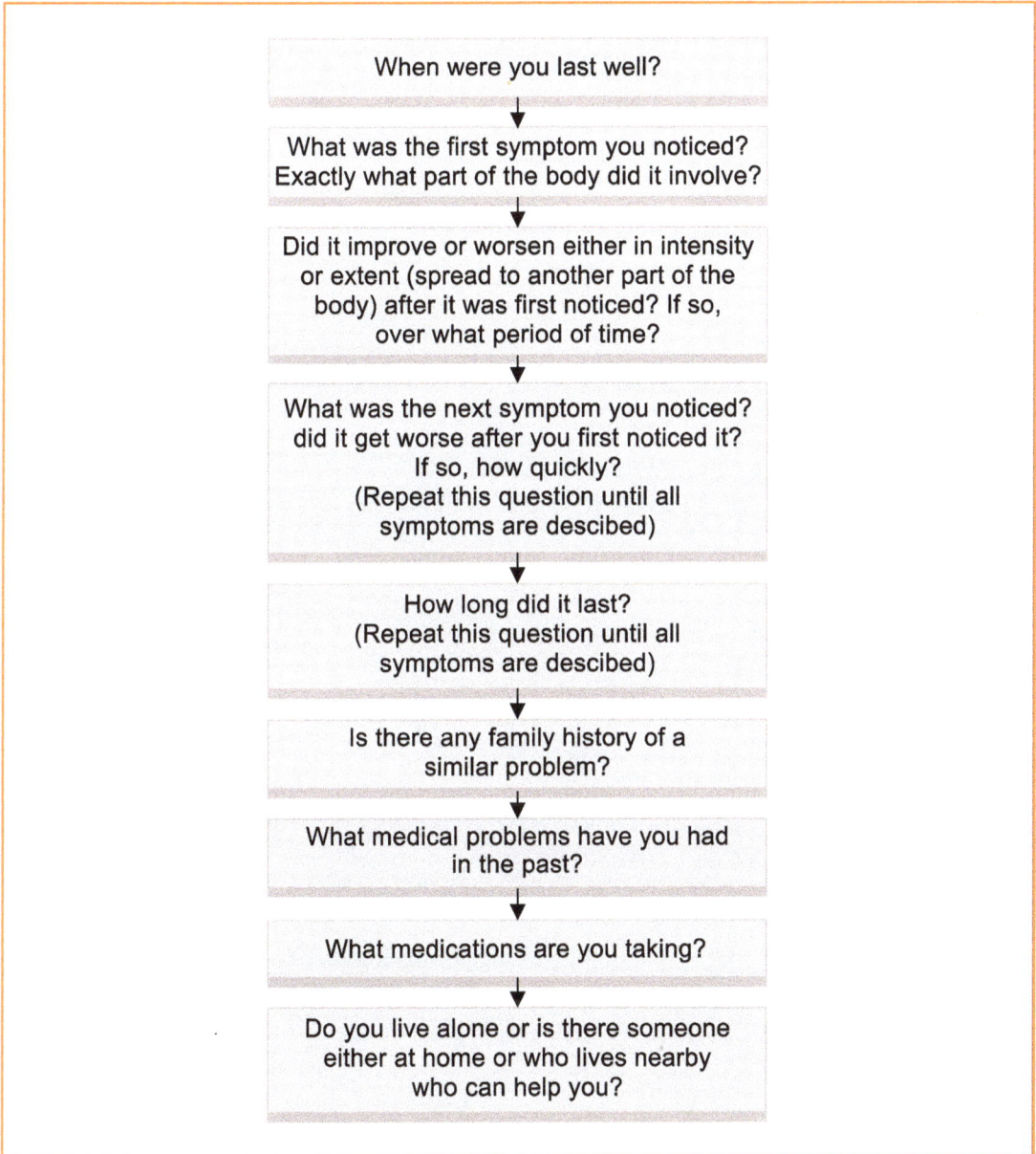

**Figure 2.2** A suggested method of asking questions of patients who have a monophasic illness

Unfortunately, this latter aspect does require prior knowledge and experience. Although he comments that this is a pattern he recognises, his technique of taking the history reflects the principles espoused in this chapter.

We have already pointed out that it is impossible to learn how to elicit a good history by reading a textbook. It is hoped that students armed with the information in this chapter will find their time on the wards taking histories from patients with neurological disorders more rewarding.

# References

1   Spencer J. Learning and teaching in the clinical environment. *BMJ* 2003;326(7389): 591–594.

2   Sackett DL, Haynes RB, Tugwell P. Clinical diagnostic strategies. In: Sackett DL, Haynes RB, Tugwell P, editors. *Clinical epidemiology: A basic science for clinical medicine*. 1st edn Boston: Little, Brown and Company; 1985. p. 11.

3   International Headache Society. The international classification of headache disorders, 2nd edn. *Cephalgia* 2004; 24:24–37.

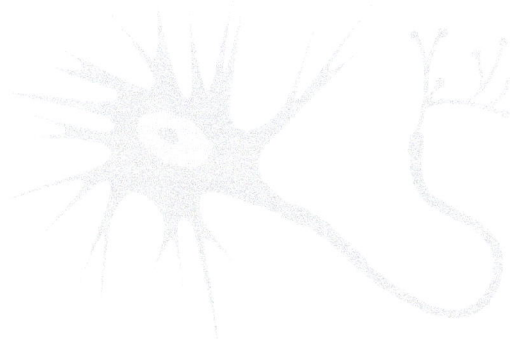

# Neurological Examination of the Limbs

Learning how to perform a neurological examination requires repeated practice. Practice without understanding how to examine the various aspects of the nervous system and how to interpret the findings is akin to practising golf without having had lessons – potentially useless. This chapter describes how to examine the limbs and interpret the findings. It is very difficult to learn how to examine from a textbook. A video of the technique is on the website.

Apart from a few pathognomonic signs that distinguish one disease from another, for example, the tremor, rigidity, and bradykinesia implicating Parkinson's disease with involvement of the substantia nigra or basal ganglia, in most instances the neurological examination does not establish the aetiology or cause of the problem. It simply localises the part of the nervous system affected by the pathological process.

The principal purpose of the examination is to determine whether the patient has **lower motor neuron (LMN)** signs or, more specifically, signs that indicate involvement of the peripheral nervous system (anterior horn cells, nerve roots, brachial or lumbosacral plexus, peripheral nerve, neuromuscular junction or muscle) or **upper motor neuron (UMN)** signs that indicate involvement of the central nervous system (brain, cerebellum and spinal cord). These were briefly discussed in Chapter 2 and are discussed in more detail in this chapter (see Table 3.1).

Although there are many ways to examine a patient, the following method is used by many neurologists and is the one recommended by this author.

## The Motor Examination

The Examination of the Motor System Involves:
- inspecting for wasting and fasciculations in the muscles
- looking for changes in tone and reflexes
- testing strength
- checking the plantar responses.

The examination should start with inspection for wasting and fasciculations. This author then examines the tone, followed by strength, then the reflexes and the plantar responses. The exact order is not important. Having said this if the tone is increased then I know I am looking for UMN signs.

49

Many examiners will perform a screening test of the upper limbs by observing patients elevating their arms and holding them horizontally straight out in front, initially with their eyes open and then subsequently closed (see Figure 3.1). The palms can be turned either down or up – it does not matter – although occasionally having the palms turned upwards seems a more sensitive technique[1]

The arm(s) will:

- drift downwards if there is weakness
- drift upwards and often outwards if there is a proprioceptive or parietal lobe problem
- oscillate up and down with a cerebellar disturbance if the patient is asked to elevate the limbs briskly, which can be missed if the movement is too slow.

---

If the history has been obtained using the method discussed in chapter 2 then the nature and distribution of the symptoms should provide a clue as to whether we will find upper or lower motor neuron signs

The pathology is always at the level of the LMN signs and at or above the upper limit of the UMN signs

In most instances the examination does NOT establish the diagnosis it merely localises the site of the pathology within the nervous system

---

**Table 3.1**

|  | **Upper motor neuron lesion** | **Lower motor neuron lesion** |
|---|---|---|
| **Wasting** | Usually, no wasting but there may be mild wasting with long-standing problems | No wasting in the very early stages but usually associated with significant wasting |
| **Power** | Weakness of extensor muscles in the arms* and flexor muscles in the legs** | The pattern of weakness reflects that part of the LMN that is affected |
| **Tone** | Increased +/– clonus | Decreased |
| **Reflexes** | Increased | Decreased or absent |
| **Plantars** | Up-going (extensor) | Down-going |
| **Sensory findings** | Sensory level | Focal sensory from a nerve root, plexus, or peripheral nerve |

* In the arms initially, wrist and finger extension are weak and then as the weakness increases in severity shoulder abduction and then elbow extension become weak.

**In the legs hip flexion is the first to become weak followed by foot dorsiflexion and then knee flexion. The tone may not be increased, and the reflexes can be absent in acute spinal cord lesions referred to as spinal shock. Clonus is a series of involuntary repetitive movements of the ankle, up and down, induced by suddenly pushing the foot upwards while the leg is extended [1]. The test is less painful if it is performed with the knee slightly flexed.

**Table 3.1** The neurological findings in upper versus lower motor neuron lesions

---

1   Personal Observation

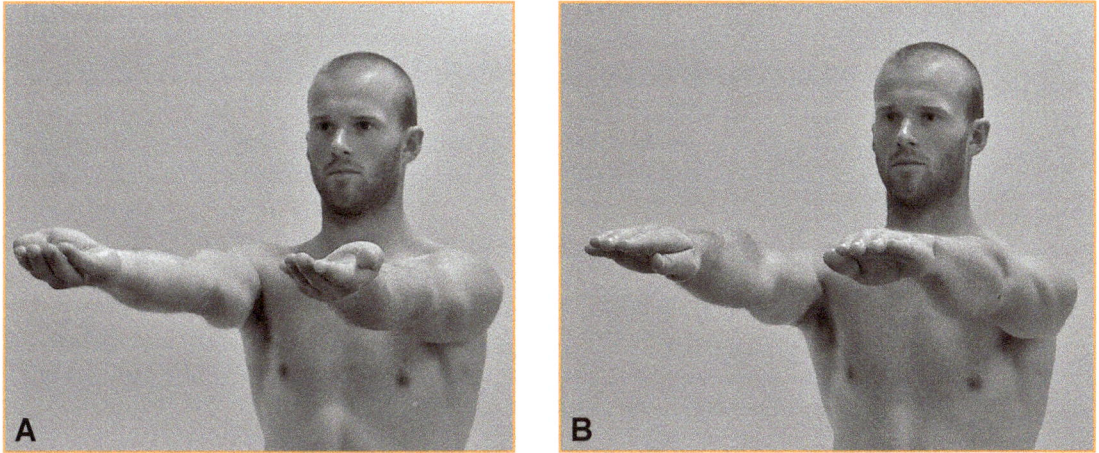

**Figure 3.1** Screening test of the upper limbs with hands outstretched: **A** with palms up; **B** with palms down

# Inspection for Wasting and Fasciculations

The muscles of the upper arm, forearm, hand, thigh, anterior tibial compartment, and calves are examined for wasting and/or fasciculations. Fasciculations are visible spontaneous contractions or twitching of muscle fibres that are innervated by a single motor unit [1]. It may be necessary to spend several minutes carefully examining the muscles to detect fasciculations. It is easy to be certain that wasting is present when it is very severe, but with milder degrees of wasting one is less certain that there is a lesion involving the peripheral (LMN) nervous system.

Some patients are very thin, and inexperienced clinicians may incorrectly suspect wasting when examining the small muscles of the hands, particularly in older patients. If the wasting affects one arm or one leg a comparison can be made with the contralateral limb.

The muscles, if wasted, will lose their rounded convex appearance, and appear flattened or even concave.

The reliable signs of muscle wasting are:
- loss of the visible bulge that occurs when the thumb is adducted towards the index finger – the 1st dorsal interosseous muscle. (Figure 3.2)
- prominence of the anterior border of the tibia – tibialis anterior muscle
- prominence of the spine of the scapula – supraspinatus and infraspinatus muscles
- scalloped appearance just above the patella as if a bite has been taken out of the muscle – quadriceps.

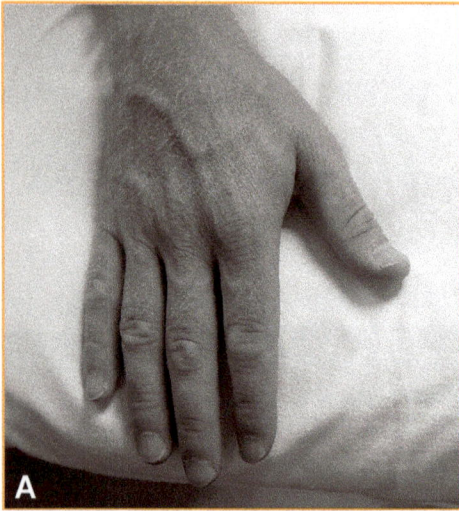

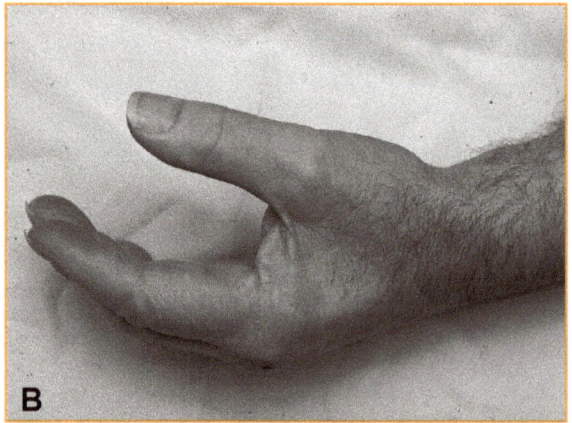

**Figure 3.2** The first dorsal interosseous muscle: A no wasting; B wasting

## Looking for Changes in Tone

There are two different ways to test for tone, depending on whether the problem is affecting the motor system or the extrapyramidal system.

The tone is tested using quick movements when the motor system is being assessed.

## Testing Tone due to an Upper Motor Neuron Problem

It is important to first check with the patient whether a quick movement of the arm or leg would cause pain.

Arms. The tone is tested with the forearm semi-pronated, and the elbow flexed at 90° (Figure 3.3A). The examiner holds the elbow with one hand and then places the other hand in the hand of the patient as if they were shaking hands. The test is performed with quick supination of the forearm. If there is an increased tone, there will be a discernible catch. Very occasionally, when the tone is markedly increased, repetitive contractions may occur, and this is referred to as clonus.

Legs. The tone is tested with the leg lying flat on the bed, slightly externally rotated and with the knee flexed very slightly. The examiner places their hands behind the leg just above the knee and attempts to quickly elevate the leg. If there is increased tone, the heel will lift off the bed. The leg may lift off the bed in patients who are very anxious and who find it difficult to relax – slight external rotation of the leg before the quick movement helps in this situation and eliminates the false impression of increased tone in anxious patients. The other test for increased tone in the legs is ankle clonus, where the leg is slightly flexed at the knee with the ankle plantar-flexed. The examiner places one hand behind the knee and grasps the foot with the other hand and forcibly dorsiflexes the foot. Repetitive contractions while the examiner holds the foot in dorsiflexion is a sign of increased tone, referred to as ankle clonus.

# Testing Tone Related to an Extrapyramidal Problem

To test the upper limbs (Figure 3.3B), the forearm and hand are pronated, and the examiner holds the middle of the forearm with one hand and holds the hand of the patient in a monkey grip. The patient's hand is compressed into the wrist as the wrist is slowly flexed and extended. This technique will elicit the classical cog-wheel rigidity seen with *extrapyramidal problems*. The sensitivity of this test can be increased using Jendrassik's manoeuvre. This involves contracting muscles in another part of the body. This can involve clenching their teeth, although the method I prefer is to ask the patient to clench their fist on the opposite hand, then raise their arm above their head and finally to shake their head to and fro. This increases the tone (and will also enhance reflexes) by countering some of the normal descending inhibitory brainstem inputs to the reflex arc.

To test the lower limbs, the leg is flexed at the knee and the examiner holds the leg behind the knee. Using the other hand, the examiner grasps the foot and slowly dorsiflexes and plantarflexes the ankle, looking for the cog-wheel rigidity. The two techniques for testing tone are demonstrated on the DVD.

---

If the signs are not what one would expect from taking the history, then the diagnosis should be reviewed and the whole process should be repeated to confirm both the history and findings.

This approach is far more rewarding than ordering many investigations.

---

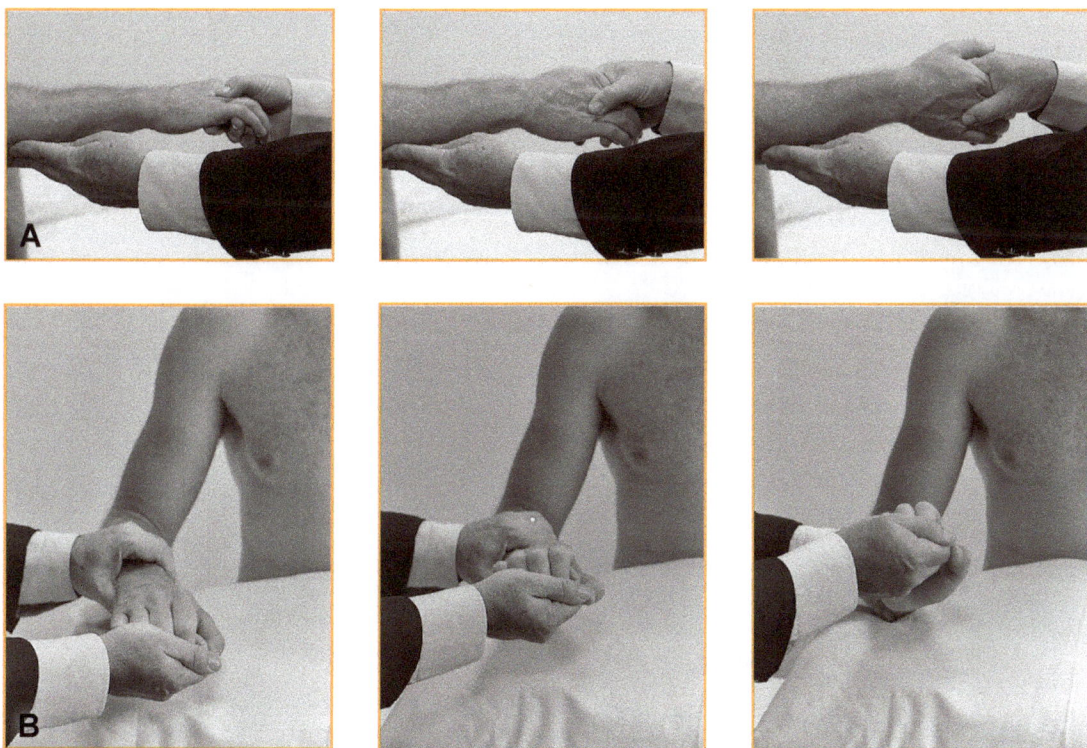

**Figure 3.3** How to test tone in the upper limbs: A motor system; B extrapyramidal system

# Testing Muscle Strength

Use simple language that the patient can understand. The extent of muscle testing can be varied, depending on whether the history suggests a UMN problem or an LMN problem. In patients with involvement of the central nervous system or corticospinal tract, specific patterns of weakness occur and these are discussed below. In patients with focal weakness with or without focal sensory loss, suggesting a LMN problem, it is important to examine strength by commencing in that part of the limb that the patient describes as weak. The examiner then tests every single muscle of the affected limb to establish the pattern of weakness and, from this, the anatomical basis for the weakness and the site of the pathology within the peripheral nervous system can be determined. The 5*3*5 (chapter 11) and the 2*2*4 (chapter 12) rules assist the non-neurologist to diagnose all peripheral nerve and nerve root problems causing weakness in the arm and leg respectively.

The following technique is recommended when examining muscle strength. The muscle/muscle group, nerve-related to that muscle/muscle group, the nerve root(s), and the action of the muscle [2] are listed in each section below. Experienced neurologists have memorised the neuroanatomy; inexperienced clinicians can record the pattern of weakness and consult a textbook of neuroanatomy, the illustrations in Chapter 1 or alternatively use the 5*3*5 rule and the 2*2*4 rules for examining the upper (chapter 11) and lower (chapter 12) limbs respectively and consult the relevant tables.

# Upper Limbs
## Muscles around the shoulder

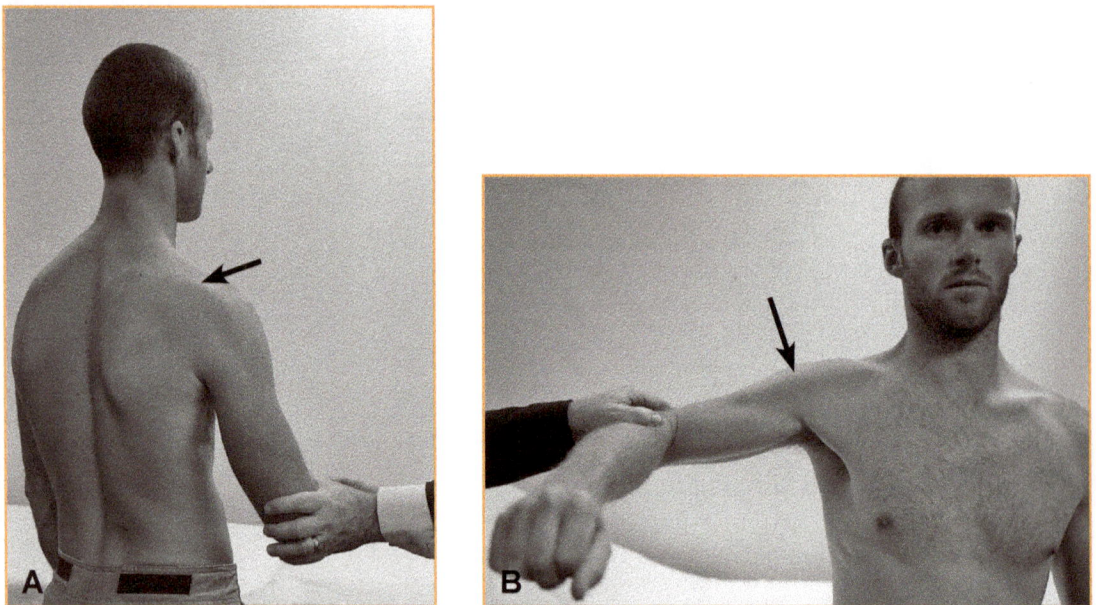

**Figure 3.4** Testing of the **A** supraspinatuss and **B** deltoid muscles (abduction of the shoulder)

**Figure 3.4A**

| | |
|---|---|
| **Muscle** | Supraspinatus |
| **Nerve supply** | Suprascapular nerve |
| **Nerve root** | C5 – 6 |
| **Action** | Initial abduction of shoulder to 30° |

**Figure 3.4B**

| | |
|---|---|
| **Muscle** | Deltoid |
| **Nerve supply** | Axillary nerve |
| **Nerve root** | C5 – 6 |
| **Action** | Abduction of shoulder beyond 30° |

To test the supraspinatus (Figure 3.4A) the elbow should be abducted from the side of the body to approximately 30°, the examiner places a hand over the elbow and pushes the elbow towards the trunk while the patient tries to resist.

To test the deltoid muscle (Figure 3.4B) the elbow should be abducted from the side to 90°, the examiner places a hand over the upper arm just above the elbow and pushes downwards while the patient attempts to resist.

**Figure 3.5**

| | |
|---|---|
| **Muscle** | Infraspinatus |
| **Nerve supply** | Suprascapular nerve |
| **Nerve root** | C5 – 6 |
| **Action** | External rotation of the shoulder |

To test the infraspinatus the elbow is kept by the side, the forearm is flexed at 90° and the hand is semi-pronated (Figure 3.5). The examiner places a hand over the middle of the back of the forearm and attempts to internally rotate the forearm towards the body as the patient resists.

**Figure 3.6**

| | |
|---|---|
| **Muscle** | Subscapularis |
| **Nerve supply** | Nerve to subscapularis |
| **Nerve root** | C5 – 7 |
| **Action** | Internal rotation of the shoulder |

To test subscapularis the elbow is kept by the side, the forearm is flexed at 90° and the hand is semi-pronated (Figure 3.6). The examiner places a hand on the middle of the forearm and attempts to prevent internal rotation of the forearm.

**Figure 3.7**

| | |
|---|---|
| **Muscle** | Serratus anterior |
| **Nerve supply** | Nerve to serratus anterior |
| **Nerve root** | C5 – 7 |
| **Action** | Anchoring the scapular to the chest wall |

There is a rare entity called winging of the scapular that is the result of damage to the nerve to the serratus anterior (see Chapter 1). The patient is instructed to stand in front of a wall, with the elbows slightly flexed and the palms on the wall (Figure 3.7). They are then instructed to push as hard as they can, and the scapular should not lift off the chest wall. If it does the muscle is weak, resulting in 'winging of the scapula'.

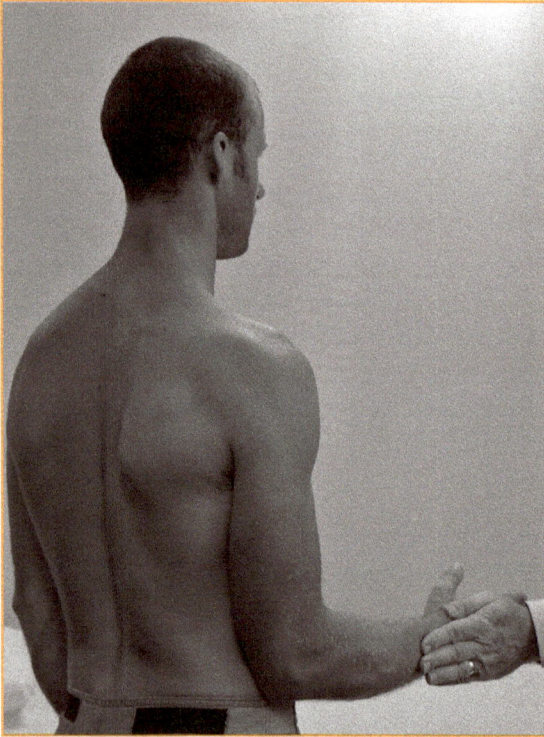

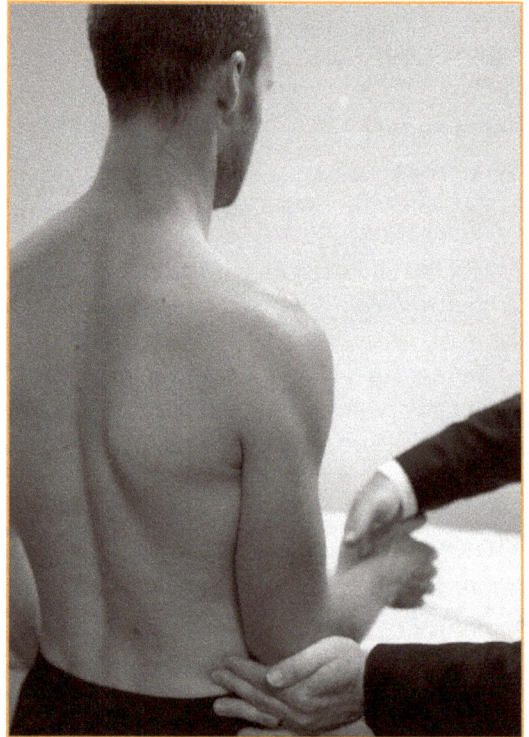

**Figure 3.5** Left Testing of the infraspinatus (external rotation of the shoulder) and right **Figure 3.6** Testing of the subscapularis (internal rotation of the shoulder)

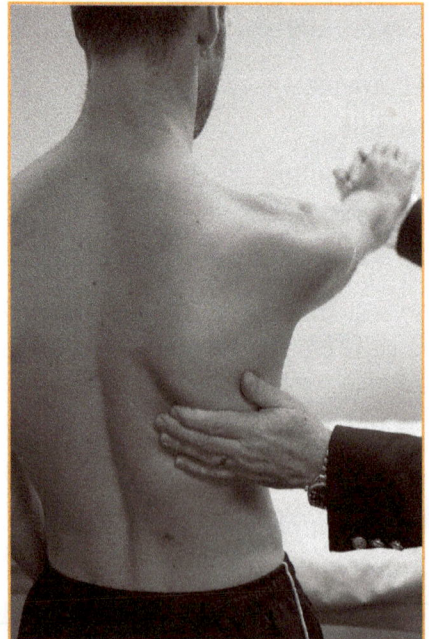

**Figure 3.7** Testing of the serratus anterior

# Muscles around the elbow

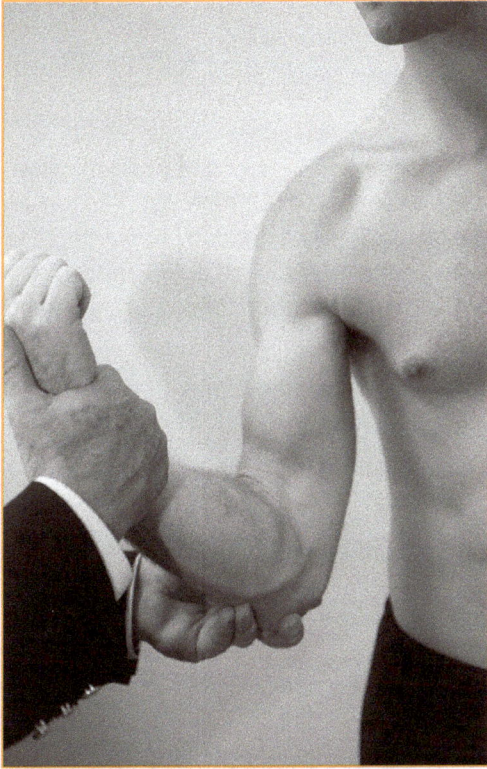

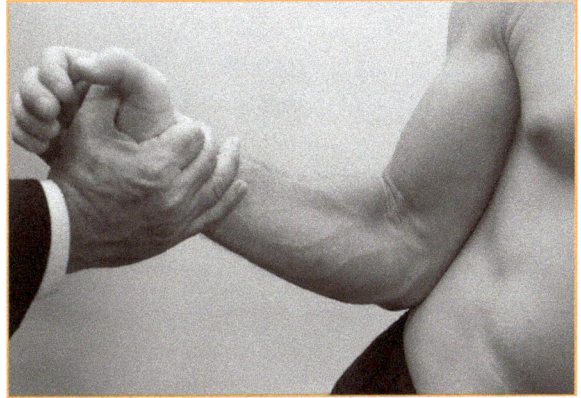

**Figure 3.8** Left Testing elbow flexion with the forearm supinated (biceps) and right **Figure 3.9** testing elbow flexion with the elbow semi-pronated (brachioradialis)

| **Figure 3.8** | |
|---|---|
| **Muscle** | Biceps and brachialis |
| **Nerve supply** | Musculocutaneous nerve |
| **Nerve root** | C5 – 6 |
| **Action** | Elbow flexion with the palm of hand pointing to the ceiling |

The elbow is bent at 90° with the forearm supinated i.e., the palm pointing towards the ceiling (Figure 3.8). The examiner grasps the elbow with the left hand and the wrist with the right hand and attempts to prevent further flexion of the elbow.

| **Figure 3.9** | |
|---|---|
| **Muscle** | Brachioradialis |
| **Nerve supply** | Radial nerve |
| **Nerve root** | C6 |
| **Action** | Elbow flexion with palm pointed to the wall |

The elbow is flexed at 90° with the forearm semi-pronated i.e., palm pointed to the wall (Figure 3.9). The examiner places the left hand under the elbow and the right hand on the wrist and attempts to prevent further flexion of the elbow.

**Figure 3.10**

| Muscle | Triceps Figure 3.10 |
| --- | --- |
| Nerve supply | Radial nerve |
| Nerve root | C5 – 7 |
| Action | Elbow extension |

The elbow must be only slightly flexed (as little as 20–30° from the fully extended position) when testing extension (Figure 3.10a). If the elbow is fully flexed (figure 3.10B), this will result in an apparent weakness of the triceps when it is strong. If the elbow is fully extended, subtle degrees of weakness may be missed. The examiner places the left hand over the anterior aspect of the elbow and the right hand under the wrist and attempts to prevent the patient from straightening their elbow.

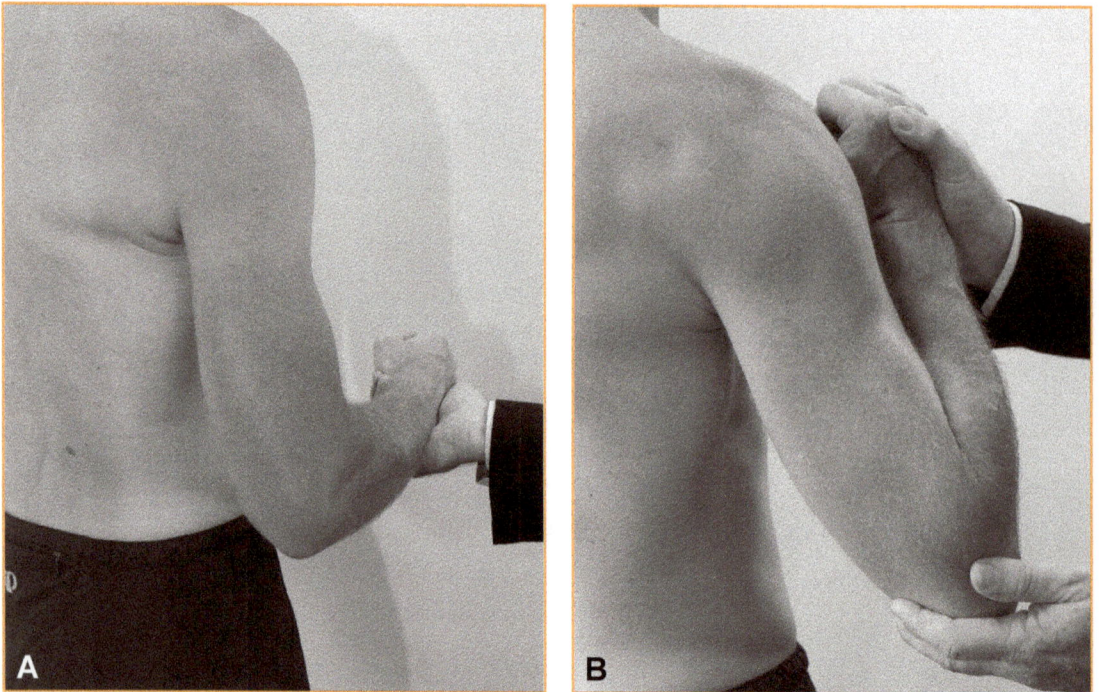

Figure 3.10 Testing of the triceps (elbow extension): **A** correct method; **B** incorrect method

# Muscles in the forearm

**Figure 3.11 A and B**

| Muscle | Extensor digitorum, extensor carpi ulnaris, extensor carpi radialis longus and brevis and extensor digiti minimi |
| --- | --- |
| Nerve Supply | Radial |
| Nerve Root | C7 |
| Action | Extension of wrist and fingers |

The patient is instructed to extend their wrist and the examiner places the back of their hand on the back of the patient's hand and attempts to flex the wrist while the patient resists (Figure 3.11). Similarly, the patient is asked to extend their fingers and the examiner places the back of their fingers across the patient's fingers. The 5th digit of the examiner's hand lies over the patient's metacarpophalangeal joints while the second digit of the patient's hand is beneath the metacarpophalangeal joints of the examiner. Using this technique both the examiner and the patient can exert a full effort if strength is normal.

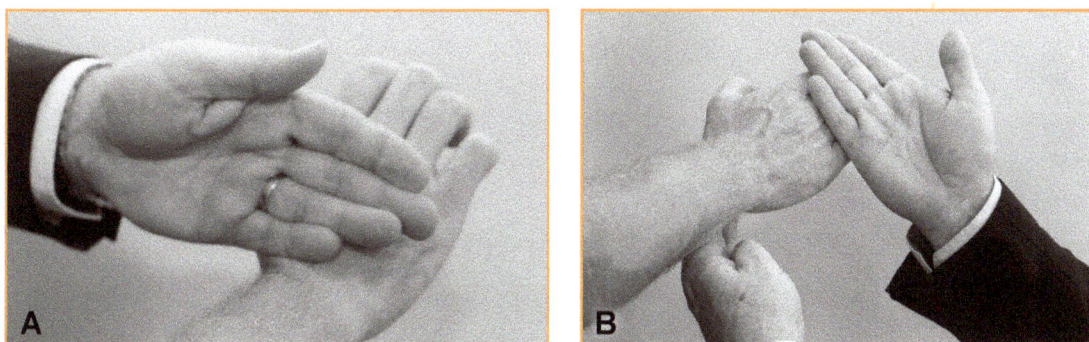

**Figure 3.11** Testing wrist (**A**) and finger (**B**) extension (the extensor digitorum longus, extensor pollicis longus, extensor carpi radialis and extensor carpi ulnaris)

**Figure 3.12**

| | |
|---|---|
| **Muscle** | Interossei and Lumbricals |
| **Nerve supply** | Ulnar nerve |
| **Nerve root** | C8 – T1 |
| **Action** | Finger abduction |

The patient is instructed to spread the fingers apart and the examiner attempts to push them together by pressing on the base of the fingers close to the metacarpophalangeal joints (Figure 3.12). Using this technique, the patient should be able to resist very firm pressure whereas, if the examiner pushes against the tips of the fingers, even patients with normal strength cannot resist.

**Figure 3.13**

| | |
|---|---|
| **Muscle** | Abductor pollicis brevis |
| **Nerve supply** | Median nerve |
| **Nerve root** | C7 – 8 |
| **Action** | Abduction of the thumb |

The patient's palm is supinated and the patient is instructed to point the thumb up towards the ceiling (Figure 3.13) while the examiner pushes down on either the base or the proximal phalanx of the thumb.

**Figure 3.14**

| Muscle | Flexor pollicis longus |
|---|---|
| **Nerve supply** | Median nerve (anterior interosseous branch) |
| **Nerve root** | C8 – T1 |
| **Action** | Flexion of the distal phalanx of the thumb |

The patient is instructed to bend the tip of the thumb while the examiner tries to straighten the patient's thumb (Figure 3.14). Normal patients should be able to resist very firm pressure.

**Figure 3.15**

| Muscle | Flexor digitorum profundus |
|---|---|
| **Nerve supply** | Median nerve (anterior interosseous branch) |
| **Nerve root** | C8 – T1 |
| **Action** | Flexion of distal interphalangeal joints of the 2nd and 3rd digit. |

The examiner places the left hand over the palm and palmar surfaces of the patient's 2nd and 3rd fingers to prevent flexion at the metacarpophalangeal and proximal interphalangeal joints (Figure 3.15). The patient is instructed to bend the tips of the 2nd and 3rd digits while the examiner tries to straighten them using the tips of the 2nd and 3rd digits of the right hand. Normal patients can resist very firm pressure.

**Figure 3.16**

| Muscle | Flexor digitorum profundus |
|---|---|
| **Nerve supply** | Ulnar nerve |
| **Nerve root** | C8 – T1 |
| **Action** | Flexion of distal interphalangeal joints of the 4th and 5th digits |

The examiner places the left hand over the palm and palmar surfaces of the patient's 4th and 5th fingers to prevent flexion at the metacarpophalangeal and proximal interphalangeal joints (Figure 3.16). The patient is instructed to bend the tips of the 4th and 5th digits while the examiner tries to straighten them using the tips of the 2nd and 3rd digits of their right hand. Normal patients can resist very firm pressure.

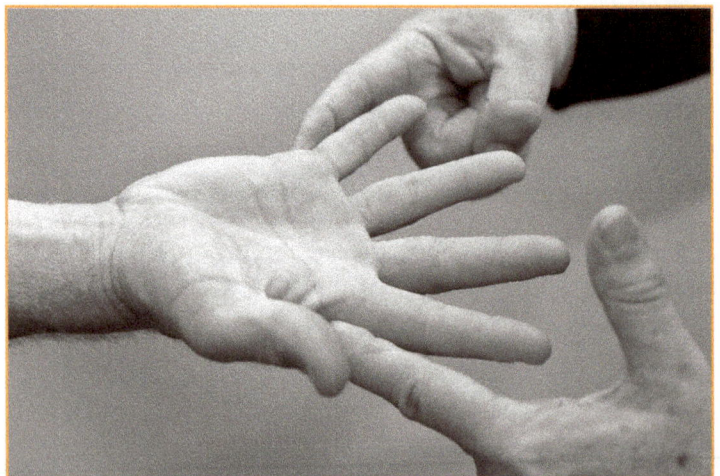

**Figure 3.12** Testing finger abduction (interossei and lumbricals)

**Contrarian Thought**

The neurological observation chart advises testing handgrip. This is one of the last muscle groups that will become weak in patients with an upper motor problem causing weakness. It would be far better to test wrist and finger extension, the very first muscles in the upper limb to become weak.

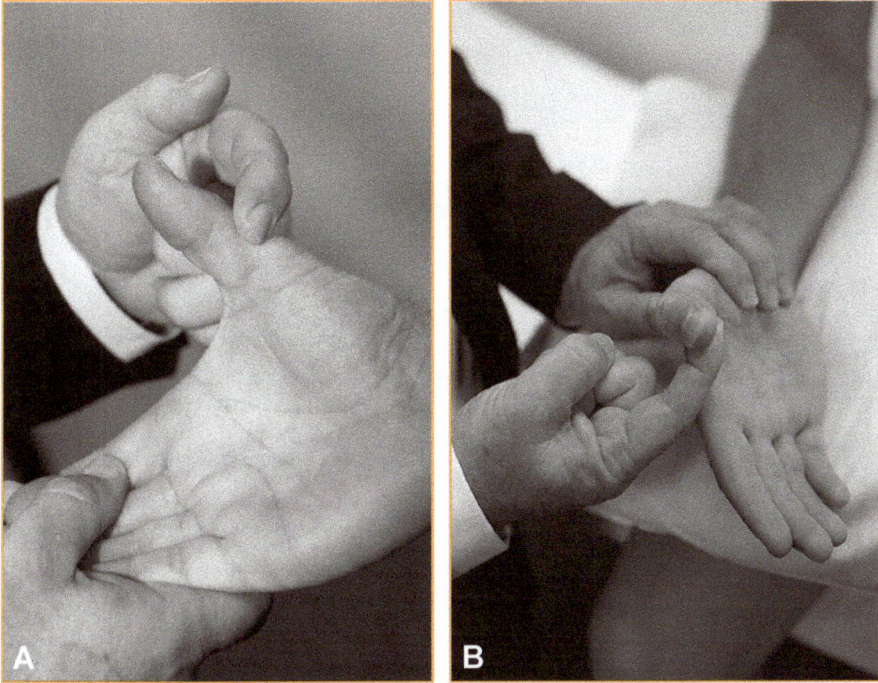

**Figure 3.13 and 3.14** Testing of abduction(A) and Flexion (B) of the thumb (abductor pollicis brevis)

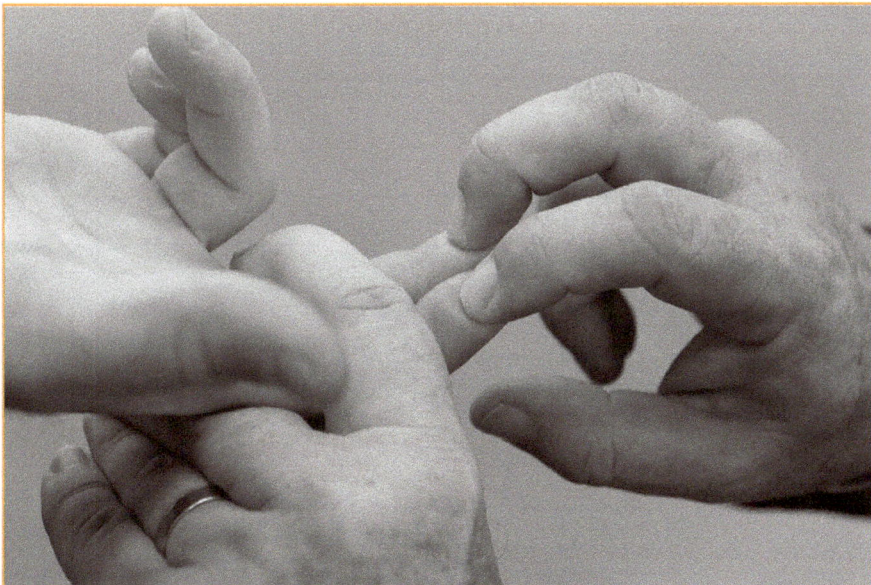

**Figure 3.15** Testing flexion of the 2nd and 3rd digits

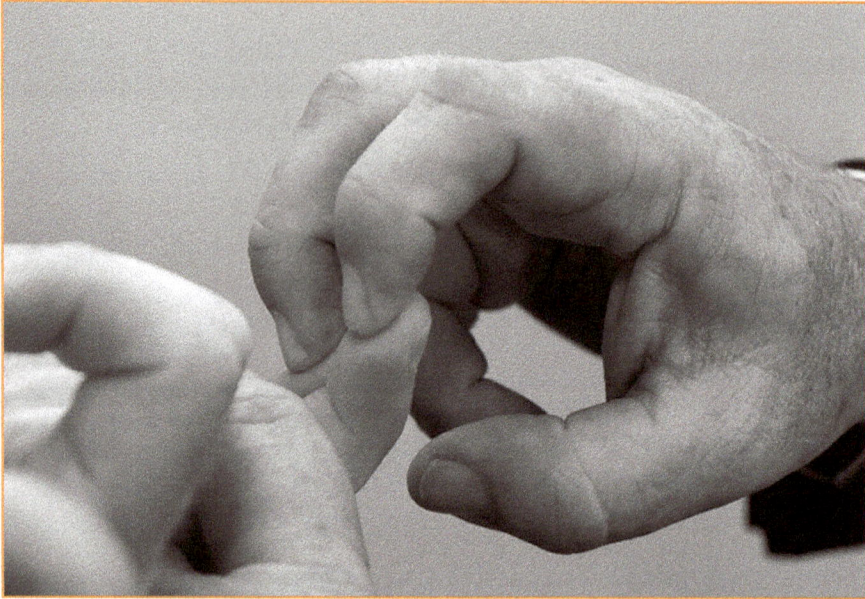

**Figure 3.16** Testing flexion of the 4th and 5th digits

Table 3.2 lists the muscles/muscle groups, nerves, and nerve roots of the upper limbs.

| Table 3.2 Muscles, muscle groups, nerve supply and nerve root innervation in the upper limbs | | |
|---|---|---|
| Muscle/muscle group | Nerve | Nerve root |
| Supraspinatus | Suprascapular | C4–6 |
| Infraspinatus | Suprascapular | C5–6 |
| Subscapularis | Nerve to subscapularis | C 5–7 |
| Deltoid | Axillary | C5–6 |
| Serratus anterior | Nerve to serratus anterior | C5–7 |
| Biceps | Musculocutaneous | C5–6 |
| Triceps | Radial | C6–8 |
| Brachioradialis | Radial | C5–7 |
| Extensor carpi radialis | Radial | C6–7 |
| Extensor carpi ulnaris | Posterior interosseous | C7–8 |
| Extensor digitorum | Posterior interosseous | C7–8 |
| Extensor pollicus longus | Posterior interosseous | C7–8 |
| Abductor pollicus brevis | Median | C8–T1 |
| Abductor digiti minimi | Ulnar | C8–T1 |
| Flexor digitorum profundus | Median (2nd and 3rd digits) | C8-T1 |
| Flexor digitorum profundus | Ulnar (4th and 5th digits) | C8-T1 |

# Lower Limbs
## Muscles around the hip and knee

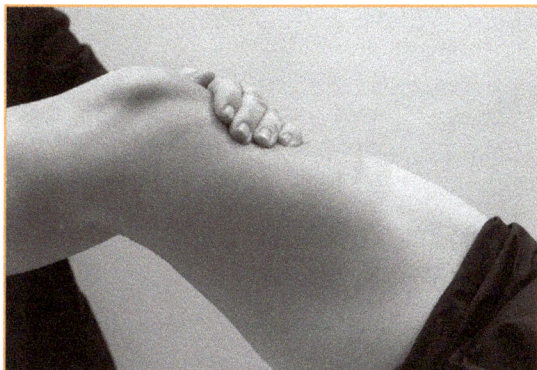

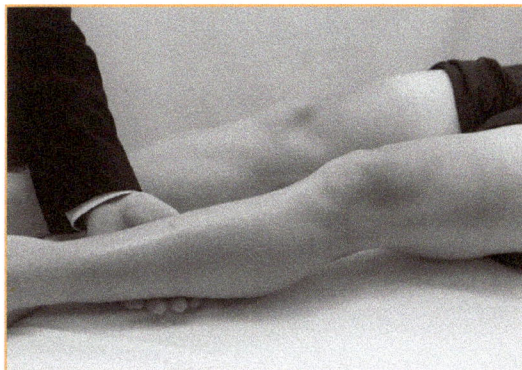

**Figure 3.17** Testing of hip flexion and **Figure 3.18** hip extension

**Figure 3.17**

| | |
|---|---|
| **Muscle** | Iliopsoas and Quadriceps |
| **Nerve supply** | Iliopsoas nerve and Femoral nerve |
| **Nerve root** | L2 – 4 |
| **Action** | Hip flexion |

The patient is instructed to lift their leg straight up off the bed to approximately 30–40° and keep it elevated (Figure 3.17). The examiner then places their hand over the thigh just above the knee and pushes down as hard as they can while instructing the patient to resist. Patients of all ages, except perhaps the very elderly and frail, can prevent the examiner from pushing the leg downwards.

**Figure 3.18**

| | |
|---|---|
| **Muscle** | Gluteus maximus |
| **Nerve supply** | Inferior gluteal nerve |
| **Nerve root** | L5 – S1 |
| **Action** | Hip extension |

The patient is instructed to keep the leg and the heel on the surface of the bed (Figure 3.18). The examiner places a hand under the leg, just below the calf, and attempts to lift the leg up off the bed instructing the patient to keep the heel on the bed to prevent the leg from being elevated.

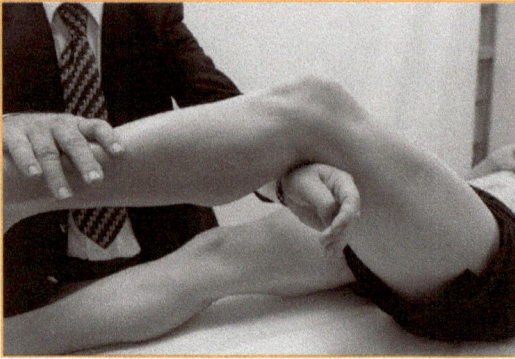

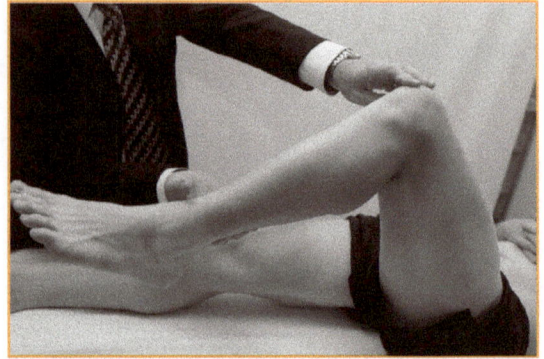

**Figure 3.19** Testing of knee extension and **Figure 3.20** knee flexion

**Figure 3.19**

| | |
|---|---|
| **Muscle** | Quadriceps |
| **Nerve supply** | Femoral nerve |
| **Nerve root** | L2 – 4 |
| **Action** | Knee extension |

The patient's leg is elevated, and the knee slightly bent (figure 3.19). The examiner places the left arm behind the knee and the right hand on the shin. As they attempt to bend the knee, the patient is instructed to straighten their leg and not allow it to be bent.

Testing of hip abduction is not particularly useful because it tests more than one muscle and one nerve and multiple nerve roots at the same time. It is never affected in isolation. On the other hand, hip adduction can be weak with damage to the obturator nerve (L2–4), for example, complicating obstetric procedures.

**Figure 3.20**

| | |
|---|---|
| **Muscle** | Biceps femoris, semimembranosus, semitendinosus |
| **Nerve supply** | Sciatic nerve |
| **Nerve root** | L5 – S1 |
| **Action** | Knee flexion |

The patient is instructed to bend the knee to approximately 90° with the heel just off the bed (Figure 3.20). The examiner places the left hand on the kneecap and the right hand just below the calf. The patient is instructed to bend the knee and not allow it to be straightened.

# Muscles around the ankle

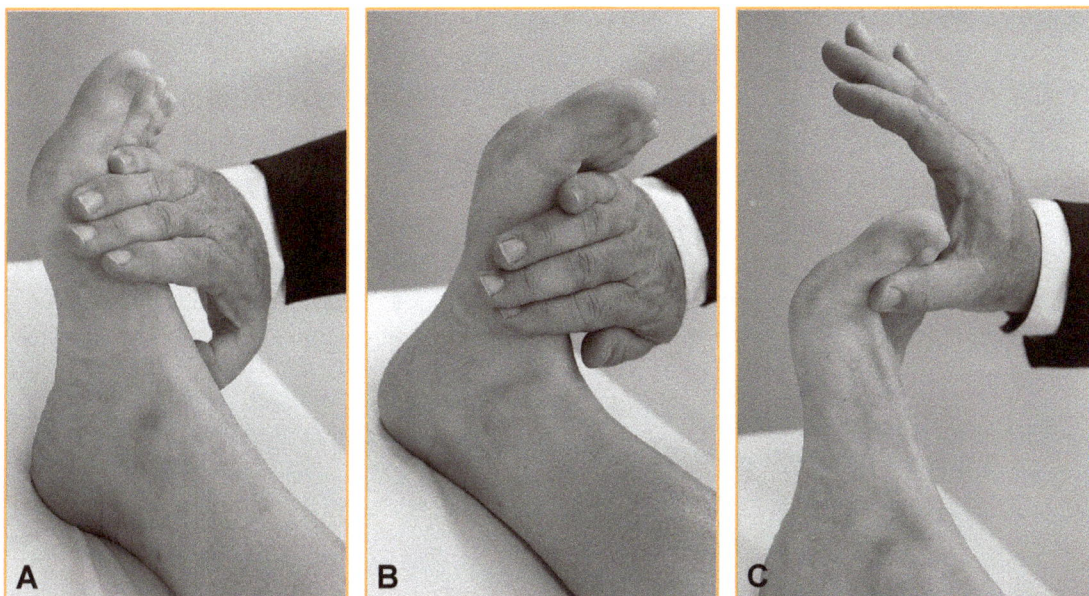

**Figure 3.21** Testing of dorsiflexion of the foot: **A** and **B**; **C** of the big toe

| | |
|---|---|
| **Muscle** | Tibialis anterior, Extensor hallucis longus |
| **Nerve supply** | Deep branch of the Common peroneal nerve (Common fibular nerve) |
| **Nerve root** | L5 – S1 |
| **Action** | Dorsiflexion of the foot |

The patient is instructed to bring the foot up towards the nose (Figure 3.21B). The examiner places a hand over the dorsal aspect of the foot and pushes downwards while the patient attempts to prevent the foot from being pushed downwards. Subtle degrees of weakness may be missed using this technique. A more sensitive method is for the patient to have the ankle in a neutral position, neither plantarflexed nor dorsiflexed (Figure 3.21A). The examiner places a hand over the dorsal aspect of the foot and asks the patient to lift the foot towards the nose while the examiner pushes down firmly on the foot. An even more sensitive technique is to have the patient bend the big toe up towards their nose while the examiner pushes on the toe at the level of the metatarsophalangeal joint (Figure 3.21C). Remember, however, as the sensitivity of testing is increased the specificity decreases, and a mild degree of weakness may be interpreted as abnormal when in fact it is a normal finding for a patient of that age.

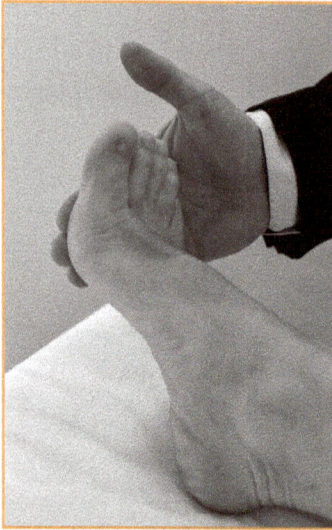

Figure 3.22 Testing of plantar flexion of the foot

**Figure 3.22**

| | |
|---|---|
| **Muscles** | Medial and lateral Gastrocnemii, Soleus |
| **Nerve supply** | Tibial nerve |
| **Nerve root** | L5 – S1 |
| **Action** | Plantar flexion of the foot |

The examiner places the palm of their hand over the ball of the foot and the patient is instructed to push down as hard as they can while the examiner attempts to push the foot upwards (Figure 3.22).

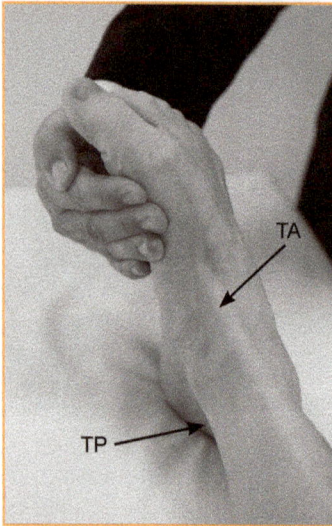

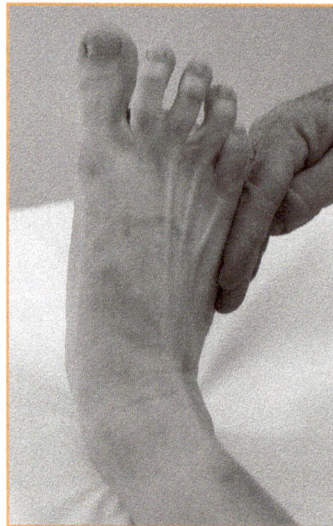

Figure 3.23 Testing inversion and **Figure 3.24** inversion of the ankle

**Figure 3.23**

| | |
|---|---|
| **Muscle** | Tibialis anterior and Tibialis posterior |
| **Nerve supply** | Tibial nerve + Deep branch Common peroneal Nerve (Common fibular nerve) |
| **Nerve root** | L5 |
| **Action** | Inversion of the ankle |

The examiner places the palm of a hand on the medial aspect of the foot and instructs the patient to turn the foot inwards and not to allow it to be turned outwards while the examiner attempts to turn the foot out laterally and observes the tibialis anterior and tibialis posterior tendons in front and behind the medial malleolus, respectively. These tendons can be palpated if they are not visible (Figure 3.23).

It is very important to test inversion and eversion of the ankle in a patient who has a foot drop. This is discussed further in Chapter 11. In essence, testing these two muscles helps to differentiate between a deep branch common peroneal nerve lesion, peripheral neuropathy and an L5 radiculopathy.

**Figure 3.24**

| | |
|---|---|
| **Muscle** | Peroneus longus and brevis |
| **Nerve supply** | Deep branch of the common peroneal nerve (Common fibular nerve) |
| **Nerve root** | L5 |
| **Action** | Eversion of the foot |

The examiner places the palm of a hand on the lateral aspect of the foot and instructs the patient to turn the foot outwards and prevent it being turned inwards while the examiner attempts to push the foot in medially (Figure 3.24).

**Table 3.3** Muscle groups, nerve supply and nerve root innervation in the lower limbs

| Muscle group | Nerve | Nerve root |
|---|---|---|
| Hip flexion | Femoral | L2–4 |
| Hip extension | Superior and inferior gluteal | L5–S1 |
| Knee extension | Femoral | L2–4 |
| Knee flexion | Sciatic | L5–S 1 |
| Foot dorsiflexion | Deep branch of common peroneal | L4–5, S1 |
| Plantar flexion | Posterior tibial | L5–S1 |
| Eversion of foot | Superficial peroneal | L5–S1 |
| Inversion of foot | Posterior tibial and deep branch of common peroneal | L4–5 |

The 5*3*5 rule for examining the muscles of the upper limb is described in chapter 11.

# Looking for changes in reflexes

Testing the reflexes should be easy, however, many factors can influence the reflexes:
- If the patient is anxious the reflexes can give the appearance of being abnormally brisk.
- Reduced or absent ankle reflexes are almost the norm in the elderly patient.
- Sometimes in teenagers, it can be difficult to elicit the upper limb and knee reflexes and yet curiously the ankle reflexes are well preserved. I have no explanation for this curious phenomenon.
- If the limb is not in the correct position and the joint is not relaxed, this can give the impression of reduced reflexes.

As with all aspects of the neurological examination, one needs to interpret the findings in the context of the history and other neurological signs.

The upper limb reflexes are best tested with the patient sitting, if possible, with a pillow on their lap and the arms resting comfortably on that pillow. The lower limb reflexes are best tested with the patient lying flat (Figure 3.25).

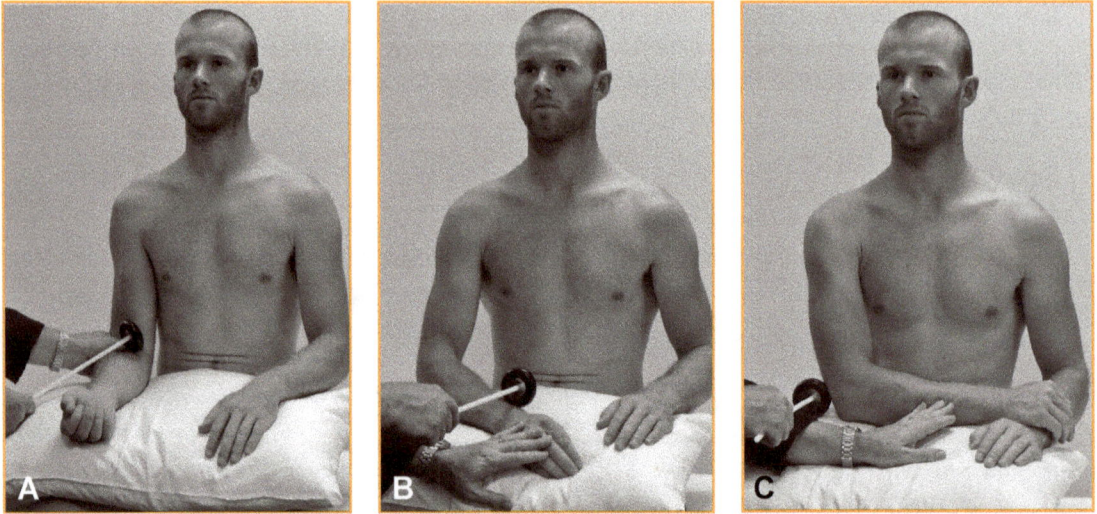

**Figure 3.25A** How to test the reflexes in the upper limbs.

**A** Biceps: The thumb or fingers of one hand are placed over the biceps tendon and the examiner's fingers are struck with the tendon hammer.

**B** Brachioradialis: The brachioradialis tendon can be struck directly or else the examiner can place a finger or two over the tendon and strike their own fingers.

**C** Triceps: This is best tested with the patient's arm folded across their body and the triceps tendon struck directly.

Table 3.4 lists the limb reflexes and their nerve root supply. The primary nerve root supply is the figure outside the brackets.

| Table 3.4 The limb reflexes and the nerve root supply | |
|---|---|
| **Reflex** | **Nerve root supply** |
| Biceps | C 5(6) |
| Brachioradialis | C (5)6 |
| Triceps | C (5,6)7 |
| Knee jerk | L 2,3,4 |
| Ankle reflex | S 1 |

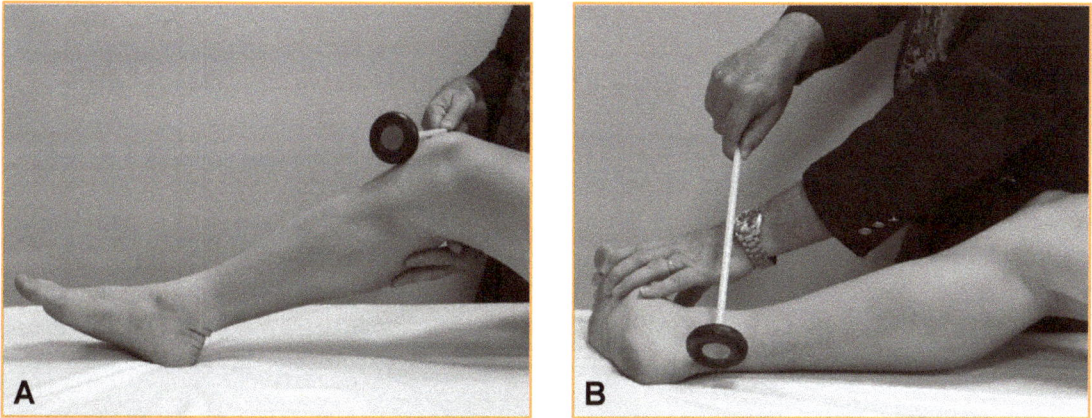

**Figure 3.25** How to test the reflexes in the lower limbs.

**A** Knee reflex: The knee should be at approximately 45° and the patella tendon struck directly.

**B** Ankle reflex: Externally rotate the leg, have the ankle slightly plantarflexed, and strike the Achilles tendon directly.

# The Sensory Examination

The primary sensory modalities tested in the clinical setting include:
- vibration
- proprioception
- pain
- temperature
- light touch.

Sensory testing can be difficult and, at times, confusing because of inconsistent responses. Some simple techniques that can help reduce this problem are described below and demonstrated on the website.

It is probably irrelevant whether sensory testing commences with vibration, proprioception, pain, or temperature. I prefer to start with proprioception, then vibration. I am then holding a cold tuning fork that I can use to test temperature sensation, finally the most challenging modality to test, pain sensation.

Anticipating what sensory abnormalities will be found based on the *nature and distribution of symptoms* described in the history influences the method of examination, particularly where to start looking for the sensory signs. If the patient complains of altered sensation in a particular part of the body, it is appropriate and sensible to examine sensation in that region. Suppose there were no sensory symptoms in the history. In that case, the most suitable technique for testing sensation will depend on whether the history and motor examination suggest a central nervous system or a peripheral nervous system problem.

# Vibration and Proprioception

To test vibration sense, use a 128-Hz tuning fork. The tuning fork should be vibrating intensely and be placed over the patient's big toe or index finger (Figure 3.26). The intensity of the vibration is reduced gradually by running the examiner's fingers slowly up the tuning fork until it stops vibrating or until the patient states they can no longer feel any vibration. This gradual reduction in the intensity of vibration increases the sensitivity of the testing. Still, it is essential to remember that elderly patients often have reduced or absent vibration sense in the feet and ankles. In younger patients, vibration can be detected in the toes almost to the point where the tuning fork stops vibrating. In the hands, patients of all ages can appreciate vibration over the dorsal aspect of the distal phalanx of the finger. However, once again, older patients may have a very slight reduction in vibration sense.

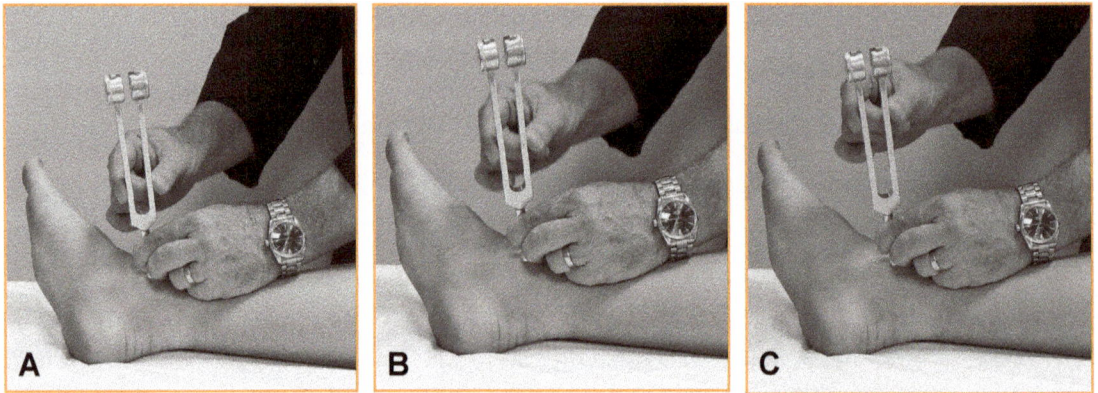

**Figure 3.26** How to test vibration

**A**, **B**, **C**: The examiner's finger is moved slowly up the tuning fork, gradually reducing the intensity until the patient states they can no longer feel the vibration.

Proprioception is tested by moving the index finger or big toe up or down while holding the digit on its side, initially showing the patient which way is up and which way is down. Then ask the patient to close their eyes and say which way the toe or finger is being moved (Figure 3.27). The digit should be moved two or three times in the same direction because some patients guess, and guesses may coincide with the direction of movement if the digit is alternately moved up and then down. The movement amplitude will again depend on the patient's age, with older patients typically losing appreciation of minor degrees of movement. A very slight movement in the range of 1 or 2 mm can be detected in the index finger, although the range may be slightly greater for older patients. The normal range of movement that can be detected in the big toe is 3 to 4 mm.

If the impairment of proprioception is very severe (and this is rare), there may be impairment at the ankle and wrist or even the knee and elbow. This assessment of the severity of proprioceptive and vibration loss adds nothing to localising the pathology. Once there is impairment of these modalities in a limb, one is dealing with peripheral neuropathy or a central nervous system problem on the ipsilateral side of the spinal cord or the contralateral side of the brain. Abnormalities in these modalities rarely occur with single nerve or nerve root lesions.

As the sensitivity of testing increases the specificity decreases. In these circumstances, the patient may appear to have impairment of vibration sense when in fact, it is a normal finding in a patient of that age.

Although proprioception can be tested on the face by pulling the cheek or earlobe up or down while the patient's eyes are closed, this is rarely done.

Abnormalities of vibration and proprioception virtually never occur proximally in a limb if they are not present distally.

# Pain, Temperature and Light Touch

The pain, temperature and light touch sensations are particularly useful for mapping areas of sensory loss.

- *Temperature sensation* is tested using a cold object such as the tuning fork. Patients with cold feet may not appreciate that the object is cold, and this can produce an 'apparent alteration' of temperature sensation confined to the feet in a circumferential pattern up to where the limb becomes warm when in fact sensation is normal. Pain sensation will be normal in this area of 'seemingly altered' temperature sensation. If the feet are very cold, temperature sensation should be tested using a warm object.
- *Pain sensation* is tested using a commercially available sharp object or alternatively a toothpick. Hypodermic needles are too sharp, often cause bleeding and should not be used. Pain sensation is probably the most challenging modality to test. It is subjective and very dependent on how hard the sharp object is pressed into the skin. Repeated rapid stimuli (2–3) in one spot, initially with a blunt object such as the tip of the finger and then with a sharp object, helps to reduce this variability. This technique is demonstrated on the website.
- Testing *light touch* does not help differentiate whether the pathology affects a particular pathway. Both the spinothalamic tract and the pathways carrying vibration and proprioception transmit light touch sensation. Testing light touch can be beneficial when the other sensory signs are confusing. A helpful technique is to gently stroke with the fingers of one hand the skin in an area of normal sensation on the same limb while using the other hand's fingers to stroke the skin in the area of suspected abnormal sensation. One then slowly moves from the site of abnormal sensation until the patient says the feeling is the same. It may be necessary to do this repeatedly to confirm the findings.

When testing pain, temperature, or light touch, if an altered sensation is detected, the examination continues to test that same modality in all four directions away from the original area of abnormal sensation until the full extent of sensory loss is established. The pattern of sensory loss is then compared with the figures in Chapter 1.

---

When an area of abnormal sensation is found, it is imperative to extend the examination in all four directions from where the initial sensory loss is detected until the exact extent of the sensory loss is determined.

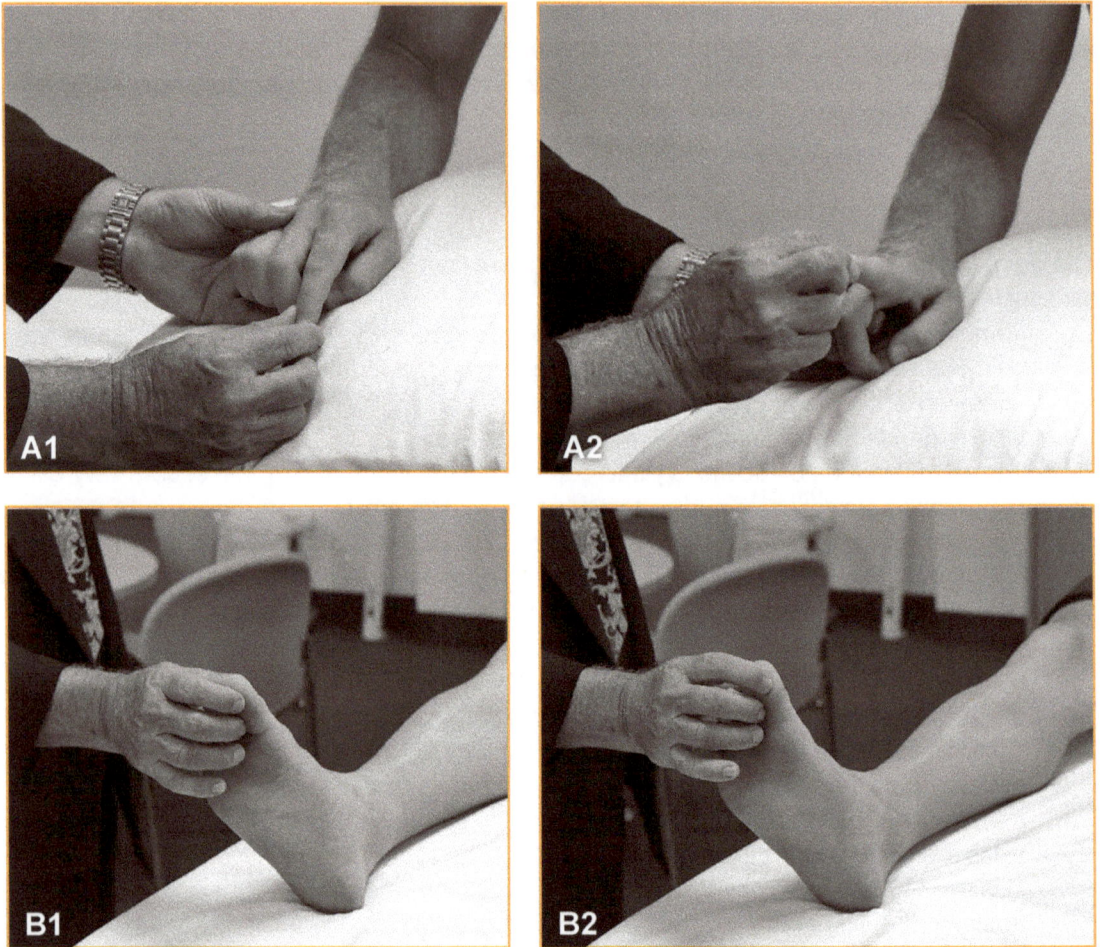

**Figure 3.27** How to test proprioception in the hand (**A**) and foot (**B**). The examiner grasps the top and bottom of the big toe rather than grasping the sides of the toe, as is traditionally taught.

## Sensory Loss Due to a Central Nervous System Lesion

When the history suggests that the problem may involve the central nervous system or spinothalamic tract, the most appropriate method to test pain, temperature, and light touch sensation is to commence testing over the tips of the fingers or toes. If an abnormality is detected, the stimulus is moved quickly up the arm or leg until normal sensation is found. The anterior and posterior aspects of the limb should be tested, ensuring that testing crosses the skin supplied by multiple individual nerves and multiple individual nerve roots. The sensory loss should be higher up on the back than on the front of the trunk because the area of skin supplied by the thoracic nerve roots is higher on the back than on the chest or abdomen (see Figures 1.11 and 1.12). A horizontal band of sensory abnormality around the trunk is indicative of a non-organic problem. Suppose the sensory loss extends up the leg and trunk. In that case, the sensation is then tested on the inside of the upper arm (T2), down the medial aspect of the forearm (C8), across the fingers from the little finger (C8), 3rd digit (C7) to the thumb (C6) and up the lateral aspect of the forearm (C6) and upper arm (C5) onto the neck (C2–4) and if necessary, to the face (trigeminal nerve) and the occipital region of the head (C2–3).

- Lesions in different parts of the central nervous system will produce different patterns of loss of pain, temperature, and touch sensations.
- Lesions involving the spinothalamic tract of the central nervous system will produce abnormal pain and/or temperature sensation affecting:
- The whole of the contralateral leg if the lesion is in or above the thoracic spinal cord
- The contralateral arm and leg if the lesion is in or above the upper cervical spinal cord or brain stem below the level of the pons where the 5th nerve nucleus is situated.
- If the pathology is above the 5th nerve nucleus, abnormal pain and temperature sensation will affect the contralateral face, arm, and leg.
- Suppose the pathology is at the level of the lateral pons or medulla in the brain stem. This can result in ipsilateral impairment of pain and temperature sensation on the face with contralateral impairment in the arm and leg.
- Alterations of pain and temperature affecting the whole of one side of the body indicate that the lesion is above the pons but cannot determine the exact site of the pathology, and it is the associated symptoms and signs that will localise the pathology more accurately.

Syringomyelia (a cyst within the central region of the spinal cord) in the cervical spinal cord can result in a suspended sensory loss affecting the upper trunk and upper limbs and, if the lesion extends into the lower brainstem, also involve the trigeminal nerve causing sensory loss on the face commencing in front of the ear and extending forward in an onion-skin pattern. This is because the syrinx affects the nerve fibres conveying pain and temperature sensation in the centre of the spinal cord, and these nerve fibres enter the spinal cord via the dorsal root ganglion, cross the midline and push the nerve fibres from the lower part of the body out laterally so that a syrinx in the centre of the cord will affect the spinothalamic tract fibres from the upper part of the body closest to the syrinx first (see Figure 3.28).

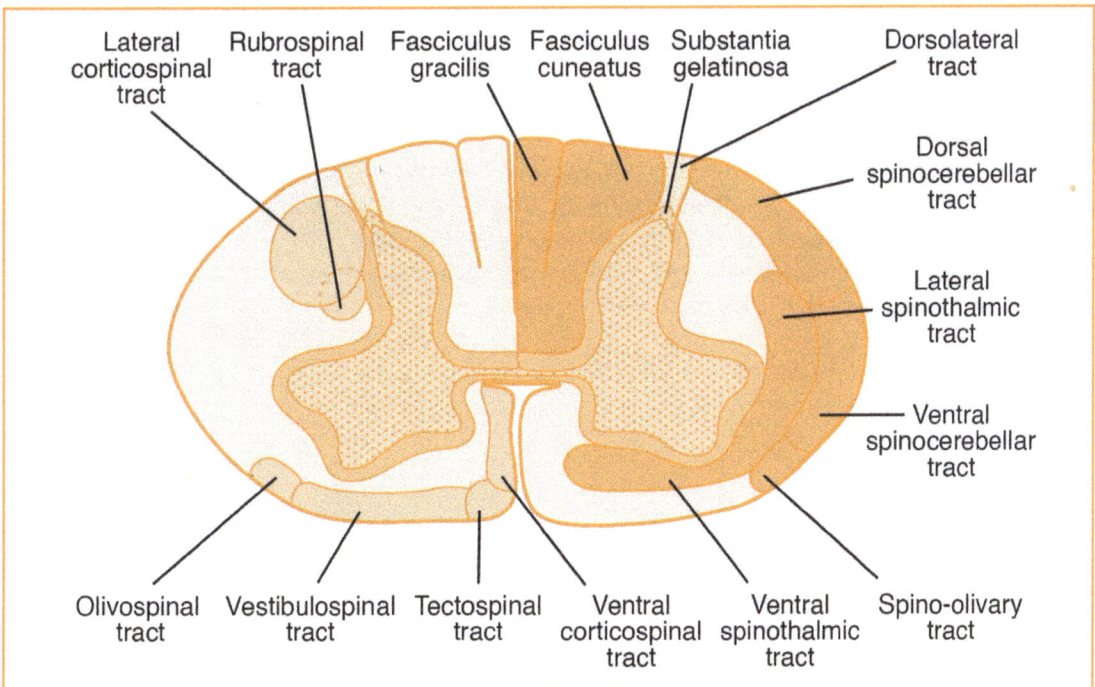

**Figure 3.28** Cross-section of the spinal cord showing the pathways; the lateral spinothalamic tract conveys pain and temperature, and the sacral nerve fibres are medial in the tract and the thoracic and cervical fibres are lateral.

## Sensory Loss Due to a Peripheral Nervous System Lesion

If a peripheral nervous system problem is suspected but there are no sensory symptoms, sensory testing should commence in the area where weakness is found. If there are sensory abnormalities, they will reflect whether the sensory nerve root, plexus or peripheral nerve(s) are affected, and the pattern will be different depending on what part of the peripheral nervous system is involved. It is not uncommon for inexperienced examiners to commence sensory testing partway up the foot or hand. If pain, temperature, and a light touch sensation are not tested on the very tips of the toes and fingers, subtle degrees of peripheral sensory loss that occur in patients with for example a peripheral neuropathy can be missed.

## Examining Cerebellar Function

Coordination test. The patient alternately touches their nose with their index finger and then the examiner's finger held at arm's length from the patient. It is important to ensure that the patient is not anchoring their upper arm against their torso, as this can mask ataxia in the upper limb. To test the lower limbs the patient whilst lying flat on a couch or bed elevates their leg high up off the bed and then places the heel as accurately as possible on the opposite kneecap. This initial movement is the most important to observe, although many examiners will then test the heel sliding down the shin. This latter technique at times can obscure subtle ataxia because the heel can be anchored against the shin. These two tests are referred to as finger-to-nose and heel-to-shin testing.

In patients with midline cerebellar disturbance, finger-to-nose and heel-to-shin testing may be normal as these largely reflect the cerebellar hemispheres. Heel-to-toe testing is performed where a patient is asked to walk in a straight line placing the heel of one foot in front of the toes of the other foot.

A third technique is rapidly alternating movements. The patient is asked to tap the back of the hand, alternating with the palm and the back of the opposite hand, repeatedly for 10 seconds. For the lower limbs, rapid alternating movement is best tested by having the patient place their toes and the ball of their foot on the floor and tap their heel up and down rapidly. This causes less discomfort I the front to the shin than tapping the toes up and down with the heel on the ground. The first method can be performed for much longer than the latter.

Finally, patients with cerebellar disturbance may have nystagmus when the external ocular movements are tested. This is discussed in Chapter 4.

# Clinical Cases

The following cases illustrate how the pattern of involvement can be used to localise the lesion.

## Lesions in the central nervous system

**Case 3.1** A 60-year-old female with leg weakness and difficulty with micturition

A 60-year-old female presents with gradual onset of weakness in both legs and recent-onset difficulty with micturition. The arms are not affected. The motor examination of the lower limbs reveals the patient has an UMN pattern of weakness in the leg(s), with weakness confined to hip flexion and dorsiflexion of the feet, increased tone and reflexes and extensor plantar responses, indicating the involvement of the motor pathway (meridian of longitude) within the central nervous system and not the peripheral nervous system. There is reduced pain and temperature sensation involving both legs up onto the abdomen to the level of the umbilicus anteriorly and 3-4 cm higher on the back (the parallel of latitude).

Based on these motor findings, it can be inferred that the lesion is above the level of L1 (first lumbar).

The incontinence suggests a spinal cord problem.

The altered pain and temperature sensation reflect involvement of the spinothalamic tract up to the level of T10 (the umbilicus). A sensory level (the upper limit of sensory loss) also points to a spinal cord problem. This sensory level is the parallel of latitude as it points to the level in spinal cord. A mid-thoracic spinal cord problem in a middle-aged to elderly female is a meningioma until proven otherwise.

**Case 3.2** A 76-year-old man with leg weakness and arm pain

A 76-year-old-man presents with 6 months of progressive weakness in both legs and 3 weeks of pain and numbness down the lateral aspect of his right forearm into the 1st and 2nd digits. When examined he has UMN signs in the legs thus the lesions must involve the motor pathway (meridian of longitude) above the level of L1. The pain and sensory symptoms in his arm are in the distribution of the C6 nerve root, this is the parallel of latitude the lesion must be in the cervical region because the pathology is always at the level of the LMN. He had a C5-6 disc prolapse compressing the C6 nerve root and the spinal cord at that level. This assumes that the patient is suffering from a single disease entity and not multiple diseases.

## Lesions in the peripheral nervous system

**Case 3.3** A 45-year-old man with weakness and numbness in both legs

A 45-year-old man presents with **progressive** weakness in both lower legs causing foot drop and numbness affecting the top and bottom of both feet up to just above his ankles. His arms are not affected. He has weakness of dorsiflexion, inversion, eversion and plantarflexion of both feet, absent ankle reflexes, reduced tone and loss of pain and temperature sensation in a circumferential pattern to 8 cm above his ankles.

The distal weakness in both lower legs is beyond the distribution of any single nerve or nerve root and thus affects multiple nerves and together with reduced tone and absent reflexes are LMN signs, thus the problem must be between the anterior horn cell and the muscle.

The presence of sensory symptoms excludes the anterior horn cell, motor nerve roots, neuromuscular junction, and muscle as the site of the problem. The altered sensation is also beyond the distribution of any single nerve or nerve root and thus affects multiple nerves.

This is the pattern of peripheral neuropathy.

---

**Case 3.4** A 25-year-old female with weakness and numbness in her left hand

A 25-year-old female presents with the gradual onset of weakness in her left hand and numbness affecting the medial 1½ fingers on both the palmar and dorsal aspects.

The examination reveals wasting of the muscle between the thumb and index finger (the 1st dorsal interosseous) and selective weakness of finger abduction and finger adduction without involvement of the APB muscle of the hand. In addition, there is weakness of flexion of the distal phalanges of the medial two but not the lateral two digits.

The weakness of the small muscles of the hand and the long flexors of the medial two digits points to an ulnar nerve lesion at the elbow, a common site for compression of the nerve.

The sensory loss affecting both the palmar and dorsal surface of the medial 1½ digits and the medial aspect of the hand up to the wrist is also within the distribution of the ulnar nerve and because it affects the dorsal aspect this tells us the problem is proximal to the wrist because the dorsal ulnar cutaneous nerve arises several cm above the wrist.

Thus, the pattern of weakness and sensory loss indicates that this is an ulnar nerve lesion at the elbow. If there was just sensory loss without weakness all we could say is that the lesion is above the wrist, most likely at the elbow but we cannot be 100% certain.

---

# References

1   *Dorland's pocket medical dictionary*. 21st edn Philadelphia: WB Saunders Company; 1968.

2   Williams PL, et al. *Gray's anatomy*. 37th edn London: Churchill Livingstone; 1989.

3   Rosenblum ML, Levy RM, Bredesen DE. *AIDS and the nervous system*. New York: Raven Press; 1988, 410.

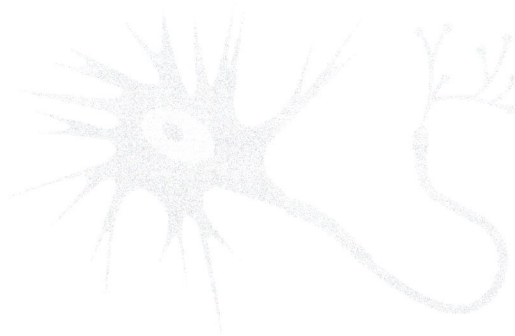

# The Cranial Nerves and Brainstem

The first section of this chapter will describe the anatomy, the techniques for examining the individual cranial nerves and the more common abnormalities encountered. The second part will discuss the novel 'Rule of 4 of the Brainstem' first published in 2005[1] that greatly simplifies localising the problem within the brainstem, in particular understanding brainstem stroke syndromes.

## Olfactory (1st) Nerve

### Anatomy

The receptors for smell are in the nasal passages. Afferent fibres pass into the skull through a multitude of small holes, called the cribriform plate, in the base of the skull situated beneath the frontal lobes in the anterior cranial fossa. The olfactory nerves thus formed pass backwards under the frontal lobes to the temporal lobes and olfactory cortex on the same side.

### Method of Testing

It is best to use items that are familiar to most people, such as perfume or coffee (coffee may be more suitable because some patients may have a perfume allergy). With the eyes closed the patient is asked to recognise the odour in each nostril separately while the other is occluded.

This is not a particularly useful test because the most frequent cause of anosmia (loss of the sense of smell) is the common cold. Anosmia can also occur following severe head injuries when the olfactory nerves are torn at the floor of the anterior cranial fossa. The nerve can be compressed by a sub frontal meningioma and the loss may be unilateral. Rarely, permanent anosmia can develop without any obvious cause (idiopathic) or following an influenza-like illness.

# Optic (2nd) Nerve and Visual Pathway
## Anatomy

The visual pathways together, with the visual field abnormalities produced by lesions at certain sites along the pathway, are illustrated in Figure 4.1. Note that the lateral retina radiates back to the occiput on the same side via the optic nerve, chiasm, and optic radiation, while the fibres from the medial retina cross at the optic chiasm and radiate to the opposite occipital lobe. The left occipital lobe receives fibres from the left lateral retina and the right medial retina (i.e. the right visual field), while the opposite is the case for the right occipital lobe.

An optic nerve lesion will produce a visual field loss in one eye. The optic chiasm lies above the pituitary gland and beneath the hypothalamus and is subject to compression from the pituitary and hypothalamic tumours. Lesions of the optic chiasm will produce a bitemporal field loss. Optic radiation or occipital lobe problem will result in a contralateral visual field loss, either hemianopia (loss of one-half of the visual field) or a quadrantanopia (loss of one-quarter of the visual field).

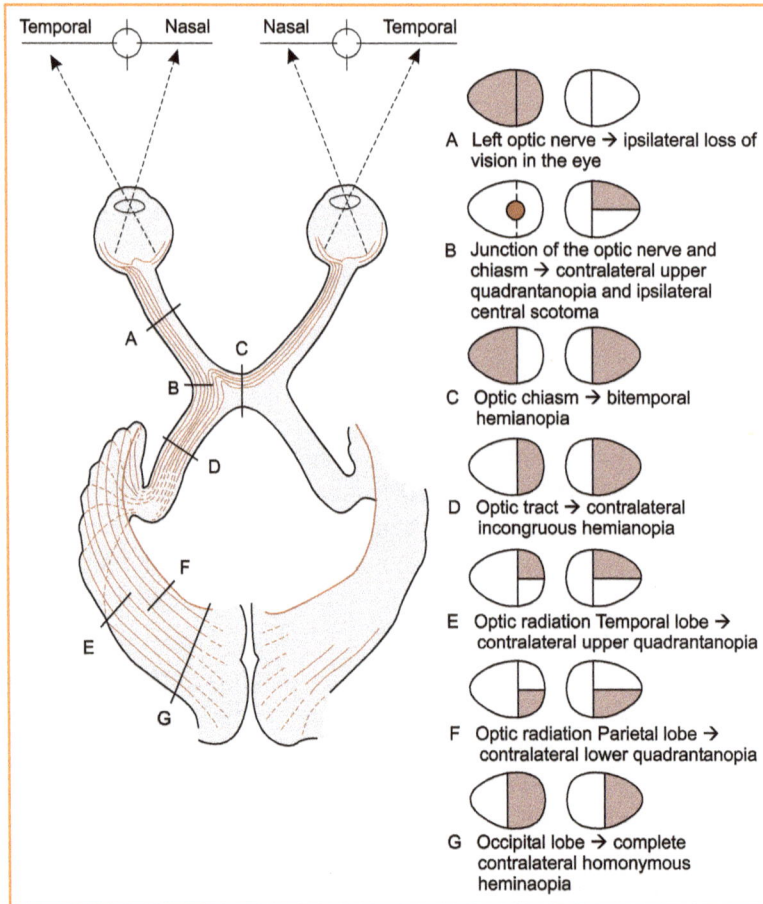

**Figure 4.1** The drawing on the left represents the visual pathway; the drawings on the right are the visual abnormalities that occur at the relevant sites along the pathway. Reproduced from Principles of Neurology, 3rd edn, by RD Adams and M Victor, 1985, McGraw–Hill Book Company, Figure 12.2, p 1186 [2]

Note: Ipsilateral refers to the left and contralateral to the right.

# Methods of Testing
## Visual Acuity

The visual acuity in each eye is assessed with glasses on (corrected) and glasses off (uncorrected) using a Snellen chart (see Figure 4.2). In patients with a neurological problem, it is preferable to check the acuity corrected to remove any ocular refractive error contributing to visual impairment. In the absence of glasses, impaired vision due to a refractive error can be corrected by asking the patient to look through a small hole in a piece of cardboard or paper. This will improve the vision if the impairment is related to a refractive error in the eye.

## Colour Vision

The Ishihara charts (Figure 4.3) are used to check colour vision. Colour blindness is most often hereditary, and there are two distinct patterns of impairment:

- If the patient is a protanope colour blindness is characterised by a defective perception of red and confusion of red with green or bluish-green.
- If the patient is a deuteranope, colour blindness is characterised by insensitivity to green.

Pathological colour blindness indicates disease in the optic nerves and can occur even in the absence of prior visual symptoms, typically with a demyelinating optic neuropathy associated with multiple sclerosis.

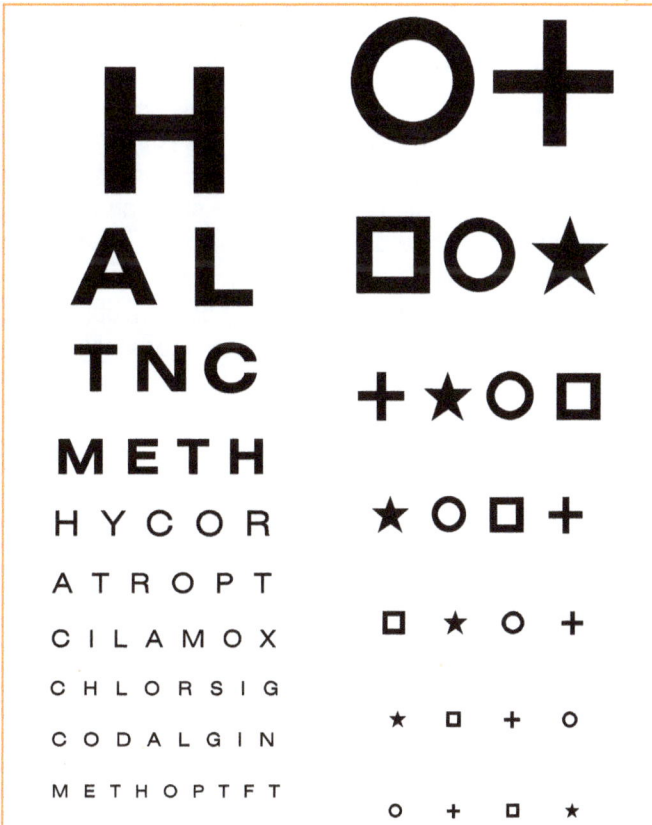

**Figure 4.2** Snellen visual acuity chart

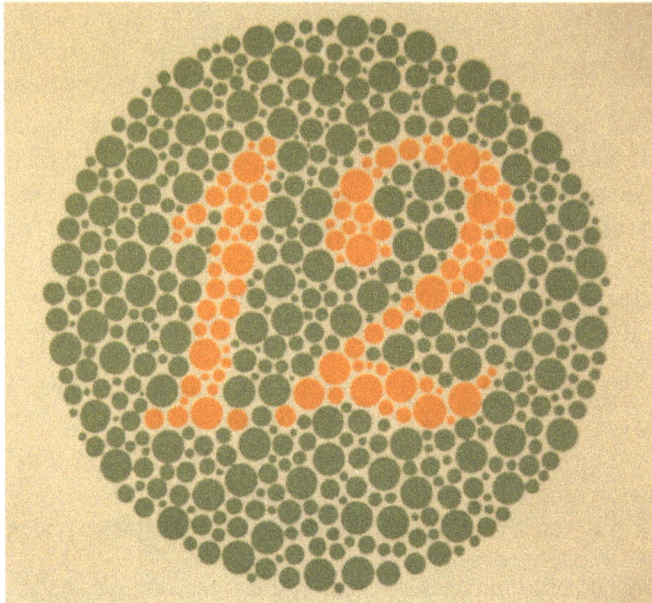

**Figure 4.3** Ishihara sample chart

## Vision
## Severe Visual Field Loss:

**Quadrantanopia, Hemianopia, Visual Inattention**

A simple screening test that will detect a severe visual field loss, such as a quadrantanopia (loss of vision in the same quarter of the visual field in both eyes) or hemianopia (loss of vision in the same half of the visual field of both eyes), is to move a finger in the peripheral vision in both upper and then both lower visual fields. If with double simultaneous stimulation the patient cannot see the moving finger in one of the fields, the problem is either a visual field loss or visual inattention. Visual inattention is the inability to see objects moving in both visual fields simultaneously, although the moving object can be seen if each visual field is tested separately.

To differentiate between these two possibilities, the examiner's finger is moved in one visual field at a time slowly from lateral to medial aspect of the field. If the visual disturbance is a loss of vision, the finger will not be seen until it reaches the midline. On the other hand, if the visual problem is inattention the single moving finger will be seen in the areas of vision where it could not initially be seen with double simultaneous stimuli. Once again, this is the principle of testing from the area of abnormality until normality is found to define the exact pattern of impairment.

## Subtle Visual Field Defects

## Central Scotoma

To detect more subtle defects of the visual fields at the bedside a 4-mm red pin is used. In this test, the examiner holds the pin at a distance midway between himself and the patient. The visual field of the examiner is used as the normal control. The visual fields are tested with the patient covering the left eye, for example, while the examiner covers their right eye, directly opposite the patient's closed eye. The patient and the examiner look directly into each other's eye and in this way the examiner can tell if the patient's eye is moving during the test. Initially, the 4-mm red pin is placed in the centre of the visual field to detect if there is a loss of central vision, a central scotoma. If there is a loss of vision in the centre, the pin is moved slowly away in each of the 4 quadrants in turn until it is visualised by the patient, establishing the size of the central scotoma. This indicates a lesion of the fovea in the eye.

## Enlarged Blind Spot

An enlarged blind spot occurs with a lesion of the optic discs (either optic neuritis or papilloedema). To detect an enlarged blind spot, the examiner slowly moves the 4-mm red pin out laterally from the centre at the level of the equator of the eye until the blind spot is detected. Once found, the examiner moves the pin-up, down, medially, and laterally until the size of the patient's blind spot is established and compared with that of the examiner.

## Subtle Hemianopia, Quadrantanopia or Bitemporal Hemianopia

To test the visual fields for subtle hemianopia, quadrantanopia or bi-temporal hemianopia, the examiner moves the pin slowly from the periphery to the midline in each of the 4 quadrants asking the patient to indicate when the red pin is first noticed. If a loss is detected with this technique, the pin is then moved slowly from the area of abnormal vision to normal vision to establish the exact pattern of visual loss. Testing the visual fields individually with the 4-mm red pin will NOT detect visual inattention, nor will it detect an optic nerve problem unless you are examining the blind spot.

A Goldman Perimeter or Bjerum Screen is used to formally test the visual fields.

# Examination of the Optic Fundi

The patient is instructed to look straight ahead, preferably at a small dot or mark on the wall. The examiner approaches from the side at about 30–45° lateral to the midline until a retinal blood vessel is visualised and this is traced back to the optic disc (Figure 4.4). The blood vessels can be traced outwards from the optic disc to detect any abnormality. To examine the fovea (central vision), the patient looks directly at the ophthalmoscope with the intensity of the light reduced.

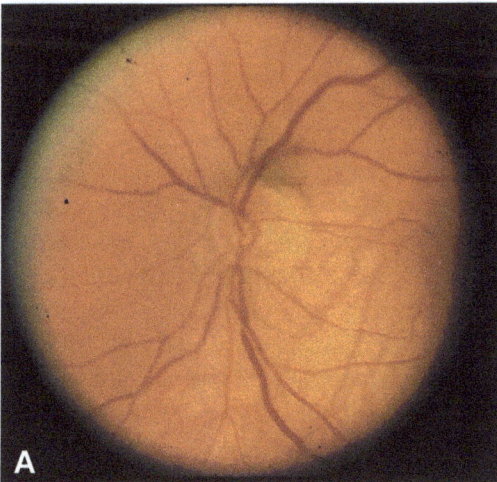

**Figure 4.4** A Normal optic disc

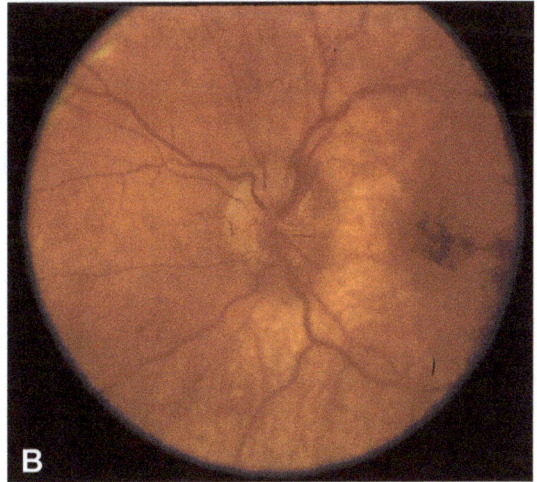

**Figure 4.4 B** Papilloedema

The visual acuity is normal unless the papilloedema is chronic, and the blind spot is enlarged. The visual fields are otherwise normal. The pupillary responses are normal.

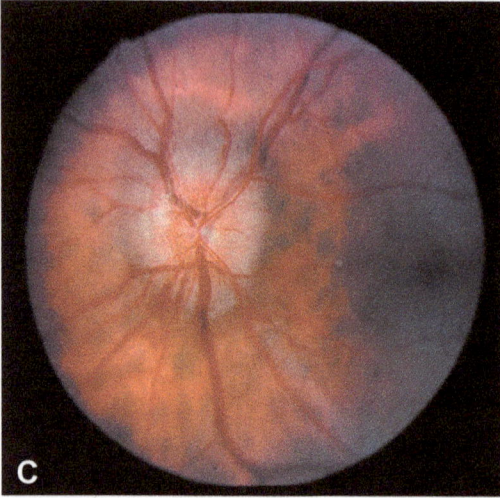

**Figure 4.4 C** Acute optic neuritis

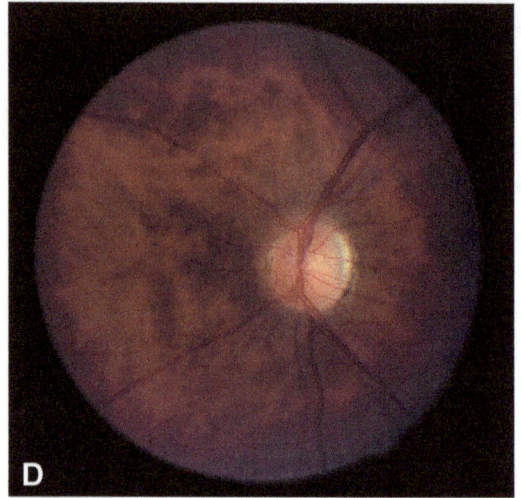

**Figure 4.4 D** Long-standing optic neuritis with pallor of the optic disc

In optic neuritis the visual acuity is markedly impaired; colour vision is abnormal if the patient can read the chart (severe visual impairment will prevent the patient from seeing the numbers on the chart). The blind spot is enlarged. The direct pupillary response is slow and there is a Marcus–Gunn pupillary phenomenon (the pupil contracts promptly when the light is shone in the normal eye and when the light is shone in the abnormal eye the pupil initially dilates and then slowly contracts). Retrobulbar neuritis is the term applied to an inflammatory optic nerve lesion within the optic nerve but not affecting the optic nerve head, the part of the optic nerve that is visualised on examination of the fundus. In this situation, the visual acuity and colour vision are impaired, the visual field defect is usually a central scotoma although it may be a diffuse, lateral, superior, or inferior defect. The fundus looks normal [3].

The visual acuity is reduced, colour vision is abnormal, and a Marcus–Gunn pupillary phenomenon is present (see 4C for an explanation of this abnormality).

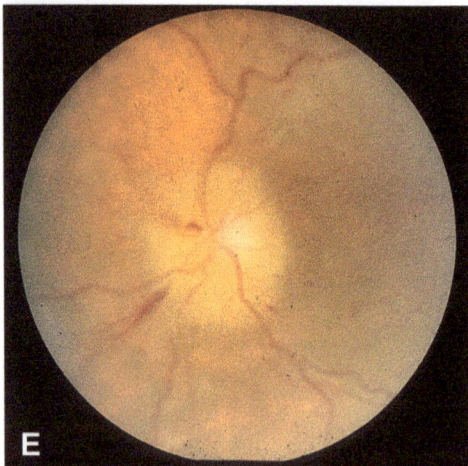

**Figure 4.4** E Anterior ischaemic optic neuropathy (AION)

Anterior ischaemic optic neuropathy (AION) is the most common cause of acute optic neuropathy among older persons. It can be non-arteritic (nonarteritic anterior ischaemic optic neuropathy [NAION]) or arteritic, the latter being associated with giant cell arteritis. Visual loss usually occurs suddenly, or over a few days at most, and it is usually permanent. The optic disc is pale and swollen and there are flame haemorrhages.

# 3rd, 4th, and 6th Cranial Nerves.

## Anatomy

The 3rd and 4th cranial nerves are in the midbrain, the 6th cranial nerve is in the pons. They are connected to each other by a pathway called the median longitudinal fasciculus. The median longitudinal fasciculus also connects to the vestibular pathway and the proprioceptive fibres in the upper cervical spine.

## Methods of Testing

This section discusses the cranial nerves that innervate the muscle that move the eyes and discusses the pupil reflex. It describes the more common abnormalities seen in clinical neurology.

Figure 4.5 shows normal eye movements and the primary direction of pull of each of the extra-ocular muscles. Figures 4.7, 4.8, 4.9 and 4.10 illustrate the common abnormalities of ocular movements: a 3rd and 6th nerve palsy, an internuclear ophthalmoplegia and a Horner's syndrome, respectively.

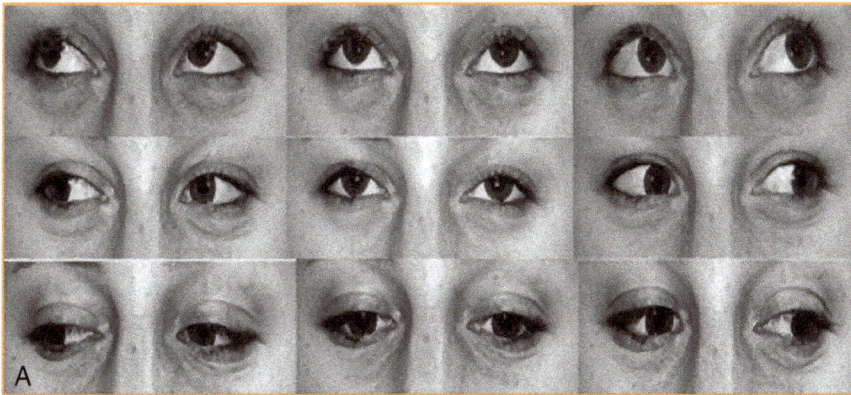

| Looking right and up<br>Right SR, Left IO | Looking up<br>Right SR+IO<br>Left SR + IO | Looking left and up<br>Left SR + Right IO |
|---|---|---|
| Looking right and down<br>Right IR + left SO | Looking down<br>Right IR+SO<br>Left IR + SO | Looking left and down<br>Left IR + right SO |

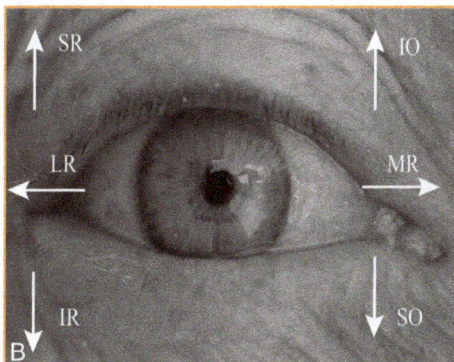

**Figure 4.5 A** Normal full ocular movements all directions

**B** The direction of action of the individual ocular muscles in the right eye IO = inferior oblique, IR = inferior rectus, LR= lateral rectus MR = medial rectus, SO = superior oblique, SR = superior rectus

Note: It is important to examine up gaze in the primary position (looking straight ahead) and also in the direction of action of each ocular muscle as shown.

When a patient complains of diplopia it is important to clarify whether they are seeing double as some patients use the term 'double vision' to describe blurred vision. Once diplopia is confirmed, the next step is to enquire whether the diplopia is horizontal or vertical. Horizontal diplopia occurs with lesions in the pons, 6th nerve palsies and an internuclear ophthalmoplegia while vertical diplopia occurs with lesions in the midbrain, 3rd, or 4th nerve palsies. Internuclear ophthalmoplegia is when the eye on the side of the lesion in the brainstem fails to adduct and there is nystagmus in the contralateral eye as it looks outwards (refer to Figure 4.9).

## Methods of examining eye movement

The examiner stands in front of the patient and observes the eye movements.

The patient is requested to look up as a check for impairment of up gaze. This is a common finding in older patients but it may also represent a supranuclear gaze palsy, which refers to impairment of eye movements due to pathology above the cranial nerve nuclei that innervate the extraocular muscles.

The patient is asked to look to the right and then to the left while the examiner observes the eyes to see that there is a full range of horizontal eye movements and observes if any nystagmus is present.

The patient is instructed to look up and then down when the eye is fully abducted towards the lateral aspect of the eye and then when it is fully adducted towards the nose.

## Testing patients with diplopia

If the patient complains of double vision there are two methods of determining the cause.

1  **Cover testing** The patient is asked to look towards an object and, if diplopia occurs, the eyes are covered one at a time and the patient is asked to say whether the image closest or furthest away from the midline disappears. The image that is furthest from the midline is the abnormal one and the impaired muscle is in the covered eye. It is often difficult for the patient to be certain which image disappears.

2  An easier and in my opinion a more reliable method is to use red-green glasses (Figure 4.6) and a torch. The patient is asked to identify which colour (red or green) is furthest from the midline in patients with horizontal diplopia and furthest from the equator with vertical diplopia. The light that is furthest from the midline is the abnormal one and reflects the muscle that is affected. For example, in Figure 4.7 showing a left 3rd nerve palsy, when the patient is looking to the right the green image would be furthest to the right indicating weakness of the left medial rectus muscle. If the patient had a left 6th nerve palsy, the green image would be furthest from the midline when they look left.

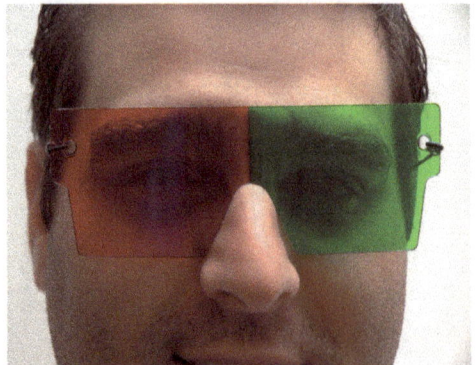

**Figure 4.6** Red-green glasses to examine patients with diplopia

# Oculomotor (3rd) Nerve
## Anatomy

The 3rd nerve nucleus is in the midbrain close to the midline, and the nerve exits the brainstem at the junction of the midbrain and pons just lateral to the midline (see Figure 1.6). It then crosses the subarachnoid space and, after traversing the cavernous sinus, it enters the orbit through the superior orbital fissure. The posterior communicating artery lies close to the nerve and this artery is a common site for berry aneurysm formation which can cause a 3rd nerve palsy.

The 3rd nerve supplies the following muscles:
- levator palpebrae superioris, one of the two muscles that elevate the eyelid
- medial rectus (MR) that adducts the eye towards the nose
- superior rectus (SR) and inferior rectus (IR) that cause the eye to look up and down, respectively, when the eye is in abduction (looking laterally).

## Method of Testing

Stand in front of the patient and hold an object up in front of their eyes. A finger is fine but a torch is better. Ask the patient to follow your finger/torch as you move it with their eyes and not moving their head. Move your finger/torch to one side and then whilst the eyes are looking to that side move your finger/torch up and then down testing one and then the other eye. Then move your finger/torch to the other side and once again move it up and then down. One is looking for the range of movement, asking if the patient sees double and looking for nystagmus. A word of caution, if you go beyond binocular vision (too far to one side) then you may induce nystagmus that is physiological and not indicative of disease. The simple way to avoid this is to use a torch and look for the reflection in both eyes, if it is only in one eye you have gone too far

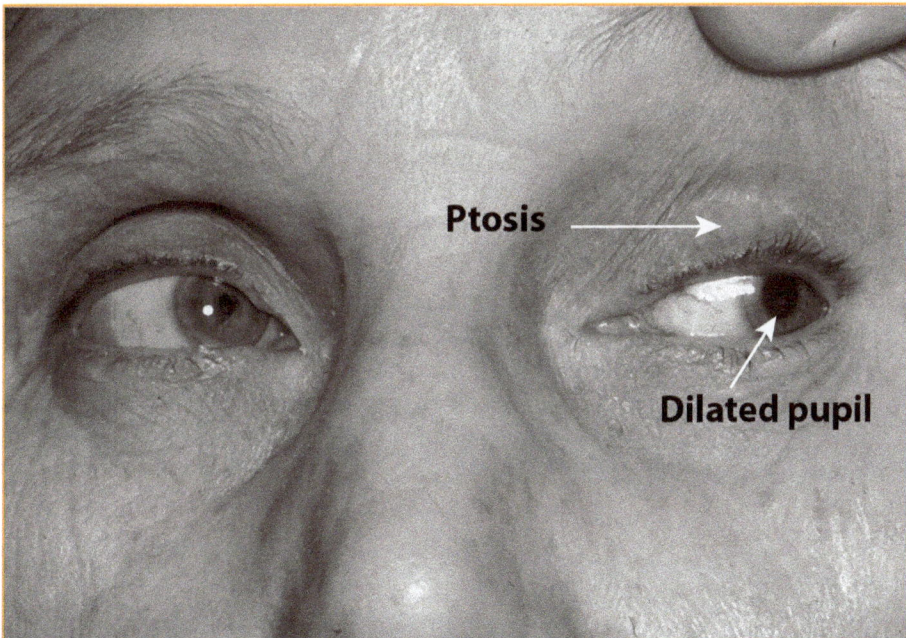

**Figure 4.7** A left 3rd nerve palsy affecting the pupil

The pupil is dilated due to the involvement of the parasympathetic fibres that constrict the pupil. The left eye cannot be elevated due to weakness of the superior rectus muscle. The other muscles that are affected but not illustrated are the medial and inferior rectus muscles and the inferior oblique. The left eyelid is being elevated to show the eye. In a 3rd nerve palsy, the ptosis is severe and usually covers the entire eye. If the pupil is not affected this is referred to as a 'pupil-sparing 3rd nerve palsy' and is most often related to infarction of the 3rd nerve, most often seen in patients with diabetes.

# Trochlear (4th) Nerve
## Anatomy

The 4th nerve nucleus is in the paramedian midbrain. The fibres of the 4th nerve cross the midline in the posterior aspect of the midbrain and emerge adjacent to the crus cerebri (Figure 1.6). The 4th nerve passes through the cavernous sinus and enters the orbit via the superior orbital fissure. It supplies the superior oblique (SO) muscle that depresses the eye when it is in the adducted position and internally rotates the eye when it is looking laterally (abducted) and down. Fourth nerve palsies are commonly associated with lesions of the other oculomotor nerves due to their proximity in the cavernous sinus and orbit; an isolated 4th nerve palsy is rare but can be congenital in origin or the result of trauma.

## Method of Testing

The trochlear nerve is tested by asking the patient to look towards the nose and then down. However, if the patient also has a 3rd nerve palsy and cannot adduct the eye towards the nose, the method of testing the 4th nerve is to ask the patient to look laterally and then down. If the 4th nerve is intact there will be internal rotation of the eye as it looks down; if the 4th nerve is impaired the eye will not internally rotate.

# Abducent (6th) Nerve
## Anatomy

The 6th cranial nerve nucleus lies within the pons (encircled by the 7th cranial nerve). It exits the pons laterally at the junction of the pons and medulla ( Figure. 1.6, chapter one). It crosses the subarachnoid space, passes through the cavernous sinus, and enters the orbit via the superior orbital fissure to supply the lateral rectus (LR) muscle. The proximity between the 6th nerve nucleus and the 7th nerve within the pons means it is very unusual to have an isolated 6th nerve lesion with a problem in the pons[1]. Most often a 6th nerve palsy indicates a lesion directly affecting the nerve, but occasionally it can be a false localising sign due to raised intracranial pressure. A 6th nerve palsy results in an inability to abduct (move the eye laterally within the orbit) the eye fully (Figure 4.8).

---

1   Foville's Syndrome is a rare brainstem lesion causing a LMN 7th cranial nerve palsy, contralateral hemiparesis, and an ipsilateral gaze palsy [9-10] due to a lesion affecting the motor pathway and the horizontal gaze centre in the pons that is adjacent to the 6th nerve nucleus.

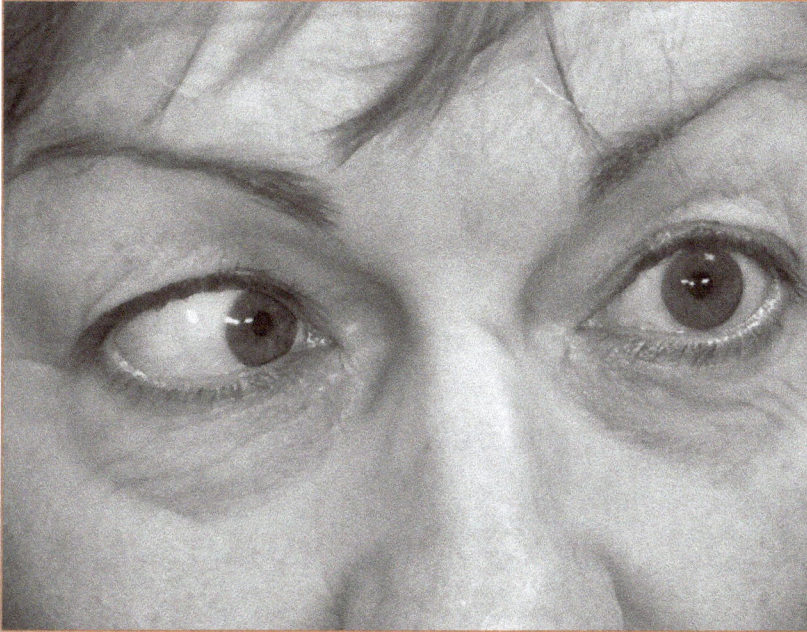

**Figure 4.8** A left 6th Nerve Palsy

The patient is looking to the left and the left eye does not go past the midline with a complete 6th nerve palsy and may pass the midline but not reach the lateral aspect of the orbit with a partial 6th Nerve palsy.

## Method of Testing

1. The patient is asked to look to the left, testing the left lateral rectus.
2. The patient is asked to look to the right, testing the right lateral rectus.

# Internuclear Ophthalmoplegia

## Anatomy

The median longitudinal fasciculus (MLF) is the pathway that connects the 3rd, 4th, and 6th nerves. There is one on each side close to the midline connecting the 3rd and 4th cranial nerve nuclei in the midbrain, down to the 6th nerve nucleus in the pons. A unilateral internuclear ophthalmoplegia (INO) is a common stroke syndrome in older patients with hypertension and diabetes. A unilateral or bilateral INO can be a manifestation of multiple sclerosis.

## Method of Testing

The patient is asked to look to the right or left. One would observe failure of adduction of the medial rectus muscle on one side with or without leading eye nystagmus in the eye looking laterally. The lesion is always on the side that fails to adduct. (Figure 4.9)

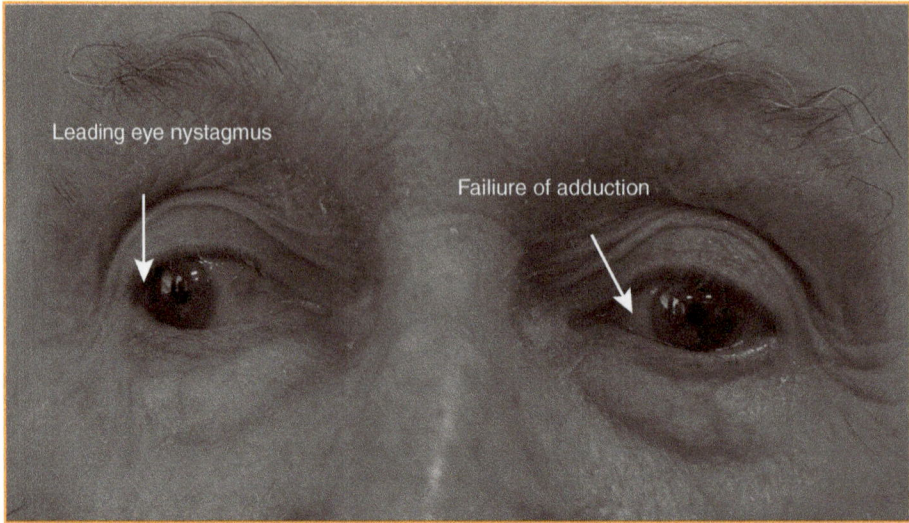

**Figure 4.9** Left internuclear ophthalmoplegia

Note the failure of adduction of the left eye. There is often but not always nystagmus in the opposite abducting (on this occasion the right) eye, termed leading eye nystagmus.

## Abnormalities of the Pupil

The pupil is innervated by parasympathetic fibres that constrict and sympathetic fibres that dilate the pupil. The parasympathetic fibres are on the surface of the 3$^{rd}$ nerve and a dilated pupil results when these are affected. A constricted pupil occurs when the sympathetic fibres are affected. This may occur anywhere along the pathway from their origin in the sympathetic ganglion at the level of the 1st and 2nd thoracic nerve roots up through the neck, where the fibres are closely related to the internal carotid artery, into the cranium, where the fibres are adjacent to the carotid siphon of the internal carotid artery, into the orbit via the superior orbital fissure. Sympathetic fibres also innervate the eyelid. Impairment of the sympathetic pathway will result in mild ptosis and a constricted pupil, known as Horner's syndrome (Figure 4.10). Other signs of a Horner's syndrome that are more subtle and more difficult to elicit are enophthalmos (the eye is partially withdrawn into the eye socket) and reduced or absent sweating (anhidrosis) on that side of the face.

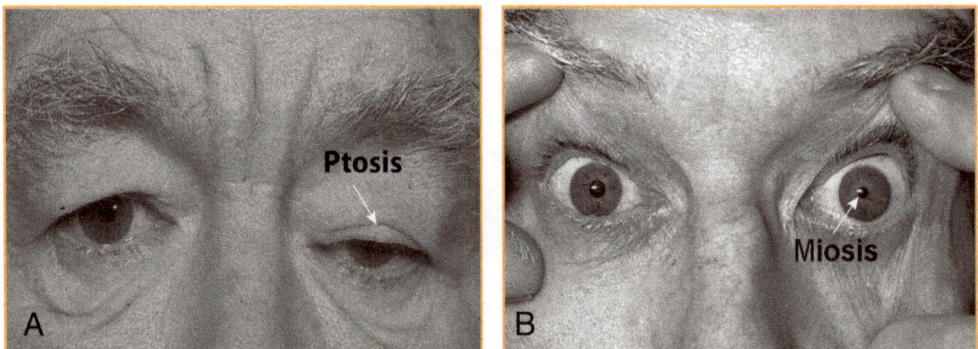

**Figure 4.10 A** Horner's syndrome with partial ptosis (drooping of the eyelid). **B** small pupil (miosis) with the eyelid elevated to show the pupil

# Trigeminal (5th) Nerve
## Anatomy

The trigeminal nerve has motor fibres that supply the ipsilateral pterygoid and masseter muscles (the muscles that push open and pull closed the jaw, respectively) and sensory fibres that supply sensation to the anterior one-third to two-thirds of the scalp, forehead, cheek, and jaw on the same side, but not the angle of the jaw (Figure 4.11). The motor fibres are only rarely affected by disease whereas there are many causes of sensory loss on the face. It is important to differentiate between altered sensation on the face due to a trigeminal nerve lesion and a quintothalamic tract lesion (the pathway between the 5th cranial nerve nucleus and the thalamus). The angle of the jaw is spared and the sensory loss affects only the anterior one-third to two-thirds of the scalp with a trigeminal nerve (peripheral nervous system) sensory problem whereas, with a quintothalamic tract (central nervous system) lesion, the sensory loss will extend over the entire (contralateral) scalp and face including the angle of the jaw. As this is almost invariably associated with spinothalamic tract involvement, the sensory loss will also affect the neck, arm, and leg on the same side.

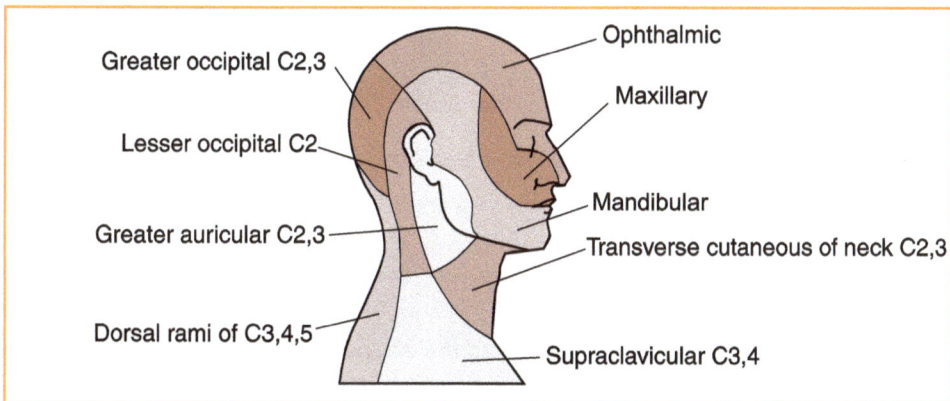

**Figure 4.11** The sensory areas ophthalmic, maxillary, and mandibular supplied by the 5th cranial nerve Reproduced from Gray's Anatomy, 37th edn, edited by PL Williams et al, 1989, Churchill Livingstone, Figure 7.242 [4]

## Method of Testing

Whether testing pain, light touch, or temperature sensation, test the forehead, cheek, and jaw on each side. To test sensation on the face, I use a toothpick for pain, cotton wool for light touch and the cold tuning fork for temperature sensation. If an area of abnormality is found, continue to test up over the forehead, across to the midline, back towards the ear and down to below the jaw until you find normal sensation, and the precise distribution of the sensory loss will be determined.

The corneal reflex is tested with cotton wool (not paper as it may abrade the cornea). Approach the eye from the side to avoid blinking due to the visual stimulus and touch the lateral aspect of the cornea (not the sclera) gently. The afferent pathway is the 1st division of the trigeminal nerve; the efferent pathway is the facial nerve resulting in eye closure. A similar reflex is the nasal tickle reflex. Tickle the inside of the nose with cotton wool: the afferent pathway is the 1st division of the trigeminal nerve; the efferent pathway is the facial nerve. A normal corneal and nasal tickle response evokes forced eye closure bilaterally.

The motor component is tested by asking the patient to protrude the jaw (pterygoid muscles). If it is normal it will protrude in the midline; if there is an abnormal 5th motor nerve the jaw will deviate towards the side of the weak muscle – the side of the lesion. Another technique is to gently push the jaw to the right and then to the left; an inability to resist indicates a contralateral 5th motor nerve lesion. To test the masseter muscles the patient is requested to clench the jaw while the examiner places both hands over the muscles to feel for the contraction (Figure 4.12). If there is an abnormality the muscle cannot be felt to contract beneath the fingers.

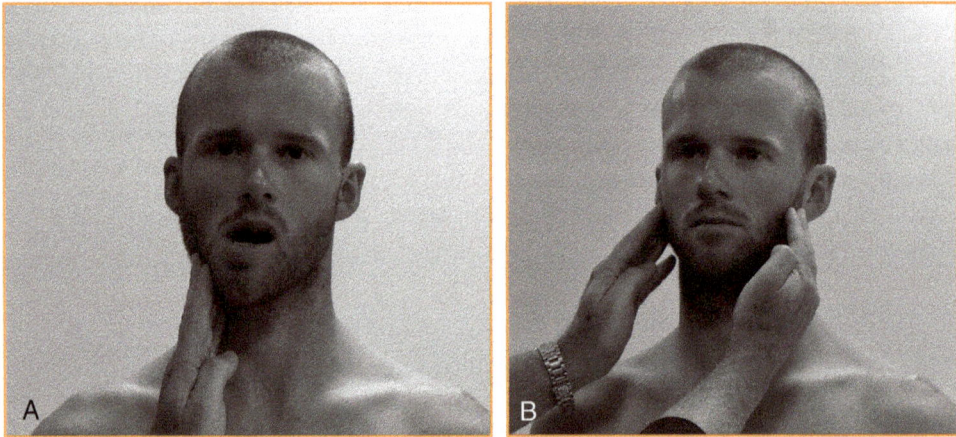

**Figure 4.12** The technique for testing the **A** pterygoid and **B** masseter muscles

# Facial (7th) Nerve

## Anatomy

The facial nerve nucleus is in the lateral pons of the brainstem. The nerve fibres hook around the 6th nerve nucleus and exit the pons laterally close to the 8th nerve (Figure 1.6, chapter one). The nerve then passes across the subarachnoid space and exits the skull via the facial canal and passes through the parotid gland to supply the facial muscles of the forehead, around the eye (orbicularis oculi), the cheek and around the mouth (orbicularis oris). A branch leaves the nerve before the canal and supplies the stapedius muscle in the middle ear (the nerve to stapedius); if it is affected, for example in a patient with a Bell's palsy, it causes hyperacusis (increased sensitivity to noise) in the ear. Another branch, the lingual nerve, supplies the sense of taste to the anterior two-thirds of the tongue; if affected it causes altered taste on the ipsilateral side of the tongue.

## Method of Testing

Facial movements are tested by asking the patient to show their teeth, close their eyes tightly and then open them wide. This latter command will cause elevation of the eyebrows and differentiates a lower motor from an upper motor facial weakness. The frontalis muscle controls the movement of the forehead and has bilateral innervation from the facial nerve. Thus, with an upper motor neuron problem, the patient can still wrinkle the forehead and raise the eyebrows whereas, with a lower motor problem, they cannot. Figure 4.13 shows the difference between upper and lower motor problems.

The most common lesion affecting the facial nerve is a Bell's palsy. This typically produces a LMN weakness on the same side of the face and is often, but not invariably, associated with ipsilateral hyperacusis (increased hearing in that ear) and altered taste.

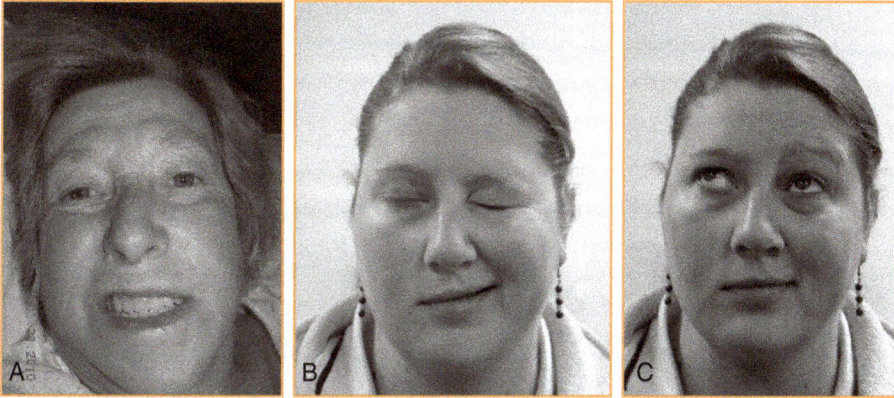

Figure 4.13 **A** an upper motor neuron facial weakness (note the patient can elevate both sides of the forehead);**B & C** Lower motor neuron 7th nerve palsy with an inability to smile, close the eye fully and wrinkle the ipsilateral forehead

# Auditory and Vestibular (8th) Nerve
## Anatomy

The 8th cranial nerve has two components, the auditory or cochlear (hearing) nerve and the vestibular (balance) nerve (Figure 4.14). The nerve emerges from the ear canal in the cerebellar–pontine angle, pierces the dura mater (the thick membrane surrounding the brain, just beneath the bone) and transverses the subarachnoid space. It enters the brainstem in the lateral pons where the vestibular and auditory nuclei are situated.

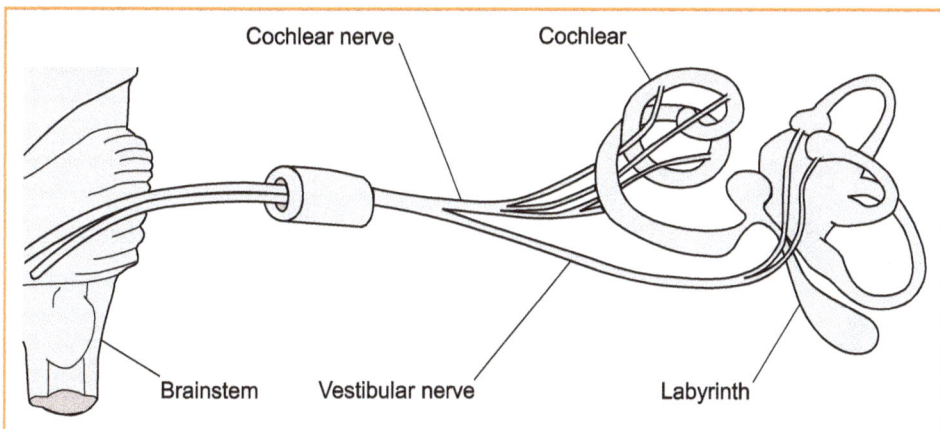

Figure 4.14 The vestibular pathway. Reproduced and modified from Clinically Oriented Anatomy, 4th edn, by KL Moore and AF Dalley, 1999, Lippincott Williams & Wilkins, Figure 7.82, p 975 [5]

## Method of Testing

The external ear canal is examined first to ensure it is not occluded by wax, and to visualise the eardrum. There are many ways to test hearing, including:

1. Rustle the patient's hair that is just above the ear between your fingers.
2. Hold a mechanical watch close to the ear.
3. Whisper numbers in one ear while occluding the opposite ear.

If there is hearing impairment, then it is useful to perform the Weber test and Rinne test using a 256-Hz tuning fork. In the Weber test, the ringing tuning fork is placed in the midline of the forehead. If there is a conduction defect (middle ear problem), the noise will be heard in that ear; on the other hand, if there is an 8th nerve deafness, the noise will be heard in the opposite ear. In the Rinne test, the tuning fork is placed next to the ear and subsequently on the mastoid process. Bone conduction (on the mastoid) is louder than air conduction (next to the ear) when deafness is due to a conduction problem. An easy way to remember the features of these two tests is for the examiner to occlude their external canal and test themselves. Occluding the external canal simulates a conduction defect (Figure 4.15).

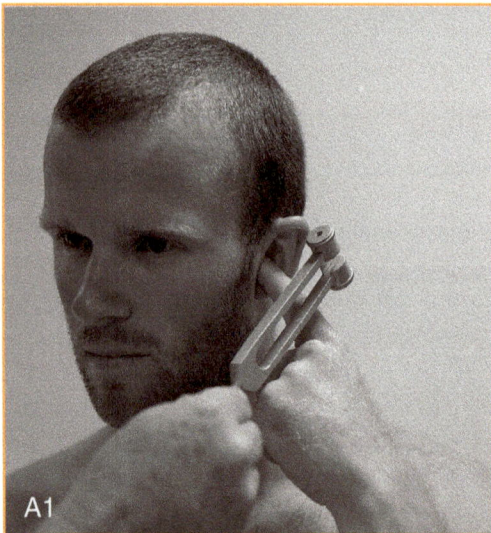

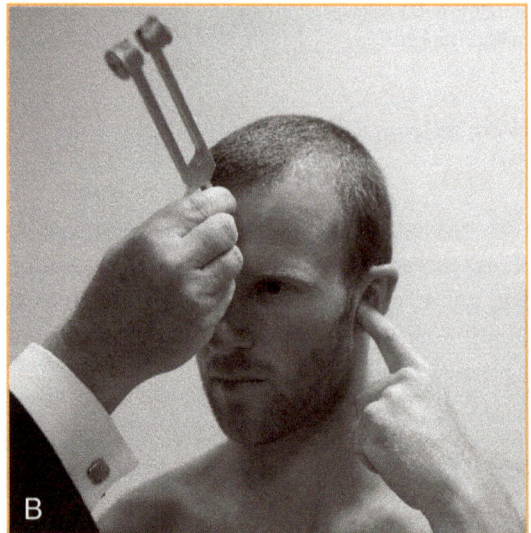

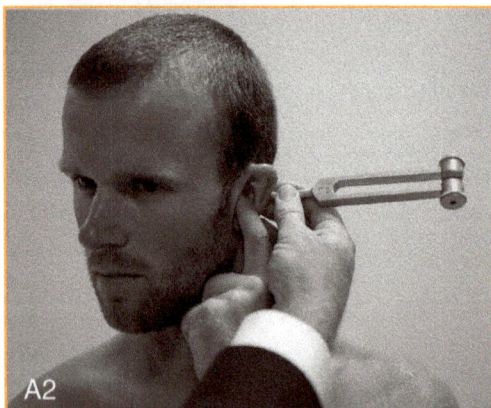

**Figure 4.15 A** – Tuning fork Rinne's test and simulation with the ear occluded
**B** – Tuning fork Weber's test and simulation with the ear occluded

# Vertigo and the Vestibular Pathway

If a patient has the sensation that the head or room is spinning (vertigo), the problem must affect the vestibular pathway (Figure 4.14), which runs from the inner ear to the cerebellum or vestibular nuclei in the brainstem and up to the vestibular cortex in the temporal lobe. Practically speaking, most cases of vertigo relate to inner ear problems and, to a lesser extent, cerebellar or brainstem lesions; they are very rarely due to more central pathology. Associated deafness and tinnitus coinciding with vertigo (and not a preexisting unrelated problem) indicate a problem in the ear while other neurological symptoms such as diplopia, dysarthria, dysphagia, weakness, or sensory disturbance point to a problem in the brainstem. Vertigo due to problems in the ear or vestibular nerve is referred to as peripheral vertigo whilst vertigo related to the brainstem or cerebellar problems is referred to as central vertigo. Vertigo is discussed in Chapter 7, 'Episodic disturbances of neurological function'.

# Glossopharyngeal (9th) Nerve

## Anatomy

The glossopharyngeal nerve nucleus lies in the lateral part of the medulla; the nerve emerges from the medulla, traverses the subarachnoid space, and exits through the jugular foramen in the base of the skull. It supplies sensation to the soft palate and pharynx, together with taste to the posterior two-thirds of the tongue.

# Method of Testing

The gag reflex is an unpleasant test and is only recommended as part of the examination when the patient complains of dysphagia. The pharynx is touched with a blunt object such as a spatula. The patient experiences a choking sensation. The soft palate will rise to the opposite side if there is a 10th cranial nerve (the efferent arc of the gag reflex) problem. The reflex will be absent if there is a 9th cranial nerve (the afferent arc of the gag reflex) problem.

# Vagus (10th) Nerve

## Anatomy

The vagus nerve nucleus lies in the lateral aspect of the medulla; the nerve emerges laterally and traverses the subarachnoid space to exit through the jugular foramen at the base of the skull. It then descends from the neck to the thorax and abdomen.

## Method of Testing

The patient is requested to say 'ah' and movement of the soft palate is observed. If there is a problem with the vagus nerve, the palate will deviate to the opposite side as it is pulled upwards by the normal muscle (Figure 4.16). This can also be observed with the gag reflex, described above.

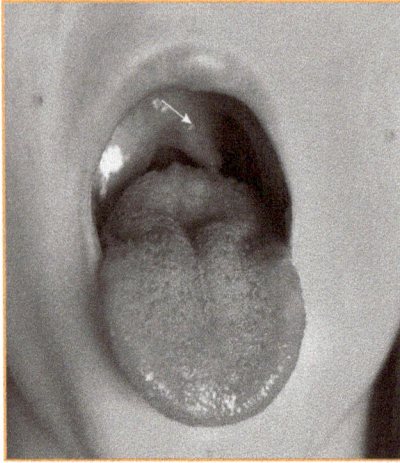

**Figure 4.16** Deviated palate to the left indicating a right-sided palatal weakness (as the muscle is a pulling and not a pushing one, thus the normal muscle pulls the palate up and to the same side)

# Accessory (11th) Nerve

## Anatomy

The accessory nerve nucleus also lies in the lateral medulla and the nerve exits adjacent to the lateral aspect of the pyramids of the motor pathway or corticospinal tract and traverses the subarachnoid space to exit through the jugular foramen in the base of the skull. After it exits the jugular foramen it is joined by the spinal component that derives fibres from the C2–C4 nerve roots to innervate the sternocleidomastoid and trapezius muscles. The spinal accessory nerve is prone to iatrogenic injury with posterior dissection of the neck.

## Method of Testing

The patient turns the head to one side and the examiner observes the sternocleidomastoid muscle on the opposite side (as the muscle pulls the sternum and mastoid closer together). To test the trapezius, the patient shrugs the shoulders against resistance (Figure 4.17).

**Figure 4.17** Method of testing the **A** sternocleidomastoid and **B** trapezius muscles

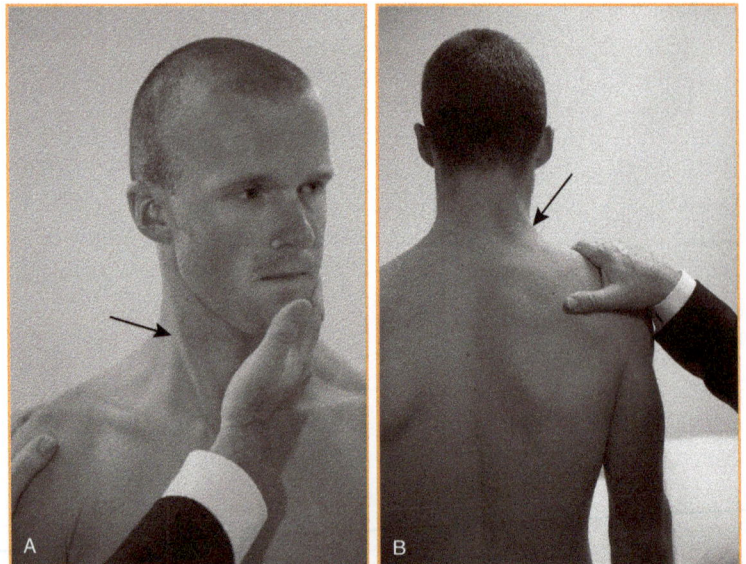

# Hypoglossal (12th) Nerve

## Anatomy

The hypoglossal nerve nucleus lies adjacent to the midline of the medulla and the nerve emerges from the anterior aspect of the medulla just laterally to the pyramids of the medulla and traverses the subarachnoid space to exit through the hypoglossal canal in the base of the skull to supply the muscle of the ipsilateral half of the tongue.

## Method of Testing

The patient is asked to protrude the tongue and, as the muscle pushes the tongue forward, the tongue will deviate towards the paralysed side (Figure 4.18).

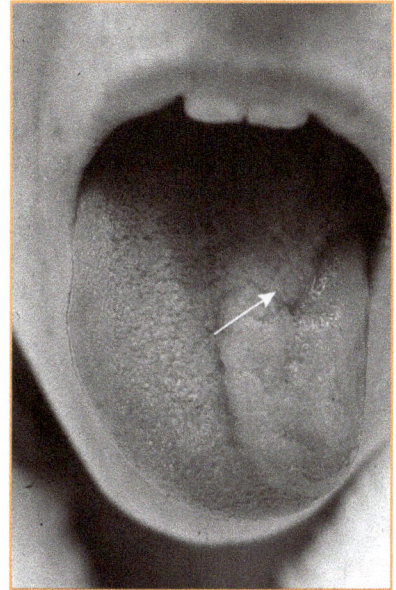

**Figure 4.18** Wasting and deviation of the protruded tongue to the left due to a left 12th (hypoglossal) nerve palsy

The website demonstrates the techniques for examination of the cranial nerves.

# The 'Rule of 4' of the Brainstem

The most common disorder to affect the brainstem is cerebrovascular disease. The following discussion entitled the 'Rule of 4' is a simplified method for understanding the brainstem and the various vascular syndromes. This has been previously published in the Internal Medicine Journal [1], Practical Neurology and [7] and Notfall und Rettungsmedizin [8]

The brainstem contains a bewildering number of structures with curious names such as superior colliculi, inferior olives, various cranial nerve nuclei and the medial longitudinal fasciculus. In reality, a neurological examination can only test a few of these structures. The 'Rule of 4' recognises this and describes only those parts of the brainstem that can be examined clinically. The blood supply of the brainstem is such that there are paramedian branches and long circumferential branches (the anterior inferior cerebellar artery 'AICA,' the posterior inferior cerebellar artery 'PICA' and the superior cerebellar artery 'SCA'). Involvement of the paramedian branches results in paramedian brainstem syndromes and involvement of the circumferential branches results in lateral brainstem syndromes. Occasionally, medial, or lateral brainstem syndromes occur with ipsilateral vertebral occlusion.

# The 4 rules of the 'Rule of 4'

**Rule 1** There are 4 structures in the 'midline' (the paramedian aspect of the midbrain adjacent to the midline) beginning with **M**:

- **M**otor nucleus
- **M**edian longitudinal fasciculus

- **M**edial lemniscus
- **M**otor pathway (corticospinal tract)

**Rule 2** There are 4 structures to the side (lateral) beginning with **S**:

- **S**pinocerebellar pathway
- **S**pinothalamic pathway
- **S**ensory nucleus of the 5th cranial nerve
- **S**ympathetic pathway

**Rule 3** The 4 cranial nerves in the medulla, 4 in the pons and 4 above the pons with 3 and 4 in the midbrain in ascending order are:

**Medulla**

- **12th** Hypoglossal nerve
- **11th** Accessory nerve
- **10th** Vagus nerve
- **9th** Glossopharyngeal nerve

**Pons**

- **8th** Auditory and Vestibular nerve
- **7th** Facial nerve
- **6th** Abducent nerve
- **5th** Trigeminal nerve

**Above the pons**

- **4th** Trochlear
- **3rd** Oculomotor nerve

The 3rd and 4th nerves are in the midbrain, the 2nd or ocular nerve and the 1st olfactory nerve are outside the midbrain and are not part of this rule of 4.

**Rule 4** The 4 motor nuclei that are in the midline (just to the side of the midline-paramedian) are those that divide (numerically) equally into 12, except for 1 and 2 i.e. 3,4 6 and 12 (5, 7, 9, 10 and 11 are the cranial nerves that are in the lateral brainstem):

- **3rd** Oculomotor nerve
- **4th** Trochlear nerve
- **6th** Abducent nerve
- **12th** Hypoglossal nerve

Figure 4.19 depicts a cross-section of the brainstem at the level of the medulla, but the concept of 4 lateral and 4 medial structures also applies to the pons; only the 4 medial structures relate to the midbrain. Figure 4.20 shows the location of the 12 cranial nerves and figure 4.21 shows the vertebrobasilar blood supply.

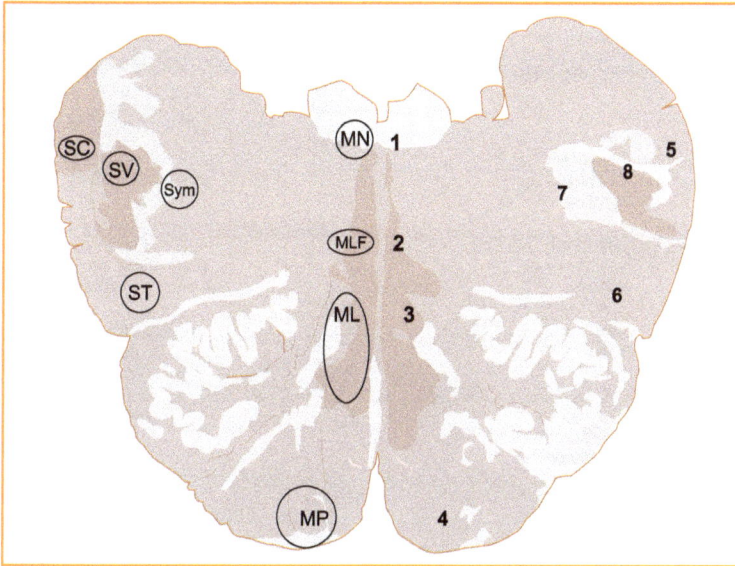

**Figure 4.19** Cross-section of the brainstem (in this case the medulla, but the same 'Rule of 4' applies to the pons) showing the 4 midline structures and the 4 structures in the lateral (side) aspect of the brainstem. Adapted from Gray's Anatomy, 34th edn, by E Davies et al, 1967, Longmans, Figure 813, p 1011 [6] The sizes of the coloured areas do not represent the actual anatomical size but have been made large enough to see and label. Abbreviations:1 MN = motor nucleus (3, 4, 6 or 12); 2 MLF = median longitudinal fasciculus; 3 ML = medial lemniscus; 4 MP = motor pathway (corticospinal tract); 5 SC = spinocerebellar; 6 ST = spinothalamic, 7 SY = sympathetic; 8 SV = sensory nucleus of Vth cranial nerve.

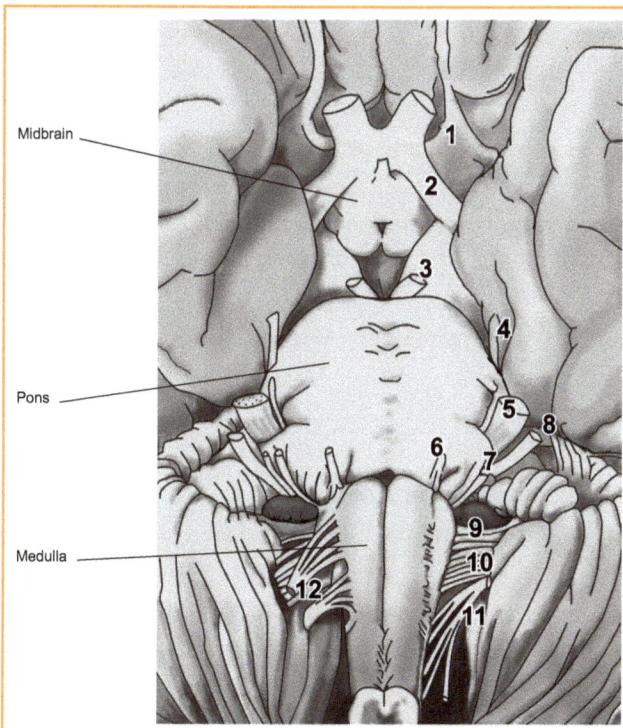

Figure 4.20 shows the ventral aspect of the brainstem and the emerging cranial nerves from the midbrain, pons, and medulla.

**Figure 4.20** The ventral aspect of the brainstem and its blood supply. The individual cranial nerves (numbered) in the medulla, pons, and midbrain (parallels of latitude) are shown. The large arteries that cause lateral brainstem/cerebellar strokes and the paramedian perforators that cause medial brainstem strokes are also shown. Adapted from Gray's Anatomy, 34th edn, by E Davies et al, 1967, Longmans, Figure 806, p 1003. 1 = olfactory; 2 = ophthalmic; 3 = oculomotor; 4 = trochlear; 5 = trigeminal; 6 = abducent; 7 = facial; 8 = auditory; 9 = glossopharyngeal; 10 = vagus,; 11 = spinal accessory and 12 = hypoglossal

The next section discusses the abnormalities produced by each of these structures in the brainstem.

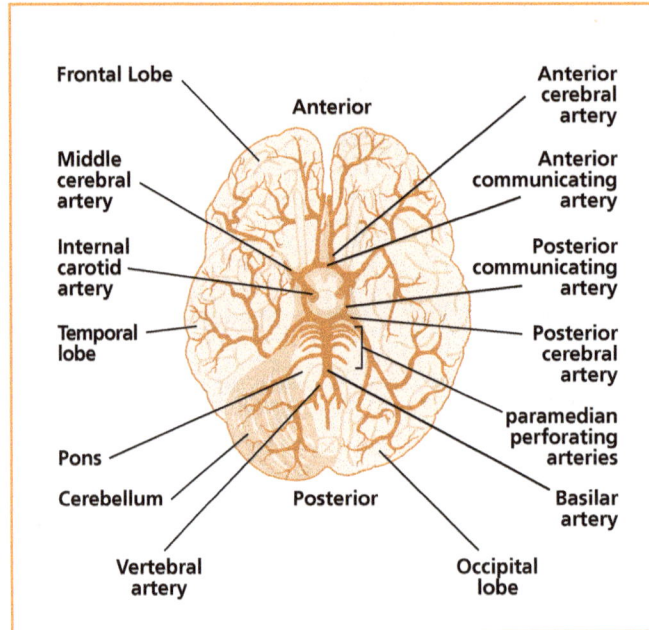

Figure 4.21 The undersurface of the brain including the ventral aspect of the brainstem, showing the cerebral circulation

The clinical features seen with problems affecting these structures are:

## The 4 Medial Structures

1. The **M**otor pathway (corticospinal tract): contralateral weakness of the arm and leg if the problem is above the mid pons the contralateral face will also be weak in an upper motor neuron pattern.

2. The **M**edial lemniscus: contralateral loss of vibration and proprioception affecting the arm and leg

3. The **M**edial longitudinal fasciculus: ipsilateral internuclear ophthalmoplegia (failure of adduction of the ipsilateral eye towards the nose and nystagmus in the opposite eye as it looks laterally)

4. The **M**otor nucleus and nerve: ipsilateral loss of the cranial nerve that is affected (3rd, 4th, 6th or 12th)

## The 4 Lateral Structures

1. The **S**pinocerebellar pathways: ipsilateral ataxia of the arm and leg

2. The **S**pinothalamic pathway: contralateral alteration of pain and temperature affecting the arm, leg and often the trunk

3. The **S**ensory nucleus of the 5th cranial nerve (a long vertical structure that extends in the lateral aspect of the pons down into the medulla): ipsilateral alteration of pain and temperature on the face in the distribution of the 5th cranial nerve (Figure 4.11)

4. The **S**ympathetic pathway: ipsilateral Horner's syndrome, i.e. partial ptosis, and a small pupil (miosis)

# The 4 Cranial Nerves in the Medulla

1. **9th** (glossopharyngeal): altered taste, ipsilateral loss of pharyngeal sensation
2. **10th** (vagus): dysphagia, ipsilateral palatal weakness
3. **11th** (spinal accessory): often asymptomatic ipsilateral weakness of the trapezius and sternocleidomastoid muscles
4. **12th** (hypoglossal): dysarthria, difficulty chewing, ipsilateral weakness of the tongue

The 12th cranial nerve is the motor nerve in the midline of the medulla. Although the 9th 10th and 11th cranial nerves have motor components, using the simple rule that they do not divide evenly into 12, they are thus not motor nerves in the midline.

# The 4 Cranial Nerves in the Pons

1. **5th** (trigeminal): ipsilateral alteration of pain, temperature, and light touch on the face back as far as the anterior 2/3 of the scalp and sparing the angle of the jaw, absent corneal response.
2. **6th** (abducent): horizontal diplopia, ipsilateral weakness of abduction (lateral movement) of the eye
3. **7th** (facial): lower motor neuron ipsilateral facial weakness
4. **8th** (auditory): ipsilateral deafness

The 6th cranial nerve is the motor nerve in the pons. The 7th is a motor nerve but it also carries pathways of taste and, using the Rule of 4, it does not divide equally into 12 and thus it is not a motor nerve. The vestibular portion of the 8th nerve is not included to keep the concept simple and to avoid confusion. Nausea, vomiting, and vertigo occur with the involvement of the vestibular connections in the lateral medulla.

# The 4 Cranial Nerves above the Pons

1. **1st** (olfactory): altered smell not in midbrain
2. **2nd** (optic): altered unilateral visual not in midbrain
3. **3rd** (oculomotor): vertical diplopia, impaired adduction, elevation, and depression of the ipsilateral eye with or without a dilated pupil; the eye is turned out and slightly down
4. **4th** (trochlear): vertical diplopia, head tilted to the same side and the eye unable to look down when it is looking in towards the nose

The 3rd and 4th cranial nerves are the motor nerves in the midbrain.

The motor and sensory pathways pass through the entire length of the brainstem and can be likened to 'meridians of longitude' while the various cranial nerves can be regarded as 'parallels of latitude.' If you can establish where the meridians of longitude and parallels of latitude intersect, you have established the site of the lesion.

Using these rules a medial brainstem syndrome will consist of the 4 M's + the relevant motor cranial nerve (3rd, 6th, or 12th) and a lateral brainstem syndrome will consist of the 4 S's + either the 9th, 10th and 11th cranial nerves if in the medulla or the 5th, 7th, and 8th cranial nerves if in the pons.

# Medial (Paramedian) Brainstem Syndromes

Let us assume that the patient you are examining has a brainstem problem (most often a stroke). If you find UMN weakness in the arm and the leg on one side then you know the patient has a contralateral medial brainstem syndrome because the motor pathway is paramedian and crosses at the level of the foramen magnum (at the decussation of the pyramids, where the brainstem meets the spinal cord). The involvement of the motor pathway is the 'meridian of longitude.' Refer to Figure 4.22 for a summary of the signs. So far, the lesion could be anywhere in the medial aspect of the brainstem although, if the face is also affected, it has to be above the mid pons, the level of the 7th nerve nucleus.

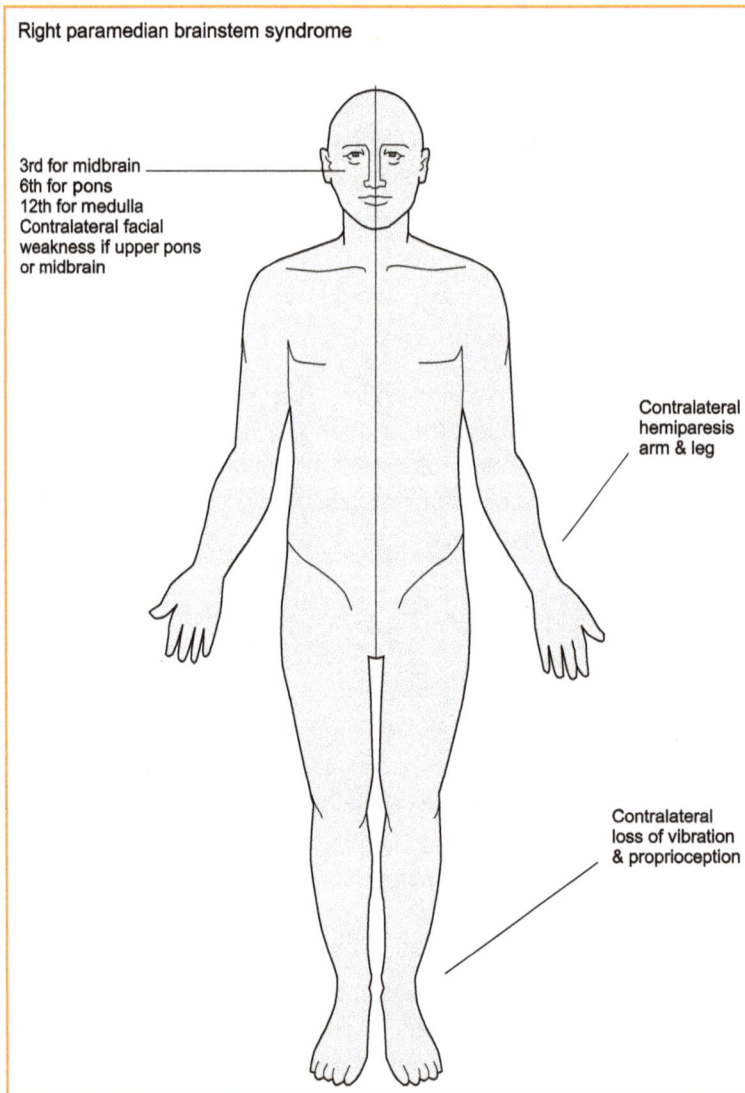

Right paramedian brainstem syndrome

3rd for midbrain
6th for pons
12th for medulla
Contralateral facial
weakness if upper pons
or midbrain

Contralateral
hemiparesis
arm & leg

Contralateral
loss of vibration
& proprioception

**Figure 4.22** The signs seen in medial (paramedian) brainstem syndromes.

The motor cranial nerve, 'the parallel of latitude,' indicates whether the lesion is in the medulla (12th), pons (6th) or midbrain (3rd). Remember that the cranial nerve palsy will be ipsilateral to the side of the lesion and contralateral to the hemiparesis. If the medial lemniscus is also affected, you will find a contralateral (the same side affected by the hemiparesis) loss of vibration and proprioception in the arm and leg as the posterior columns also cross at or just above the level of the foramen magnum. If no cranial nerve is affected it is impossible to localise the site of the pathology, although if it is brainstem problem it is most frequently in the pons.

The median longitudinal fasciculus (MLF) is usually not affected when there is a hemiparesis as the MLF is further back in the brainstem. The MLF can be affected in isolation, a 'lacunar infarct', resulting in an ipsilateral internuclear ophthalmoplegia, with failure of adduction (movement towards the nose) of the ipsilateral eye and leading eye nystagmus on looking laterally to the opposite side of the lesion in the contralateral eye. If the patient has the involvement of the left MLF, when asked to look to the left the eye movements would be normal, but on looking to the right the left eye would not go past the midline while there would be nystagmus in the right eye as it looked to the right.

# Lateral Brainstem Syndromes

Once again, we are assuming that the patient you are seeing has a brainstem problem, most likely a vascular lesion. The 4 S's or 'meridians of longitude' will indicate that you are dealing with a lateral brainstem problem, and the cranial nerves or 'parallels of latitude' will indicate whether the problem is in the lateral medulla or lateral pons. Refer to Figure 4.23 for a summary of the signs.

A lateral brainstem infarct will result in:

- ipsilateral ataxia of the arm and leg due to the involvement of the spinocerebellar pathways
- contralateral alteration of pain and temperature sensation due to involvement of the spinothalamic pathway
- ipsilateral loss of pain, temperature and light touch sensation affecting the face within the distribution of the sensory nucleus of the trigeminal nerve
- An ipsilateral Horner's syndrome with partial ptosis and a small pupil (miosis) is due to the involvement of the sympathetic pathway.

The power, tone and reflexes should all be normal. So far all we have done is localise the problem to the lateral aspect of the brainstem. By adding the relevant 3 cranial nerves in the medulla or the pons we can localise the lesion to one of these regions of the brain.

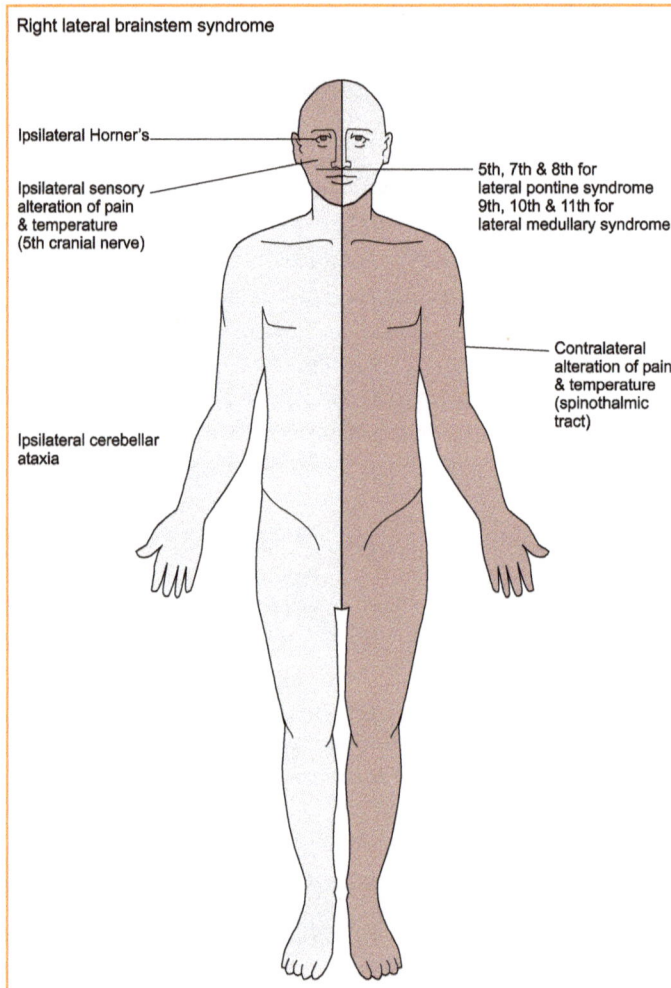

**Figure 4.23** The signs with lateral brainstem syndromes. Note: Trapezius weakness is rarely seen in lateral medullary lesions.

The lowest 4 cranial nerves are in the medulla and the 12th nerve is in the midline so that the 9th, 10th, and 11th will be in the lateral aspect of the medulla. When these are affected the result is dysarthria and dysphagia with an ipsilateral impairment of the gag reflex and the palate will pull up to the opposite side when the patient is asked to say ahh. Occasionally, there may be a weakness of the ipsilateral trapezius and/or sternocleidomastoid muscle. This is the lateral medullary syndrome, usually due to occlusion of the ipsilateral vertebral or posterior inferior cerebellar artery.

The next 4 cranial nerves are in the pons and the 6th nerve is the motor nerve in the midline, so that the 5th, 7th, and 8th are in the lateral aspect of the pons. When these are affected there will be ipsilateral LMN facial weakness, weakness of the ipsilateral masseter and pterygoid muscles (muscles that open and close the mouth) and occasionally ipsilateral deafness. A tumour such as an acoustic neuroma in the cerebellopontine angle will result in ipsilateral deafness, facial weakness, and impairment of facial sensation; there may also be ipsilateral limb ataxia if it compresses the ipsilateral cerebellum or brainstem. The sympathetic pathway is usually too deep to be affected.

If there are signs of both lateral and medial brainstem syndrome, one needs to consider a basilar artery problem, possibly an occlusion.

In summary, if one can remember:

- 4 structures in the midline commencing with the letter M
- 4 structures in the lateral aspect of the brainstem commencing with the letter S
- the lower 4 cranial nerves are in the medulla
- the middle 4 cranial nerves are in the pons
- the first 4 cranial nerves are above the pons, with the 3$^{rd}$ and 4$^{th}$ in the midbrain
- the 4 motor nerves that are in the midline are the 4 that divide evenly into 12 (except for 1 and 2), i.e. the 3rd, 4th, 6th, and 12th.

Then you will be able to diagnose brainstem stroke syndromes.

**Another way to remember:**
In a patient with a hemiparesis the lesion will be in the paramedian region of the brainstem and the 3rd, 6th and 12th will localise it to the midbrain, pons, or medulla, respectively.

A lateral medullary syndrome is four "S's" + 9th, 10th, and 11th!

# References

1 Gates P. The rule of 4 of the brainstem: A simplified method for understanding brainstem anatomy and brainstem vascular syndromes for the non-neurologist. *Intern Med J* 35 (4) (2005) 263–266.

2 Adams R.D.; Victor M.. *Principles of neurology*. (1985) McGraw–Hill Book Company: New York. 1186.

3 Gerling J.; Meyer J.H.; Kommerell G.. Visual field defects in optic neuritis and anterior ischemic optic neuropathy: Distinctive features. *Graefes Arch Clin Exp Ophthalmol* 236 (3) (1998) 188–192.

4 Williams P.L.; et al. *Gray's anatomy*. 37th edn (1989) Churchill Livingstone: London.

5 Moore K.L.; Dalley A.F. *Clinically oriented anatomy*. 4th edn (1999) Lippincott Williams & Wilkins: Maryland.

6 Davies E.; et al. *Gray's anatomy*. 34th edn (1967) Longmans. 1011, Figure 813.

7 Gates P. Work out where the problem is in the brainstem using 'the rule of 4'. *Pract Neurol* 2011; 11(3): 167-72.

8 Gates P. Recognising brainstem problems in the emergency department using the rule of 4 of the brainstem. *Notfall + Rettungsmedizin* 2015; 18(5): 364-9.

9 Silverman, I. E., et al. (1995). "The crossed paralyses. The original brain-stem syndromes of Millard-Gubler, Foville, Weber, and Raymond-Cestan." *Arch Neurol* 52(6): 635-638.

10 Foville, A. (1858). "Note sur une paralysie peu connue de certains muscles de l'oeil, et sa liaison avec quelques points de l'anatomie et la physiologie de la protub\l=e'\ranceannulaire." *Bull Soc Anat Paris*. 33: 393-414.

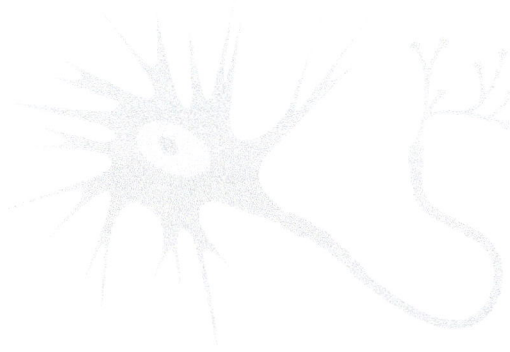

# The Cerebral Hemispheres and Cerebellum
## Assessment of Higher Cognitive Function

Although subtitled 'Assessment of higher cognitive function', this chapter will not deal with the very complex neuropsychological testing in patients with impairment of cognitive function. Instead, this chapter discusses a simplistic assessment of language disturbances and some very basic higher cortical functions, particularly the parietal lobes, that enable localisation of the site of the pathology when taking the neurological history and examining the patient.

This simple approach involves terms such as primary pathways and secondary association areas. There is no evidence that the parietal lobes are 'hard-wired' in such a manner. Symptoms from lesions in a part of the nervous system do not necessarily reflect the function of that part; the symptoms may arise from either a loss of specific functions or functional overactivity of the portions of the brain that remain intact [1]. The higher cortical functions are the parallels of latitude within the cerebral hemisphere.

---

The pathology is always at the level of the parallel of latitude (LMN signs).

---

More comprehensive discussions can be found in the major textbooks [1–3]. Figure 5.1 is a lateral view of the cerebral hemispheres and the cerebellum. The frontal, parietal, occipital and temporal lobes and the various functions of those lobes are shown.

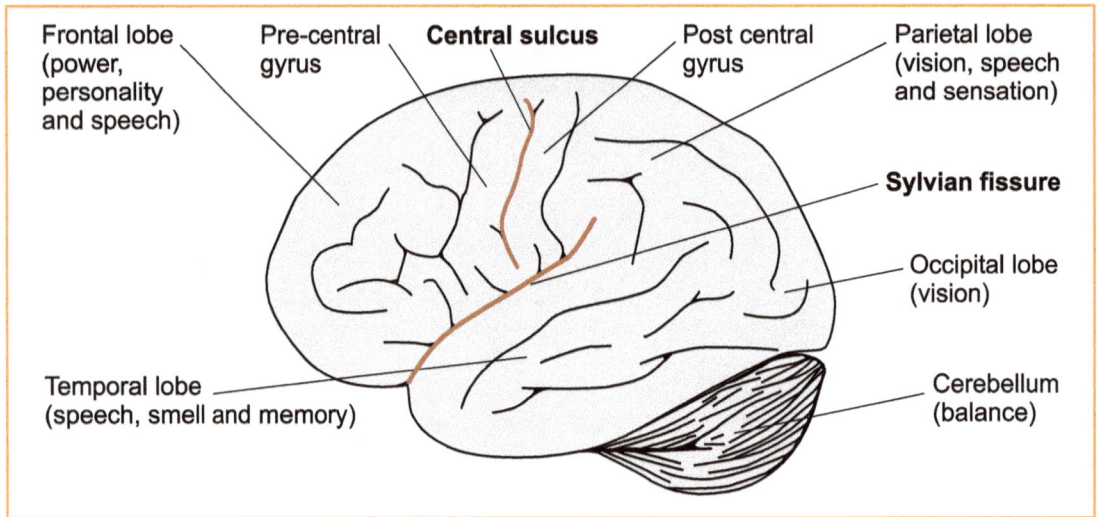

**Figure 5.1** A lateral view of the brain and a brief description of the common functions associated with the specific lobes of the brain. *Note:* The central sulcus separates the frontal lobe and the parietal lobe.

# The Frontal Lobes

Patients should be suspected of having a problem in the frontal lobe if they present with one of the following:
- contralateral weakness
- changes in personality or behaviour
- difficulty walking in the absence of any weakness or sensory symptoms in the legs (a condition referred to as apraxia of gait)
- non-fluent dysphasia (dominant hemisphere only).

## Contralateral Weakness

The area just in front of the central sulcus, the pre-central gyrus (Figure 5.1), is the origin of the motor fibres that innervate the muscles on the opposite side of the body. This pathway is the corticospinal tract. The corticospinal pathway crosses the midline at the level of the foramen magnum, the junction of the lower end of the brainstem and the upper end of the cervical spinal cord. Lesions affecting the pre-central gyrus will result in a contralateral hemiparesis affecting the face, arm, and leg, although one limb may be weaker. The clues that the hemiparesis is due to a lesion in the frontal lobe are:
- Conjugate deviation of the eyes away from the side of the weakness and towards the side of the lesion. The frontal lobe controls conjugate deviation of the eyes to the opposite side.
- Non-fluent dysphasia with dominant hemisphere lesions.
- Cortical sensory signs due to associated involvement of the parietal lobe on that side

Rarely, an irritative lesion can cause a contralateral hemiparesis with the eyes deviated to the side of the weakness and away from the side of the pathology. This mimics a pontine lesion in the brainstem where there is an area responsible for conjugate deviation of the eyes to the same side.

# Changes to Personality or Behaviour

The pre-frontal region is the area of the frontal lobes anterior to the motor cortex and the motor speech area. Diseases affecting this region of the frontal lobe result in changes to personality or behaviour best summarised by the phrase 'they are not themselves'.

These patients can lose spontaneity and initiative and appear apathetic and depressed or, at the other end of the spectrum, patients can appear to 'have a short fuse'. In this situation, patients can become aggressive and violent, even after a trivial incident. This is sometimes seen following a head injury. Patients with frontal lobe pathology can develop an elevated mood and behave inappropriately, such as the vicar's wife who began to tell dirty jokes and who was subsequently diagnosed with a meningioma (a benign tumour) in the frontal lobe.

If the olfactory tracts that lie beneath the frontal lobe are also affected, there can be an associated unilateral or bilateral anosmia (loss of the sense of smell).

An inability to perform acts voluntarily or to make decisions is seen in patients with pre-frontal problems and is termed abulia, reflecting pathology in the medial aspect of the frontal lobes. Abulia sometimes occurs with a subarachnoid haemorrhage (bleeding into the subarachnoid space) related to a ruptured berry aneurysm on the anterior communicating artery complicated by vasospasm of the anterior cerebral artery.

# Difficulty Walking

Frontal lobe pathology can present with an apraxia of gait. The history is one of progressive difficulty walking in the absence of any weakness, sensory disturbance, ataxia, or extrapyramidal dysfunction to account for the difficulty walking. It is as if the patient has forgotten how to walk. Gait apraxia is discussed in Chapter 13. This is often confused with Parkinson's disease.

Frontal lobe signs, referred to as *primitive reflexes* because they are present in normal babies, may or may not be present in patients with frontal lobe pathology. These include:
- a *grasp reflex*, where the patient involuntarily grasps an object (usually the examiner's hand) placed in the palm of their hand.
- a *positive palmo-mental reflex*, where the palm is stroked and there is retraction of the ipsilateral chin.
- a *pout reflex*, where the patient purses the lips when a stimulus is applied to them.

Although changes in personality and behaviour may be one of the presenting symptoms of dementia, severe depression can produce a similar clinical picture termed 'pseudodementia'.

# The Parietal Lobes

Patients with parietal lobe problems may present in several ways:
- Speech disturbance such as fluent dysphasia or if Wernicke's area in the posterior temporal lobe is affected, the patient may appear to be confused (discussed below).
- Disturbances of vision in the contralateral visual field.
- Lost or disorientated even in a familiar environment.
- A concerned relative brings the patient for an assessment. This occurs as some patients are not aware of any problems.

Visual disturbances can occur in both dominant and non-dominant hemisphere involvement; dysphasia is a feature of the dominant hemisphere; being lost, disoriented and unaware that anything is amiss are very typical features of the non-dominant hemisphere.

In both the dominant and non-dominant hemispheres, visual pathways pass through on their way to the occipital lobe, and sensory pathways terminate in the parietal lobe. If the so-called 'primary pathway' is affected, there will be a contralateral loss of function. No loss of function occurs if the 'primary pathway' is intact. If the 'secondary association areas' are affected, a contralateral inattention with double simultaneous stimuli where the patient is not aware of the stimulus on one side when the other side is stimulated in the same manner simultaneously.

| Table 5.1 The clinical features with lesions of the dominant and non-dominant parietal lobes | | |
|---|---|---|
| | **Dominant** | **Non-dominant** |
| Primary sensory pathway* | Contralateral sensory loss | Contralateral sensory loss |
| Secondary association area for sensation* | Contralateral sensory inattention | Contralateral sensory inattention |
| Primary visual pathway* | Contralateral loss of vision ** | Contralateral loss of vision** |
| Secondary association area for vision* | Contralateral visual inattention | Contralateral visual inattention |
| Cortical signs* | Graphaesthesia, 2-point discrimination and stereognosis | Graphaesthesia, 2-point discrimination and stereognosis |
| Speech | Fluent dysphasia | Dysarthria |
| Other | Gerstmann's syndrome (RAAF) | "Lost in space" |

\*  Sensory and visual symptoms and the unique parietal cortical signs are common to both the dominant and non-dominant parietal lobes.

\*\* Either loss of vision in the opposite visual field (hemianopia) or loss of vision in the upper or lower aspect of the visual field on the opposite side (quadrantanopia).

Speech disturbance (dysphasia) and the term RAAF (an abbreviation for the **R**oyal **A**ustralian **A**ir **F**orce) is a way to remember the features of problems in the dominant hemisphere. The term 'lost in space' is an easy way to remember the characteristics of non-dominant parietal lobe problems (Table 5.1). RAAF refers to the clinical findings seen in dominant parietal lobe problems and, in its pure form, is called Gerstmann's syndrome (for an explanation of RAAF, see 'Gerstmann's syndrome' below).

# Abnormalities of Vision

- Contralateral loss of vision. The optic radiation from the contralateral visual field passes through the parietal lobe to the occipital lobe (Figure 5.1). If the 'primary pathway' is affected, there will be a loss of vision on the contralateral side. A lower quadrantanopia if only the parietal lobe is affected, but often the optic radiation fibres in the temporal lobe are also affected causing a contralateral homonymous hemianopia. The visual field disturbance is identical in both eyes.

- Contralateral visual inattention. If the 'primary visual pathways' are preserved, but the so-called 'secondary association areas' are affected, visual inattention will occur. This is elicited with double simultaneous stimuli. The patient cannot appreciate the visual stimulus in one visual field, when the examiner simultaneously moves a finger on each of their hands in both the right and left visual field. The patient can see both the finger in the left and right visual fields when moved one at a time.

# Abnormalities of Sensation

Although abnormalities of sensation may be detected in patients with parietal lobe problems, they are not always symptomatic.

- Contralateral loss of sensation affecting the primary sensory modalities of vibration and proprioception, pain, and temperature
- Contralateral sensory inattention where the patient cannot appreciate sensation on one side of the body when the stimulus is applied simultaneously to both sides
- Unique parietal sensory phenomena
  - Impairment of 2-point discrimination
  - Impaired stereognosis
  - Impaired graphaesthesia

The sensory pathways from the body terminate in the contralateral post-central gyrus of the parietal lobe. If the 'primary sensory pathway' is affected a loss or impairment of vibration and proprioception will occur on the opposite of the body. These sensory modalities are affected by cortical and deep hemisphere parietal lobe problems. A loss or impairment of pain and temperature sensation is seen with deep hemisphere but not cortical parietal lobe problems.

If the 'primary pathways' are not affected, but the 'secondary association areas' are involved the resulting abnormality will be a loss of appreciation of sensation elicited with double simultaneous stimulation termed sensory inattention. Here, the examiner applies the same stimulus to both sides of the body simultaneously. This is done by gently stroking the skin on both limbs simultaneously with a finger. Patients with sensory inattention do not notice the sensory stimulus on the contralateral side of the body to the pathology when both sides are stimulated simultaneously but can appreciate the sensory stimulus when only one side is stimulated.

Although abnormalities of vibration and proprioception can occur in cortical lesions, their presence does not localise the problem to the cortex. When the primary sensory modalities of pain, temperature, vibration, and proprioception are normal or only mildly affected, it is possible to perform more detailed sensory testing looking for abnormalities seen with contralateral parietal cortical lesions. The three cortical signs consist of:

1. Impairment of **stereognosis**: the patient cannot appreciate the shape and size of an object, for example, a pen or a coin, placed in the affected hand without looking at it. Proprioception must not be affected; otherwise, the inability to identify the object would reflect impairment of the proprioceptive pathway and not necessarily the contralateral parietal cortex.
2. Impairment of **graphaesthesia**: the patient cannot identify a number drawn or a letter on the palm of the contralateral affected hand without looking. The drawing must be more than 4 cm in size. It is best to draw on the palm while the patient watches. The patient then

closes their eyes and asked to identify another number drawn on the palm. It is easier for patients to identify numbers if their palm faces them and not the examiner. If light touch is severely impaired, abnormal graphaesthesia may occur and not indicate a cortical problem.

3. Impairment of **2-point discrimination**: an inability to distinguish two points from one. This can be tested on any part of the body. The normal distance between the two points varies greatly from 1 mm on the tip of the tongue to 20–30 mm on the dorsum of the hands and feet [1]. The most useful site to test 2-point discrimination is on the fingertips, where the normal distance is 3–5 mm. It is prudent to test the opposite hand (if it is normal) to determine the distance between the two points in this particular patient, as this can vary from patient to patient depending on their age.

The above sensory and visual abnormalities occur with pathology in either the dominant (usually left) or non-dominant hemisphere with the three cortical signs contralateral to the side of the pathology.

# The Dominant Hemisphere

In addition to the sensory and or visual abnormalities with or without the three cortical sensory signs described above, patients with dominant hemisphere lesions may have a speech disturbance termed dysphasia and some or all of the signs of Gerstmann's syndrome.

## Disturbances of Speech

Clinicians use abnormalities of speech to localise the problem within the nervous system. On the other hand, speech therapists assess speech differently and more from the therapeutic point of view. A simplified approach is shown in Figure 5.2.

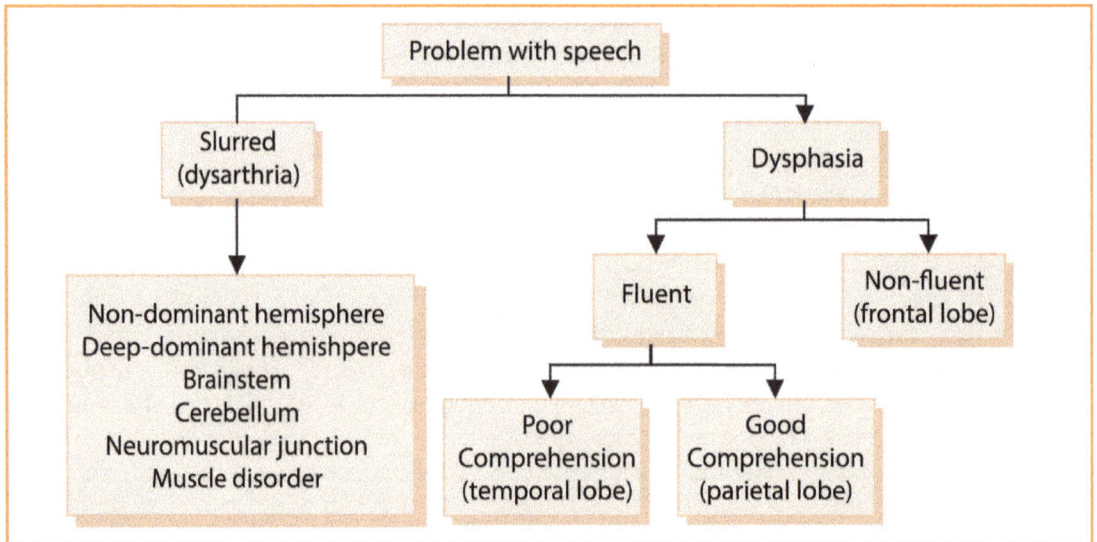

**Figure 5.2** Simplified approach to speech disturbances.

Dysarthria refers to difficulty in speaking because of impairment of the organs of speech or their nerve supply [4]. Dysarthria occurs with problems in the frontal lobes, parietal lobes, cortex or deep within the subcortical white matter of either the dominant or non-dominant hemisphere.

Dysarthria also occurs with brainstem and cerebellar problems, disorders of the 9th,10th and 12th cranial nerves, disorders of the neuromuscular junction or even diseases affecting the face, tongue, or palatal muscles. Although experienced neurologists may differentiate between the various types of dysarthria, this is difficult for non-neurologists.

- Dysphasia is an impairment of the ability to understand and use the symbols of language, both spoken and written [4]. Aphasia is a total loss of speech. Aphasia and dysphasia occur with dominant hemisphere problems (Figure 5.3). The dominant hemisphere is the left in 90% of right-handed people and 50% of left-handed people.

The simplest classification to understand is the one that reflects the abnormality of speech encountered: non-fluent (C) or fluent with (A) or without (B) comprehension difficulties.

A. If the pathology is in the posterior aspect of the dominant temporal lobe (area A, Figure 5.3), the patient has word deafness. They cannot monitor their speech or understand what is said to them. The patient will appear to be very confused. Speech is fluent with literal (letters) and verbal (words) paraphasic errors. Paraphasic errors are where letters of some words or entire words are replaced by other letters or words. An example of a literal paraphasic error is 'mouse' instead of 'house', and an example of a verbal paraphasic error is 'the sky is brown' instead of blue. Non-existent words, referred to as neologisms, are invented. An example of a neologism is 'rumpstle'. As patients cannot monitor their speech, the words are often out of sequence, described as a word salad.

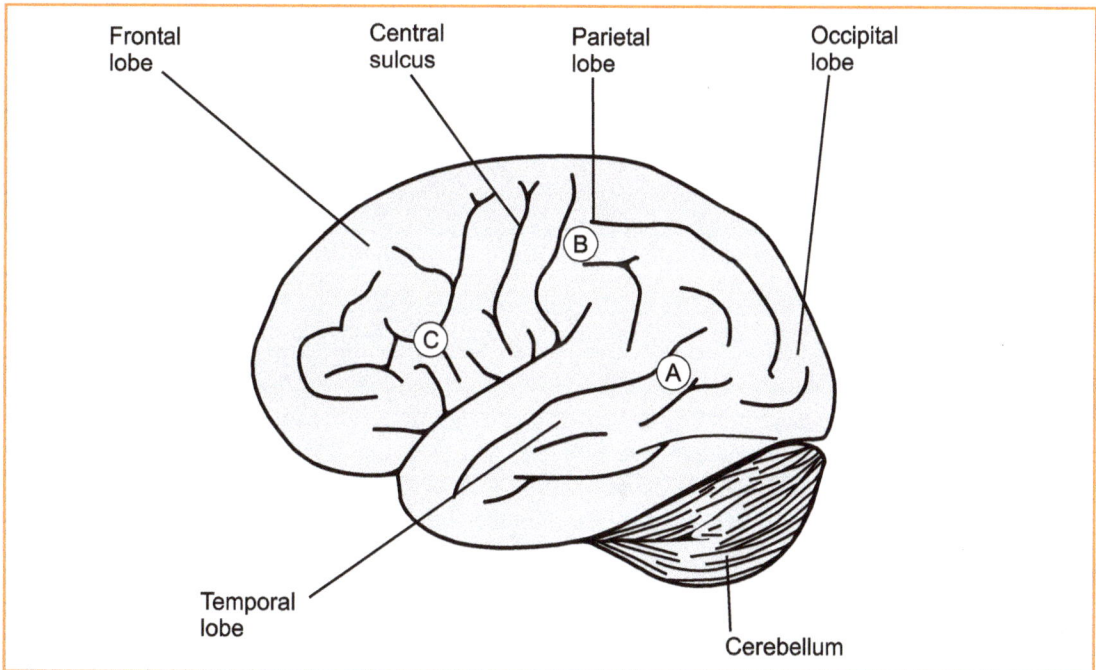

**Figure 5.3** Lateral view of the dominant hemisphere showing the three main areas where pathological processes can produce the more commonly encountered types of dysphasia. The different type of dysphasia have many different names. These are: A Temporal lobe: fluent, sensory, receptive, Wernicke's aphasia; B Parietal lobe: fluent, amnestic, nominal aphasia; C Frontal lobe: non-fluent, motor, expressive, Broca's aphasia. Note: In this illustration, the sites for speech are not strictly anatomically correct, but are simply located within the relevant lobe.

**B.** If the pathology lies within the parietal lobe (area B, Figure 5.3) and behind the central sulcus the speech will be fluent. The patient can understand the spoken word and they can monitor their own speech. There are occasional literal and verbal paraphasic errors, but neologisms and word salad are not a feature. These patients have a curious deficit. They are unable to name objects, thus the term nominal dysphasia. They struggle to name the object and yet can often describe how its used. This type of dysphasia may be a disconnection syndrome [1].

**C.** The frontal lobe area involved with the production of speech (area C, Figure 5.3) is close to the motor strip. Thus a frontal lobe speech disorder is almost invariably associated with a contralateral hemiparesis (partial weakness) or hemiplegia (total weakness). The patient can understand what is being said, they know exactly what they want to say but are unable to produce the words. They are not mute, which is the inability to produce sound. They give the appearance of having a stutter of variable severity reflecting the severity of the underlying speech disturbance. The patient frequently becomes very frustrated at the inability to express themselves. If the examiner shows the patient a pencil, for example, and asks them to name the object, the patient can be seen to be struggling to express the correct word. If the examiner correctly names the object, the patient will nod in agreement.

Patients who are unable to speak cannot produce written language, even in the absence of paralysis of the arm. If all three areas are affected, a total or global dysphasia is the result. In this situation, the patient may be able to understand or utter a few words but is unable to follow simple commands and unable to read or write.

There are several disconnection syndromes that produce speech disturbances. These include conduction aphasia, pure word deafness and pure word blindness, to name just a few. These are believed to result from lesions affecting the association pathways joining the primary receptive areas to the language areas and not from lesions affecting the cortical language areas. A detailed discussion of these seldom encountered speech abnormalities is beyond the scope of this book but can be found in textbooks [1–3].

## Gerstmann's Syndrome

Gerstmann's syndrome refers to a constellation of abnormal neurological findings reflecting involvement of the dominant parietal lobe when they occur in isolation. In clinical practice the four features that Gerstmann described almost invariably occur in association with visual and speech disturbance. A simple way to remember the clinical features of Gerstmann's syndrome is to recall the abbreviation for the Royal Australian Air Force, RAAF. The abnormalities consist of:

*   **R**ight to left confusion – unable to distinguish the right from the left side
*   **A**graphia – inability to write
*   **A**calculia – inability to perform simple arithmetic (e.g. 13 – 7 = 6)
*   **F**inger agnosia – inability to identify the correct finger.

The patient is asked to identify the second or third digit of one hand to test finger agnosia. The side of the hand should not be tested simultaneously as this could be confused with an inability to distinguish right from left.

# The Non-Dominant Hemisphere
## 'Lost in Space'

The non-dominant hemisphere is the right hemisphere in 90% of right-handed and 50% of left-handed patients. The simple method for remembering the abnormalities that occur in lesions of the non-dominant parietal lobe is the phrase 'lost in space'. This consists of neglect of one side of the body, usually the left side as the right hemisphere is the non-dominant hemisphere in most patients. The patient may present with an inability to dress, referred to as *dressing apraxia*, often only placing one arm in the sleeve of their coat. Strictly speaking, this is not true dressing apraxia, but the patient does have difficulty dressing because they are neglecting one side. True dressing apraxia, where patients cannot dress is a feature of dominant parietal lobe lesions. They may neglect to shave or apply makeup on one side of their face. This neglect can be so severe that the patient may not know that their arm and leg are weak, so called *anosognosia*. Rarely, some patients may not even recognise the limb(s) as their own, *autotopagnosia*. These abnormalities are often associated with visual field disturbances, visual or sensory inattention, and hemiparesis if the frontal lobe is involved.

There are a variety of tests that can demonstrate this neglect or 'lost in space'. These include bisecting a line, drawing a map of the country, and placing the capital cities on the map or drawing a house, a bicycle, a daisy, or a clock face. Invariably, one side of the illustration is not completed; some examples are shown in Figure 5.4.

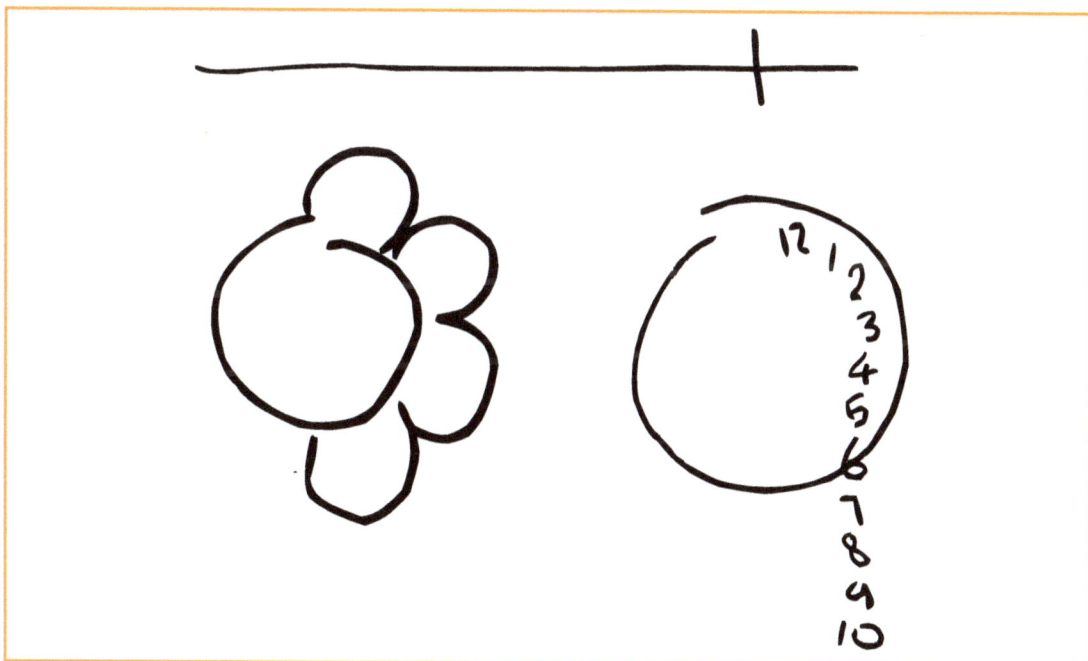

**Figure 5.4** Diagrams that patients with left-sided neglect draw. The circles are usually incomplete. The numbers on a clock face or the petals on a daisy are missing down the left side. The left half of a line is neglected so that, when requested to divide the line in half, the patient draws a line through the right half of the line.

These patients present in a state of bewilderment or are brought to medical attention by a concerned relative. The patient is unaware that anything is the matter. These patients become lost in their own homes. They arise at night to go to the bathroom, and as they walk down the hallway, the bathroom is on the left-hand side of their body and is not 'seen'. On their way back to the bedroom, they see the bathroom because it is on the right-hand side of their body, the side that they are not neglecting. Another example is a patient who suddenly cannot find their way home even though they have driven the same route home for 20 years.

The terms *inattention* and *neglect* are often confused by students. Inattention is rarely symptomatic and is elicited with bilateral simultaneous visual or sensory stimuli. Neglect is a more severe form of inattention that results in significant symptoms and disability.

A variety of *apraxia's* are seen in patients with parietal lobe dysfunction. Apraxia is an impairment of using objects correctly without any apparent physical disability that would prevent them from doing so. Apraxia can be elicited by requesting the patient demonstrate how to use a toothbrush, hammer, or comb [1–3]. These are described more fully at the end of this chapter.

# The Occipital Lobes

The presenting symptoms of occipital lobe pathology include:
- **Visual loss**. The occipital lobes are the termination of the visual pathways and are essential for visual perception and recognition. The pathway is illustrated in Figure 4.1. Lesions of the occipital lobe cause a congruent contralateral homonymous hemianopic visual field loss. Cortical blindness can result from bilateral occipital lobe lesions. Patients are unaware that they are blind and behave as if they can see, a condition called Anton's syndrome or cortical blindness. The pupillary light reflexes are preserved, the eyes and fundi are normal to examination.
- **Prosopagnosia**. Very occasionally, patients may present with prosopagnosia. This is an inability to recognise themselves in a mirror or the faces of other people. It is almost invariably associated with a visual field abnormality, usually an upper quadrantanopia.
- **Visual illusions**. Termed metamorphopsia, are distortions of size, form or colour. Objects may seem too small (micropsia) or too large (macropsia).
- **Visual hallucinations**. Both unformed and formed, arise from the occipital lobe or the junction between the occipital and temporal lobes. Formed visual hallucinations include objects, animals, or people, but these may be distorted, either larger or smaller than normal. Unformed visual hallucinations involve flashing lights, colours, stars, circles or squares and reflect occipital lobe pathology.

# The Cerebellum

Disorders of the cerebellum were initially described in the latter part of the 19th century and early 20th century [5, 6]. Babinski recognised the impairment of rapid alternating movements and referred to this as dys- or adiadochokinesis [6].

The classic presenting features with disorders of the cerebellum include:
- **Intention tremor** is a slow, high-amplitude (easily visible) tremor of the extremities (e.g., arm, leg) that <u>occurs at the end of a purposeful movement</u>. It is elicited by asking the patient to touch your outstretched finger and their nose backwards and forwards. In the

legs, it is elicited by asking the patient to lift their leg up high and place their heel accurately on their knee. The tremor appears as the heel approaches the knee.

- **Ataxia** or incoordination of voluntary movement. Patients are unsteady when they walk. Typically, with midline cerebellar pathology, they walk with a wide-based gait. They cannot walk heel to toe (the test for intoxication). Pathology affecting the cerebellar hemispheres produces ataxia of the ipsilateral arm and leg. It is tested in the upper limbs by asking the patient to touch their nose and then your finger held at arms-length in front of them. Ensure that your finger is far enough away from the patient so that they have to extend their arm fully; if it is not, the patient can anchor their arm against the chest wall and disguise any ataxia. In the lower limbs, ataxia is tested by asking the recumbent patient to lift their leg high in the air and then place their heel accurately on their kneecap and slide it down their shin. Ensure the patient does not disguise the ataxia by stabilising their heel on the inner aspect of the shin. The ataxia is evident as the patient's finger approaches the examiner's finger or their nose and as the heel approaches the kneecap.

- **Oscillopsia** Patients with cerebellar disorders may develop involuntary jerking of the eyes called nystagmus. The symptom of nystagmus is oscillopsia. This is where objects appear to move spontaneously. Nystagmus may be present with the eyes in the midline, otherwise, it is elicited by asking the patient to look up, down and to each side. Best tested using a torch to ensure you do not go beyond binocular vision.

- **Vertigo** true vertigo with either the room or head-spinning is a common symptom in patients with cerebellar pathology. It is central vertigo that will persist when patients lie on one side and only resolve when they roll over to the other side. Like all vertigo, it is worse with head movement.

- **Dysarthria** with cerebellar dysfunction is slow and slurred, or the words are broken up into syllables, so-called scanning dysarthria. This latter form of dysarthria is characteristic of cerebellar pathology. Another very descriptive term is explosive speech because the words are very soft and, at other times, very loud.

Cerebellar function is also tested by performing rapid alternating movements. In the upper limbs, ask the patient to tap the back and then the palm of their hand on their other hand. The patient taps their heel up and down on the floor in the lower limbs. If impaired the movement will be irregular.

# The Temporal Lobes

Patients presenting with symptoms related to temporal lobe pathology are less common than those with frontal, parietal, or occipital lobe involvement. Symptoms include:
- fluent dysphasia
- visual field defects
- auditory, visual, olfactory, and gustatory hallucinations
- memory problems.

Fluent dysphasia has already been discussed. The visual field defect is a contralateral homonymous upper quadrantanopia. Hallucinations are discussed in Chapter 8. Although the temporal lobes are involved with vestibular function, vertigo is rare with temporal lobe pathology; it may be the aura of a seizure originating in the temporal lobe.

# Disturbances of memory

Memory includes three basic mental processes:
1. **Registration:** The ability to perceive, recognise, and establish information in the central nervous system.
2. **Retention:** The ability to retain registered information.
3. **Recall:** The ability to retrieve stored information at will.

Short-term (immediate) memory is the reproduction, recognition or recall of perceived material within a period of up to 30 seconds after presentation.

Long-term memory can be divided into recent and remote. Recent memory involves events occurring during the past few hours, the past few months. Remote or distant memory is events that occurred in past years.

## Transient Global Amnesia

Transient global amnesia (TGA) is not uncommon. The diagnostic criteria include the episode being witnessed and involving anterograde amnesia. The patient must not have any neurological signs or deficits, features of epilepsy, or recent head injury. Finally, the episode must resolve within 24 hours [7]. These patients appear bewildered; they keep asking the same questions repeatedly because they are unable to lay down new memory. Patients remain alert and attentive, and cognition is not impaired. However, they are disoriented in time and place. In all other respects, they are normal. The duration of attacks is usually 1–8 hours but should be less than 24 hours. After the attack resolves, the period of amnesia shrinks with a permanent memory loss of variable duration from just a short period at the commencement of the episode to the entire episode.

The aetiology of this condition is unknown. Unilateral or bilateral punctate lesions in the lateral aspect of the hippocampal formation have been demonstrated by diffusion-weighted MRI (dwMRI), not in the hyperacute phase but at 48 hours [8].

The difficulty with TGA is the lack of a gold-standard test to confirm the diagnosis. Several other conditions can present with abrupt onset of a memory disturbance, including Wernicke–Korsakoff syndrome, cerebral ischaemia in the posterior circulation affecting the medial aspect of both temporal lobes, subarachnoid haemorrhage, cerebral angiography, head injury and epilepsy. Establishing a diagnosis from the clinical features is not difficult if the episode has been witnessed, as most other conditions are associated with other neurological symptoms or signs.

## Dementia

Dementia is a global deterioration in intellectual function, in particular short-term memory. However, remote memory is usually also significantly impaired in patients with dementia than non-demented persons of comparable age. There is impairment of abstract thinking, judgment, other cortical functions, and personality changes.

There are many causes of dementia, and many others are incompletely understood. The diagnosis is based on clinical features, with very few tests available to confirm the diagnosis.

A detailed discussion of dementia is beyond the scope of this chapter. A more detailed discussion can be found in Chapter 14.

# Dementia versus Pseudodementia

Patients with severe depression may present with features suggesting possible dementia. This is pseudodementia. The predominant complaint is impaired memory. However, during the history taking, it becomes obvious that the patient can usually remember the details of the illness and that there is no other alteration in intellectual function.

# Testing Higher Cognitive Function

Higher cognitive function (HCF) consists of memory, orientation, concentration, language, stimulus recognition (examined by tests for agnosia), and performance of learned skilled movements (examined by tests for apraxia).[4]

The Mini-Mental State Examination [9] ,the St Louis University Mental Status Exam (SLUMS)[1] and the Montreal Cognitive Assessment (MoCA)[2] are standardised, widely accepted tests to screen for cognitive impairment. They examine orientation in detail and then briefly touch on registration and recall, attention/concentration, language, and constructional abilities. They can be administered in 5–10 minutes. They are screening tests that may indicate the need for more extensive testing. Details are given in Appendix A.

# Some Rarer Abnormalities of Higher Cognitive Function

## Agnosia

Agnosia is the inability to recognise and identify objects or persons. The more common types of agnosia are:

- **Auditory agnosia** – the inability to recognise the significance of sounds (dominant temporal lobe)
- **Finger agnosia** – the loss of ability to indicate one's own or another's fingers (dominant parietal lobe)
- **Tactile agnosia** – the inability to recognise familiar objects by touch or feel (parieto-temporal cortices, possibly including the 2nd somatosensory cortex)
- **Visual agnosia** – the inability to recognise objects by sight (posterior occipital and or temporal lobe(s) in the brain)
- **Prosopagnosia** – the inability to recognise faces of people well known or newly introduced to the patient (mesial cortex of occipital and temporal lobes)
- **Anosognosia** – the inability to recognise that a part of the body is affected by the disease (non-dominant parietal lobe).

---

1  https://www.slu.edu/medicine/internal-medicine/geriatric-medicine/aging-successfully/assessment-tools/mental-status-exam.php

2  www.mocatest.com

# Apraxia

Apraxia is a disorder of skilled movement. It is not related to weakness, akinesia, deafferentation, abnormal tone or posture, movement disorders such as tremors or chorea, intellectual deterioration, poor comprehension, or uncooperativeness [10]. It is one of the best localising signs of the mental status examination and predicts disability. The more common forms of apraxia are listed below, together with the most common site of the pathology.

- **Sensory (ideational) apraxia** – loss of the ability to make proper use of an object due to the lack of perception of its purpose (dominant posterior temporoparietal junction)
- **Constructional apraxia** – the individual fails to represent spatial relations correctly in drawing or construction (non-dominant parietal lobe)
- **Ideomotor apraxia** – simple single acts can be performed but not a sequence of acts (dominant parietal lobe and the premotor cortex)
- **Dressing apraxia** – difficulty in orienting articles of clothing with reference to the body; the obvious test is to ask the patient to put on a piece of clothing (non-dominant parietal lobe if one side is neglected but dominant if the patient has no idea how to dress).

# Wernicke–Korsakoff encephalopathy

The reason for including Wernicke–Korsakoff syndrome in this book is that although rare, it is preventable and treatable. Thiamine should be administered to all confused patients before they are given glucose, as glucose worsens the effects of thiamine deficiency

Wernicke encephalopathy [11, 12] is the clinical triad of confusion, ataxia, and nystagmus (or ophthalmoplegia). At autopsy, punctate haemorrhages are seen in the grey matter around the 3rd and 4th ventricles and the aqueduct of Sylvius. Korsakoff syndrome or amnestic disorder is the inability to learn new information while other higher cognitive functions are retained. Lack of motivation, lack of insight, a flat affect and denial of difficulties are common. Spontaneous speech is minimal. Confabulation (false memories which the patient believes to be true) may occur in the early stages but usually disappears with time. These patients are severely disabled and are usually incapable of independent living. The syndrome is due to thiamine (vitamin B1) deficiency related to malnutrition and is very common in patients suffering from alcoholism.

The onset is over days to weeks and, although all the features can develop simultaneously, the initial manifestation is often ataxia followed later by confusion. The nystagmus is both vertical and horizontal and often associated with bilateral 6th nerve palsies. The truncal ataxia can be so severe it renders the patient unable to walk. Limb ataxia, dysarthria and intention tremor are rare.

# References

1   Adams RD, Victor M. *Principles of neurology*. New York: McGraw–Hill Book Company; 1985, 1186.

2   Rowland LP, editor. *Merritt's textbook of neurology*. Vol 11ePhiladelphia, PA: Lippincott Williams & Wilkins; 2005.

3   Wilson JD, editor. *Harrison's principles of internal medicine*. 12th edn New York: McGraw–Hill; 1991.

4   *Dorland's pocket medical dictionary*. 21st edn Philadelphia: WB Saunders Company; 1968.

5   Holmes G. The cerebellum of man: Hughlings Jackson lecture. *Brain* 1939;62:1.

6   Babinski J. De l'asynergie cerebelleuse. *Rev Neurol* 1899;7:806.

7   Hodges JR, Warlow CP. Syndromes of transient amnesia: Towards a classification. A study of 153 cases. *J Neurol Neurosurg Psychiatry* 1990;53(10):834–843.

8   Sedlaczek O, et al. Detection of delayed focal MR changes in the lateral hippocampus in transient global amnesia. *Neurology* 2004;62(12):2165–2170.

9   Folstein MF, Folstein SE, McHugh PR. "Mini-mental state". A practical method for grading the cognitive state of patients for the clinician. *J Psychiatr Res* 1975;12(3):189–198.

10  Heilman KM, Rothi LJG. Apraxia. *Heilman KM, Valenstein E (eds). Clinical neuropsychology*. Oxford: Oxford University Press; 1993. p. 141–163.

11  Thomson AD, et al. Wernicke's encephalopathy revisited. [translation of the case history section of the original manuscript by Carl Wernicke 'Lehrbuch der Gehirnkrankheiten fur Aerzte and Studirende' (1881) with a commentary]. *Alcohol* 2008;43(2):174–179.

12  Pearce JM. Wernicke–Korsakoff encephalopathy. *Eur Neurol* 2008;59(1–2):101–104.

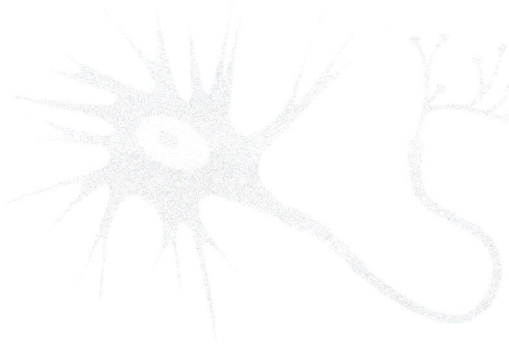

# After the History and Examination, what to do next?

After completing the history and examination, the next step is influenced by the following factors:
- Diagnostic certainty
- The availability of tests to confirm or exclude specific diagnoses
- The potential complications of those tests
- The severity and level of urgency in terms of the consequences of not diagnosing and treating a particular illness promptly
- The benefit versus risk profile of any potential treatment
- The presence of any social factors or past medical history that might influence a course of action or therapy.

This chapter will discuss each of these aspects and how they affect the course of action.

## Level of Certainty of Diagnosis

There are three possible scenarios:
1. A particular diagnosis seems obvious.
2. One specific diagnosis is not apparent, and there are several possible diagnoses.
3. You have no idea what is wrong with the patient.

## A Particular Diagnosis Seems Certain

In most instances, the diagnosis is apparent. In the general/family practice setting, almost 90% of diagnoses are established after the history and examination. [1] In one outpatient clinic, this figure was 73% (history 56% and examination 17%) in patients with cardiovascular, neurological, respiratory, urinary, and other miscellaneous problems. [2] In patients with neurological problems, the initial diagnosis is less obvious and is correct in only 60% of patients presenting to an emergency department. [3] When the diagnosis is apparent, the appropriate course of action is to initiate investigations to confirm the diagnosis. Tests also need to exclude alternative diagnoses with potentially more severe adverse outcomes. A management plan needs to be instituted, taking into account factors in the past, social and medical drug history that would influence management in this particular patient.

**A word of caution**: being certain *is potentially the most dangerous scenario*. Doctors are firmly anchored by their initial diagnoses [4] (see Case 6.1) and are at risk of closing their minds to possible alternatives, often in the presence of clinical features or results from investigations that should raise doubt about the diagnosis.

---

**Case 6.1** An incorrect initial diagnosis

A 65-year-old patient with confusion and headache was treated for herpes zoster (HZV) meningoencephalitis because the CSF contained HZV DNA. The CSF findings of a very high white cell count and protein level and very low glucose level were most atypical for HZV meningoencephalitis. The patient was failing to respond to the appropriate treatment for HZV. The positive test for DNA in the CSF should not have been interpreted as proving herpes zoster meningoencephalitis. It was related to the presence of herpes zoster ophthalmicus. [5] The patient had malignant meningitis.

---

Doctors recognise patterns of familiar problems from critical cues. [6] More experienced doctors appear to weigh their first impressions more heavily and risk closing their minds early on in the diagnostic process than those less experienced. [7] Even experienced clinicians may be unaware of the correctness of their diagnoses when they initially make them. [8] If tests are available to confirm the diagnosis, it is appropriate to perform them, provided the patient is informed of the risks. When reviewing the results be aware of the **sensitivity, specificity,** influence of the prevalence of the disease on the **positive predictive** and **negative predictive value.** (see below). [9]

If there are no tests the diagnosis is a clinical one, one can proceed cautiously with management. In this setting, it is essential to monitor the response to therapy. A lack of response to treatment or the emergence of unexpected side effects[1] is often a clue that the diagnosis is incorrect. Conversely, *a response to therapy does not prove the diagnosis*. This author has seen patients with vertebral artery dissection, viral meningitis and pituitary cysts 'respond' to treatment for migraine.

# Several Possible Diagnoses

It is imperative to keep the diagnostic options open by making provisional diagnoses while keeping alternatives in mind. Be circumspect and take action to minimise the possibility of missing other critical diagnoses. [10] Once again, if tests can differentiate one particular diagnosis from another, it would be appropriate to perform those tests. If a specific diagnosis cannot be confirmed following the investigations, the approach is similar to that discussed in the following section.

# You Have No Idea What is Wrong

In the setting of uncertainty, there are several possible courses of action. A *particularly useful strategy is to start again:* take a more detailed history and repeat the examination.[2] Starting again is the recommended approach when you have no idea what the diagnosis is. In this situation performing many tests is often misleading because of the sensitivity and specificity of tests.

---

1  personal observation

2  recommended in 1985 to the author by the late Dr Arthur Schwieger, neurologist and, to this day, remains one of the most powerful clinical tools available

If you have obtained a detailed history but still have no idea what is wrong with the patient, there are several options, including:

- Wait and see
- Undertake investigations
- Seek a second opinion
- Consult a textbook
- Search for an answer on the internet.

These various approaches have relative merits and deficiencies.

# Wait and See

In resolving uncertainty, time is a potent diagnostic tool. The idea is to wait for a while, anticipating that the diagnosis becomes clear or the patient gets better. [10,11] If the patient is already showing signs of improving spontaneously, it is reasonable to wait and see in the hope that the problem will resolve completely, accepting that we never knew the diagnosis. It is crucial to inform the patient to make contact should the symptoms recur in this setting. The effective use of this approach requires considerable skill, however. Often in this situation, a doctor may order unnecessary tests in the hope that a diagnosis may be established; most often, it is not. If the 'wait and see' approach is adopted, it is essential to:

- inform the patient that there is uncertainty
- advise them of the possible outcomes
- recommend that they report immediately should symptoms worsen or if new symptoms develop.

Shared medical decision making is a process in which patients and providers consider outcome probabilities and patient preferences and reach a healthcare decision based on mutual agreement. Shared decision making is best employed when there is medical uncertainty. [12] However, it is essential to consider that not all patients wish to be involved in shared medical decisions. [13]

# Undertake Investigations

In most cases, some tests can confirm or exclude a particular disease. It is essential to understand the concepts of the sensitivity, specificity, and the influence of disease prevalence on the tests. The critical questions to ask when considering investigations include:

- In what way will the results, whether positive or negative, alter the management of this patient?
- What is the risk of undertaking the test?

There is a more detailed discussion of investigations later in this chapter.

There are some diseases where the diagnosis is based entirely on the clinical features as there are no currently available tests to confirm the diagnosis. A prime example is migraine.

When there are several possible diagnoses, or when one has no idea what the diagnosis might be, performing numerous tests in the hope of making a diagnosis is a wonderful way of giving the illusion that something valuable is being done. Often one is simply stalling or buying time. It is a tactic that many clinicians use in the hope that a diagnosis will be made by a test result (unlikely), the illness will progress so that the diagnosis will become apparent or the patient's problem will resolve (most likely outcome).

A reasonable approach is to <u>think of the worst-case scenario</u> (the most serious diagnosis that the symptoms could represent, a diagnosis that if missed could result in an adverse outcome) and proceed accordingly.

# Obtain a Second Opinion

Although doctors prefer to obtain information from journals and books, they often consult colleagues to get answers to clinical and research questions. [14], [15] Even for doctors whose first choice of information source was the medical literature – either books or journals – the most frequent second choice was consultations. [14]

In a study of 254 referrals seen by a neurologist there was a significant change in diagnosis in 55%, and in management in nearly 70%. [16]

There are several ways of obtaining a second opinion:
- An 'informal consultation with a colleague'
  - Telephone advice
  - The 'curbside' conversation in the corridor without actually seeing the patient
  - Presenting at meetings and seeking several opinions, often but not invariably with the patient at the meeting
- The 'formal second opinion' by referring the patient to a colleague.

# Telephone advice

Telephoning a colleague for advice is very common. General Practitioners frequently call specialists for advice, specialist to specialist is rarer. The recipient of the call faces a challenging situation. Providing the correct advice depends on an accurate history and examination findings. An experienced clinician often knows the particular questions to ask and can decide if and when they should see the patient. It is probably wiser for an inexperienced clinician to formally arrange to see the patient in consultation. If one cannot be sure, it is best to err on the side of seeing the patient as soon as possible.

# Corridor or curbside consultation

'Corridor or curbside consultation' is another oft used approach. [17] Unfortunately, and sometimes with dire consequences, this is used by medical practitioners to seek informal advice about their medical problems. An excellent curbside consultation model is to say what you know and what you don't know. Then you hope the person you are consulting with will treat you with respect. [17] Requesting doctors who could not present relevant information, frame a clear question or answer consultant questions in a well-informed manner were generally asked to refer the patient for a formal opinion. Perley et al. [17] commented that these unspoken rules govern curbside consultation interactions, and negative consequences result when the rules are misunderstood or not observed.

Once again, the correct advice depends on being given accurate information. The neurologist providing advice will want to know the mode of onset and progression of the symptoms of the current illness, the EXACT nature and distribution of the symptoms and the abnormal neurological signs if present. It is difficult for inexperienced clinicians to perform detailed neurological examinations

Still, there should be no reason why, as outlined in Chapter 2, 'The neurological history', an inexperienced clinician cannot obtain a detailed history. Finally, the neurologist would want information about the social, past and drug history that may influence any subsequent course of action.

## Clinical meetings

"Second opinions" are often sought in clinical meetings for a diagnosis and or treatment. There is the perception that one is obtaining multiple opinions. Presenting a case at a clinical conference can be a valuable tool if one of the participants identifies the problem. In a more complex case, what is said in meetings is very different from what is said in a formal consultation. The advice obtained in clinical meetings should be viewed with circumspection. A brain biopsy is often recommended in clinical meetings but not often performed despite the recommendation.[3]

## The formal second opinion

The formal second opinion is probably the most effective method of dealing with diagnostic or therapeutic uncertainties. *There is no shame in asking a colleague to see the patient for a second opinion.* If you do, it can be a learning experience; if you do not and the patient perceives a lack of progress, they will independently seek a second opinion, and you will miss out on a learning opportunity. If a patient requests a second opinion, NEVER hesitate to arrange one.

Remember, a second opinion is simply that; you are the clinician caring for the patient and the 'buck stops with you'. You must decide if the second opinion is helpful or not and act accordingly – this may include obtaining a third opinion!

## Consult a Textbook

Yet another approach is to consult textbooks. This is useful if you are looking at the clinical features of a particular disease(s) or learning what investigations would be appropriate. However, therapy evolves so rapidly that recommendations in textbooks are soon out of date.

## Search the Internet

An increasingly popular and useful strategy is to search the Internet. [18–20] Patients frequently look for answers on the internet. [21] In the author's own experience, many patients bring the results of their searches to the consultation. In one study [19], Google made the correct diagnosis in 58% of the cases in the New England Journal of Medicine clinical-pathological conferences. In a comparison of PubMed, Scopus, Web of Science and Google Scholar, the keyword search function of PubMed was superior. While Google Scholar could retrieve the most obscure information, its use was marred by inadequate and less frequently updated citation information. [22] Searching in Google Scholar can be refined by adding + emedicine to the search. [23] For example, 'trigeminal neuralgia' yields 48,000 'hits' while 'trigeminal neuralgia + emedicine' retrieves 478 references.[4] Many medical practitioners and researchers

---

3  Personal observation

4  12 years alter the number of hits are 84,100 and 460 respectively. In google the number of hits is a staggering 10,800,000 but with +emedicine on 62!

remain sceptical. [24] Twisselmann stated that the jury is still out on whether searching for symptoms on the internet is the way forward for doctors and consumers. [25]

The author frequently consults the internet, even during the formal consultation.[5] It is a useful way to look for any new advances in therapy, provide information to the patient or referring practitioner by adding the abstracts and references to the letter, or even search for an obscure diagnosis (see Case 6.2).

| **Case 6.2** A trumpet player with nasal escape |
|---|
| This example illustrates how searching the internet can be very useful. A young trumpet player developed nasal escape of air after 30 minutes of playing and could not continue to play. The symptoms took too long to develop and persisted for too long after cessation of playing to be related to myasthenia gravis. Three ENT surgeons had seen her and said there was nothing wrong! A quick search of 'trumpet player and nasal escape' revealed the diagnosis of a very rare condition termed velopharyngeal incompetence. [26] |

An online information retrieval system [27] was associated with a significant improvement in the quality of answers provided by clinicians to typical clinical problems. In a small proportion of cases, the use of the system produced errors. [27] Many doctors do not yet use just-in-time to immediately solve complex patient problems despite ready access to the internet. Instead, they continue to rely on consultation with colleagues. [28, 29] One major obstacle is the time it takes to search for information. Other difficulties primary care doctors experience is formulating an appropriate search question, finding an optimal search strategy, and interpreting the evidence. [29]

Computer programs aid paediatricians diagnose rare congenital syndromes in children. [30] Other computer-aided software systems for diagnosing neurological diseases exist. [31, 42] In the USA, the National Institute of Health has established the Undiagnosed Disease Program[4] to aid individuals whose conditions have eluded medical diagnosis. Such software will always be dependent upon the information provided by the user. One of the issues when searching the internet is the reliability of the information. Government websites and national organisations (identified by the URL ending in .org) are the most accurate (80.9% and 72.5% respectively). Sadly, university and other educational websites are not that accurate, (50.2%) but certainly more accurate than blogs and websites of individuals (25.7% and 30.3% respectively). {Rehman, 2012 #2707} The National Institute on Ageing has a webpage that provides a checklist of seven questions to assist in assessing the reliability of online health information.[6] An alternative is to ask for the assistance of a librarian to help refine your search question[7].

# Availability of Tests to Confirm or Exclude Certain Diagnoses

This section discusses the general principles of investigations or tests. Essentially it will cover why tests give the 'wrong' or unexpected result and what to do when this occurs. Many excellent books discuss the interpretation of tests in great detail. [32–34]

---

5   https://www.genome.gov/Current-NHGRI-Clinical-Studies/Undiagnosed-Diseases-Program-UDN
6   https://www.nia.nih.gov/health/online-health-information-it-reliable
7   I have used this method with great success on many occasions.

# Understanding and interpreting test results
## Sensitivity, Specificity, Positive and Negative Predictive Values

To understand how to interpret investigations correctly, you need to understand some basic principles. All tests have associated sensitivity, specificity, positive and negative predictive values. The prior likelihood influences them that the disease is present in a particular patient. The usefulness of a test is very dependent on the prior probability that a patient has a specific disease, i.e. the prevalence of the disease.

- **Sensitivity** refers to how good a test is at correctly identifying people who have the disease.
- **Specificity** is concerned with how good the test is at correctly excluding people who do not have the condition.
- **Positive predictive value** refers to the chance that a positive test result will be correct.
- **Negative predictive value** is concerned only with negative test results.

**Table 6.1** The influence of sensitivity (90%) and specificity (80%) of a test result for 100 patients with the suspected diagnosis

|  | Positive Test | Negative Test |
|---|---|---|
| Patient has disease | 90 | 10 |
| A patient does not have the disease | 20 | 80 |

**Table 6.2** The effect of a 50% likelihood that the patient has a disease and the influence of the sensitivity and specificity on the number of correct diagnoses (n = 100)

|  | Positive Test | Negative Test |
|---|---|---|
| Patient has disease | 45 | 5 |
| A patient does not have the disease | 5 | 45 |

**Table 6.3** The number of positive and negative test results when the likelihood of a particular diagnosis is low (10%), i.e. doing tests to exclude rare conditions causes more problems than it solves (n = 100)

|  | Positive Test | Negative Test |
|---|---|---|
| Patient has the disease | 9 | 1 |
| A patient does not have the disease | 18 | 72 |

For any diagnostic test, the positive predictive value will fall as the prevalence of the disease decreases, whilst the negative predictive value will rise. In practice, since most diseases have a low prevalence, even when the tests we use have good sensitivity and specificity, the positive predictive value may be very low.

Table 6.1 shows the results of a test with a sensitivity of 90% and a specificity of 80% (this is the sensitivity and specificity of many tests). When the test is performed on 100 patients with the suspected diagnosis, 10 patients with the diagnosis will have a negative test while 20 patients who do not have that particular diagnosis will have an incorrect positive test. The ideal test would be one with 100% sensitivity and 100% specificity, but this does not occur.

The pre-test likelihood of a patient having a particular diagnosis dramatically influences how a test result should be interpreted. Table 6.2 shows the results of testing 100 patients when only

50 of them have the diagnosis. Using the same sensitivity and specificity, a positive test will detect 45 patients with the disease. (90% of 50) However, the test will also be positive in 10 (20% of 50) patients who do not have the disease! This is referred to as a false positive test.

If the prior probability of a particular diagnosis being present is even lower, the results are more dramatic. If the patient is very unlikely to have the disease, say a 10% chance (i.e. 10 in every 100 patients tested), with the same sensitivity and specificity of 90% and 80%, respectively, a positive result will correctly identify nine of the ten patients with the disease but will incorrectly diagnose 18 patients without the disease. (90% of 10 = 9 and 20% of 90 = 18). The rarer the problem, the more certain we can be that a negative test excludes that disease but less certain that a positive test indicates an abnormality (see Table 6.3).

In this setting, a negative test in the presence of a strong suspicion of a diagnosis may lead inexperienced clinicians to dismiss that diagnosis. The antithesis of this is a patient being incorrectly diagnosed with a particular illness because of a false positive test.

The variability in the prevalence of a particular disease between one study and another means that predictive values found in one study do not apply universally. [35] A common practice of inexperienced doctors is to repeat borderline abnormal tests simply because the result is 'outside the normal range' even when the test result is irrelevant to the clinical problem. It is better to discuss the result with the relevant pathologist or radiologist in this situation.

## Incidental and Irrelevant Findings on Tests:

An 'incidentaloma' is an abnormal finding on a test that is unrelated to the patient's presenting problem. Incidentalomas are common with medical imaging. One common example is the asymptomatic degenerative disease in the cervical, thoracic, or lumbar spine that occurs with advancing age. Other examples are the asymptomatic lacunar cerebral infarct or an unidentified bright object on an MRI scan in a patient investigated for headaches. Often, only experience gives us the confidence to ignore such incidental findings.

## Why and What to do When Tests Give the Wrong Result

Although the sensitivity and specificity of investigations largely explains why tests may be negative or positive in the wrong setting, a test may also be negative (not detect the problem) for several other reasons. Patients with intermittent disturbances of neurological function will invariably have normal tests between events. The test will only be positive if the examiner happens to capture an event and, if episodes are infrequent, this is unlikely. Symptoms can also precede the development of abnormalities with currently available investigations. Common examples include carpal tunnel syndrome and acute inflammatory demyelinating peripheral neuropathy with normal nerve conduction studies in the early stages. Another example is patients with a cerebral infarct. The initial CT scan of the brain can be normal for several hours after the onset of the infarction.

Other causes of 'negative tests' are when the test is directed to the wrong part of the body and an ordered test that is not suitable for detecting abnormalities in that region. For example, a patient may have difficulty walking with a normal CT scan of the lumbosacral spine when they have a cervical or thoracic spinal cord problem. CT scan of the thoracic spine is not a sensitive enough test for detecting abnormalities in this region.

Tests' relative 'fallibility' emphasises the importance of a detailed history and examination. If you are confident that a patient has a particular diagnosis, then a negative test should not dissuade you from that diagnosis. The corollary of this is a positive test should not imply a diagnosis if the symptoms and signs are not consistent with that diagnosis.

# The Possible Complications of Tests

There are very few tests that are not associated with risk. Venesection is perfectly safe in close to 100% of patients but rarely can be associated with injury to a nerve that can result in long-term pain and dysaesthesia. Although this complication is infrequent (<0.02% [36]), the result can be very distressing.

When ordering any investigation, it is important to consider the potential complications of the test and the seriousness of the illness being investigated. A patient with a life-threatening illness might be willing to consider a potentially life-threatening investigation if it could make a significant difference. On the other hand, a patient with symptoms without a disability would be concerned about any investigation that might cause harm.

The patient should be informed of the risks versus benefits of the procedure beforehand.

# How Quickly Should Tests be Performed?

This is discussed below in the section severity and urgency. It is imperative to consider the potential consequences of a particular illness not being promptly diagnosed and treated.

## The Possible Consequences of a Particular Illness not Being Diagnosed and Treated

In everyday clinical practice, knowledge of a condition's natural history would dictate how quickly one would investigate and treat the patient. Patients presenting comatose or with status epilepticus (a seizure that lasts more than 30 minutes or recurrent seizures without return of consciousness between seizures) require urgent intervention.

The difficulty arises in the patient with a neurological problem when there is uncertainty about the diagnosis. There is very little literature that can guide us in this setting. Scoring tools for priority setting for general surgery and hip and knee surgery were useful but were not particularly good for MRI scanning. [37] The discussion below contains observations made by this author during more than 40 years of clinical practice as well as observations from colleagues who were asked specifically, 'What do you think constitutes an urgent problem?'

*The overriding principle is to consider the worst-case scenario.* It is prudent to consider the most serious possible diagnosis that, if left untreated, could result in significant morbidity or mortality. This will dictate the 'level of urgency' and how promptly a doctor should act. For example if cerebral ischaemia is a possibility, investigations should be undertaken with minimal delay.

Experienced clinicians can often accurately assess the level of urgency in a particular clinical setting. This may well relate to their level of expertise and 'having seen it before'. On the other hand they use the tempo of the illness (the rapidity of development of symptoms and signs) to dictate how quickly they should act.

- *Rapidly evolving weakness* dictates immediate action.
- Although not all patients with *symptoms related to the spinal cord* have urgent neurological problems, disorders in this region can result in devastating neurological deficits. The degree of recovery depends on the severity of the spinal cord lesion. [38] The investigations should be prompt if one suspects spinal cord disease.[5] One would suspect a spinal cord problem in patients with bilateral leg weakness, particularly if there is associated sphincter disturbance or mid-thoracic back pain.

- Similarly, patients with *symptoms related to the brainstem* such as diplopia, dysphagia, and vertigo, particularly if combined with ataxia or limb weakness, should be investigated as a matter of urgency.
- Patients with *recurrent symptoms within a short time* should also be dealt with as a matter of urgency. As a general rule, symptoms of weakness are more likely to imply significant neurological problems than isolated sensory symptoms.
- Similarly, *symptoms associated with loss of function* are more likely to be significant than symptoms without functional loss. Patients with multiple symptoms without loss of function, particularly if associated with non-neurological symptoms, are less likely to have a severe illness requiring urgent intervention. Transient symptoms lasting seconds are also unlikely to be of any significance. One study found that higher numbers of physical symptoms and the complaint of pain were indicators of possible non-organic disease. [39]

Table 6.4. summarises urgent and non-urgent presentations. A simple rule is: 'if in doubt, do not hesitate to ask for help'.

| Table 6.4 Some urgent and non-urgent clinical presentations | |
|---|---|
| **Very urgent** | **Less urgent** |
| LOC | Symptoms lasting seconds |
| Status epilepticus | Symptoms without functional loss |
| Recurrent symptoms within a short period | Isolated sensory symptoms |
| Rapidly progressive symptoms | Intermittent symptoms affecting multiple organ systems as well as the nervous system |

## The Benefit Versus Risk of a Potential Treatment

All medical interventions, whether pharmacological or surgical, can cause harm.

- Most patients can tolerate most drugs with few or no side effects. When a diagnosis is established, the appropriate treatment choice would primarily be dictated by the knowledge that one particular therapy has greater efficacy than another.
- On the other hand, if there are several treatments with equal efficacy, the choice of therapy would then depend on the risk profile and the patient's willingness to consider particular side effects. For example, two or three drugs could be used to treat epilepsy; the drugs that may cause weight gain or interfere with the oral contraceptive pill would be most unacceptable to a young female patient.
- In the setting where the diagnosis is uncertain, and one is instituting empirical therapy, it is important to inform the patient of the perceived benefits of the therapy prescribed and alert the patient to the potential risks of that therapy. More importantly, carefully monitor the response to therapy and be willing to reconsider the diagnosis and choice of therapy. I send by email or print and give the patient the information about the drug from the MIMS[8] manual.

---

8   The acronym, MIMS, was derived from the original publication (1963) which was called Monthly Index of Medical Specialties

# Social Factors and Past Medical Problems that may Influence a Course of Action or Treatment

In Chapter 2, we cautioned against using the past medical history, family history and social history to make a diagnosis. Once a diagnosis is established, however, the subsequent management of the patient is very much influenced by their past medical history, their social circumstances and, more importantly, the drugs they are currently taking.

- Ten to thirty per cent of hospital admissions are due to iatrogenic drug-related problems. [40, 41] Computer software programs can alert clinicians to the potential drug interactions and should be used when prescribing a new medication[9].
- Other medical problems may have a major impact on subsequent management. They can limit the therapeutic options as a choice of therapy could be contraindicated in that condition. An example of this is a history of asthma in patients with migraine, preventing the use of non-selective beta-blockers.
- Similarly, an elderly patient who has the support of a spouse and family can be managed at home instead of a patient who has no support and who develops an illness that would prevent them from living independently.

# References

1   Crombie DL. Diagnostic process. *J Coll Gen Pract* 1963;6:579–589.

2   Sandler G. Costs of unnecessary tests. *BMJ* 1979;2(6181):21–24.

3   Moeller JJ, et al. Diagnostic accuracy of neurological problems in the emergency department. *Can J Neurol Sci* 2008;35(3):335–341.

4   Berner ES, et al. Clinician performance and prominence of diagnoses displayed by a clinical diagnostic decision support system. *AMIA Annu Symp Proc* 2003:76–80.

5   Gregoire SM, et al. Polymerase chain reaction analysis and oligoclonal antibody in the cerebrospinal fluid from 34 patients with varicella-zoster virus infection of the nervous system. *J Neurol Neurosurg Psychiatry* 2006;77(8):938–942.

6   Coughlin LD, Patel VL. Processing of critical information by physicians and medical students. *J Med Educ* 1987;62(10):818–828.

7   Eva KW, Cunnington JP. The difficulty with experience: Does practice increase susceptibility to premature closure?. *J Contin Educ Health Prof* 2006;26(3):192–198.

8   Friedman CP, et al. Do physicians know when their diagnoses are correct? Implications for decision support and error reduction. *J Gen Intern Med* 2005;20(4):334–339.

9   Loong TW. Understanding sensitivity and specificity with the right side of the brain. *BMJ* 2003;327(7417):716–719.

10  Hewson MG, et al. Strategies for managing uncertainty and complexity. *J Gen Intern Med* 1996;11(8):481–485.

11  Sloane PD, et al. Introduction to clinical problems. In: Sloane PD, Slatt LM, Ebell MH, Jacques LB, Smith MA, editors. *Essentials of family medicine*. Philadelphia: Lippincott Williams & Wilkins; 2007. p. 126.

---

9  I routinely use the MIMS interact program in my medical software patient management system. It frequently detects potential interactions between the drugs the patient is already taking ever before I enter the new drug I am prescribing.

12  Frosch DL, Kaplan RM. Shared decision making in clinical medicine: Past research and future directions. *Am J Prev Med* 1999;17(4):285–294.

13  Levinson W, et al. Not all patients want to participate in decision making. A national study of public preferences. *J Gen Intern Med* 2005;20(6):531–535.

14  Haug JD. Physicians' preferences for information sources: A meta-analytic study. *Bull Med Libr Assoc* 1997;85(3):223–232.

15  Campbell EJ. Use of the telephone in consultant practice. *BMJ* 1978;2(6154):1784–1785.

16  Roberts K, et al. What difference does a neurologist make in a general hospital? Estimating the impact of neurology consultations on in-patient care. *Ir J Med Sci* 2007;176(3):211–214.

17  Perley CM. Physician use of the curbside consultation to address information needs: Report on a collective case study. *J Med Libr Assoc* 2006;94(2):137–144.

18  Maulden SA. Information technology, the internet, and the future of neurology. *Neurologist* 2003;9(3):149–159.

19  Tang H, Ng JH. Googling for a diagnosis — use of Google as a diagnostic aid: Internet-based study. *BMJ* 2006;333(7579):1143–1145.

20  Yu H, Kaufman D. A cognitive evaluation of four online search engines for answering definitional questions posed by physicians. *Pac Symp Biocomput* 2007:328–339.

21  Shuyler KS, Knight KM. What are patients seeking when they turn to the Internet? Qualitative content analysis of questions asked by visitors to an orthopaedics web site. *J Med Internet Res* 2003;5(4):e24.

22  Falagas ME, et al. Comparison of PubMed, Scopus, Web of Science, and Google Scholar: Strengths and weaknesses. *FASEB J* 2008;22(2):338–342.

23  Taubert M. Use of Google as a diagnostic aid: Bias your search. *BMJ* 2006;333(7581):1270; author reply 1270.

24  Rapid responses. Googling for a diagnosis — use of Google as a diagnostic aid: Internet-based study. 2006. Available: www.bmj.com/cgi/eletters/333/7579/1143 (1 Dec 2009).

25  Twisselmann B. Use of Google as a diagnostic aid: Summary of other responses. *BMJ* 2006;333(7581):1270–1271.

26  Conley SF, Beecher RB, Marks S. Stress velopharyngeal incompetence in an adolescent trumpet player. *Ann Otol Rhinol Laryngol* 1995;104(9 Pt 1):715–717.

27  Westbrook JI, Coiera EW, Gosling AS. Do online information retrieval systems help experienced clinicians answer clinical questions?. *J Am Med Inform Assoc* 2005;12(3):315–321.

28  Bennett NL, et al. Information-seeking behaviors and reflective practice. *J Contin Educ Health Prof* 2006;26(2):120–127.

29  Coumou HC, Meijman FJ. How do primary care physicians seek answers to clinical questions? A literature review. *J Med Libr Assoc* 2006;94(1):55–60.

30  Pelz J, Arendt V, Kunze J. Computer-assisted diagnosis of malformation syndromes: An evaluation of three databases (LDDB, POSSUM, and SYNDROC). *Am J Med Genet* 1996;63(1):257–267.

31  Computer-aided diagnosis software for neurological diseases. 2007. Available: http://www.flintbox. com/technology.asp?page=3087&IID=MCU (1 Dec 2009).

32  Sackett DL, et al. *Evidence-based medicine. How to practice and teach EBM*. Toronto: Churchill Livingstone; 2000, 261.

33  Greenhalgh T. *How to read a paper. The basics of evidence-based medicine*. 2nd edn London: BMJ; 2001, 222.

34  Sackett DL, Haynes RB, Tugwell P. *Clinical epidemiology: A basic science for clinical medicine*. Boston: Little, Brown; 1985, 370.

35  Altman, D.G. and J.M. Bland, *Diagnostic tests 2: Predictive values*. BMJ, 1994. 309(6947): p.102.

36  Newman BH, Waxman DA. Blood donation-related neurologic needle injury: Evaluation of 2 yeas' worth of data from a large blood center. *Transfusion* 1996;36(3):213–215.

37 Noseworthy TW, McGurran JJ, Hadorn DC. Waiting for scheduled services in Canada: Development of priority-setting scoring systems. *J Eval Clin Pract* 2003;9(1):23–31.

38 Catz A, et al. Recovery of neurologic function following nontraumatic spinal cord lesions in Israel. *Spine* 2004;29(20):2278–2282:discussion 2283.

39 Fitzpatrick R, Hopkins A. Referrals to neurologists for headaches not due to structural disease. *J Neurol Neurosurg Psychiatry* 1981;44(12):1061–1067.

40 Koh Y, Fatimah BM, Li SC. Therapy-related hospital admission in patients on polypharmacy in Singapore: A pilot study. *Pharm World Sci* 2003;25(4):135–137.

41 Courtman BJ, Stallings SB. Characterisation of drug-related problems in elderly patients on admission to a medical ward. *Can J Hosp Pharm* 1995;48(3):161–166.

42 Centogene. Centogene the Rare Diseases Company. https://www.centogene.com/.

# Websites

The following are websites that illustrate how to search the Internet for medical information:

PubMed Tutorial: http://www.nlm.nih.gov/bsd/disted/pubmed.html

Google Web Search Help Centre:

http://www.google.com/support/bin/static.py?page=searchguides.html&ctx=advanced&hl=en

UC Berkeley Library Internet Searching Tutorial:

http://lib.berkeley.edu/TeachingLib/Guides/Internet/FindInfo.html

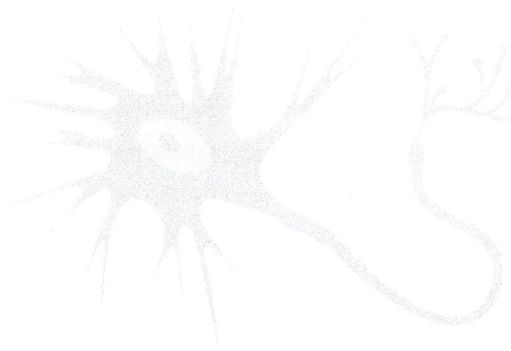

# Episodic Disturbances of Neurological Function

The assessment of patients with intermittent disturbances of neurological function is one of the most interesting and challenging aspects of clinical neurology. One needs to be an amateur detective like Sherlock Holmes, whom Arthur Conan Doyle modelled on Dr Joseph Bell, one of his teachers at the medical school of Edinburgh University. Dr Bell was a master at observation, logic, deduction, and diagnosis. [1]

This chapter discusses the various causes of episodic disturbance of neurological function. Epilepsy and cerebrovascular disease are briefly mentioned and discussed in more detail in later chapters. Vertigo is covered in this chapter as it is often an episodic disturbance, but mainly because it seemed to fit better in this chapter than in any other.

Patients with intermittent disturbances are rarely, if ever, seen during the episode. Therefore, *the diagnosis is almost entirely dependent on obtaining a very detailed history*. As the symptoms are episodic, these patients usually do not have any abnormal neurological signs and investigations rarely, if ever, yield a diagnosis.

---

If you have only 30 minutes, spend 29 on the history, one on the examination and none on tests. Sometimes a diagnosis is not possible when the patient is first seen. Provided you are convinced that a delay in diagnosis would not lead to a serious adverse outcome, give the patient a list of things to observe that will help clarify the diagnosis.

---

Sometimes a diagnosis is not possible when the patient first presents. A very useful technique is to send the patient away with a list of things to observe and record. This often leads to the diagnosis. However, this technique can only be employed if the episodes are likely to be benign, and the patient is advised to avoid activities that could result in harm should an event recur during that activity. For example, where there is a suspicion of epilepsy, patients should be advised not to drive, go swimming, have a bath alone etc.

# The History: A Different Approach

Most inexperienced clinicians simply ascertain the nature of the symptoms. They do not determine their exact distribution, the mode of onset and progression of every symptom, particularly in relation to the other symptoms, nor the circumstances under which symptoms occur, which often provides the vital clue to the diagnosis.

The recommended method of taking a history is different from that described in Chapter 2, 'The neurological history'. It is far more useful to ask the patient to provide a detailed account of several individual episodes.

It is more rewarding to obtain a blow-by-blow description from the patient or any eyewitness of several individual episodes, rather than asking the patient to summarise what happens when they have a 'turn'. Often it is the circumstances under which the episode occurs that provides the vital clue to the diagnosis.

As you take the history question the patient or eye-witness about the symptoms:
1. immediately before the episode (pre-ictal)
2. during the event (ictus)
3. after the event (post-ictal).

*Note:* The strict definition of the term ictus is a stroke, blow or sudden attack, but it is used here to mean the event or episode.

## A Suggested Method of History Taking

A suggested approach is to ask the following questions:
1. Tell me about the last episode you had: what were you doing at the time it commenced?
2. What was the very first symptom that you noticed?
3. From the moment you first noticed that symptom, was it at its most severe or did it become more intense or spread to involve other parts of the body?
4. If it did worsen, how long did it take to spread or reach maximum intensity?
5. How long did it last?
6. What was the next symptom that you noticed?
7. How long after the first symptom did it commence?
8. Was the initial symptom showing signs of improving or worsening before this symptom began?
9. How long did this symptom take to develop in terms of maximum intensity or extent of involvement of the body?
10. And then what happened is the very best question to ask repeatedly.

Keep asking questions in this manner until the entire episode has been described and there is a clear understanding of the exact nature and distribution of every symptom and the time course of every symptom during the episode. Then ask the patient to describe other episodes using the same technique.

The value of such a painstaking approach is highlighted by the following cases seen by the author over the years.

# Single Episode of Symptoms

> **Case 7.1** A 20-year-old man with epilepsy.
>
> The referral letter read:
> Dear Doctor,
> Thank you for seeing this 20-year-old man with epilepsy. He walked into a video games parlour, noticed a strange smell, and was witnessed to have an epileptic seizure with incontinence of urine.
> Dr' Too Quick'
>
> On the surface, this does appear to be an epileptic seizure preceded by an olfactory aura (see Chapter 8) The word 'aura', is used to describe the initial symptom(s) of a seizure, often referred to as the warning symptoms. However, this doctor was too quick in jumping to the diagnosis of epilepsy and used only the nature of the symptoms to make a diagnosis, recalling that some seizures are associated with an altered smell. The correct diagnosis was apparent when a detailed history was obtained. His initial symptom was light-headedness that persisted and worsened over several minutes. He went on to feel hot and sweaty, his visioned darkened. He knew he was going to faint and last recalls thinking he needed to go outside. His next recollection was awakening on the floor and being told he had had a seizure. He had a seizure secondary to a syncopal episode in a games parlour that stank!

> **Case 7.2** A 38-year-old right-handed woman presented with an inability to speak
>
> A 38-year-old right-handed woman presented with the sudden onset of an inability to speak lasting approximately 30 seconds. She knew what she wanted to say but was unable to express any words (a non-fluent dysphasia, (Chapter 5). Despite her young age the patient was initially thought to have had an episode of cerebral ischaemia and underwent an urgent cerebral angiogram (pre-MRI and CT angiography era) that demonstrated a left frontal meningioma.
>
> The non-fluent dysphasia indicated the involvement of the frontal speech area in the dominant hemisphere. The fact that she was right-handed meant it was most likely (90% chance) in the left hemisphere. The sudden onset suggested a vascular, mechanical, or electrical problem. A more detailed history established that, in addition to the inability to speak, the patient had noticed that the jaw had clenched shut involuntarily during the episode. This is a positive phenomenon and indicates that the problem was a focal seizure affecting the speech cortex related to the meningioma and not a transient ischaemic attack (TIA). Positive phenomena such as transient jaw clenching does not occur with cerebral ischaemia.

# Recurrent Transient Symptoms

In patients with recurrent episodes of transient neurological symptoms, establish whether all episodes were identical or whether the symptoms varied from one episode to another by asking: 'Are all your turns the same or are some different to the others?' If the episodes varied, it is more rewarding to ask about several individual episodes. This is most relevant in some patients with epilepsy who may have multiple types of seizures (Chapter 8). If the events were all identical, it is possible to use the approach of asking the patient to imagine they were having an episode right now in front of you and using the questioning technique described above to obtain a detailed description of every symptom. This approach could miss the diagnosis when the circumstances under which these episodes occurred provide the vital clue to the diagnosis. This is highlighted by the next two cases.

> **Case 7.3** A 56-year-old woman who has had three episodes of *"vertebrobasilar insufficiency"*.
>
> Dear Dr,
> Thank you for seeing this 56-year-old woman who has had three episodes of vertebrobasilar insufficiency. In all three episodes, there was weakness in all four limbs, true vertigo with the room spinning, double vision and slurred speech. In two of the episodes, she lost consciousness.
> Yours sincerely,
>
> **A more detailed history obtained the following facts**
> On the first occasion, the patient was walking up a flight of stairs and the symptoms developed as she reached the top. She kept walking and, as she walked out of the stairwell, she lost consciousness. The second episode occurred while the patient was walking up over an overpass. The symptoms subsided when she stopped walking at the top of the overpass and, on this occasion, she did not blackout. The third episode was identical to the first and once again occurred after the patient climbed a flight of stairs.

Note in case 7.3 the same error: only the nature of the symptoms was obtained. The weakness in all four limbs combined with true vertigo (the room spinning), diplopia (double vision) and dysarthria (slurred speech) points to the involvement of the brainstem. The intermittent nature of the symptoms combined with the age of the patient suggests the diagnosis of vertebrobasilar insufficiency (VBI, i.e. transient cerebral ischaemia in the posterior circulation). To the experienced clinician, the transient loss of consciousness (LOC) in two of the episodes is atypical and would raise doubts about this being primarily related to cerebral vascular disease. (LOC is extremely rare in patients with VBI.

A more detailed history obtained the vital clue. The detailed description of the three individual events given above revealed that they all occurred with exertion and cerebral ischaemia related to vascular disease does not occur in such a predictable manner.[1] Examination of the patient demonstrated severe aortic stenosis, and the explanation for her symptoms was exercise-induced hypotension due to poor cardiac output with initial selective involvement of the posterior circulation causing the focal symptoms and the subsequent global cerebral ischaemia resulting in LOC. Syncope, chest pain and shortness of breath are the three classical symptoms of aortic stenosis. Symptoms such as those that occurred in this patient are very unusual.

The patient described in Case 7.4 alerted this author to the importance of obtaining a blow-by-blow description of each of the episodes. She had recently been discharged from the hospital without a clear diagnosis and after having undergone extensive investigation over 2 weeks. The patient was an 85-year-old woman who would be called in the trade 'a poor historian'.

> **Case 7.4** An 85-year-old woman unable to give a clear history
>
> *Good morning, Mrs. S. Could you please tell me about your funny turns?*
> 'They are terrible, doctor, I feel awful.'
> *Could you be a little more specific as to what happens?*
> 'I feel dizzy in the head and unwell and then I do not remember what happens.'
> *What do you mean by dizzy?*
> 'It is awful, doctor, I feel terrible.'
> *Can you describe to me what you mean by dizzy?*
> 'It's a terrible feeling in my head.'
> *How long have you had them for?*
> '6 months.'

---

1 Except in the very rare instance of subclavian steal syndrome where stenosis of the left subclavian artery proximal to the vertebral artery means that the left arm "steals" blood from the brainstem when it is exercising

It was evident after 10 minutes that the initial line of questioning was getting nowhere and that a different approach was required. The remainder of the consultation went along the following lines.

| Case 7.4 The alternative approach of asking about individual episodes |
|---|
| *Can you tell me about the last episode you had?*<br>'Yes doctor, it was terrible, it was awful.'<br>*I understand that it was terrible but what were you doing at the time it happened?*<br>'I was watching television.'<br>*What time of day?*<br>'Just before lunch about midday.'<br>*And then what happened?*<br>'I stood up to change the TV channel.'<br>*And then what happened?*<br>'That terrible turn, doctor, where I felt awful and dizzy in the head and then I don't remember what happened after that except I was on the floor in front of the TV.'<br>*Can you tell me how long you felt dizzy before you blacked out?*<br>'I don't think it was very long but I am not sure.'<br>*How long were you out to it?*<br>'I do not know but the same TV show was on so it could not have been very long.'<br>*Were you aware of anything the matter with you when you came to?*<br>'No.'<br>*And then what happened?*<br>'I crawled to my bed and went to sleep.'<br>*Can you tell me about another episode? What were you doing when it started?*<br>'I was having lunch.'<br>*What time of day?*<br>'About 12.30 pm.'<br>*And then what happened?*<br>'I stood up to go to the sink and that awful thing happened again.' |

After the patient described two episodes it became clear that every episode occurred about midday and only when she stood up. Six months beforehand she had been placed on prazosin, a drug for hypertension with postural hypotension a recognized side effect. Her blood pressure fell from 170/100 lying to 110/65 standing and her symptoms resolved upon cessation of this drug.

In each of these four cases, the crucial clue(s) were missed because a very detailed history was not obtained.

---

In patients with episodic disturbances of function, it is not only the nature and distribution of the symptoms but also the time course of the individual symptoms in relation to each other, the duration of each symptom and of the whole episode. In some cases, it is the circumstances under which they occur that differentiates the various possible diagnoses.

# A Novel Approach to Intermittent Disturbances

There are many ways to classify intermittent disturbances of neurological function. The traditional approach is to classify them according to the aetiology or underlying pathological basis. On the other hand, the simplest classification from the clinical point of view depends on what can readily be observed during episodes and is shown in Figure 7.1. Patients:

- fall (or slump if seated) or do not fall
- have a 'blackout' or they do not, whether they fall or not
- may or may not experience abnormal movements under any of these circumstances
- may experience episodes that vary in duration from seconds to minutes or even hours.

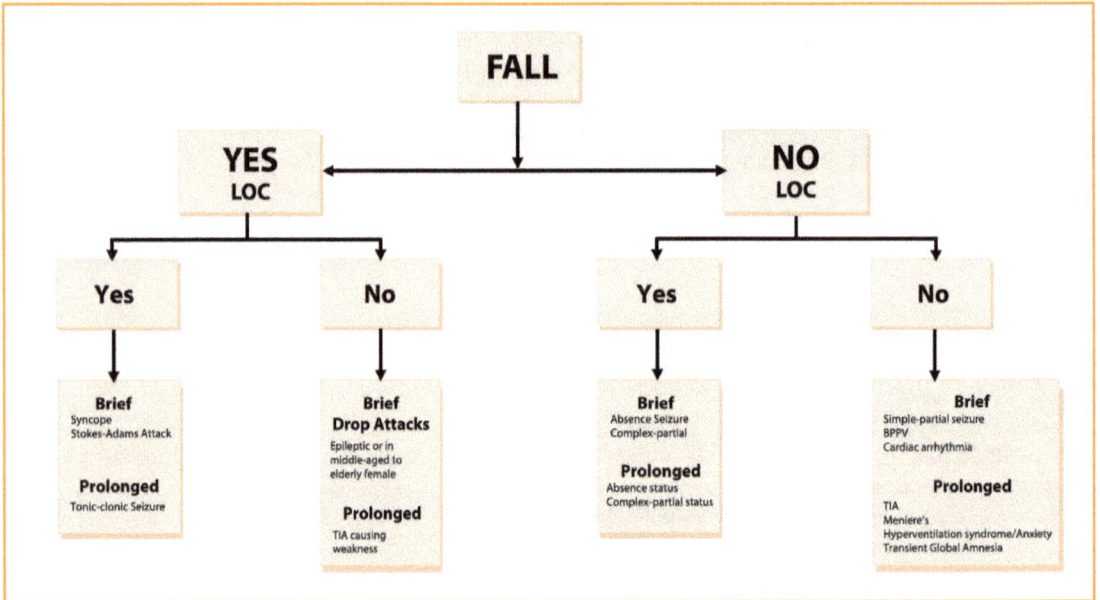

**Figure 7.1** A suggested approach to intermittent disturbances. Brief=seconds to a few minutes, LOC=loss of consciousness, prolonged=many minutes to hours or even days

The various causes of intermittent disturbances can be differentiated along these lines.

Most episodes in patients who fall with or without LOC are brief. The exceptions are:

- the very rare, prolonged tonic-clonic seizure lasting many minutes
- syncope with a prolonged aura
- a head injury with LOC complicating the fall, whatever the cause.

If the head injury is more severe, retrograde (occurring before the LOC) amnesia may give the impression that the episode has lasted for a longer time simply because the patient cannot recall what happened.

In patients with 'funny turns' where there is no fall or LOC, a significant variation of the duration and or the nature of the symptoms from one episode to another is very suggestive of a psychological disturbance.

Most intermittent disturbances result from one of the mechanisms illustrated in Figure 7.2.

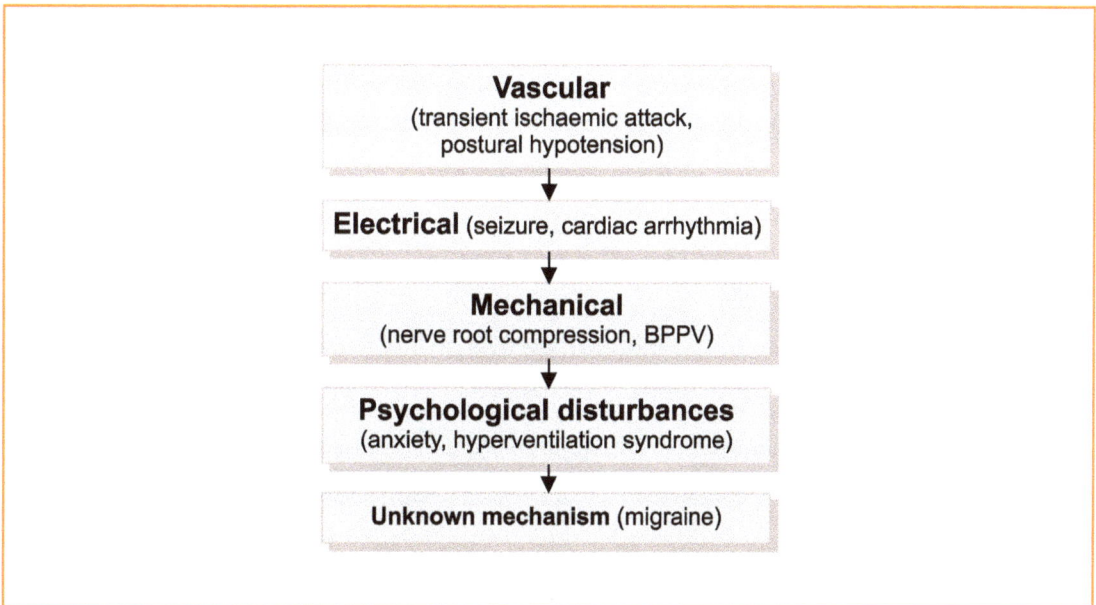

**Vascular**
(transient ischaemic attack,
postural hypotension)

↓

**Electrical** (seizure, cardiac arrhythmia)

↓

**Mechanical**
(nerve root compression, BPPV)

↓

**Psychological disturbances**
(anxiety, hyperventilation syndrome)

↓

**Unknown mechanism** (migraine)

**Figure 7.2** Basic mechanisms underlying intermittent disturbances of function BPPV= benign paroxysmal positional vertigo

# Episodic Disturbances with Falling
## Falling with Loss of Consciousness

| Table 7.1 Causes of transient loss of consciousness with falling | | |
|---|---|---|
| **Common causes** | **Less common causes** | **Very rare causes** |
| Syncope<br>Tonic–clonic seizures<br>Stokes–Adams attack or other arrhythmias<br>Postural hypotension | Sudden and<br>Severe gastrointestinal haemorrhage<br>Subarachnoid haemorrhage<br>Intracerebral haemorrhage<br>Sudden unilateral carotid occlusion<br>Massive pulmonary embolism<br>Aortic stenosis | Obstructive hydrocephalus<br>Colloid cyst 3rd ventricle<br>Idiopathic hypertrophic subaortic stenosis<br>Pulmonary hypertension |

The four most common causes of transient LOC with falling are shown in the 1st column of Figure 7.3. A complete summary of the numerous causes of transient LOC associated with a fall is listed in Table 7.1. Table 7.2 summarises the main clinical features of the common causes. Note that all are brief.

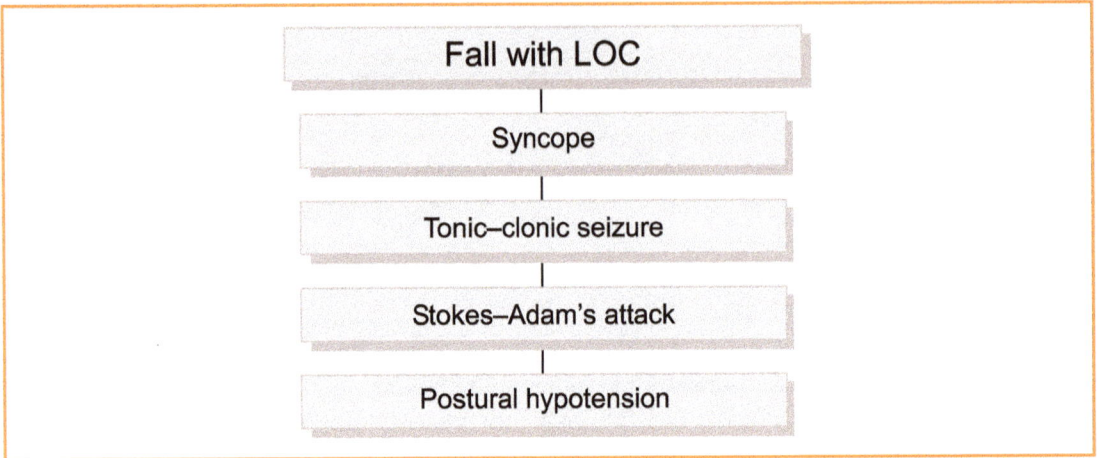

**Figure 7.3** The four most common causes of transient loss of consciousness with falling

---

It does not require experience, just patience and time, to obtain a detailed history in patients with episodic disturbances of function. Obtain a blow-by-blow description of episodes with particular attention to:
- the circumstances under which they occur
- the nature and distribution of the symptoms
- the time course of each and every symptom both individually and in relation to each other.

---

**Table 7.2** The main pre-ictal, ictal, and post-ictal features of the four most common causes of a fall with loss of consciousness

| Type of event | Pre-ictal | Ictal | Post-ictal | Duration |
|---|---|---|---|---|
| Syncope | Seconds to minutes | LOC, no abnormal movement | No drowsiness or confusion | 2–3 minutes |
| Tonic-clonic seizure | Aura (if present) lasting seconds | LOC + abnormal movements | Drowsy and confused | Ictus 2–3 minutes Drowsiness many minutes longer in older patients |
| Stokes–Adams attack | None | LOC, no abnormal movements | No drowsiness or confusion | Seconds (< 1 minute) |
| Postural hypotension | Seconds to 1 minute | LOC, no abnormal movements | No drowsiness or confusion | < 1 minute |

## Syncope

Syncope is also referred to as fainting, vasovagal or neurocardiogenic syncope.

Although syncope can afflict anyone of any age it tends to occur more commonly in young adults. [2] The patient is almost invariably standing, occasionally sitting and very, very rarely in a recumbent position. There is often, but not always, a trigger such as pain, alcohol, stressful situation, the sight of blood or being in a hot crowded environment.

- **Immediately before ictus:** There are several warning (pre-ictal) symptoms that increase in intensity over a period lasting between 30 seconds and 2 minutes after they first appear. These warning symptoms are referred to as pre-syncope and include light-headedness, nausea and feeling hot and clammy. If the symptoms worsen the patient becomes sweaty, their vision darkens and their hearing dims.
- **During ictus:** The patient subsequently loses consciousness (ictus), the eyes are closed, they are very pale and there are no abnormal movements unless the patient suffers a secondary seizure that usually consists of a very brief tonic seizure lasting less than 20 seconds. In some patients syncope, can occur with little or no warning, mimicking a Stokes–Adams attack (see below). Patients with a shorter duration of warning symptoms may suffer traumatic injuries. [3]
- **After ictus:** The patient rapidly regains consciousness (within 10–30 seconds) and, although they wonder what has happened, they are neither confused nor drowsy and can continue a sensible conversation almost immediately after the episode, even when there has been a brief secondary seizure. The patient can have a 2nd episode if they stand up too quickly after the 1st episode.

Unlike epilepsy, many patients who suffer from syncope can prevent LOC by lying or sitting down quickly when they experience the warning symptoms. This is an important diagnostic clue. Where there is uncertainty advise the patient to lie down immediately when the episode next occurs to see if LOC can be prevented by elevating the legs so that they are above the level of the head. There is a very rare condition in elderly patients where syncope can be related to carotid sinus sensitivity. [4]

## Some Notes of Caution

1. Patients and eyewitnesses often have difficulty estimating time, and 'funny turns' always seem to last longer than they do.
2. Pallor by itself is not overly useful, as patients are invariably described as being pale or a dreadful colour with all types of funny turns of differing causes. Having said this, extreme pallor associated with sweating is very suggestive of a cardiovascular cause.
3. Feeling the pulse quickly is very difficult, even for people who are trained such as medical practitioners and nurses; the apparent absence of a pulse does not necessarily imply an arrhythmia.
4. Eyewitnesses and patients often interpret having no recollection of the event as post-ictal confusion.
5. Regarding confusion, it is very important to clarify what observers and patients mean when they say the patient was confused after the episode.

## Tonic-Clonic Seizure

Only a few brief principles are discussed here, as Chapter 8 deals with the subject of epilepsy in detail.

- **Immediately before ictus:** The pre-ictal phase or aura if present is very brief, lasting only a few seconds. In patients with primary generalised epilepsy there is no warning before they lose consciousness with a tonic-clonic seizure.
- **During ictus:** The patient will fall to the ground if standing. They are unconscious with brief stiffening of the limbs (tonic phase) lasting 10–20 seconds followed by jerking

(clonic phase) of the limbs lasting on average 5–30 seconds. The duration of impaired consciousness is brief. Most tonic-clonic seizures last approximately 1 minute, although they can last as long as 10 minutes. [5] The eyes are usually open during the seizure and observers often say the eyes rolled up into the top of the head. The patient may bite their lip, cheek or tongue and they may suffer incontinence of urine and/or faeces during the tonic phase of the seizure.

- **After ictus:** The post-ictal period is associated with drowsiness and confusion lasting from 30 seconds to several minutes. [5] The period of post-ictal drowsiness and confusion may be as long as 24 hours or even up to 1 week following prolonged seizures and in older patients. [6]

## Stokes–Adam's Attack

This predominantly occurs in the elderly, although very rarely Stokes–Adam's attacks can occur in younger patients. These episodes are usually related to a bradyarrhythmia or complete heart block, although similar symptoms can occur with a tachyarrhythmia if it results in sudden hypotension. [7]

- **Immediately before ictus:** There is no warning.
- **During ictus:** The patient suddenly finds themselves on the ground, wondering what has happened. They do NOT recall falling. The period of impaired consciousness (ictus) is very brief, usually only a matter of seconds, certainly less than 1 minute. [8]
- **After ictus:** There is no post-ictal confusion, although the patient is bewildered as to what happened to them they can converse without difficulty.

Patients who lose consciousness due to a tachyarrhythmia may experience rapid palpitations, either just before the LOC or at other times, without losing consciousness. The presence of rapid palpitations at the time of the event provides a possible clue to an underlying cardiac cause for the transient LOC. The period of impaired consciousness may be longer if the patient suffers a head injury as a result of the fall.

## Postural Hypotension with Loss of Consciousness

This is the fourth most common cause of a fall associated with LOC. A *vital* clue is that, if the patient resumes a sitting or recumbent posture quickly, LOC may be prevented. Postural hypotension is suspected if episodes occur when the patient assumes an upright posture (e.g. stands up from sitting or lying).

- **Immediately before ictus:** The 'pre-ictal symptoms are the initial symptoms of the event and are similar to those seen with syncope.
- **During ictus:** The LOC, if it occurs, is momentary. If standing the patient will fall, if sitting they will slump in the chair. No abnormal movements occur.
- **After ictus:** There is no post-ictal confusion.

The diagnosis can be confirmed by measuring the blood pressure and pulse while lying and standing. The blood pressure falls and the pulse either increases or does not change at all depending on the aetiology of the postural hypotension. The commonest cause is drug-induced postural hypotension and in this case, the blood pressure may not fall if it is measured several hours after the patient has taken the drug. The clue that the problem may be drug-induced is that the episodes occur at a similar time of the day, usually within a few hours of the patient taking the medication.

The other causes of transient LOC listed in Table 7.1 are very rare and are usually obvious because of the associated symptoms or circumstances elicited with a very detailed history. Syncope due to aortic stenosis, idiopathic hypertrophic subaortic stenosis and pulmonary hypertension is precipitated by exertion. With these conditions, LOC can be avoided if the patient stops exercising with the very first symptom. There may also be associated dyspnoea with or without chest pain. Subarachnoid and intracerebral haemorrhage or a colloid cyst of the third ventricle will have associated severe explosive headache and vomiting. Pulmonary embolism causing a fall with LOC will be associated with severe chest pain, dyspnoea and severe hypotension. Gastrointestinal haemorrhage will be associated with haematemesis and/or melaena. The melaena may not be apparent when the patient is initially assessed.

## Falling Without Loss of Consciousness

Some patients will experience a fall and not lose consciousness. There are three common causes as shown in Figure 7.4.

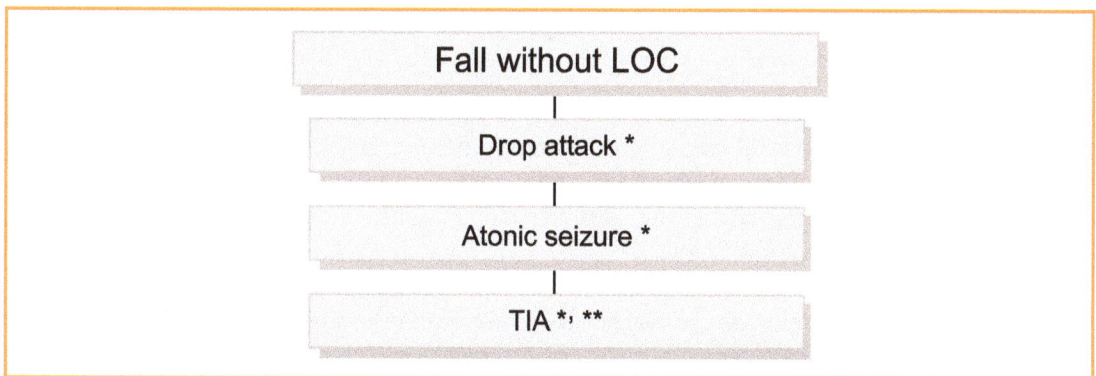

**Figure 7.4** Causes of a fall without loss of consciousness. TIA = transient ischaemic attack, brief = seconds to less than two minutes, prolonged = many minutes to hours. Note: patients with a TIA will fall only if the episode results in weakness of the legs or the neurological symptoms are associated with severe vertigo. More commonly patients with VBI do not experience loss of consciousness nor do they fall (see later in this chapter for more on TIA)

## Drop Attacks

Drop attacks occur for as yet no obvious reason in middle-aged to elderly females.
- **Immediately before ictus:** There is no warning.
- **During ictus:** The patient suddenly feels their legs go out from underneath them. The patient can recall falling. The fall or ictus is very brief, lasting only a matter of seconds. The patient does not lose consciousness and may or may not feel themselves falling.
- **After ictus:** There are no post-ictal symptoms unless the patient has been injured in the fall or is elderly with some physical disability. The patient can arise immediately and resume normal activities. In these episodes, a patient may suffer serious injuries.

These falls may well relate to the same mechanisms that causes syncope in the elderly. [9] Drop attacks also occur in patients with advanced Meniere's disease, [10] although if less severe the patient may simply experience an acute loss of balance without falling. Drop attacks are clinically identical to atonic seizures except that the latter is extremely rare in adults.

## Atonic Seizure

Atonic seizures commence in childhood and continue into adulthood. They are seen in patients with Lennox–Gastaut syndrome. These patients suddenly fall or feel as if they are thrown to the ground.

- **Immediately before ictus:** There is no warning.
- **During ictus:** Very rarely there may be a momentary myoclonic jerk of the limbs preceding the sudden fall. The ictus is brief, usually lasting only seconds, or occasionally up to 1 minute. If an attack lasts for 1 minute there may be an associated LOC. No abnormal movements. Atonic seizures rarely, if ever, occur as an isolated phenomenon and are almost invariably associated with other types of seizures (Chapter 8).
- **After ictus:** There are no symptoms.

# Episodic Disturbances Without Falling and Loss of Awareness

Most people interpret loss of consciousness as a dramatic event with profound impairment of consciousness and collapse. In patients with impaired consciousness without falling perhaps a better term would be loss of awareness, where 'the lights are on but no one is at home' or, as a farmer once commented about his son, 'there are no sheep in the top paddock for 30 seconds'.[2] The patient remains sitting, standing or lying. They simply go off the air for a short period, unresponsive to external stimuli.

Figure 7.5 shows the more common intermittent disturbances of neurological function associated with a loss of awareness but no fall. The duration of the episodes is usually brief, seconds to less than 2–3 minutes unless the patient develops status epilepsy.

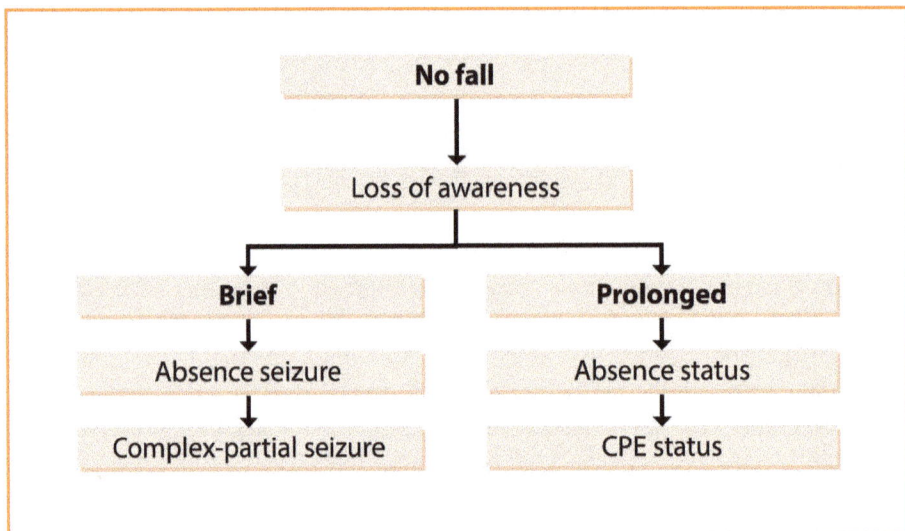

**Figure 7.5** Intermittent disturbances without falling brief = seconds to less than 2–3 minutes CPE=complex-partial epilepsy.

2   Two descriptions from relatives of patients with absence and complex-partial seizures

# Brief Episodes

## Absence Seizure

Absence epilepsy is almost exclusively a problem in childhood. Very rarely it may present in adulthood, but in the form of recurrent absence seizures termed absence status (Chapter 8).

- **Immediately before ictus:** There is no warning.
- **During ictus:** The ictus is very brief, usually 4–9 (range 1–44) seconds. [11] During the seizure, the eyes are open and the patient stares into space without any abnormal movements apart from frequent blinking.
- **After ictus:** No symptoms, the patient behaves as if nothing had happened (unless driving, cycling, or operating machinery where the seizure may result in an accident).

## Complex–Partial Seizure

- **Immediately before ictus:** Most but not all patients with complex–partial seizures will experience brief pre-ictal symptoms (aura) lasting seconds. The nature of the symptoms during the aura reflects the site of origin of the seizure within the brain and is discussed in Chapter 8.
- **During ictus:** During the ictus, the patient remains in the same posture, stares into space and is unresponsive for approximately 1–3 minutes. Very rarely, complex–partial seizures can last up to 16 minutes. [5] Minor abnormal movements, especially of the mouth (lip-smacking), termed automatisms are not uncommon.
- **After ictus:** There is a period of post-ictal confusion lasting several minutes, occasionally much longer.

# Prolonged Episodes

Non-convulsive status epilepsy (NCSE) causes prolonged episodes lasting hours to days. [12] It presents with confusion rather than unresponsiveness. Patients in NCSE may exhibit a wide range of clinical presentations including subtle memory deficits, bizarre behaviour, psychosis, or coma. Absence status and complex partial status are the two primary types of NCSE. This is discussed in more detail in Chapter 8.

## Absence Status Epilepsy

There are no pre-ictal symptoms of absence status epilepsy. This manifest as a prolonged period of depression of the mental state that may not be noticed by eyewitnesses because it is mild. Often there is associated repetitive blinking.

## Complex–Partial Status Epilepsy

Complex–partial status epilepsy manifests as a fluctuating mental state with confusion related to repeated typical and at times atypical complex–partial seizures, with or without clearing of consciousness between the episodes. [13] Prolonged confusion and episodic stereotyped repetitive automatisms with fluctuating impairment of consciousness lasting days have also been described. [12]

# No Loss of Consciousness and No Fall

Some intermittent disturbances are not associated with either loss of consciousness (awareness) or falling. Figure 7.6 shows the more common intermittent disturbances of neurological function that are not associated with a fall or loss of awareness (consciousness), distinguishing brief from prolonged episodes. The diagnosis is based on the duration of the episode as well as the nature of the symptoms. In this setting, some problems produce symptoms lasting hours and occasionally days.

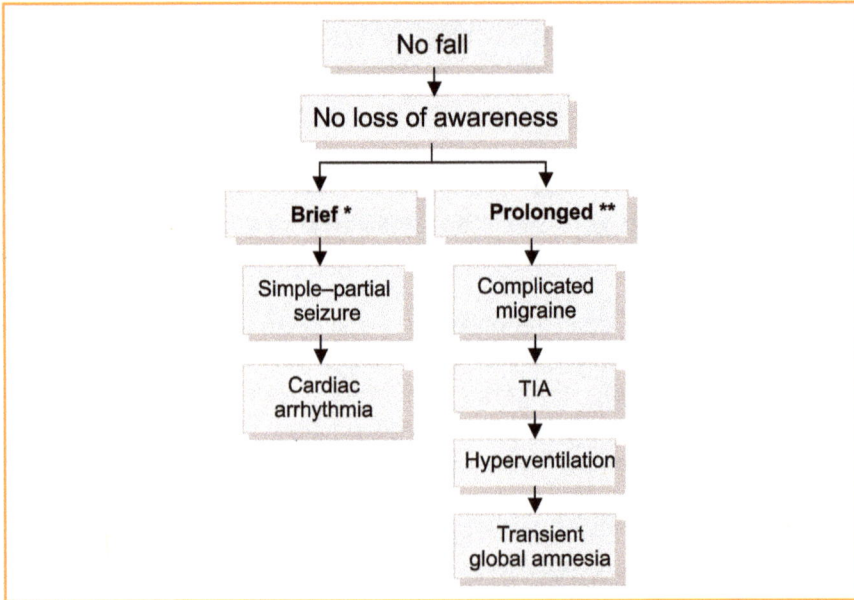

**Figure 7.6** Causes of episodic disturbances without a fall or loss of consciousness TIA = transient ischaemic attack, brief = seconds to less than two minutes, prolonged = many minutes to hours

# Brief Episodes

## Simple–Partial Seizure

Simple-partial seizures are unusual in that there is no loss of awareness and the patient is able to describe the stereotyped symptoms that they experience.

- **Immediately before ictus:** There are no pre-ictal symptoms
- **During ictus:** The ictus consists of brief stereotyped episodes lasting 30 seconds to 3 minutes, rarely up to 8 minutes [5] There is no loss of awareness and in most instances, the patient can continue normal activities during the episode but often chooses to halt them momentarily until the symptoms pass. The patient can describe all the symptoms. The nature of the symptoms reflects the site of origin within the cerebral hemisphere.
- **After ictus:** There is no post-ictal confusion or drowsiness.

## Cardiac Arrhythmia

Cardiac arrhythmias can cause neurological symptoms without loss consciousness or falling. The presence of palpitations at the time of the symptoms is a vital clue although not all patients will be aware of palpitations, although if these occur they are a valuable clue to the underlying diagnosis. The main arrhythmias are complete heart block (CHB) and ventricular tachycardia (VT), and rarely supraventricular tachycardia (SVT).

- **Immediately before ictus:** There are no symptoms.
- **During ictus:** Although a patient presenting with palpitations with or without dyspnoea or chest pain presents little difficulty, many patients experience the symptoms related to hypotension secondary to the arrhythmia without being aware of the altered cardiac rhythm and in the absence of dyspnoea or chest pain. Here the diagnosis can present some difficulty, as the symptoms are non-specific and include light-headedness, nausea, sweating, blurred vision, and a sensation of feeling unwell. The *one potential clue* is that these symptoms, which seem like hypotension, unlike postural hypotension or syncope may occur in the recumbent or sitting posture.
- **After ictus:** There are no symptoms.

# Prolonged Episodes

## Complicated Migraine

Complicated migraine is discussed in more detail in Chapter 9. In essence, the symptoms come on gradually over minutes to less than 2 hours in 97% of patients. [14] and persist on average for 24 hours but may persist for days [15] *The most important diagnostic feature, and the one that differentiates migraine from cerebral ischaemia, is the partial or complete resolution of the initial or early symptoms before the later symptoms have either appeared or fully evolved.* In contrast, in cerebral ischaemia the symptoms are either of maximum intensity and distribution at onset or a cumulative neurological deficit develops with a stroke in evolution (Chapter 10). No symptom improves before the stroke or TIA reaches its maximum severity. The second clue is that the symptoms spread from their original site to other parts of the body, reflecting the spreading cortical depression of Leão. This is typically seen with the visual aura of migraine where the scotoma or photopsia enlarge and moves across the visual field. Focal seizures can spread as can cerebral ischaemia. The clue to a seizure is the presence of positive phenomena and with cerebral ischaemia is the cumulative deficit discussed above. The third clue is that the aura of migraine typically develops over 5 or more minutes and, when there is more than one symptom, they occur in succession. [16]

> The partial or complete resolution of the initial or early symptoms before the later symptoms have either appeared or fully evolved is pathognemonic for migraine

# Transient Ischaemic Attack (TIA) including Vertebrobasilar Insufficiency (VBI)

The great majority of patients with cerebral ischaemia, even those with widespread symptoms of VBI such as diplopia, dysarthria, visual loss and motor and sensory symptoms, can describe their symptoms and have not lost consciousness or awareness. The exception is the very rare patient with VBI where there is medial temporal lobe or thalamic involvement with amnesia for the event. [17] If the degree of weakness is severe patients with a TIA may fall if they are standing.

- **Immediately before ictus:** There are no clear-cut pre-ictal symptoms, although some patients describe being off-colour in the preceding few days.
- **During ictus:** The 'ictal' symptoms last from minutes to hours (by definition up to 24 hours, but usually 3–4 hours [18]). The nature of the symptoms depends on the vascular territory affected (carotid versus vertebrobasilar, large vessel versus small vessel). This is discussed in more detail in Chapter 10, 'Cerebrovascular disease'.
- **After ictus:** There are no obvious post-ictal symptoms.

# Hyperventilation Syndrome

Hyperventilation syndrome is a very common clinical problem that is often under-recognised.[3] Hyperventilation syndrome is characterised by a variety of somatic symptoms induced by physiologically inappropriate hyperventilation and usually reproduced in whole or in part by voluntary hyperventilation. [19] There is no pre-ictal or post-ictal phase.

- **Immediately before ictus:** There are no symptoms.
- **During ictus:** The symptoms gradually increase in intensity and then fluctuate in severity as the episode continues. The ictus consists of light-headedness that increases in severity over minutes and persists for hours, fluctuating in intensity. There are often, but not invariably, associated symptoms with a sense of heaviness in the chest. Chest pain can occur but is rare and is usually described as a sense of tightness. Occasionally, patients complain of shortness of breath; more often they complain of an inability to get enough air into their lungs, which is often associated with dryness of the mouth. I have seen the very rare patient who has described true vertigo with a sense of spinning. There may or may not be peripheral or perioral paraesthesia, that at times can be unilateral leading to a concern that these are stroke symptoms.
- **After ictus:** There are no symptoms.

Patients may have a background history of tension headache and neck discomfort, but in many cases, hyperventilation is not necessarily associated with recent provocative stress. [21] Some patients develop this problem after attending relaxation classes where they are instructed to take deep breaths to relax![4] The symptoms can be reproduced by asking the patient to take deep breaths (not panting) for 2–5 minutes. Alternatively, blood gases measured during an episode should reveal a low carbon dioxide ($CO_2$) level.

---

3   Personal observation
4   Personal observation

Everyone will develop giddiness or dizziness when they hyperventilate.
Therefore it is imperative to confirm that the patient's symptoms have been reproduced exactly. If the symptoms are not reproduced, the clinician should maintain a healthy scepticism about the diagnosis of hyperventilation syndrome

If the symptoms are not reproduced, the clinician should maintain a healthy scepticism about the diagnosis of hyperventilation syndrome. If the patient's symptoms are not reproduced exactly, and yet the symptoms strongly suggest hyperventilation, it is worthwhile sending the patient away with instructions to slow their breathing (see below) as soon as symptoms commence. In many instances when it is hyperventilation syndrome the symptoms will resolve more rapidly with the patient slowing their breathing. The patient is instructed to return for further evaluation if the symptoms do not resolve. Treatment by breathing in and out of a paper bag, although effective, is embarrassing and impractical. A far more practical method is for the patient to breathe in and then exhale holding their breath for 15 or 20 seconds, repeating this procedure until the symptoms subside. This may take several minutes. It is easier to hold the breath after expiration than inspiration. The aim is to allow the $CO_2$ level to return to normal, having been lowered by hyperventilation.

# Transient Global Amnesia

Transient global amnesia (TGA) was first described in 1956 [22] and is a curious clinical syndrome characterised by the abrupt onset of severe anterograde amnesia. [23] It lasts several hours and is seen most often in the middle-aged or elderly. These patients are often not aware of any problems and are brought to medical attention by a concerned relative or an observer. During the attack, the patient remains alert and communicative but keeps asking the same questions over and over again. Their identity is preserved and there are no focal neurological or epileptic features. Apart from short-term memory loss, the patient behaves as if nothing else is wrong; they can talk, walk etc. The ability to lay down new memories gradually recovers as the period of amnesia shrinks. There is often a residual amnesia for events near the onset of the episode.

There are strict criteria for the diagnosis of TGA: [24]
1. The attack must be witnessed if it is to be diagnosed with a degree of certainty. Clear-cut anterograde amnesia must be present during the attack.
2. Clouding of consciousness and loss of personal identity must be absent.
3. The cognitive impairment must be limited to amnesia.
4. There should be no accompanying focal neurological symptoms.
5. Epileptic seizures must be absent.
6. Attacks must resolve within 24 hours and patients with recent head injury or known active epilepsy are excluded.

Other causes of the acute amnestic syndrome include head injury, subarachnoid haemorrhage, Wernicke–Korsakoff syndrome and carbon monoxide poisoning. The associated symptoms of these other causes should enable easy differentiation from TGA.

151

# Vertigo

| Table 7.3 Central versus peripheral vertigo | | |
| --- | --- | --- |
| **Feature** | **Central vertigo** | **Peripheral vertigo** |
| **Deafness and tinnitus** | Absent | May be present |
| **Inability to stand** | Yes | Yes/No |
| **Dysarthria, diplopia** | Yes | No |
| **Findings with the Hallpike manoeuvre** | | |
| **Delayed onset of vertigo** | None | 2-40 seconds |
| **Severity of vertigo** | Mild | Severe |
| **Symptoms fatigue*** | No | Yes |
| **Symptoms habituate**** | No | Yes |
| **Duration of nystagmus** | >1 minute | Minute<1 |
| *Fatigue refers to the abatement of vertigo and nystagmus after provocation while the head is still in the position that precipitated the symptoms **Habituation refers to a lessening the severity of the symptoms with repeated Hallpike testing Nystagmus is a rapid, involuntary, oscillator emotion of the eyeball note: vertigo is precipitated by the Hallpike manoeuvre in both central and peripheral lesions. The bottom five rows refer to the differing findings on the Hallpike manoeuvre | | |

Dizziness and giddiness are very non-specific terms that are commonly used by patients to describe their symptoms. Four types of dizziness have been defined: vertigo, pre-syncope, disequilibrium, and others. [25] Vertigo is a false sensation that the body or the environment is moving (head or room spinning). This is true vertigo and indicates a problem within the peripheral vestibular system (labyrinth or vestibular nerve) or the central vestibular connections in the brainstem or cerebellum. Table 7.3 lists the distinguishing features of central vertigo and peripheral vertigo as described by Swartz and Longwell. [26] Cerebellar infarction is discussed in greater detail in Chapter 10.

Vertigo essentially presents either as an acute severe episode or as recurrent attacks over months to years. Whatever the cause, vertigo is almost invariably associated with variable degrees of nausea and vomiting. Figure 7.7 shows the more common causes of vertigo. The two main causes of *acute severe vertigo* are 'acute vestibulopathy' (vestibular neuronitis, labyrinthitis) and cerebellar infarction. [27]

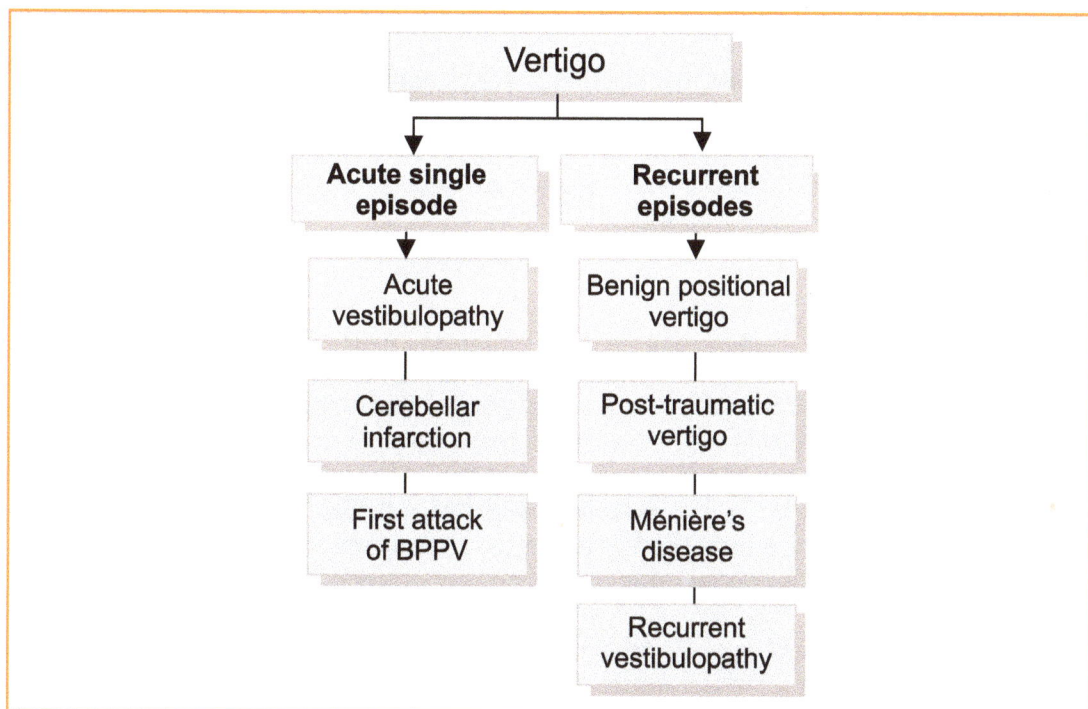

**Figure 7.7** The more common causes of vertigo and BPPV = benign paroxysmal positional vertigo

Apart from cerebellar infarction, most conditions that cause vertigo do not have 'gold standard' tests to confirm the clinical diagnosis. Ménière's disease also lacks a diagnostic test but the syndrome is well defined so the term has been retained.

As an isolated symptom, vertigo is most often peripheral in origin (inner ear or vestibular nerve including the entry zone in the brain stem) with benign positional vertigo, post-traumatic positional vertigo, acute vestibular neuronitis and Ménière's disease accounting for 93% of patients with vertigo presenting to primary care physicians. [28] Very occasionally vertigo is central in origin, affecting the vestibular connections within the brainstem, but there are almost always other neurological symptoms and/or signs referable to the brainstem such as diplopia, slurred speech weakness or sensory symptoms.

A sensation of imbalance (likened to being on a ship) may relate to the vestibular system and may represent a less severe form of vertigo. Patients use terms such as giddiness and dizziness to refer to this sense of imbalance. However, the more one deviates from the true definition of vertigo as a spinning sensation (either of the head or environment), the less one can be certain that the symptoms represent involvement of the vestibular pathway. In patients who complain that they are unsteady, it is important to clarify whether there is an associated sensation of giddiness (suggesting either hypotension or a vestibular pathway cause for the instability) or a problem with their legs in the absence of giddiness. The latter may be due to diseases affecting the central or peripheral nervous system and not involving the vestibular system. Rarely, vertigo can result from new spectacles or the sudden onset of diplopia due to an extraocular muscle paresis.

## Acute Single Episode

Although the two conditions discussed in this section are monophasic illnesses, they are important causes of vertigo and it seems appropriate to include them in this chapter with the other causes of vertigo that result in episodic symptoms. In theory, patients with an initial attack of benign paroxysmal positional vertigo could present as an acute single episode; in reality, these patients rarely if ever present after the first episode.

## Acute Vestibulopathy

The use of the term 'vestibulopathy' reflects the unknown aetiology of this clinical syndrome and as already explained, is preferred to the terms 'labyrinthitis' or 'vestibular neuronitis' which imply a site of pathology and an infective or inflammatory process that is not proven. [29] By definition vestibular neuritis (or neuronitis) is confined to the vestibular system and hearing is unaffected, whilst labyrinthitis is a process that is thought to affect the inner ear as a whole or the 8th nerve as a whole and where hearing may be reduced or distorted in tandem with vertigo. [30]

- **Immediately before ictus:** There may be an antecedent upper respiratory infection. In some patients, a vague sense of imbalance may precede by some hours to days the more severe vertigo.
- **During ictus:** Vertigo typically develops slowly over hours, is severe for a few days and then subsides over a few weeks. Nausea and vomiting are marked but there is no tinnitus or deafness. The patients prefer to lie completely immobile on the side opposite to the affected ear as the slightest movement exacerbates vertigo. There is unidirectional nystagmus with the fast phase to the unaffected ear. The nystagmus can be suppressed by visual fixation (asking the patient to stare at an object). Examination of one retina with the ophthalmoscope, while the other eye is covered, can elicit nystagmus as this removes visual fixation. Other than nystagmus there are no focal neurological symptoms or signs.
- **After ictus:** Some patients can have residual non-specific post-ictal giddiness and imbalance that lasts for months. Benign paroxysmal positional vertigo may develop as a sequela.

## Cerebellar Infarction/Haemorrhage

- **Immediately before ictus:** There are no 'pre-ictal' symptoms.
- **During ictus:** Onset is sudden if ischaemic or over many minutes if related to haemorrhage. 'Ictal' symptoms last for days. Although the patient may present with severe vertigo, cerebellar infarction or haemorrhage should be suspected in patients who present with:
  - severe nausea and vomiting
  - and inability to stand (Chapter 10).

Unlike acute vestibulopathy, the patient is unable to stand. When there is associated dysarthria, diplopia and limb ataxia, the diagnosis of a central cause for the vertigo is apparent.

- **After ictus**: Residual symptoms will occur if recovery is incomplete.

In both cerebellar infarction and acute vestibulopathy, the vomiting may be so severe and repeated that a Mallory–Weiss tear in the lower end of the oesophagus may occur and haematemesis may be the presenting symptom. It is not uncommon for these patients to be misdiagnosed with an acute gastrointestinal problem and admitted under the gastroenterology unit. The presence of severe vertigo or an inability to stand in these patients should alert the clinician to the correct diagnosis.

The head impulse test [34] detects severe unilateral loss of semicircular canal function clinically. It can distinguish between vestibular neuritis and cerebellar infarction as it is normal in a patient with cerebellar infarction but abnormal in a patient with vestibular neuritis or acute vestibulopathy. The head thrust test consists of holding the patient's face with both hands with the patient's head turned to one side slightly past the midline and then rapidly thrusting it to just past the midline on the opposite side. The patient is asked to fixate on a distant object. When the subject's head is turned to the side of the lesion, the vestibular ocular reflex is deficient and the eyes will move with the head so that they no longer fixate on the point in the distance. A CT scan will detect haemorrhage but may be normal in the early hours after an infarct. An MRI scan will detect the infarction earlier.

# Recurrent Attacks of Vertigo
# Benign Paroxysmal Positional Vertigo

Benign paroxysmal positional vertigo (BPPV) was first described in detail by Barany in 1921. [35] This usually, but not invariably, occurs in the middle-aged to elderly where it is related to small deposits of calcium on the hair cells in the vestibule. Positional vertigo can also occur after a head injury or an acute vestibulopathy.

- **Pre-ictal:** There are no warning (pre-ictal) symptoms.
- **During ictus:** Patients describe paroxysms of true vertigo precipitated by head movement such as:
  - looking up to get something out of a cupboard or off the clothesline
  - bending over to tie shoelaces or to pick up an object
  - getting in and out of bed
  - lying down
  - rolling over in bed
  - turning their head quickly
- **After ictus:** There are usually no symptoms.

Although vertigo may be precipitated by all of these actions, in some patients only one or two of these head movements precipitate vertigo. The symptoms are brief, lasting less than 2 minutes. Although nausea may occur, vomiting is rare. There are no other symptoms such as tinnitus (ringing in the ears), deafness, diplopia, dysarthria, slurred speech, blindness (termed amaurosis) weakness or sensory symptoms. Symptoms are present most days for weeks and occasionally months. Patients will notice good and bad days and on bad days there are repeated episodes in a day. The moment the patient gets out of bed they know if they are in for a good or bad day depending upon the appearance or not of symptoms. The crucial diagnostic clue is that the patient is free of vertigo when lying or sitting perfectly still.

The symptoms and the associated delayed onset of nystagmus that abates with the maintenance of a fixed posture can be precipitated by the positioning test or Hallpike manoeuvre: [36]

1. The examiner should describe to the patient what the test involves and reassure them that it is safe and painless, but that it may reproduce their symptoms and make them very giddy. The patient should be reassured that they will not be allowed to fall off the examination couch.
2. Ask the patient to sit on an examination couch so that when they lie down the head is over and below the end of the couch. The movement has to be quick and the examiner needs

to ensure that the patient does not suffer from back or neck problems before doing this procedure. Ensure that the back and neck are supported during the procedure.

3. When this test is performed the patient will want to close their eyes but must be encouraged to keep them open so that the nystagmus can be seen. Commence with the head looking to one side and then rapidly lie the patient down from the sitting position. If the problem is benign positional vertigo affecting the right ear, there is the delayed onset of a fast phase clockwise (as the patient sees it, anti-clockwise from the examiner's perspective) torsional nystagmus with the affected right ear dependent or lower.

4. To complete the procedure the patient is returned to the seated position and the eyes are observed for reversal in the direction of the nystagmus, in this case, fast-phase anticlockwise nystagmus. The nystagmus settles within 30 seconds if the patient stays still in that position. [36]

The rationale behind this is the observations of Schuknecht and Ruby who described small deposits of calcium (otoconia) on the hair cells, most often within the posterior semi-circular canals, as the cause of this problem. [37] These deposits are flushed out of the semi-circular canals using the Epley manoeuvre or particle/canalith repositioning manoeuvre. The condition can be cured in 80% of patients, using the Canalith Repositioning Procedure or Epley manoeuvre. [38] This requires identification of whether it is the right or left ear in which the problem occurs and this is not always possible, particularly if the patient is having a good day and the Hallpike manoeuvre is negative. If one cannot provoke vertigo with the Hallpike manoeuvre, one cannot cure it with the Epley manoeuvre. In these circumstances the options are to bring the patient back on a bad day or recommend that they deliberately precipitate the symptoms many times in the morning and the evening until the problem resolves, using the Brandt–Daroff exercises. [39] This problem can recur on more than one occasion months or even years later.

## Ménière's Disease

The term Ménière's disease is used to define the classic triad of:

1. vertigo of vestibular origin
2. tinnitus and progressive hearing impairment (cochlear symptoms)
3. aural pressure.

Ménière's disease is manifested by episodic true vertigo associated with nausea and vomiting lasting longer than 1 hour and usually a few hours, together with a sense of fullness in the ear. Tinnitus may occur, and *transient deafness during the attack that improves following the episode is a pathognomonic* (this is a term that indicates that only one condition can cause the problem) symptom of Ménière's that occurs in two-thirds of patients. [40] The tinnitus and deafness may persist for days. The symptoms increase in intensity over several minutes and may continue to increase for up to half an hour. There may be a further period of up to half an hour of a sense of instability before the onset of the severe true vertigo with a sense of rotation. The patient prefers to lie still with the affected ear uppermost, but vertigo persists even if the patient remains motionless. This condition recurs at variable intervals, as frequently as several attacks within a week or none for some years. *Two episodes of vertigo in 1 day are incompatible with the diagnosis of Ménière's.* Repeated attacks usually lead to progressive hearing loss over many years. In the early stages tinnitus, hearing impairment and/or fullness in the ear may appear before the onset of the first vertigo attack and vertigo can occur without tinnitus and deafness. [41]

Three stages are identified in Ménière's disease:

- **Stage I**. In the early phase, the predominant symptom is vertigo, characteristically rotatory or rocking, associated with nausea or vomiting. The episode is often preceded by an aura of fullness or pressure in the ear or on the side of the head and usually lasts from 20 minutes to several hours. Between the attacks hearing reverts to normal and examination of the patient during this period of remission invariably shows normal results.
- **Stage II**. As the disease advances the hearing loss becomes established but continues to fluctuate. The deafness is sensorineural and initially affects the lower pitches. The paroxysms of vertigo reach their maximum severity and then tend to become less severe. The period of remission is highly variable, often lasting for several months.
- **Stage III**. In the last stage of the disorder, the hearing loss stops fluctuating and progressively worsens; both ears tend to be affected so that the prime disability is deafness. The episodes of vertigo diminish and then disappear, although the patient may be unsteady, especially in the dark. [42]

## Recurrent Vestibulopathy

Essentially, patients have recurrent *isolated vertigo* of unknown cause and without headache, neurological or auditory symptoms. Patients experience recurrent episodes of vertigo, with nausea and vomiting lasting hours or sometimes days. [43] These episodes occur at variable intervals and do not display the features of Ménière's syndrome, such as transient deafness and tinnitus during the attacks, and patients do not subsequently develop deafness. The precise aetiology of these episodes has not been established. At the time of writing, there is a strong body of opinion that considers these episodes to be migrainous. [44–50] The increased incidence of migraine in patients with vertigo and vice versa and the response to 'migraine therapy' is cited as evidence for the link between migraine and vertigo. Diagnostic criteria have been proposed. [47] The evidence is circumstantial and, as there is no gold standard diagnostic test for migraine or migrainous vertigo, the episodes have been referred to as recurrent vestibulopathy.

# Fleeting Symptoms

Patients are occasionally encountered who describe fleeting symptoms lasting only 1 or 2 seconds. There may be a momentary sensation of impending LOC, particularly when a person is relaxed, referred to as the blip syndrome. [51] There may be transient symptoms of pain such as ice-pick headache (Chapter 9) or there may be transient sensory symptoms. These often defy explanation and are benign, and all investigations are normal.[5]

---

5   Personal observation

# References

1    Official website of the Sir Arthur Conan Doyle Literary Estate, 2006. Available: http://www. sherlockholmesonline.org/Biography/index.htm (14 Dec 2009).

2    Sheldon RS, Sheldon AG, Connolly SJ, et al. Age of first faint in patients with vasovagal syncope. *J Cardiovasc Electrophysiol* 2006;17:49–54.

3    Ammirati F, Colivicchi F, Velardi A, et al. Prevalence and correlates of syncope-related traumatic injuries in tilt-induced vasovagal syncope. *Ital Heart J* 2001;2:38–41.

4    Brignole M, Alboni P, Benditt D, et al. Guidelines on management (diagnosis and treatment) of syncope. *Eur Heart J* 2001;22:1256–1306.

5    Jenssen S, Gracely EJ, Sperling MR. How long do most seizures last? A systematic comparison of seizures recorded in the epilepsy monitoring unit. *Epilepsia* 2006;47:1499–1503.

6    Godfrey JW, Roberts MA, Caird FI. Epileptic seizures in the elderly. II: Diagnostic problems. *Age Ageing* 1982;11:29–34.

7    Johansson BW. Long-term ECG in ambulatory clinical practice. Analysis and 2-year follow-up of 100 patients studied with a portable ECG tape recorder. *Eur J Cardiol* 1977;5:39–48.

8    Harbison J, Newton JL, Seifer C, et al. Stokes Adams attacks and cardiovascular syncope. *Lancet* 2002;359:158–160.

9    Kenny RA, Traynor G. Carotid sinus syndrome – clinical characteristics in elderly patients. *Age Ageing* 1991;20:449–454.

10   Kentala E, Havia M, Pyykko I. Short-lasting drop attacks in Ménière's disease. *Otolaryngol Head Neck Surg* 2001;124:526–530.

11   Sadleir LG, Farrell K, Smith S, et al. Electroclinical features of absence seizures in childhood absence epilepsy. *Neurology* 2006;67:413–418.

12   Escueta AV, Boxley J, Stubbs N, et al. Prolonged twilight state and automatisms: A case report. *Neurology* 1974;24:331–339.

13   Ellis JM, Lee SI. Acute prolonged confusion in later life as an ictal state. *Epilepsia* 1978;19:119–128.

14   Pryse-Phillips W, Aube M, Bailey P, et al. A clinical study of migraine evolution. *Headache* 2006;46:1480–1486.

15   Kelman L. Pain characteristics of the acute migraine attack. *Headache* 2006;46:942–953.

16   Kirchmann M. Migraine with aura: new understanding from clinical epidemiologic studies. *Curr Opin Neurol* 2006;19:286–293.

17   Akiguchi I, Ino T, Nabatame H, et al. Acute-onset amnestic syndrome with localized infarct on the dominant side – comparison between anteromedial thalamic lesion and posterior cerebral artery territory lesion. *Jpn J Med* 1987;26:15–20.

18   Crisostomo RA, Garcia MM, Tong DC. Detection of diffusion-weighted MRI abnormalities in patients with transient ischemic attack: Correlation with clinical characteristics. *Stroke* 2003;34:932–937.

19   Lewis RA, Howell JB. Definition of the hyperventilation syndrome. *Bull Eur Physiopathol Respir* 1986;22:201–205.

20   Saisch SG, Wessely S, Gardner WN. Patients with acute hyperventilation presenting to an inner-city emergency department. *Chest* 1996;110:952–957.

21   Fejerman N. Nonepileptic disorders imitating generalized idiopathic epilepsies. *Epilepsia* 2005;46(Suppl 9): S80–S83.

22   Courjon J, Guyotat J. [Amnesic strokes.]. *J Med Lyon* 1956;37:697–701.

23   Fisher CM, Adams RD. Transient global amnesia. *Acta Neurol Scand* 1964;40(Suppl 9): S1–S83.

24   Hodges JR, Warlow CP. Syndromes of transient amnesia: Towards a classification. A study of 153 cases. *J Neurol Neurosurg Psychiatry* 1990;53:834–843.

25   Drachman DA, Hart CW. An approach to the dizzy patient. *Neurology* 1972;22:323–234.

26  Swartz R, Longwell P. Treatment of vertigo. *Am Fam Physician* 2005;71:1115–1122.

27  Halmagyi GM. Diagnosis and management of vertigo. *Clin Med* 2005;5:159–165.

28  Hanley K, O'Dowd T. Symptoms of vertigo in general practice: A prospective study of diagnosis. *Br J Gen Pract* 2002;52:809–812.

29  Ryu JH. Vestibular neuritis: An overview using a classical case. *Acta Otolaryngol Suppl* 1993;503:25–30.

30  Silvoniemi P. Vestibular neuronitis. An otoneurological evaluation. *Acta Otolaryngol Suppl* 1988;453:1–72.

31  Fukuda T. The stepping test: Two phases of the labyrinthine reflex. *Acta Otolaryngol* 1959;50:95–108.

32  Brandt TH, Dieterich M. Different types of skew deviation. *J Neurol Neurosurg Psychiatry* 1991;54:549–550.

33  Safran AB, Vibert D, Issoua D, et al. Skew deviation after vestibular neuritis. *Am J Ophthalmol* 1994;118:238–245.

34  Halmagyi GM, Curthoys IS. A clinical sign of canal paresis. *Arch Neurol* 1988;45:737–739.

35  Barany R. Diagnose von Krankheitserscheinungen im Bereiche des Otolithenapparates. *Acta Otolaryng* 1921;2:434–437.

36  Dix MR, Hallpike CS. The pathology, symptomatology, and diagnosis of certain common disorders of the vestibular system. *Proc R Soc Med* 1952;45:341–354.

37  Schuknecht HF, Ruby RR. Cupulolithiasis. *Adv Otorhinolaryngol* 1973;20:434–443.

38  Epley JM. The canalith repositioning procedure: For treatment of benign paroxysmal positional vertigo. *Otolaryngol Head Neck Surg* 1992;107:399–404.

39  Brandt T, Daroff RB. Physical therapy for benign paroxysmal positional vertigo. *Arch Otolaryngol* 1980;106:484–485.

40  Havia M, Kentala E, Pyykko I. Hearing loss and tinnitus in Ménière's disease. *Auris Nasus Larynx* 2002;29:115–119.

41  Tokumasu K, Fujino A, Naganuma H, et al. Initial symptoms, and retrospective evaluation of prognosis in Ménière's disease. *Acta Otolaryngol Suppl* 1996;524:43–49.

42  Saeed SR. Fortnightly review: Diagnosis and treatment of Ménière's disease. *BMJ* 1998;316:368–372.

43  Lee H, Sohn SI, Jung DK, et al. Migraine and isolated recurrent vertigo of unknown cause. *Neurol Res* 2002;24:663–665.

44  Maione A. Migraine-related vertigo: Diagnostic criteria and prophylactic treatment. *Laryngoscope* 2006;116:1782–1786.

45  Eggers SD. Migraine-related vertigo: Diagnosis and treatment. *Curr Neurol Neurosci Rep* 2006;6:106–115.

46  Neuhauser HK, Lempert T. Diagnostic criteria for migrainous vertigo. *Acta Otolaryngol* 2005;125:1247–1248.

47  Neuhauser H, Leopold M, von Brevern M, et al. The interrelations of migraine, vertigo, and migrainous vertigo. *Neurology* 2001;56:436–441.

48  Gupta VK. Migraine-related vertigo: The challenge of the basic sciences. *Clin Neurol Neurosurg* 2005;108:109–110:reply 111–112.

49  Lempert T, Neuhauser H. Migrainous vertigo. *Neurol Clin* 2005;23:715–730:vi.

50  Brantberg K, Trees N, Baloh RW. Migraine-associated vertigo. *Acta Otolaryngol* 2005;125:276–279.

51  Lance JW. Transient sensations of impending loss of consciousness: The "blip" syndrome. *J Neurol Neurosurg Psychiatry* 1996;60:437–438.

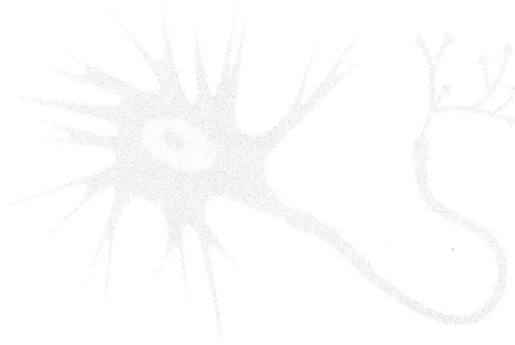

# Seizures and Epilepsy

| Key Terms | |
|---|---|
| **Seizure:** | A sudden change in behaviour due to an abnormal firing of nerve cells in the brain. Symptoms of cerebral dysfunction resulting from paroxysmal discharges of neurons involving the cerebral cortex. |
| **Epilepsy:** | Recurrent seizures. |
| **Ictus:** | Strictly defined as a blow or sudden attack, it is another term used to describe a seizure |
| **Aura:** | The brief warning that may precede the actual seizure |
| **Déjà vu:** | is the experience of feeling sure that one has witnessed or experienced the same sensation before |
| **Jamais vu:** | A feeling of unfamiliarity, a sense of seeing the situation for the first time, |
| **Post-Ictal:** | The time immediately after the seizure |

This chapter is a brief discussion of the clinical aspects of epilepsy; it does not discuss pathophysiology. The numerous classification schemes [1-4] will not be addressed as it is inevitable that these will continue to evolve.

In clinical practice, it is more useful to divide seizures based on what happens to the patient and what can be witnessed.

The basic principles of clinical assessment and management of patients suffering from a suspected seizure or epilepsy (recurrent seizures) are discussed. This chapter is not a comprehensive discussion of epilepsy; more detailed information can be found in numerous wonderful textbooks. [5-7]

Drug treatment is discussed in Appendix C. However, it will continue to evolve rapidly; thus, any discussion in a textbook will be very rapidly out of date. Links to neurology and epilepsy-related websites are included in chapter 15. These websites will provide the reader with up-to-date information that a textbook cannot provide.

# Clinical Features of Epilepsy

The clinical manifestations of epilepsy are highly variable and depend on the origin of the seizures within the central nervous system. However, there are specific characteristics of all forms of epilepsy that are independent of any classification scheme.

**Epilepsy (apart from the very rare reflex epilepsies) is:**
- An episodic disturbance
- With or without warning (aura)
- Brief
- Largely unpredictable
- Stereotyped clinical manifestations from one episode to the next
- ± Positive phenomena (not loss of function)
- ± Impaired consciousness or awareness
- ± A period of post-ictal (after the event) confusion

Epilepsy is an **episodic disturbance** of function with variable frequency from a single seizure in a lifetime to many episodes per day. Apart from reflex epilepsy (see below), attacks are **unpredictable** and can occur any time of the day or night and under any circumstance. Some patients may experience a brief warning (**aura**) lasting second only prior to the ictus. Unless a patient has more than one type of seizure, each episode is identical or almost identical **(stereotyped)** in terms of what occurs, although the duration may vary from one seizure to another. If a patient suffers from multiple types of seizures, each will have its stereotypical features. Episodes are **brief,** usually less than 1 to 3 minutes (even tonic-clonic seizures), rarely 5-10 minutes. [8] There are characteristic **positive phenomena,** i.e., abnormal movements or sensations such as smell, taste, sensory, psychic, or visual. A loss of function such as paralysis or sensory loss is NOT a feature during a seizure but may follow a seizure. This phenomenon is referred to as Todd's palsy (see below).

If post-ictal confusion and drowsiness are prolonged, this may be due to hypoxia during the seizure. It may also indicate a disease process, such as hypoglycaemic coma or infections such as meningitis and encephalitis that could cause prolonged confusion. The duration of post-ictal confusion and drowsiness is generally longer in older patients.

# The Principles of Management

- Confirmation that the patient has suffered a seizure
- Establish the type(s) of seizure(s)
- Assess the frequency of seizures
- Identify any precipitating causes
- Establish the aetiology
- Decide whether to treat or not
- Choice of the appropriate drug and dose
- Monitoring the response to therapy
- Lifestyle advice
- Consider surgery if drug therapy fails to eliminate seizures
- If and when to withdraw therapy in 'seizure-free patients

# Confirming the Patient has had a Seizure or Suffers from Epilepsy

Epilepsy is an intermittent disturbance of neurological function. Therefore, unless the seizures are frequent, it is unlikely that the clinician, routine electroencephalography (EEG) or even video-EEG telemetry will witness or capture an actual event. The diagnosis, therefore, is almost entirely dependent on the neurological history. If there is an eyewitness to the episode(s), question them; otherwise, ask the patient what they recall.

As many seizures are associated with a loss of consciousness, this will be limited to what happened before and after the ictus. The best technique in patients with suspected seizure(s) is to obtain a blow-by-blow description of the individual episode or several episodes. Concentrate on the periods immediately before (pre-ictal), during (ictus) and after (post-ictal) the event. The correct diagnosis depends on establishing the exact duration and nature of the symptoms occurring during each of these 3 phases. The alternative diagnoses that may be confused with epilepsy were covered in chapter 7.

> In patients with suspected seizure(s), the best history taking technique is to obtain a blow-by-blow description of the episode or several episodes.

Several helpful questions are discussed below.

## Useful questions to the patient.

*What were you doing just before the episode?* The precipitating factors or circumstances when the episode occurs often provide a vital clue in terms of aetiology, such as the flashing lights in a discotheque with photosensitive epilepsy or a seizure secondary to syncope during venesection.

*Was there any warning? If so, what was the exact nature of this warning, and how long did it last?* A brief warning or aura lasting only seconds is typical of epilepsy; a more prolonged warning would point to a possible alternative diagnosis.

*What was your next recollection? Can you establish how long this was after the episode commenced?* A short period of lost time, 10 minutes at most 20 minutes, is more in keeping with epilepsy.

*When you came to, were you aware of anything the matter?* A period of post-ictal drowsiness or confusion in the absence of a head injury strongly suggests epilepsy.

*Did you injure yourself?* An injury is non-specific, but a dislocated shoulder occasionally occurs with tonic-clonic seizures. An injury indicates a fall, thus reducing the number of diagnostic possibilities, as discussed in chapter seven.

*Did you bite your tongue or cheek during the episode, lose control of your bladder or bowels?* These occur with tonic-clonic seizures.

*Have you ever had any unexplained motor vehicle accidents?* An explanation may be a seizure without warning.

***When you're watching a television program that you are interested in or conversing with a person, do you ever miss parts of the program or conversation?*** An affirmative answer to this suggests the possibility of minor absence or complex-partial seizures that the patient may not have noticed. However, when patients are just sitting in front of the television, it would be not uncommon for lack of concentration to miss parts of the program. On the other hand, if it interrupts a program that the patient is particularly interested in, it is more likely to be a minor seizure

***Do people accuse you of being a daydreamer?*** It is not uncommon for children and adolescents to be thought of as daydreamers when in fact they have been having unrecognised minor seizures. It is also not unusual for children and teenagers to daydream, so interpret the answer to this question with caution. If the patient has suffered from repeated episodes, establish if every episode is identical or whether there may be different types of seizures. Detailed questioning of several other events is necessary.

***Have you ever been able to prevent one of these episodes? If so, how?*** It is possible to avert the seizure secondary to syncope or hypotension if the patient assumes a recumbent posture immediately after they experience the 1st warning[1].

## Useful Questions of an Eyewitness or Relative.

Some patients can suffer unrecognised seizures for many years, [9] particularly children and teenagers thought to be daydreaming. Relatives may have witnessed many episodes and not recognised them as seizures. A useful sequence of questions includes:

***What was the patient doing at the time the episode commenced?***

***What was the first thing that you noticed, and how long did it last?***

***What was the next thing that you noticed, and how long did it last?***

***What was the next thing that you noticed, and how long did it last?***

Keep asking this question until the whole episode has been described. More specific questions include:

***During the episode, was the patient able to hear what you were saying or were they out to it or switched off?*** If the answer is no, this indicates a loss of awareness, suggesting a generalised seizure or complex-partial seizure.

***Did you see any excessive blinking or abnormal chewing movements of the mouth?*** These occur with absence and complex-partial seizures, respectively.

***Have you ever seen the patient suddenly interrupt what they were doing and stare into space, where their eyes were open, but they did not respond to you?*** If the answer is yes, this is in keeping with absence or complex-partial seizures.

It is often helpful to question more than one eyewitness or relative as one individual may not have observed all the details. When seeing a patient with suspected epilepsy or a seizure, more is gained by picking up the telephone and ringing a family member or eyewitness rather than undertaking investigations.

1   Very rarely patients with epilepsy can suppress a seizure.

> 🔑
> As a rule, the longer the duration, the more complex and varied the behaviour during an episode and the more varied the symptoms from one episode to the next the less likely one is dealing with a seizure disorder

# Epilepsy in the Elderly

It is a common misconception that epilepsy is a childhood disease. This statement is true with absence (petit-mal) seizures that are rarely seen in adults. If they occur in adults, the presentation is with absence status epilepsy. Other types of seizures happen in the elderly, and the incidence increases with increasing age, as shown in figure 8.1. Elderly patients with epilepsy most often present with complex partial seizures with a higher recurrence rate than the younger population. The episodes are often difficult to diagnose since they show atypical symptoms, particularly prolonged post-ictal symptoms, including memory lapses, confusion, altered mental status, and inattention. [10]

Although there is a continuing incidence of seizures throughout life, they are more common in the first five years. There is also a higher incidence in the 70 to 80-year-old age group. [11]

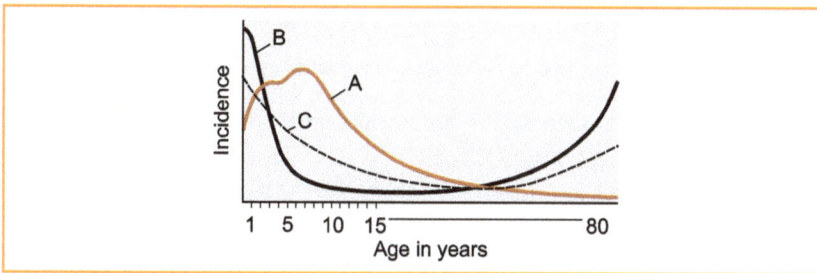

**Figure 8.1 Incidence of epilepsy with age** (Reproduced *Anderson, VE: Family studies of epilepsy. In Genetic Basis of the Epilepsies. Edited by VE Anderson, WA Hauser, JK Penry and CF Sing. New York: Raven Press, 1982, pp 103-112.* [11]) [2]

> 🔑
> Seizures can occur in any age group and of either sex.

# Establish the Type(s) of Seizure(s)

The International League Against Epilepsy (ILAE) has altered the classification of seizures and epilepsy syndromes. [108] The ILAE advocates (a) establishing the type of the individual seizure(s) (generalised, focal, or unknown), (b) the type of epilepsy (focal, generalised, combined focal and generalised and unknown) and (c) the epilepsy syndrome. The next step is to establish the aetiology of epilepsy/seizures (structural, genetic, infectious, metabolic, immune, and unknown)

---

2  The caption was incorrect in the 1st edition. Although the illustration is in Engels book [12] is was reproduced from Andersons book chapter. [11]

and assess any co-morbidities. Generalised epilepsy includes absence, myoclonic, atonic, tonic and tonic-clonic seizures. An interictal (between seizures) EEG can show generalised spike-wave activity in patients with primary generalised epilepsy.

The clinical manifestations of the more common types of seizures are discussed. More detail can be found in textbooks. [12–14] In clinical practice, the more common seizures are:

- Tonic-clonic (previously called grand-mal)
- absence and (previously called petit-mal)
- complex-partial seizures. (previously called temporal lobe)

Less common are:
- simple-partial (now called Focal Onset Aware)
- myoclonic
- clonic
- tonic
- atonic and
- benign rolandic seizures.

Although the traditional approach is to classify seizure as focal vs generalised or primary (no apparent cause) vs secondary, the simplest and the most useful way to characterise the various types of seizures in terms of making a diagnosis is based on what is witnessed during an episode and divide them into:

1. Seizures that cause the patient to fall with or without loss of consciousness and

2. Seizures that are not associated with a fall with or without loss of consciousness (awareness) See figures 8.2 and 8.43

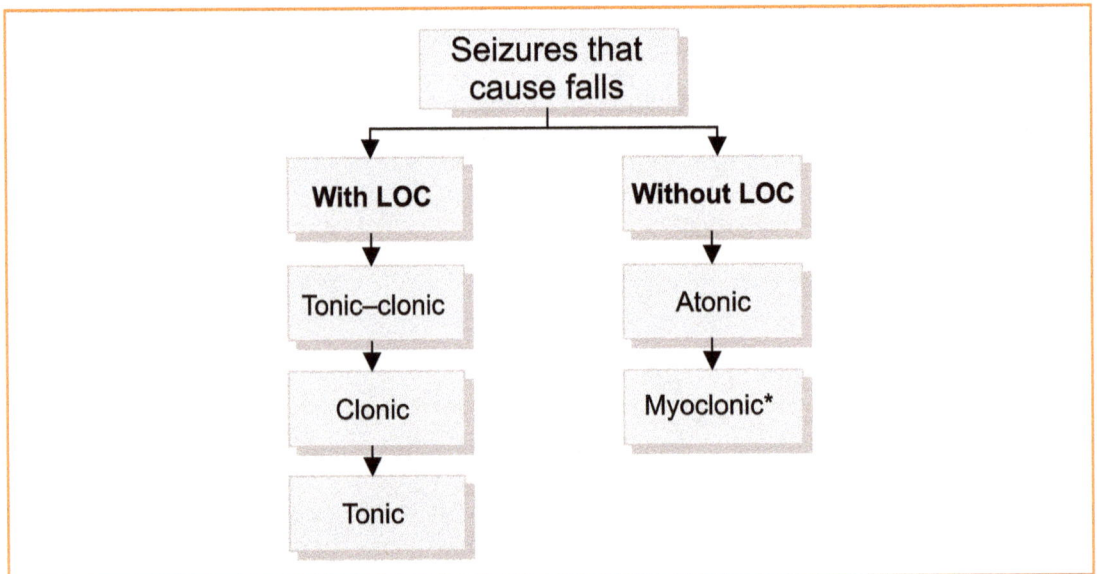

**Figure 8.2** Seizures that result in a fall with or without loss of consciousness * A fall will result if the patient is standing and the myoclonus affects the legs. Patients with brief focal myoclonic seizures do not fall if seated. Abbreviations LOC = loss of consciousness. The new terminology is in appendix C.

# Tonic-Clonic Seizures (Generalised Onset-Motor-Tonic-Clonic)

A tonic-clonic seizure will cause the patient to fall to the ground with or without warning (an aura). They are rigid with their teeth clenched, arms and legs extended, and eyes open. At times arms may be flexed instead of extended. Many eyewitnesses describe the eyes as rolling up into the top of the head, which means that the eyes are open. This tonic phase is brief, usually less than 30 seconds, followed by repetitive jerking (clonic phase) of the arms and legs, also brief, less than 1 or 2 minutes although may be prolonged, anything up to 10 minutes. Seizures may last longer if the patient develops recurrent (status epilepsy) seizures without recovering consciousness between seizures. There is a variable period of post-ictal confusion and drowsiness.

During a tonic-clonic seizure, the patient may bite their tongue or cheek, froth at the mouth or be incontinent of urine and or faeces. If urinary or faecal incontinence occurs, it is during the tonic phase.

Immediately following the seizure, the patient is limp, drowsy, and confused. This post-ictal confusion and drowsiness period vary depending on the seizure duration and the patient's age. The post-ictal period is longer in older adults. If seizures are brief, the duration of the post-ictal drowsiness and confusion may be less than a few minutes; with more prolonged seizures, the period of confusion can last much longer, usually less than ½ hour. In the elderly, the post-ictal period may last for several days without any obvious metabolic or infective process to account for such confusion. Very rarely, paralysis of a limb(s) follows a seizure, an entity called Todd's palsy. Once again, this tends to be more prolonged in the elderly.

# Focal Onset with Secondary Generalisation (Focal to Bilateral Seizure)

This term refers to patients who experience warning symptoms or aura before the tonic-clonic seizure. The aura (discussed below) indicates a focal onset, and the nature of the symptoms reflects the site of origin of the seizure within the cerebral hemispheres. [117]

# Tonic Seizures (Generalised Onset-Motor-Tonic)

Although these can occur at any age, they are more common in childhood. When an adult has a tonic seizure, it is usually the result of a hypotensive episode, e.g. Vasovagal syncope or a Stokes-Adams attack. Tonic contractions affect the face and limbs, resulting in flexion of the upper limbs and trunk and either flexion or extension of the lower limb; consciousness is minimally or not at all impaired. These seizures are very brief, often lasting only seconds. It is rare for these to occur in isolation, and usually, patients have other types of seizures.

# Atonic Seizures (Generalised Onset-Motor-Atonic)

Atonic seizures, also referred to as drop attacks, are rare and consist of a sudden loss of postural tone; if brief, only the head may drop, but if more severe, the person will fall to the floor, often causing injury. There may be a brief period of impaired consciousness lasting seconds only. There is no post-ictal confusion. Patients usually have other seizure types, including brief myoclonic jerks that can occur just before the atonic seizure. Most often, they also have tonic-clonic epilepsy. Drop attacks due to epilepsy mainly occur in children with the Lennox-Gastaut syndrome. This consists of multiple seizure types, including myoclonic, tonic-clonic, atonic and atypical absence seizures. There is often a degree of intellectual disability. [5]

## Myoclonic Seizures (Generalised Onset-Myoclonic)

Myoclonus is a shock-like contraction of a muscle or a group of muscles. Myoclonus occurs in people without epilepsy, often when they are just falling asleep and occasionally at any time of the day. The frequency would usually be less than once a month. In patients with myoclonic epilepsy, these myoclonic jerks are more frequent, may occur in sleep but characteristically manifest first thing in the morning on awakening. They affect the whole body or a single limb and may appear as a single jerk, or there may be repetitive jerks. There is an entity called segmental myoclonus that is not a seizure disorder. It is where a particular muscle or group of muscles supplied by a specific nerve or nerve root will have myoclonic jerks. In myoclonic seizures the patient is fully aware of what is happening. There is no aura, no loss of awareness and no post-ictal confusion, i.e., the patient, feels normal immediately before and after the event. Myoclonus induced by movement is a feature of post-hypoxic myoclonus. [15]

## Juvenile Myoclonic Epilepsy Syndrome

Juvenile myoclonic epilepsy (JME) consists of a variable combination of myoclonus, absence seizures and infrequent tonic-clonic seizures. Patients usually present between the ages of 6 and 22. It is essential to identify patients with this syndrome as they respond well to Valproic Acid and Lamotrigine, but experience increased seizures with Phenytoin and Carbamazepine. There is a lifelong predisposition to recurrent seizures without treatment. [16-17]

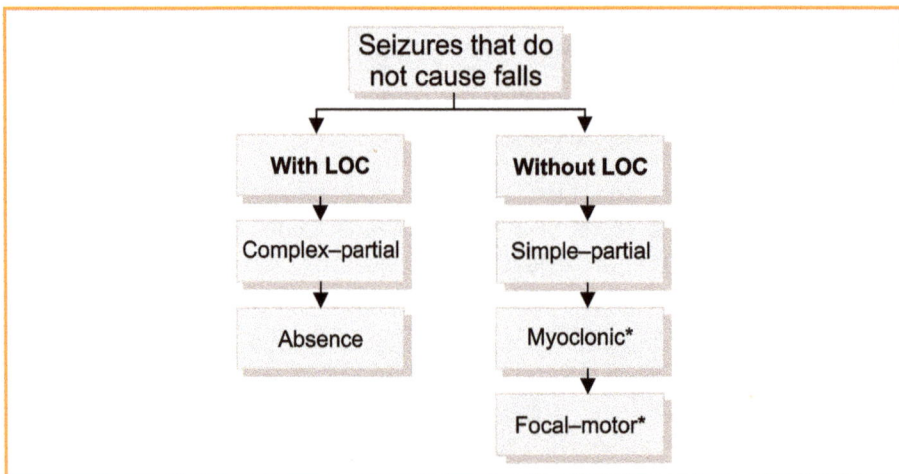

**Figure 8.3.** Seizures that do not cause a fall with or without loss of consciousness (LOC). * Patients with myoclonic or focal-motor seizures may fall if standing, but there is no LOC. (see appendix C for the new terminology).

# Complex-Partial Seizures (Focal-Onset Impaired Awareness)

Complex-partial epilepsy (CPE) was originally called temporal lobe epilepsy. However, the recognition that minor seizures that impair consciousness without causing the patient to fall may arise from the occipital, frontal or parietal lobes has led to the use of the term CPE. The new terminology is focal-onset impaired awareness.

## The Aura

The aura is brief, lasting between a few seconds and two minutes. The symptoms that occur during the aura reflect the origin of the seizure within the hemisphere. [117] Déjà vu, jamais vu, unpleasant olfactory (smell), or gustatory (taste) phenomena suggest mesial temporal sclerosis and temporal lobe origin. Vertigo, auditory (buzzing, ringing), or visual symptoms occur with lateral temporal sclerosis. Visual auras indicate occipital or parietal lobe origin. It can also be an unpleasant feeling commencing in the epigastrium and rapidly rising over a few seconds towards the head. Alternatively, it may be non-specific light headedness or an odd feeling in the head. The essential feature is that the aura is identical each time and, more importantly, very brief, usually lasting seconds only.

During the ictus of a complex partial seizure, the patient is unaware of what is happening, nor can they respond to any verbal or painful stimuli. Afterwards, they cannot relate what happened during the event. In the words of two relatives with minor seizures, "the lights were on, but no-one was at home, or there were no sheep in the top paddock". There may be involuntary movements of the mouth or limbs. The ictus lasts seconds to a few minutes and the period of post-ictal confusion can last several minutes. The patient can generally respond to outside stimuli but is disoriented and confused in the post-ictal period. [18] Complex-partial seizures most commonly arise from the temporal lobe associated with mesial temporal sclerosis.

# Absence (Petit-Mal) Seizures (Generalised Onset-Non-Motor-Typical Absence)

Absence epilepsy generally occurs in childhood and is rare in adults. Many patients presenting with their first tonic-clonic seizure, have had unrecognised absence seizures in childhood. They have been regarded as either dull or a daydreamer. [9] No warning characterises the absence seizure unless it is an atypical absence (see below). The period of impaired consciousness is brief. In one study, the average seizure duration was 9.4 seconds (range 1 to 44 seconds, SD 7 seconds); 72 seizures (26%) were shorter than 4 seconds, and 23 seizures (8%) were longer than 20 seconds. [19] The patient stares into space, they may blink, but they are unresponsive to verbal or painful stimuli. They have no recollection of what happened or what was said to them during the episode. Immediately following the ictus, the patient can resume their conversation or activity without any post-ictal confusion. It is surprising how many absence seizures patients can experience without people noticing them. Absence seizures can be induced by hyperventilation (HV). In one study of 47 children an absence seizure was induced in 83% (39/47) with hyperventilation. Of the eight children who did not have seizures provoked by HV, four were too young to perform HV. In the other four children, HV may not have been executed correctly. [19]

Suddenly interrupting their behaviour is the vital clue that differentiates absence seizures from daydreaming. They may momentarily pause unexpectedly during a conversation or a game and then appear to resume it as if nothing had happened. Many children daydream, and it can be difficult to attract their attention when watching television or playing a game on an electronic device. One common presentation of absence epilepsy is the child who has previously done well at school and then fails. Unfortunately, these children are assumed to be daydreamers and not working hard enough. The reality is that they were missing large parts of the lesson because of minor absence seizures. In the author's experience, many teachers fail to detect children in their class with minor epilepsy. Only when these children have a private tutor, the seizures are witnessed, and the correct diagnosis is made.

The EEG in absence seizures shows a characteristic 3 per second spike and wave. (Figure 8.4)

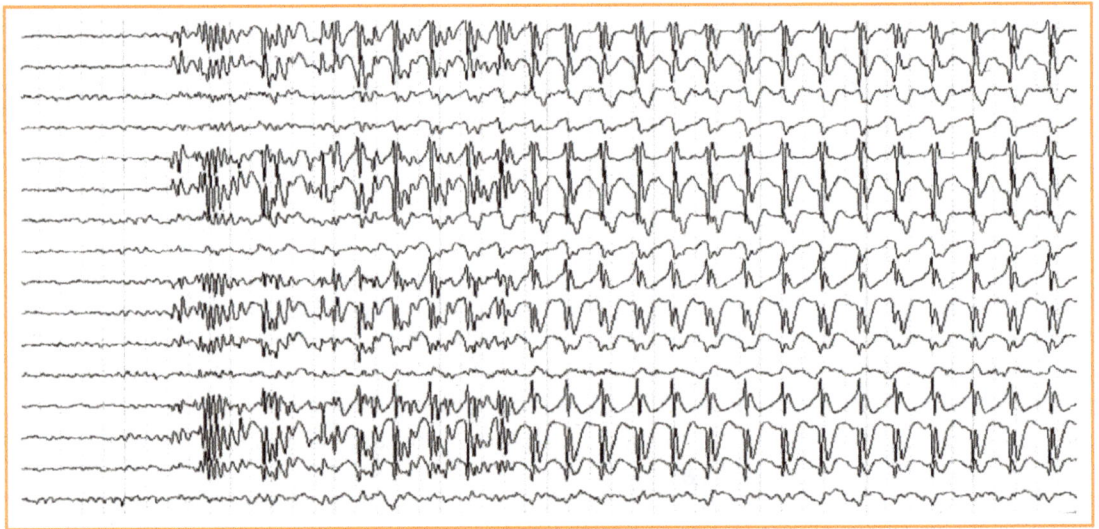

**Figure 8.4** EEG in absence epilepsy showing 3 per second spike and wave.

# Simple-Partial Seizures (Focal Onset-Aware-Non-Motor)

Simple partial (focal aware) seizures can occur at any age in either sex. They consist of a brief stereotyped sensation without loss of awareness. The patient is fully conscious of what is happening to them and can describe the whole episode from start to finish. There is no aura and no post-ictal drowsiness or confusion. Examples of this type of epilepsy are patients who experience a tingling sensation that may commence in their feet and rise to the top of the head over a matter of seconds. Some patients can experience what appears to be recurrent focal aware seizures for many years, when in fact, it was the aura to their seizure. This fact only becomes evident when they have a tonic-clonic seizure immediately following an episode. I have seen other patients diagnosed with panic attacks because their recurrent aura's were very unusual. One example was a woman who repeatedly wrung her hands for a minute or two, feeling anxious during the episode and remaining fully conscious. The vital clue was that the episodes were brief and stereotyped, the classical feature of an organic illness instead of a functional or non-organic illness. In functional illnesses, symptoms vary in duration, intensity, and content during and from one event to another.

# Focal-Motor Seizures
# (Focal Onset-Aware-Motor-Hyperkinetic)

Focal-motor seizures are very brief, usually lasting less than a minute or two. However, they can go on repetitively in patients, in which case it is termed focal motor status epilepsy. The patient is fully aware of what is going on around them. There is usually no warning. Indeed, there is no post-ictal drowsiness or confusion. Focal-motor seizures manifest as repetitive contractions of a limb(s) down one side of the body.

# Benign Focal Seizures of Childhood

There are several benign focal seizures of childhood. [20, 21] There are currently three identifiable electroclinical syndromes recognised by the International League against Epilepsy (ILAE) [22]: rolandic epilepsy, Panayiotopoulos syndrome (P.S.), common autonomic epilepsy and the idiopathic childhood occipital epilepsy of Gastaut (ICOE-G). They produce terrifying manifestations. They appear as an appendix to this chapter because they are rare. They are atypical, with symptoms lasting longer than most other seizure types.

# Febrile Convulsions

Febrile convulsions affect 2–5% of all children, usually appearing between three months and five years of age. Febrile convulsions may be provoked by any febrile bacterial or viral illness, and no specific level of fever is required to diagnose febrile seizures. It is essential to consider meningitis or encephalitis in patients presenting with seizures and fever. The risk of epilepsy following a febrile seizure is 1–6%. [23]

# Reflex Epilepsies

Reflex epilepsies although rare, are discussed to familiarise the reader with this entity. The clue to the clinical diagnosis would be the repeated precipitation of a brief stereotyped episode by a particular stimulus. One of the commonest is the tonic-clonic seizure precipitated by the stroboscope at a dance. Reflex epilepsies are syndromes in which sensory stimuli precipitate all epileptic seizures. Generalised reflex seizures are precipitated by visual light stimulation, thinking, and decision making. Numerous triggers, such as reading, writing, other language functions, startle, somatosensory stimulation, proprioception, auditory stimuli, immersion in hot water, eating, and vestibular stimulation, can induce focal reflex seizures. [24]

# Consider Possible Multiple Seizure Types

Having established that the patient has suffered a seizure, the next step is to assess for previously undiagnosed seizures. Although most patients who present with their first tonic-clonic seizure have not had other manifestations of epilepsy, with detailed questioning, it is not uncommon for patients to have had unrecognised myoclonic seizures and or minor absence or complex-partial seizures in the past. [9]

Most seizures conform to the common seizure types listed above, and the diagnosis rarely presents any difficulty. On the other hand, rare cases where the events during the ictus are most atypical can lead to an erroneous diagnosis of a non-organic event. Consider the following actual case history where the principles discussed earlier in this chapter are highlighted.

| A 25-year-old man with bizarre behaviour |
| --- |
| He had recurrent episodes lasting less than a minute or two. He had been witnessed to walk across a room and shake whoever was in the room a few times. After this, he was confused for a few more minutes and stated that he did not recall what happened. |
| Although this patient exhibited bizarre behaviour, the episodes were stereotyped, brief lasting less than 90 seconds. During the attack, there were positive phenomena in that he walked, grabbed people, and shook them; he lost awareness and was amnestic. It was followed by a short period of post-ictal confusion. Subsequent video-EEG monitoring confirmed that these episodes were complex-partial seizures. |

## Pseudoseizures

Pseudoseizures[3] are episodes of changes in behaviour that resemble epileptic seizures but are without organic cause and expected EEG changes. They are also referred to as non-epileptic seizures. Longer ictal duration, less stereotypy (the variation of the manifestations from one episode to the next) is characteristic. Other features of pseudoseizures include; asynchronous extremity movements, atypical vocalisation, alternating head movements, talking or screaming, opisthotonic posturing (arching of back) and pelvic thrusting[4].[25] An increasing frequency of 'seizures' with escalating doses of anticonvulsants should alert the clinician to this diagnoses. [26]

The management of patients with pseudoseizures can be challenging as up to 30% have epileptic seizures. Pelvic thrusting has been described as a rare manifestation of temporal lobe or frontal lobe epilepsy. [27] The diagnosis of psychogenic pseudoseizures is easier if video-electroencephalography monitoring is available. [28]

If pseudoseizures are suspected, there is one way to confirm the diagnosis. Instruct family members, nursing staff on the ward or anyone who may witness an episode to try and interrupt what is happening either by talking to the patient or using a painful stimulus, e.g., pinching the skin over the medial aspect of the elbow with ones fingernails. Organic, as opposed to pseudoseizures, cannot be interrupted.

## Assessing the Frequency of Seizures
## The Patient with their "First Seizure"

It is not uncommon to see patients with their first apparent tonic-clonic seizure, who have had a previous seizure or a long history of unrecognised minor seizures or myoclonus. [9] The patient should be asked if they have frequent involuntary brief jerking of one limb or the entire body, like when they are falling asleep. These involuntary jerks, termed myoclonus, occur infrequently, perhaps a few times per year in normal individuals. In patients with epilepsy, they occur far more

---

3   It is this author's personal experience that many females with non-epileptic seizures have suffered sexual molestation.
4   Pelvic thrusting, bicycling movements, asymmetric tonic posturing, sexual automatisms, bizarre behaviour and vocalizations can occur in frontal lobe epilepsy. The clue once again is that they are identical with every episode.

frequently and often first thing in the morning upon awakening. Although the patient is very aware of these myoclonic jerks, they interfere so little with their life that often they do not seek medical attention. Similarly, minor seizures may go undetected or undiagnosed for years. Often detailed questioning of relatives or friends using the questions described above will elicit a prior history of previously unrecognised minor seizures.

## Status Epilepsy

Status epilepticus is a seizure that "persists for a sufficient length of time or is repeated frequently enough that recovery between attacks does not occur." Both convulsive and non-convulsive status epilepsy occurs.

## Convulsive Status Epilepsy

Status tonic-clonic (convulsive) epilepsy is continuous or rapidly repeating seizures and is a medical emergency. **The treating physician should not leave the bedside until seizures cease.** There are published guidelines for the management of status epilepsy.[29-31] Guidelines are often updated, and every institution should have access to them. Patients who do not respond to initial therapy should be treated in an intensive care unit, as artificial ventilation and haemodynamic support are required.

## Non-convulsive Status Epilepsy

Non-convulsive status epilepsy is an epileptic state in which some impairment of consciousness or awareness is associated with ongoing seizure activity on the EEG. [32] It is often a sequel to convulsive status epilepsy. [32] Patients may present in a coma without any overt signs of seizure activity, [33] or present in a state of confusion during which they cannot respond to external stimuli such as talking to them to try and alter their behaviour.

## Identify Precipitating Causes for Seizures.

Identifying a reversible precipitating cause is vital as avoidance in the future can reduce the risk of subsequent seizures. Most seizures occur at any time of the day or night without a precipitating cause. Seizures can be secondary to hypotension with syncope or StokesAdams attack. They can occur with alcohol abuse or withdrawal and sedative or hypnotic drug withdrawal. In patients with epilepsy, sleep deprivation, photic stimulation, alcohol abuse [34], menstruation, and an intercurrent infective illness may predispose them to a seizure. [35] Vomiting or diarrhoea alter drug levels predisposing to recurrent seizures, and many drugs, including psychotropics, local and general anaesthetics, narcotics, antiarrhythmics and antibiotics, are recognised precipitating causes of seizures. [36] Poor compliance is one, if not the most common cause of recurrent seizures in patients on anticonvulsants. [34] Fortunately, antidepressants in therapeutic doses do not appear to trigger seizures. [114] This is important as depression is common in patients with epilepsy.

# Establishing an Aetiology

Most patients with epilepsy do not have any identifiable underlying pathology. These patients have primary generalised epilepsy. It is possible that with future advancements in the understanding of epilepsy, a cause may be identified. Focal-motor seizures, complex-partial seizures, and seizures associated with a focal neurological deficit are more likely to have identifiable pathology on imaging.[37] Seizures may occur with alcohol or drug withdrawal, infective processes within the central nervous system, drugs, benign and malignant tumours, just to mention a few possible aetiologies. Seizures can be the presenting symptom of disturbances of cardiac rhythm [38] or rarely secondary to severe pain, for example, in patients with trigeminal neuralgia.[39] Detailed lists can be found in textbooks on epilepsy. [5-7, 14, 40, 41] This means that it is impossible to be dogmatic about what investigation should be performed in an individual patient suffice to say that every effort should be made to establish a cause for their epilepsy.

---

A word of warning; the presence of a family history of epilepsy or a history of a head injury suggests that the seizure may be on a familial or post-traumatic basis, but other pathological processes need to be considered.

---

Some would argue that it is justifiable to perform medical imaging of all adult patients with tonic-clonic, complex-partial and focal motor seizures. [42], [43] Others would argue that there is currently insufficient data to justify or refute undertaking any of these tests for the routine evaluation of adults presenting with an apparent first unprovoked seizure. [43] The reality is that most patients insist on an MRI or CT scan of their brain. The yield of currently available imaging techniques is about 10%. Laboratory tests, such as blood counts, blood glucose, electrolytes (particularly sodium), lumbar puncture, and toxicology screening, may be helpful in the individual patient as determined by the specific clinical circumstances based on the history and physical and neurologic examination. Although metabolic disturbances causing seizures are rare, they are readily correctable, particularly hypoglycaemia. When a patient presents with a seizure, the most critical test to perform immediately is serum glucose to exclude hypoglycaemia. Other metabolic disturbances such as hyponatraemia, hypocalcaemia and elevated urea may cause seizures. As a general principle, these investigations are without risk, and the subsequent management is easy, and it would seem reasonable to exclude metabolic causes in all patients.

# Investigations

Current recommendations advocate an EEG, CT or MRI brain in all patients presenting with a 1st unprovoked seizure. [43] Laboratory tests, such as blood counts, blood glucose, and electrolytes, particularly sodium, lumbar puncture, and toxicology screening, may be helpful as determined by the specific clinical circumstances based on the history, physical, and neurologic examination. There is insufficient data to support or refute recommending any of these tests for the routine evaluation of adults presenting with an apparent first unprovoked seizure. [43]

# Deciding Whether to Treat or Not

In many patients with simple partial seizures, reassurance that nothing sinister is the matter suffices, and they may not wish to take medication to stop such trivial symptoms. In patients with an isolated idiopathic (unknown cause) tonic-clonic seizure, the subsequent risk of further seizures varies from study to study. In one study of children, it was 54% [44], whilst in another study of adults, there was a 27 per cent risk of recurrence at 36 months [45]. A first seizure provoked by an acute brain disturbance is unlikely to recur (3–10%), whereas a first unprovoked seizure has a 30-50% recurrence risk over the next two years.[46] The number of seizures of all types at presentation, the presence of a neurological disorder and an abnormal electroencephalogram are significant risk factors for recurrent seizures.

An abnormal EEG was defined as specific focal or generalised epileptiform or slow-wave abnormality. Individuals with two or three seizures plus a neurological disorder and or an abnormal EEG were identified as a high-risk group with a 73% incidence of recurrent episodes at five years. [47] In the same study, the recurrence rate at five years in patients with a single seizure, a normal EEG and no neurological abnormality was 39 %.[47]

In a study of immediate versus delayed treatment with currently available anticonvulsants, immediate treatment did not reduce the long-term recurrence rate. At 5-years follow-up, 76% of patients in the immediate treatment group and 77% of those in the deferred treatment group were seizure-free (difference -0.2%, 95% CI -5.8% to 5.5%). [48] Many patients elect not to take antiepileptic drug treatment after a first seizure when informed of a low risk of recurrence. [46] Therefore, it would seem reasonable not to recommend therapy in patients with an isolated tonic-clonic seizure without a positive family history, an abnormal EEG, and no pre-existing cerebral pathology. This is especially so if there was an easily reversible precipitating cause such as sleep deprivation.

The patient in this situation often decides. The question to put to the patient is, "what effect another seizure would have on their life?" The most typical reason patients state for wanting to go onto medication is that a further seizure would terrify them. However, more often, it has unacceptable social implications and the effect on their ability to drive and thus access employment influences their decision whether to take medication or not. Getting to work is a primary reason why some patients continue to drive against medical advice. [49]

Occasional patients can have two seizures many years apart. If the patient had been placed on medication after the first seizure, the clinician would have regarded the treatment as excellent when the natural history was such that the patient would not experience a second seizure for many years. In general, antiepileptic drugs (AEDs) should be offered after a first tonic-clonic seizure if:
- the patient has had previous myoclonic, absence or partial seizures
- the EEG shows unequivocal epileptic discharges
- the patient has a congenital neurological deficit
- the patient considers the risk of recurrence unacceptable

# Choosing the Appropriate Drug, Dose and Ongoing Monitoring of the Response to Therapy
## Choosing a Drug

Treatment is targeted primarily to assist the patient in adjusting psychologically to the diagnosis and maintaining as normal a lifestyle as possible, reducing or eliminating seizures and avoiding or minimising the side effects of long-term drug treatment.

Most patients with more than one seizure require prophylactic antiepileptic drug (AED) therapy. Some seizure types or epilepsy syndromes may respond to certain medications, while others may exacerbate the seizures. [50-51]

The general principle is to choose the drug with the greatest efficacy in preventing seizures, provided there is no contraindication to its use. If there are several possible drugs, then the "correct drug" is the drug the patient deems to have the least undesirable potential side effects from their perspective. e.g., the risk of weight gain or interference with the oral contraceptive are common reasons young females refuse a particular drug. Side effects are a significant reason for discontinuing an AED, particularly in the elderly. [52]

Patients can only decide when they receive detailed information regarding the proposed treatment options.

Failure of the first AED due to lack of efficacy (and not due to incorrect choice of drug, wrong dose, incorrect dosing schedule or poor compliance) implies refractoriness and trying multiple AED one after another is unlikely to be successful. [53] Thus, if the first or second monotherapy improves control but does not produce seizure freedom, another AED with different mechanisms of action should be added. Strategies for combining drugs should involve an individual assessment of the patient's seizure type and an understanding of the pharmacology, side-effects and interaction profile of the AED. [54]

An important principle when altering therapeutic regimes is to **avoid changing two things simultaneously**. It is difficult to know what has done the good or harm in this situation.

When monotherapy does not control seizures, review the diagnosis of epilepsy and check for compliance with medication. Combination therapy should be considered when treatment with two first-line AEDs has failed or when the first well-tolerated drug substantially improves seizure control but fails at maximal dosage to produce seizure freedom. The choice of drugs to use in combination should be matched to the patient's seizure type(s) and should be limited to two or at most three AED's.

Current treatment recommendations and the potential side effects of the specific drugs are in Appendix II. Links to websites that should provide more up to date information are in chapter 15.

## Choosing the Dose

Other than status epilepsy, there is no need to reach a therapeutic dose rapidly. Treatment can commence with the lowest possible dose and increase very slowly over weeks, reducing the incidence of side effects. [55, 56] The number of doses per day is dependent on the half-life of the drug, but medications prescribed more than twice a day are associated with an increased incidence of poor compliance. [57]

# Monitoring the Response

In many patients, complete freedom from seizures is not possible and sensible decisions regarding medication efficacy can only be made with careful assessment of seizure frequency. Seizure frequency has a significant impact on quality of life. [58] and although it is recommended that patients keep a diary to record the frequency of their seizures, very few do. The treating physician needs to keep detailed notes on behalf of the patient and refer to these notes when deciding if a particular anticonvulsant has effectively reduced the number of seizures. Monitoring the response to treatment at times can be extraordinarily difficult, particularly in young patients who, through embarrassment, will often deny forgetting their medication, drinking too much alcohol, or staying out all night. Technically savvy patients could be encouraged to purchase one of the many epilepsy apps to help record their seizures.

# Intractable Epilepsy

One of the significant difficulties in patients with intractable epilepsy is their failure to keep accurate records. They don't know the names of the drugs, the maximum dose tried and whether the drug was stopped due to an apparent lack of efficacy or because of side effects. The lack of efficacy may relate to an incorrect choice of drug or drug dosage and frequency of administration, i.e., giving a drug twice a day when the half-life is only 8 hours. It is helpful to show patients pictures of the specific drugs to identify the drug(s) they have taken. Unfortunately, even when they can identify the drug, they are usually unaware of the dose tried, the frequency of dosing and the reason for stopping it.

There are two reasons why it is helpful to advise patients to keep a diary of the date and time of any seizures. Firstly, one can see a decrease in the frequency of their seizures when therapy is modified. Secondly, a more important purpose is to see what time of the day the seizures occur with the timing of medication. Although compliance is better when drugs are prescribed less frequently, in patients on a twice-daily dosage regime, some patients will experience seizures in the hour or two before or within the first ½ hour after the dose because the drug's half-life is less than 12 hours. Simply increasing the individual dose in this setting results in symptoms of toxicity as the peak serum level increases but then falls below the threshold for the patient's seizures just before the next dose. The appropriate course of action is to increase the frequency of the medication if the drug has a half-life of 8 to 12 hours or change the patient to a drug that has a longer half-life.

Unfortunately, with many drugs, there is a 'honeymoon period' during the first six months of treatment where the number of seizures decreases but subsequently become just as frequent again.

# Measuring Serum Levels

Serum AED measurements are helpful when the level directly reflects efficacy; this is not the case for all drugs. Other clinical situations where AED monitoring is appropriate include checking for compliance or toxicity as a guide to adjusting the dose when another drug is added and during pregnancy, where drug levels fall in the 3rd trimester. [59]

# Advice Regarding Lifestyle
## Driving and Epilepsy

Each country has different regulations regarding driving and epilepsy. It is essential for all clinicians who care for patients with epilepsy to have a copy of their respective country's (or state's) guidelines. In more recent years, restrictions have been less stringent, reflecting the low contribution of seizures to the overall road toll. [60] In some countries, the restriction on driving is very severe whereas, in others, a more lenient approach is taken. Essentially a sufficient period needs to elapse to ensure that a recurrent seizure is unlikely to occur. In one study, patients who had seizure-free intervals > or = 12 months, had 93% reduced odds of crashing than patients with shorter intervals.

The majority (54%) of patients with epilepsy who were driving and caused an accident were driving illegally, with seizure-free intervals shorter than legally permitted. [61] Another 20% had missed an AED dose just before the crash. Patients should be told that although the risk of a seizure whilst driving is small, the potential consequences could be disastrous. It is also helpful to show patients the guidelines, explaining that the medical practitioner does not make the rules. Explain that these rules are not there to punish patients with epilepsy but protect them from hurting themselves or innocent people.

The risk of a seizure occurring whilst driving reflects the time spent driving each day. If the patient drives for only ½ an hour per day, the risk of a seizure whilst driving is much less than if they drive for 12 hours per day. The requirements are more stringent for commercial and heavy goods vehicle licenses in many countries than private motor vehicle licenses. [62]

## Pregnancy and Epilepsy

Although the increased risk of major congenital malformations in patients with epilepsy taking AED during pregnancy is possibly 2–3 times that of the average population [63], most pregnancies will result in a normal child. There is debate about the exact role of AED exposure in pregnancy and the increased risk. [64] Certain specific anticonvulsants and the use of multiple anticonvulsants (polypharmacy) may be associated with a greater risk. [65] [66, 67] Long term cognitive problems in the child may also occur. [65]

In clinical practice, many patients attend their doctor to discuss medication withdrawal when they are already 2–3 months pregnant! Any teratogenic effects will have already occurred, and it is probably unwise and essentially too late to withdraw medication at this stage of the pregnancy. The risk of uncontrolled seizures during pregnancy needs to be weighed against the risk of AED exposure. An increased risk to the mother and infant is oft quoted but finding good evidence to justify this statement is problematic. In the European Registry of Antiepileptic Drugs and Pregnancy (EURAP) study, an international antiepileptic drugs (AEDs) and pregnancy registry of 1,956 pregnancies, 58.3% were seizure-free throughout pregnancy. Seizures occurred during delivery in 60 pregnancies (3.5%), more commonly in women with seizures during pregnancy (OR: 4.8; 2.3 to 10.0). There were 36 cases of status epilepticus (12 convulsive), which resulted in stillbirth in only one case but no cases of miscarriage or maternal mortality. [68] A Cochrane review has concluded that it would seem advisable for women to continue medication during pregnancy using monotherapy at the lowest dose required to achieve seizure control based on the best currently available evidence.[65]

Some patients seek advice about ceasing their anticonvulsants before pregnancy, so the decision is more complicated. Even if the epilepsy was easily controlled, the patient must be willing to run the risk of a recurrent seizure and the subsequent consequences of altering their lifestyle, particularly driving. In general, if epilepsy has been challenging to control, an argument can be made for the patient to remain on medication throughout the pregnancy. Accumulating evidence from drug registries suggest that the lowest possible dose and avoidance of certain drugs may be appropriate. [68] [69, 70] Patients willing to consider a mid-trimester termination can have testing for significant malformations.

Some patients may experience an increased seizure frequency, whilst others have fewer seizures. [71] Occasionally patients not known to suffer from epilepsy have a tonic-clonic seizure during labour.[5] Other severe disorders need to be considered, but a detailed history will often elicit a long history of infrequent minor and previously unrecognised seizures. Most patients with epilepsy will maintain control during pregnancy. [71]

## Avoiding Hazardous Activities

Patients should be warned that in addition to risks of driving that it may be dangerous to go swimming or fishing, have a bath or walk near water if they are alone as a seizure could result in drowning. [72] Patients should also be advised not to scale heights, walk near the edge of cliffs, skydive or scuba dive.

## Surgery When Medical Therapy Fails.

Approximately one-third of patients with epilepsy are refractory to antiepileptic drug therapy; many of these patients are candidates for surgical treatment. [73] Among patients who do not respond to the first drug, the percentage who subsequently became seizure-free with a 2nd or 3rd drug is smaller (11 per cent). [53] Patients with refractory epilepsy[6] should be referred to an appropriate centre earlier than later for potential surgery. Unfortunately, less than 1% of those who could benefit are referred to comprehensive epilepsy centres for evaluation.[109] A good outcome occurs in 65% of patients with drug-resistant epilepsy. [110] The best results are seen in patients shown to have seizures arising out of a structural abnormality detected on imaging, [111]

Sophisticated imaging techniques enabling previously undetectable structural abnormalities have greatly enhanced the management of patients with refractory epilepsy. Magnetic resonance imaging (MRI) has been pivotal in evaluating patients with partial seizures. [74] High-resolution MRI can detect small neocortical lesions amenable to resection. Patients with MRI-negative partial epilepsy may be candidates for additional neuroimaging techniques, including positron emission tomography, magnetic resonance spectroscopy, and single-photon emission tomography. Peri-ictal imaging may allow the identification of the epileptogenic zone in patients with normal MRI scans. Functional MRI (fMRI), techniques such as $1^8$F-fluorodeoxyglucose ($1^8$F-FDG) imaging, tractography, magnetoencephalography, fMRI, and EE, and fMRI based on blood-oxygen-level-dependent contrast imaging signal approaches are increasingly being used to localise or lateralise language and other eloquent cortical functions. [113]

---

5    personal observation
6    A failure of adequate trials of two tolerated, appropriately chosen and used antiepileptic drug schedules (whether as monotherapies or combined) to achieve sustained seizure freedom. [112]

Macroscopic and radiological evidence of total lesional excision with isolated structural lesions such as dysembryoplastic tumours, low-grade astrocytomas, or focal vascular abnormalities is associated with excellent seizure-free outcomes. [79]

Corpus callosotomy is recommended for patients with atonic seizures. [80, 81] ]

Hemispherectomy is now a widely accepted procedure for medically refractory, catastrophic hemispheric epilepsy. The classic anatomical hemispherectomy procedure has been abandoned in favour of functional or modified hemispherectomy. [82]

---

Paients who fail 2 correctly used anticonvulsants should be referred to a comprehensive epilepsy centre.

---

Temporal lobectomy for mesial temporal sclerosis is highly effective with a randomised controlled trial, demonstrating that > 50% of the patients were seizure-free compared to 8% in the non-surgical group. [78]

In patients with refractory epilepsy, neuromodulation techniques such as vagal nerve [75], hippocampal [76] and bilateral cerebellar [77] electrical stimulation have been advocated. These techniques have reduced seizure frequency by 50%, but none have eliminated seizures.

# Whether and When to Withdraw Therapy in 'Seizure-Free' Patients.

A Patient who has been free of seizures for some time often asks whether antiepileptic drugs (AED's) can be stopped. The juvenile myoclonic epilepsy syndrome consisting of absence and myoclonic seizures with infrequent tonic-clonic seizures is a lifelong predisposition to seizures. AED should not be ceased.

In other forms of epilepsy where remission can occur, a trial off AED's is not unreasonable. The initial question to the patient must be, "what effect would a recurrent seizure have on their life". e.g., they would be unable to drive for a prescribed period. In some jurisdictions, whilst the anticonvulsant is withdrawn and for a variable period were they to suffer another seizure, impacting their life and work; if a seizure occurred in a situation where it would cause significant embarrassment or, worse still, possible injury. A minimum of 2 years free of seizures is recommended before contemplating a gradual withdrawal of medications. [83] Even when the risk of recurrence is low, there is no guarantee that they will not suffer a recurrent seizure. Recurrent seizures may occur as long as eight years off medication.[7]

In a review of 28 studies accounting for 4571 patients (2758 children, 1020 adults and a combined group of 793), most with at least two years of seizure remission, the proportion of patients with relapses during or after AED withdrawal ranged from 12 to 66%. [84]

A higher-than-average risk of seizure relapse included:

- adolescent-onset epilepsy
- partial seizures
- the presence of an underlying neurological condition and
- abnormal EEG at the time of AED withdrawal in children.[84]

---

7   Personal Observation

Most relapses occur during or within the first six months after withdrawal. [85] There is no evidence to determine the withdrawal rate [86], but reducing the dose slowly over several weeks to months would seem reasonable.

# Common Treatment Errors

In 1999 Feely [87] elegantly summarised many common treatment errors, and most of these observations apply equally as well today. They include:

1. Incorrect or incomplete identification of seizure type(s) results in the wrong treatment choice, such as confusion between brief complex-partial seizures and absences or failure to recognise juvenile myoclonic epilepsy.

2. A drug appropriate for the patient's seizure type(s) is chosen but unsuitable for that patient. E.g. Phenytoin for an adolescent female (coarsening of facial features), Valproic Acid for a woman likely to become pregnant (increased risk of congenital malformations), or Carbamazepine for a woman on the oral contraceptive pill (reduced contraceptive efficacy.

3. The diagnosis and choice of a drug are correct. However, the patient is given too low a dose (for example, only the "starting" dose is used), or the patient is given too high an amount too quickly, resulting in side effects that may not occur with a gradual increase of the dose.

4. The epilepsy is controlled, but the patient has side effects, and no change in the treatment (drug or dosage) is made.

5. The patient is seen by a specialist and referred back to the general practitioner with an appropriate recommendation regarding treatment, but when this proves ineffective, further advice is not sought.

This author would add that although a detailed explanation regarding treatment, lifestyle, etcetera is provided at the consultation time, this information is often forgotten. Therefore I send a copy of the letter to the referring doctor to all patients, especially those with epilepsy.

# The Electroencephalogram

No chapter on epilepsy would be complete without discussing the electroencephalogram (EEG).

> A NORMAL EEG does not exclude epilepsy and an ABNORMAL EEG can very occasionally be seen in patients without epilepsy.

A single inter-ictal (between seizures) EEG has a sensitivity of approximately 50% [88,89] and a specificity of 97–98%. [90,91] The sensitivity increases to 92% if a further 3 EEG's are performed. [89] Sleep deprivation increases the number of abnormal EEG's. [9, 92] Epileptiform abnormalities are more likely to be detected if the EEG is obtained within the first 24 hours after a seizure. [9] The EEG is more likely to be abnormal in patients with generalised seizures than partial seizures in adults. [9]

Prolonged EEG monitoring with or without video is helpful for patients with refractory epilepsy [93] or frequent seizures, particularly in childhood. [94] Video-EEG monitoring is very useful in patients with suspected pseudo or non-epileptic seizures. [95] An abnormal; EEG does not prove the diagnosis of epilepsy as EEG abnormalities consistent with epilepsy were detected in 3.5 % of 3726 children without epilepsy. [91].

In recent years very sophisticated invasive techniques have been devised to monitor patients. These apply to only a tiny percentage of patients with refractory seizures. Electrocorticography and intracranial EEG monitoring are used in the presurgical evaluation of patients with drug-resistant epilepsy. Electrical stimulation of the brain elicits a functional map of the eloquent cortex to outline safe boundaries for resective surgery. More detail can be found in the International Federation of Clinical Neurophysiology (IFCN) guidelines. [107]

# The Future

It is very likely that more genetic causes will be discovered, new and hopefully, more effective drugs will be developed. It is anticipated that advances in surgery will occur. Research into disease modification and possibly curing surgery is in its infancy. [115] The insertion of implantable electrodes has enabled seizure prediction algorithms to be developed and potentially prevent individual seizures with cortical stimulation. [116]

# References

1. Fisher, R.S., et al., Epileptic seizures and epilepsy: definitions proposed by the International League Against Epilepsy (ILAE) and the International Bureau for Epilepsy (IBE). *Epilepsia*, 2005. 46(4): p. 470-2.

2. Engel Jr, J. A proposed diagnostic scheme for people with epileptic seizures and with epilepsy: Report of the ILAE task force on classification and terminology. 2006 [cited; Available from: http://www.ilae-epilepsy.org/Visitors/Centre/ctf/overview.cfm.

3. Engel, J., Jr., Classifications of the International League Against Epilepsy: time for reappraisal. *Epilepsia*, 1998. 39(9): p. 1014-7.

4. Everitt, A.D. and J.W. Sander, Classification of the epilepsies: time for a change? A critical review of the International Classification of the Epilepsies and Epileptic Syndromes (ICEES) and its usefulness in clinical practice and epidemiological studies of epilepsy. *Eur Neurol*, 1999. 42(1): p. 1-10.

5. Engel Jr, J., *Contemporary Neurology Series, in Seizures and Epilepsy*, F. Plum, Editor. 1989, F.A. Davis: Philadelphia. p. 165, 203-207.

6. Shorvon, S.D., *Handbook of Epilepsy Treatment: Forms, Causes and Therapy in Children and Adults*. 2005: Blackwell Publishing. 304

7. Engel, J., et al., *Epilepsy: A Comprehensive Textbook*. 2007: Lippincott Williams & Wilkins. 3056.

8. Jenssen, S., E.J. Gracely, and M.R. Sperling, How long do most seizures last? A systematic comparison of seizures recorded in the epilepsy monitoring unit. *Epilepsia*, 2006. 47(9): p. 1499-503.

9. King, M.A., et al., Epileptology of the first-seizure presentation: a clinical, electroencephalographic, and magnetic resonance imaging study of 300 consecutive patients. *Lancet*, 1998. 352(9133): p. 1007-11.

10. Jetter, G.M. and J.E. Cavazos, Epilepsy in the elderly. *Semin Neurol*, 2008. 28(3): p. 336-41.

11. Anderson, V.E., *Family studies of epilepsy, in Genetic Basis of the Epilepsies*, V.E. Anderson, et al., Editors. 1982, Raven: New York. p. 103-112.

12. Engel, J., Jr, *Seizures and Epilepsy. Contemporary Neurology Series*, ed. F. Plum. Vol. 31. 1989, Philadelphia: F.A. Davis Company. 536.

13. Lüders, H., *Textbook of Epileptology*. 2001, Boca Raton, Florida: Taylor & Francis CRC Press. 400

14. Shorvon, S., *Handbook of Epilepsy Treatment*. 2000, Massachusetts Blackwell Publishing 248

15. Fahn, S., Posthypoxic action myoclonus: literature review update. *Adv Neurol*, 1986. 43: p. 157-69.

16. Alfradique, I. and M.M. Vasconcelos, Juvenile myoclonic epilepsy. *Arq Neuropsiquiatr*, 2007. 65(4B): p. 1266-71.

17. Auvin, S., Treatment of juvenile myoclonic epilepsy. *CNS Neurosci Ther*, 2008. 14(3): p. 227-33.

18. Caicoya, A.G. and J.M. Serratosa, Post-ictal behaviour in temporal lobe epilepsy. *Epileptic Disord*, 2006. 8(3): p. 228-31.

19. Sadleir, L.G., et al., Electroclinical features of absence seizures in childhood absence epilepsy. *Neurology*, 2006. 67(3): p. 413-8.

20. Panayiotopoulos, C.P., et al., Benign childhood focal epilepsies: assessment of established and newly recognised syndromes. *Brain*, 2008. 131(Pt 9): p. 2264-86.

21. Doose, H. and W.K. Baier, Benign partial epilepsy and related conditions: multifactorial pathogenesis with hereditary impairment of brain maturation. *Eur J Pediatr*, 1989. 149(3): p. 152-8.

22. Engel, J.J., Report of the ILAE classification core group. *Epilepsia* 2006. 47: p. 1558–68.

23. Fetveit, A., Assessment of febrile seizures in children. *Eur J Pediatr*, 2008. 167(1): p. 17-27.

24. Xue, L.Y. and A.L. Ritaccio, Reflex seizures and reflex epilepsy. *Am J Electroneurodiagnostic Technol*, 2006. 46(1): p. 39-48.

25. King, D.W., et al., Pseudoseizures: diagnostic evaluation. *Neurology*, 1982. 32(1): p. 18-23.

26. Boon, P.A. and P.D. Williamson, The diagnosis of pseudoseizures. *Clin Neurol Neurosur*g, 1993. 95(1): p. 1-8.

27. Geyer, J.D., T.A. Payne, and I. Drury, The value of pelvic thrusting in the diagnosis of seizures and pseudoseizures. *Neurology*, 2000. 54(1): p. 227-9.

28. Harden, C.L., F.T. Burgut, and A.M. Kanner, The diagnostic significance of video-EEG monitoring findings on pseudoseizure patients differs between neurologists and psychiatrists. *Epilepsia*, 2003. 44(3): p. 453-6.

29. Eriksson, K. and R. Kalviainen, Pharmacologic management of convulsive status epilepticus in childhood. *Expert Rev Neurother*, 2005. 5(6): p. 777-83.

30. Meierkord, H., et al., EFNS guideline on the management of status epilepticus. *Eur J Neurol*, 2006. 13(5): p. 445-50.

31. Riviello, J.J., Jr., et al., Practice parameter: diagnostic assessment of the child with status epilepticus (an evidence-based review): report of the Quality Standards Subcommittee of the American Academy of Neurology and the Practice Committee of the Child Neurology Society. *Neurology*, 2006. 67(9): p. 1542-50.

32. DeLorenzo, R.J., et al., Persistent nonconvulsive status epilepticus after the control of convulsive status epilepticus. *Epilepsia*, 1998. 39(8): p. 833-40.

33. Towne, A.R., et al., Prevalence of nonconvulsive status epilepticus in comatose patients. *Neurology*, 2000. 54(2): p. 340-5.

34. Bauer, J., et al., Precipitating factors and therapeutic outcome in epilepsy with generalised tonic-clonic seizures. *Acta Neurol Scand*, 2000. 102(4): p. 205-8.

35. Goulden, K.J., et al., Changes in serum anticonvulsant levels with febrile illness in children with epilepsy. *Can J Neurol Sci*, 1988. 15(3): p. 281-5.

36. Zaccara, G., G.C. Muscas, and A. Messori, Clinical features, pathogenesis and management of drug-induced seizures. *Drug Saf*, 1990. 5(2): p. 109-51.

37. Ramirez-Lassepas, M., et al., Value of computed tomographic scan in the evaluation of adult patients after their first seizure. *Ann Neurol*, 1984. 15(6): p. 536-43.

38. Phizackerley, P.J., E.W. Poole, and C.W. Whitty, Sino-auricular heart block as an epileptic manifestation; a case report. *Epilepsia*, 1954. 3: p. 89-91.

39. Garretson, H.D. and A.R. Elvidge, Glossopharyngeal neuralgia with asystole and seizures. *Arch Neurol*, 1963. 8: p. 26-31.

40. Rowland, L.P., *Merritt's Textbook of Neurology*, ed. L.P. Rowland. Vol. 11e. 2005, Philadelphia, PA 19106-3621: Lippincott Williams & Wilkins.

41. Walton, J.N., *Brain's Diseases of the Nervous System*. Eighth ed. 1977, New York: Oxford Medical Publications. 1277.

42. Practice parameter: neuroimaging in the emergency patient presenting with seizure--summary statement. Quality Standards Subcommittee of the American Academy of Neurology in cooperation with American College of Emergency Physicians, American Association of Neurological Surgeons, and American Society of Neuroradiology. *Neurology*, 1996. 47(1): p. 288-91.

43. Krumholz, A., et al., Practice Parameter: evaluating an apparent unprovoked first seizure in adults (an evidence-based review): report of the Quality Standards Subcommittee of the American Academy of Neurology and the American Epilepsy Society. *Neurology*, 2007. 69(21): p. 1996-2007.

44. Stroink, H., et al., The first unprovoked, untreated seizure in childhood: a hospital-based study of the accuracy of the diagnosis, rate of recurrence, and long term outcome after recurrence. Dutch study of epilepsy in childhood. *J Neurol Neurosurg Psychiatry*, 1998. 64(5): p. 595-600.

45. Hauser, W.A., et al., Seizure recurrence after a first unprovoked seizure. *N Engl J Med*, 1982. 307(9): p. 522-8.

46. Pohlmann-Eden, B., et al., The first seizure and its management in adults and children. BMJ, 2006. 332(7537): p. 339-42.

47. Kim, L.G., et al., Prediction of risk of seizure recurrence after a single seizure and early epilepsy: further results from the MESS trial. *Lancet Neurol*, 2006. 5(4): p. 317-22.

48. Marson, A., et al., Immediate versus deferred antiepileptic drug treatment for early epilepsy and single seizures: a randomised controlled trial. *Lancet*, 2005. 365(9476): p. 2007-13.

49. Bautista, R.E. and P. Wludyka, Driving prevalence and factors associated with driving among patients with epilepsy. *Epilepsy Behav*, 2006. 9(4): p. 625-31.

50. Verrotti, A., et al., Levetiracetam in absence epilepsy. Dev Med Child Neurol, 2008. 50(11): p. 850-3.

51. Posner, E.B. and C.P. Panayiotopoulos, The significance of specific diagnosis in the treatment of epilepsies. *Dev Med Child Neurol*, 2008. 50(11): p. 807.

52. Rowan, A.J., et al., New onset geriatric epilepsy: a randomized study of gabapentin, lamotrigine, and carbamazepine. *Neurology*, 2005. 64(11): p. 1868-73.

53. Kwan, P. and M.J. Brodie, Early identification of refractory epilepsy. *N Engl J Med*, 2000. 342(5): p. 314-9.

54. Brodie, M.J., Medical therapy of epilepsy: when to initiate treatment and when to combine? *J Neurol*, 2005. 252(2): p. 125-30.

55. Stephen, L.J., Drug treatment of epilepsy in elderly people: focus on Valproic Acid. *Drugs Aging*, 2003. 20(2): p. 141-52.

56. Hirsch, L.J., et al., Predictors of Lamotrigine-associated rash. *Epilepsia*, 2006. 47(2): p. 318-22.

57. Claxton, A.J., J. Cramer, and C. Pierce, A systematic review of the associations between dose regimens and medication compliance. *Clin Ther*, 2001. 23(8): p. 1296-310.

58. Leidy, N.K., et al., Seizure frequency and the health-related quality of life of adults with epilepsy. *Neurology*, 1999. 53(1): p. 162-6.

59. Patsalos, P.N., et al., Antiepileptic drugs--best practice guidelines for therapeutic drug monitoring: a position paper by the subcommission on therapeutic drug monitoring, ILAE Commission on Therapeutic Strategies. *Epilepsia*, 2008. 49(7): p. 1239-76.

60. Sheth, S.G., et al., Mortality in epilepsy: driving fatalities vs other causes of death in patients with epilepsy. *Neurology*, 2004. 63(6): p. 1002-7.

61. Krauss, G.L., et al., Risk factors for seizure-related motor vehicle crashes in patients with epilepsy. *Neurology*, 1999. 52(7): p. 1324-9.

62. *Austroads, Assessing Fitness to Drive*. 2003, Austroads Incorporated: Sydney.

63. Perucca, E., Birth defects after prenatal exposure to antiepileptic drugs. *Lancet Neurol*, 2005. 4(11): p. 781-6.

64. Tomson, T., E. Perucca, and D. Battino, Navigating toward fetal and maternal health: the challenge of treating epilepsy in pregnancy. *Epilepsia*, 2004. 45(10): p. 1171-5.

65. Adab, N., et al., Common antiepileptic drugs in pregnancy in women with epilepsy. Cochrane Database Syst Rev, 2004(3): p. CD004848.

66. Holmes, L.B., D.F. Wyszynski, and E. Lieberman, The AED (antiepileptic drug) pregnancy registry: a 6-year experience. *Arch Neurol*, 2004. 61(5): p. 673-8.

67. Wyszynski, D.F., et al., Increased rate of major malformations in offspring exposed to valproate during pregnancy. *Neurology*, 2005. 64(6): p. 961-5.

68. Eurap, S.G., Seizure control and treatment in pregnancy: observations from the EURAP epilepsy pregnancy registry. *Neurology*, 2006. 66(3): p. 354-60.

69. Morrow, J., et al., Malformation risks of antiepileptic drugs in pregnancy: a prospective study from the U.K. Epilepsy and Pregnancy Register. *J Neurol Neurosurg Psychiatry*, 2006. 77(2): p. 193-8.

70. Vajda, F.J., et al., Foetal malformations and seizure control: 52 months data of the Australian Pregnancy Registry. *Eur J Neurol*, 2006. 13(6): p. 645-54.

71. Seizure control and treatment in pregnancy: observations from the EURAP epilepsy pregnancy registry. *Neurology*, 2006. 66(3): p. 354-60.

72. Ryan, C.A. and G. Dowling, Drowning deaths in people with epilepsy. Cmaj, 1993. 148(5): p. 781-4.

73. Arango, M.F., D.A. Steven, and I.A. Herrick, Neurosurgery for the treatment of epilepsy. *Curr Opin Anaesthesiol*, 2004. 17(5): p. 383-387.

74. Cascino, G.D., Neuroimaging in epilepsy: diagnostic strategies in partial epilepsy. *Semin Neurol*, 2008. 28(4): p. 523-32.

75. A randomised controlled trial of chronic vagus nerve stimulation for treatment of medically intractable seizures. The Vagus Nerve Stimulation Study Group. *Neurology*, 1995. 45(2): p. 224-30.

76. Tellez-Zenteno, J.F., et al., Hippocampal electrical stimulation in mesial temporal lobe epilepsy. *Neurology*, 2006. 66(10): p. 1490-4.

77. Velasco, F., et al., Double-blind, randomised controlled pilot study of bilateral cerebellar stimulation for treatment of intractable motor seizures. Epilepsia, 2005. 46(7): p. 1071-81.

78. Wiebe, S., et al., A randomised, controlled trial of surgery for temporal-lobe epilepsy. *N Engl J Med*, 2001. 345(5): p. 311-8.

79. Shaefi, S. and W. Harkness, Current status of surgery in the management of epilepsy. *Epilepsia*, 2003. 44 Suppl 1: p. 43-7.

80. Rathore, C., et al., Outcome after corpus callosotomy in children with injurious drop attacks and severe mental retardation. *Brain Dev*, 2007. 29(9): p. 577-85.

81. Jea, A., et al., Corpus callosotomy in children with intractable epilepsy using frameless stereotactic neuronavigation: 12-year experience at The Hospital for Sick Children in Toronto. *Neurosurg Focus*, 2008. 25(3): p. E7.

82. Spencer, S. and L. Huh, Outcomes of epilepsy surgery in adults and children. *Lancet Neurol*, 2008. 7(6): p. 525-37.

83. Sirven, J.I., M. Sperling, and D.M. Wingerchuk, Early versus late antiepileptic drug withdrawal for people with epilepsy in remission. *Cochrane Database Syst Rev*, 2001(3): p. CD001902.

84. Specchio, L.M. and E. Beghi, Should antiepileptic drugs be withdrawn in seizure-free patients? *CNS Drugs*, 2004. 18(4): p. 201-12.

85. Aktekin, B., et al., Withdrawal of antiepileptic drugs in adult patients free of seizures for 4 years: a prospective study. *Epilepsy Behav*, 2006. 8(3): p. 616-9.

86. Ranganathan, L.N. and S. Ramaratnam, Rapid versus slow withdrawal of antiepileptic drugs. *Cochrane Database Syst Rev*, 2006(2): p. CD005003.

87. Feely, M., Clinical review Fortnightly review Drug treatment of epilepsy *BMJ* 1999. 318: p. 106-109

88. Marsan, C.A. and L.S. Zivin, Factors related to the occurrence of typical paroxysmal abnormalities in the EEG records of epileptic patients. *Epilepsia*, 1970. 11(4): p. 361-81.

89. Salinsky, M., R. Kanter, and R.M. Dasheiff, Effectiveness of multiple EEGs in supporting the diagnosis of epilepsy: an operational curve. *Epilepsia*, 1987. 28(4): p. 331-4.

90. Zivin, L. and C.A. Marsan, Incidence and prognostic significance of "epileptiform" activity in the EEG of non-epileptic subjects. *Brain*, 1968. 91(4): p. 751-78.

91. Cavazzuti, G.B., L. Cappella, and A. Nalin, Longitudinal study of epileptiform EEG patterns in normal children. *Epilepsia*, 1980. 21(1): p. 43-55.

92. Degen, R., A study of the diagnostic value of waking and sleep EEGs after sleep deprivation in epileptic patients on anticonvulsive therapy. *Electroencephalogr Clin Neurophysiol*, 1980. 49(5-6): p. 577-84.

93. Boon, P., et al., Interictal and ictal video-EEG monitoring. Acta Neurol Belg, 1999. 99(4): p. 247-55.

94. Watemberg, N., et al., Adding video recording increases the diagnostic yield of routine electroencephalograms in children with frequent paroxysmal events. *Epilepsia*, 2005. 46(5): p. 716-9.

95. Jedrzejczak, J., K. Owczarek, and J. Majkowski, Psychogenic pseudoepileptic seizures: clinical and electroencephalogram (EEG) video-tape recordings. *Eur J Neurol*, 1999. 6(4): p. 473-9.

96. French, J.A., et al., Efficacy and tolerability of the new antiepileptic drugs II: treatment of refractory epilepsy: report of the Therapeutics and Technology Assessment Subcommittee and Quality Standards Subcommittee of the American Academy of Neurology and the American Epilepsy Society. *Neurology*, 2004. 62(8): p. 1261-73.

97. French, J.A., et al., Efficacy and tolerability of the new antiepileptic drugs I: treatment of new-onset epilepsy: report of the Therapeutics and Technology Assessment Subcommittee and Quality Standards Subcommittee of the American Academy of Neurology and the American Epilepsy Society. *Neurology*, 2004. 62(8): p. 1252-60.

98. Glauser, T., et al., ILAE treatment guidelines: evidence-based analysis of antiepileptic drug efficacy and effectiveness as initial monotherapy for epileptic seizures and syndromes. *Epilepsia*, 2006. 47(7): p. 1094-120.

99. Appleton, R., S. Macleod, and T. Martland, Drug management for acute tonic-clonic convulsions including convulsive status epilepticus in children. *Cochrane Database Syst Rev*, 2008(3): p. CD001905.

100. Marson, A.G., et al., The SANAD study of effectiveness of valproate, lamotrigine, or topiramate for generalised and unclassifiable epilepsy: an unblinded randomised controlled trial. *Lancet*, 2007. 369(9566): p. 1016-26.

101. Marson, A.G., et al., The SANAD study of effectiveness of carbamazepine, gabapentin, lamotrigine, oxcarbazepine, or topiramate for treatment of partial epilepsy: an unblinded randomised controlled trial. *Lancet*, 2007. 369(9566): p. 1000-15.

102. Obeid, T. and C.P. Panayiotopoulos, Clonazepam in juvenile myoclonic epilepsy. *Epilepsia*, 1989. 30(5): p. 603-6.

103. Prasad, K., et al., Anticonvulsant therapy for status epilepticus. *Cochrane Database Syst Rev*, 2005(4): p. CD003723.

104. Knake, S., et al., Intravenous Levetiracetam in the treatment of benzodiazepine refractory status epilepticus. *J Neurol Neurosurg Psychiatry*, 2008. 79(5): p. 588-9.

105. Agarwal, P., et al., Randomised study of intravenous valproate and Phenytoin in status epilepticus. *Seizure*, 2007. 16(6): p. 527-32.

106. MIMS. [cited; Available from]: http://www.mims.com.au/index.php?option=com_content&task=view& id=98&Itemid=133.

107. Tatum WO, Rubboli G, Kaplan PW, et al. Clinical utility of EEG in diagnosing and monitoring epilepsy in adults. *Clin Neurophysiol* 2018; 129(5): 1056-82.

108. Scheffer IE, Berkovic S, Capovilla G, et al. ILAE classification of the epilepsies: Position paper of the ILAE Commission for Classification and Terminology. *Epilepsia* 2017; 58(4): 512-21.

109. Engel J, Jr. The current place of epilepsy surgery. *Curr Opin Neurol* 2018; 31(2): 192-7.

110. West S, Nolan SJ, Newton R. Surgery for epilepsy: a systematic review of current evidence. *Epileptic Disord* 2016; 18(2): 113-21.

111. Rugg-Gunn F, Miserocchi A, McEvoy A. Epilepsy surgery. *Pract Neurol* 2020; 20(1): 4-14.

112. Kwan P, Arzimanoglou A, Berg AT, et al. Definition of drug-resistant epilepsy: consensus proposal by the ad hoc Task Force of the ILAE Commission on Therapeutic Strategies. *Epilepsia* 2010; 51(6): 1069-77.

113. Thijs RD, Surges R, O'Brien TJ, Sander JW. Epilepsy in adults. *Lancet* 2019; 393(10172): 689-701.

114. Kanner AM. Most antidepressant drugs are safe for patients with epilepsy at therapeutic doses: A review of the evidence. *Epilepsy Behav* 2016; 61: 282-6.

115. Clossen BL, Reddy DS. Novel therapeutic approaches for disease-modification of epileptogenesis for curing epilepsy. *Biochim Biophys Acta Mol Basis Dis* 2017; 1863(6): 1519-38.

116. Cook MJ. Advancing seizure forecasting from cyclical activity data. *The Lancet Neurology* 2021; 20(2): 86-7.

117. Kumar A, Sharma S. *Complex Partial Seizure*. StatPearls. Treasure Island (FL): StatPearls Publishing Copyright © 2021, StatPearls Publishing LLC.; 2021.

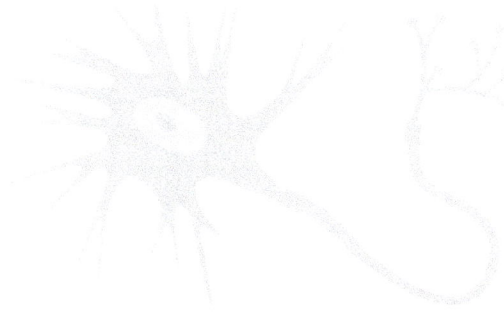

# Headache and Facial Pain

| Key Terms | |
|---|---|
| Subarachnoid haemorrhage | Haemorrhage into the subarachnoid space. |
| Photophobia | Sensitivity to light |
| Phonophobia | Sensitivity to noise |
| Aura | A peculiar sensation (visual, auditory, somatic, or gustatory disturbance) forerunning the appearance of more definite symptoms. [1] |
| Valsalva | Attempted forced expiration of air with a closed mouth and occluded nose that increases the intrathoracic pressure |
| Foramen magnum | The base of the skull, the junction of the lower aspect of the brainstem and the top of the spinal cord. |
| Chiari Malformation | A congenital malformation where the cerebellar tonsils protrude through the foramen magnum into the cervical spinal canal. |
| Pathognomonic | A sign or symptom that is so characteristic of a disease that it makes the diagnosis. |
| Photopsia | Perceived flashes of light |
| Visual obscurations | Inability to see in a particular part of the visual field for some time |

# Introduction

Headache is one of the commonest problems encountered in neurology. This chapter is not a comprehensive review of headache. The approach to the more common headache and facial pain syndromes encountered in clinical practice will be discussed. There are many excellent textbooks for more detailed information.[2-6]

The single most important question to ask a patient presenting with headache is: "from the moment you first noticed the headache how long did it take to reach maximum severity?" This is the vital clue to the likely pathology.

# chapter 9 Headache and Facial Pain

The various labels given to different types of headaches have arisen from clinicians observing recurring patterns of similar symptoms in a large number of patients in the absence of any gold standard for the diagnosis[1]. Thus, the diagnosis of the cause of most headaches or facial pain is almost entirely dependent on a detailed and accurate history because at this point there are no diagnostic tests to confirm most of the common causes of headache such as migraine, cluster & tension-type headache. Imaging techniques such as Computerized Tomography (CT) and Magnetic Resonance Imaging (MRI) detect abnormalities that can explain the clinical presentation in only 2% of cases. [7]

> "If you only have 30 minutes with a patient presenting with headache spend 29 on the history and 1 on the examination." (Quote attributed to Alfred Sahs)

Consider the following case history:

**A 26-Year-Old Man with Headache, Nausea, Vomiting, Photophobia & Phonophobia**

Write down your diagnosis or diagnoses before reading on.

Most students will say subarachnoid haemorrhage (SAH), some will say meningitis or migraine but this young man had a hangover! All four diagnoses will result in headache, nausea, vomiting and photophobia. Although fever should differentiate SAH from meningitis, migraine and hangovers and neck stiffness should raise the suspicion of SAH or meningitis. Occasionally patients with migraine complain of neck stiffness and rarely fever [8]. Similarly, if a young man had been drinking heavily, it would be wrong to assume he had a hangover if he experienced a thunderclap onset of severe generalized headache with nausea and vomiting as this is more in keeping with a SAH. This reiterates the point made in chapter two, the nature and distribution of symptoms **DO NOT** define the aetiology.

The time course (mode of onset and subsequent progression of symptoms) will differentiate between these various entities. The headache of SAH is of sudden onset reaching maximum severity within 5 minutes of onset. In contrast, the headaches of migraine, meningitis, and hangover evolve over a variable time from minutes to hours.

> In any patient suffering from a headache, establish the exact mode of onset and progression of the headache and other associated symptoms.

The International Headache Society (HIS) [9, 175] classifies headaches as:

**Primary:** Migraine, tension-type headache, cluster headache and other trigeminal autonomic cephalalgias, other primary headaches.

**Secondary:** Headache due to another disorder that resolves within three months of treatment of that disorder.

---

1 I have seen several patients over the years who have been incorrectly diagnosed with migraine when they had more sinister pathology e.g., cerebral vasculitis.

Most patients with headaches fear they may have a brain tumour. Although headache is a common symptom of a brain tumour, brain tumour as a cause of headache is extremely rare. [10] Episodic tension-type headache and migraine are the most common primary headaches. The commonest secondary causes are a hangover and fever.[11] (see table 9.1)

| Headache Type | % | 95% Confidence interval |
|---|---|---|
| Primary (non-symptomatic) | | |
| Episodic tension-type headache | 66 | 62-69 |
| Chronic tension-type headache | 3 | 2-5 |
| Migraine with aura | 6 | 5-8 |
| Migraine without aura | 9 | 7-11 |
| Idiopathic stabbing headache | 4 | 1-4 |
| External compression headache | 15 | 12-17 |
| Cold stimulus headache | 1 | 0-2 |
| Benign cough headache | 1 | 0-2 |
| Headache associated with sexual activity | 1 | 0-2 |
| Secondary (symptomatic) | | |
| Hangover | 72 | 68-75 |
| Fever | 63 | 59-66 |
| Head Injury | 4 | 2-5 |
| Disorder of the nose or sinuses | 15 | 12-17 |
| Intracranial neoplasm | 0 | |
| Metabolic Disorders | 22 | 19-25 |

**Table 9.1.** The lifetime prevalence (the number of people in a given group or population who are reported to have a disease) of various types of primary and secondary headaches. (Using the IHS criteria at the time of the study) Figures are derived from a random sample of 925 individuals from the community in Denmark. [11] External compression headache relates to compression by helmets or swimming goggles. The prevalence is likely to be similar in other countries. The terms non-symptomatic and symptomatic have also been used to describe primary vs secondary causes of headache.

# What Questions to Ask

There are 3 scenarios:
- It is the first headache that the patient has ever experienced
- It is an identical headache in a patient who suffers from recurrent headaches or
- It could be a completely different headache in a patient who has suffered from recurrent headaches.

In clinical practice, you are either dealing with a single headache (that may be the 1st of what will become recurrent headaches) or recurring headaches.

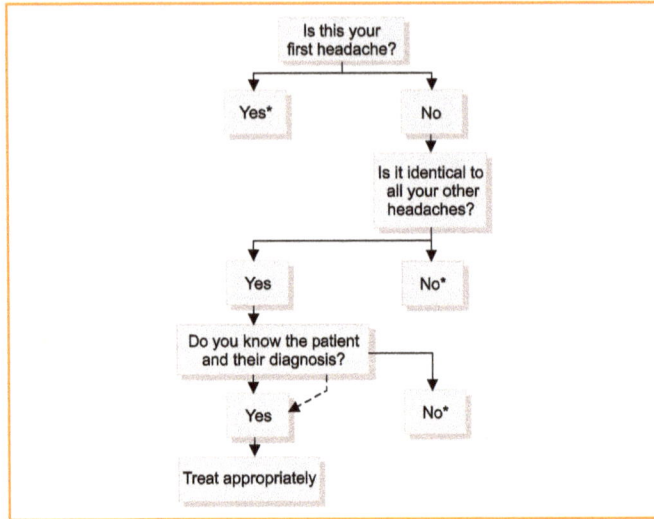

**Figure 9.1** A recommended approach when seeing a patient with a headache. The * indicates that it is important to obtain a very detailed history using the technique outlined below.

If you know the patient and their diagnosis, and the patient says the headache is identical then it is not unreasonable to treat the patient headache accordingly. On the other hand, if you do not know the patient, or if it is a different headache from that from which they have suffered in the past, you must treat this headache as if it was the first headache that they have ever experienced. When seeing patients for the first time with a prior diagnosis for their headaches **do not assume that the previous diagnosis is correct**. The lack of diagnostic tests to confirm the diagnoses in primary headaches means there is always a degree of uncertainty. Use the technique below to obtain a blow-by-blow description, like that outlined in chapter 2. Enquire as to what the patient was doing at the precise moment the headache commenced, what they had been doing just before this, the time from the onset of the headache until the headache reached its maximum severity and the exact nature, distribution, time taken to reach maximum intensity or extent of involvement of the body, duration and time taken to resolve of every associated symptom both individually and in relation to each other. Ascertaining the time taken to reach maximum intensity is the single most important question to ask as it is the vital clue as to the likely pathological process.

Classical teaching has suggested students ask whether the headache is unilateral or bilateral, constant, or throbbing, frontal, temporal, parietal, or occipital, made worse by straining, moving, or coughing, whether it awakens the patient from sleep and whether there is associated photophobia or phonophobia. *In most instances the answers to these questions are unhelpful.* As anyone who has suffered from migraines, tension-type headaches or hangovers will know most of these features are non-specific (as highlighted in the case above). Although migraine (see below) is typically unilateral, throbbing headache associated with visual, gastrointestinal, or neurological symptoms it can be bilateral, constant and is not always accompanied by any visual, neurological, or gastrointestinal symptoms. Although the pain of trigeminal neuralgia is almost exclusively unilateral, cases with bilateral pain have been described and are more likely to represent symptomatic (underlying pathology other than compression of the nerve by a vascular loop) trigeminal neuralgia. [12] Similarly, cluster headache is unilateral but even here atypical cases with bilateral headache occur.[13-15]

Virtually all headaches are exacerbated by exercise, coughing, sneezing, and straining. The exception is cluster headache where the patient often paces the floor or even hits their head on the wall to reduce the severity.

In everyday clinical practice if patients are simply asked to describe their headache(s) they often omit vital information.

The following approach is recommended when taking the history from a patient with headache:
- What were you doing at the time (circumstances) the headache first commenced?
- What had you been doing just beforehand?
- What was the first thing you noticed? How long did it take from when you first noticed this symptom until it reached its maximum severity?
- What was the next thing you noticed and how long did it take from when you first noticed this symptom until it reached its maximum severity?
- And then what happened?
- And then what happened? etc. until the entire episode is described from start to finish.

The term "and then what happened" is one of the most useful questions in patients with episodic disturbances of neurological function, it ensures the patient does not omit any details. This approach elucidates information that can be the clue to the likely underlying pathological process as discussed below.

---

A word of warning, a patient with a past history of recurrent headaches e.g. related to migraine or tension-type headache is not precluded from developing another cause such as a SAH. If the headache is not identical to those of the past, take the history as if it is the patient's first headache.

---

The following case demonstrates the value of this history-taking technique.

**Case 9.1** A 50-Year-Old Man with The Sudden Onset of Excruciatingly Severe Headache

The initial suspicion is that he may have suffered a subarachnoid haemorrhage. However, when the history was obtained using the above approach:

**What were you doing at the time the headache first commenced?**
Having a shower
**What was the first thing you noticed?**
A mild headache at the back of my head.
**How long did it take from when you first noticed this symptom until it reached its maximum severity?**
About one minute.
**then what happened?**
After the headache gradually increased over about a minute and then suddenly became excruciatingly severe and was all over my head.

This is not the history of a SAH and after further questioning, the patient admitted that he had been masturbating. The correct diagnosis was primary headache associated with sexual activity, aka benign sex headache.

---

The value of this method of obtaining histories can also be highlighted by re-examining the case scenario initially presented at the beginning of this chapter.

---

**CASE 9.2** A 26-Year-Old Man with Headache, Nausea, Vomiting and Photophobia

**What were you doing at the time the headache first commenced?**
I woke up with a headache.
**What had you been doing before?**
I was out with the lads celebrating our victory in the football match. I had drunk more than my fair share of alcohol and felt a bit under the weather when I went to bed.
**What was the first thing you noticed?**
I awoke with a headache all over my head, I felt nauseated and every time I moved, I would feel very dizzy.
**How long did it take from when you first noticed the headache until it reached its maximum severity?**
About half an hour
**then what happened?**
I got out of bed to go to the toilet, and felt worse, the bright light coming in through the bathroom window hurt my eyes, the nausea and dizziness increased
When the headache reached its maximum severity, I began to feel nauseated
**Then what happened?**
The nausea increased over the next 15 minutes
**Then what happened?**
Then I vomited several times, every time I vomited my head felt worse.
**Then what happened?**
I decided to come to the hospital for treatment.
**Have you ever had this headache before?**
No
**Is there a family history of migraine?**
No

This is a typical history of someone with either migraine or suffering from a hangover. The presence of photopsia and neurological symptoms suggests diagnosis of possible migraine. He had a hangover.

---

An alternative diagnosis becomes apparent in the next patient who on the surface initially appears to present with identical symptoms, with identical initial presenting symptoms to the case above.

---

**CASE 9.3** A 26-year-Old Man with Headache, Nausea, Vomiting and Photophobia

**What were they doing at the time the headache first commenced?**
I was sitting watching television.
**What had you been doing before?**
I was perfectly well until that time.
**What was the first thing you noticed?**
It felt as if someone had hit me over their head with an axe, I developed this very severe headache at the back and over the top of my head.
**How long did it take from when you first noticed the headache until it reached its maximum severity?**
It was at its most severe when it 1$^{st}$ started
**And then what happened?**
At the same time, I felt very nauseated and began to vomit, as I walked to the bathroom I noticed that the light coming in through the window hurt my eyes.
**then what happened?**
I decided to come to the hospital for treatment.

The diagnosis of subarachnoid haemorrhage is inescapable when the exact mode of onset and progression of the headache and associated symptoms is established.

---

**CASE 9.4** A 26-year-Old Man with Headache, Nausea, Vomiting and Photophobia

**What were you doing at the time the headache first commenced?**
I was sitting watching television.
**What had you been doing before?**
Nothing, I was perfectly well until that time.
**What was the first thing you noticed, how long did it take from when you first noticed this symptom until it reached its maximum severity and then what happened?**
I noticed flashing lights in my vision
**Where in your vision?**
They started on the left side
**Then what happened?**
They gradually enlarged and spread to the right side
**How long did they take to spread to the right side?**
Approximately 10-15 minutes.
**Then what happened?**
Just as I thought I was getting better because the trouble with my vision was resolving I developed a very severe headache all over my head.
**How long did it take from when you first noticed the headache until the headache reached its maximum severity?**
Approximately 30 minutes.
**Then what happened?**
I became nauseated and this increased over the next 15 minutes
**Then what happened?**
Then I started to vomit and I vomited several times, every time I vomited my head felt worse.
**Then what happened?**
I decided to come to the hospital for treatment.
**Have you ever had this headache before?**
No
**Is there a family history of migraine?**
No

In this patient, symptoms evolved gradually with the initial symptoms disappearing before subsequent symptoms either developed or reached their maximum intensity, a characteristic and almost pathognomonic feature of migraine. The last two questions would strengthen the diagnosis had the answer been yes, however, remember that a past or a family history of migraine is circumstantial evidence (see chapter 2).

The above discussion would suggest that taking a history from patients with headaches is easy. Unfortunately, this is not always the case. The CT scan in figure 9.2 is from a patient who was incapable of giving a detailed history because of the cognitive impairment resulting from the hydrocephalus. The patient complained of a vague headache, nondescript blurring of vision, a change in her personality (her sister's psychiatrist had diagnosed schizophrenia when her sister told him about her symptoms despite the fact that he never saw the patient). The two clues to the underlying diagnosis were the fact that her legs gave way when her brother hugged her (this would have increased intrathoracic and thus intracranial pressure) and the presence of papilloedema when examined.

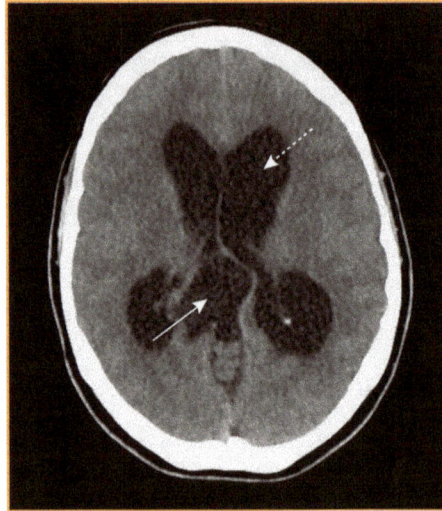

**Figure 9.2** CT scan of the brain demonstrating a large dermoid cyst (straight arrow) with secondary hydrocephalus (dotted arrow).

---

Do NOT diagnose a psychiatric problem because of an inability to obtain a history that makes sense. This could reflect cognitive impairment as a result of the underlying disease. There are some patients who are simply incapable of giving a coherent history even in the absence of any cognitive problems.

---

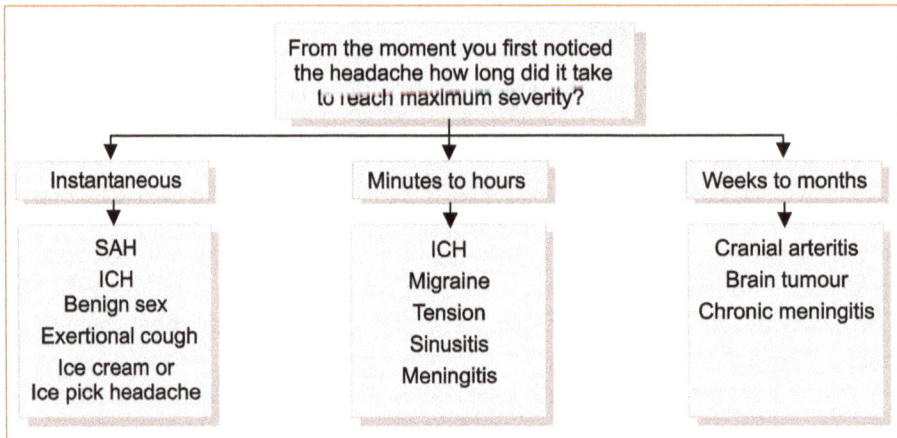

**Figure 9.3** This figure shows the three broad categories of headache.

There are many different ways to approach patients with headache. The IHS classification is into primary and secondary. In clinical practice when evaluating patients with headache there are three broad categories based on the rapidity of onset of the headache (Figure 9.3).

This chapter will initially discuss the approach to patients presenting with a single headache and then the approach to patients with recurrent headaches.

# A Single (or the first) Episode of Headache
## Sudden onset "Thunderclap Headache"

Several conditions can present with a thunderclap headache. These include:
- Intracranial Haemorrhage
  - Subarachnoid Haemorrhage
  - Intracerebral Haemorrhage
  - Intraventricular Haemorrhage
- Cough Headache – Primary cough headache
- Exertional Headache – Primary exercise headache*
- Benign Sex Headache – Primary headache associated with sexual activity*
- Ice Cream Headache – Cold stimulus headache
- Ice Pick Headache – Primary stabbing headache*
- Aseptic or viral meningitis (rarely the onset of headache can be very sudden)

All these conditions have one thing in common and that is the sudden onset of severe headache. What differentiates one from the other is the associated symptoms, the duration of the headache and to a lesser extent the circumstances under which the headache occurs. **It is important to remember that the most lethal condition NOT to miss is a Subarachnoid Haemorrhage**, which can occur under any circumstances including when patients exert themselves, coughs, sneezes or during sexual intercourse. The slight exception is the headache related to exertion or orgasm (see below). There are extremely rare causes of sudden severe headache such as a hydrocephalic attack with or without the presence of a third ventricular colloid cyst acting as a ball valve. Very rarely sudden onset headache may be the presenting symptom aseptic or viral meningitis. [16]

# Intracranial Haemorrhage
## Subarachnoid Haemorrhage

The single most important, although not the commonest cause of sudden severe headache is subarachnoid haemorrhage. A minor bleed causing a sudden headache may be the only warning of a subsequent severe and often fatal haemorrhage. Subarachnoid haemorrhage accounts for a little over 10% of patients presenting with sudden onset "Thunderclap " headache. [16] If the haemorrhage also occurs into the parenchyma of the brain there may be focal neurological symptoms. Patients often describe it as the worst headache of their life. [17]

The headache of subarachnoid haemorrhage is occipital or generalized and of sudden onset and usually reaching maximum severity within seconds, although it can be as long as 6 minutes. If the haemorrhage is of sufficient severity then there may be a transient loss of consciousness or coma, this occurs in nearly 50% of patients. [18] There is severe nausea, vomiting, photophobia, and neck stiffness. Seizures may occur. The patient is obtunded and looks extremely ill. Photopsia is NOT a feature.

However, clinical features do not always clearly separate other causes of headache from SAH. [16, 19] The presence or lack of accompanying symptoms like nausea, vomiting, photophobia and collapse at onset is not a reliable way to distinguish between SAH and benign causes for acute headache. [16]

> The moment the possibility of SAH is entertained all patients should be investigated with urgent imaging and if negative a lumbar puncture (LP) to ensure that the diagnosis of SAH is not missed.

In almost 20-40% of patients with SAH, a warning leak (minor haemorrhage) may occur 1-8 weeks before a major SAH. The headache (referred to as a sentinel headache or sentinel bleed) is often short-lived and the patient may not seek immediate medical attention.[20] Even if the patient consults a physician the headache seems so trivial that often the diagnosis is missed. [21] Some of these patients are seen some days to weeks later [20] with the story of a sudden, explosive severe headache, usually in the absence of any other symptoms. The briefer the headache, the less likely it is related to a warning bleed. Here the question arises as to whether they have suffered a SAH and how extensively they should be investigated. There is no easy answer to this question. A 3rd nerve palsy with a dilated pupil is a classic sign of a sentinel bleed.

The probability of detecting an aneurysmal haemorrhage on CT scans performed at various intervals after the ictus is [10]:

- day 0     95%
- day 3     74%
- 1 week    50%
- 2 weeks   30%
- 3 weeks   almost zero.

The probability of detecting xanthochromia with spectrophotometry in the CSF at various times after a subarachnoid haemorrhage is:[10]

- 12 hours  100%
- 1 week    100%
- 2 weeks   100%
- 3 weeks   > 70%
- 4 weeks   > 40%.

Magnetic Resonance Angiography will detect aneurysms of > 4 mm in diameter and is recommended in patients with thunderclap headache with a low index of suspicion for SAH (normal CT scan and CSF) [10] as the risk of subsequent subarachnoid haemorrhage is negligible. [22, 23] MRI however may miss aneurysms less 4 mm, CT angiography can detect aneurysms as small as 1.5 mm. [189] If the index of suspicion for SAH is high formal angiography should be performed.

> Sudden severe headache should be assumed due to SAH until proven otherwise.

## Intracerebral Haemorrhage

Patients with an intracerebral haemorrhage present with a depressed conscious state or a focal neurological deficit. [24] If the haemorrhage is small and not associated with a deficit, headache may be the only presenting symptom. The headache of intracerebral haemorrhage is often but not invariably associated with nausea & vomiting due to raised intracranial pressure. It is most often sudden in onset and of maximum severity at onset; however, it can increase in severity more slowly over minutes to hours. In this situation, the patient will usually have, depression of the conscious state and focal neurological signs.

## Intraventricular Haemorrhage

Intraventricular haemorrhage is rare and usually results from parenchymal (intracerebral) haemorrhage rupturing into the ventricle. There is an entity called primary intraventricular haemorrhage, [190] where the headache is of sudden onset and maximum intensity within seconds, it is usually associated with nausea, vomiting, photophobia, and neck rigidity. If the haemorrhage is more severe or if it leads to secondary hydrocephalus depression of the conscious state will occur. There are no focal neurological symptoms.

## Primary Cough Headache

Although cough, benign exertional, benign sex, ice cream and ice pick headache tend to recur they have one other thing in common and that is the headache is of sudden onset and therefore discussed in this section.

Anybody who has suffered from a headache knows that coughing, sneezing, or straining momentarily exacerbates the headache. Headache precipitated by coughing is referred to as cough headache. A similar headache can also be precipitated by anything that increases intrathoracic pressure such as sneezing, straining, laughing or stooping.[25] In the majority of patients with this headache, no structural pathology is present, although in as many as 25% it may be symptomatic (indicating the presence of an underlying pathology) with a significant proportion related to a Chiari malformation.[26] Primary cough headache is precipitated by coughing in the absence of any intracranial disorder. The headache is of maximum severity at onset coming on within seconds of coughing, sneezing, or straining. It is very brief, lasting only a few seconds to less than a minute. There are no associated symptoms. The headache is generalized, frontal or occipital. Recurrent headaches are the rule but usually resolve within one or two years. Cases have been described lasting up to 12 years. [25]

| Treatment of Benign Cough Headache |
| --- |
| In general, reassurance only is required. Occasionally symptomatic relief can be provided with Indomethacin or other non-steroidal anti-inflammatory drugs. [27, 28 ] |

## Benign exertional headache

The new nomenclature categorises benign exertional headache as primary exercise headache. Primary exercise headache is bilateral, throbbing headache, lasting from 5 minutes to 24 hours specifically provoked by physical exercise and not associated with any systemic or intracranial disorder.[29] A small percentage of patients with exertional headache may have structural pathology.[29] This headache is of sudden onset but not usually described as explosive. It can be generalised frontal or occipital and is precipitated by activities such as weight lifting or any other activity that causes the patient to Valsalva. Similar to coital headache there may be an antecedent dull occipital pain that increases in severity over seconds to minutes as the intensity of the exercise increases and if the person stops exerting themselves, this warning headache will subside and they will not experience the sudden severe headache. The aetiology of this headache is unknown. Recurrent episodes may occur for weeks, occasionally months.

# Benign Sex (Orgasmic or Coital) Headache

Benign sex headache, orgasmic or coital headache is now called primary headache associated with sexual activity and consists of bilateral headache precipitated by masturbation or coitus in the absence of any intracranial disorder.[30,31] The headache occurs at the moment of orgasm and is of sudden onset and is excruciatingly severe. It is predominantly occipital but may be frontal or generalized. It is brief, lasting minutes, rarely hours. There are no associated symptoms. *There is a valuable clue that is not seen with subarachnoid haemorrhage.* The patient may experience a dull pain in the occipital or sub-occipital region that increases in severity as excitement increases, subsides if they interrupt sexual activity only to recur if they become aroused again. If the patient interrupts their sexual activity and avoids orgasm this dull headache subsides without the subsequent severe explosive headache. If you can obtain this history, then the diagnosis is quite straightforward. On the other hand, if the history of this warning headache is not elicited then the major differential diagnosis, particularly if the headache lasts hours is SAH. The aetiology of this headache is unclear but it is almost invariably seen in patients who are experiencing considerable stress in their lives, and once the stress resolves, so do the headaches.

Rarely patients may experience their first subarachnoid haemorrhage when coughing, sneezing, straining, exerting themselves or during sexual intercourse.[26] Here although the headache will be explosive in onset, there will not be an antecedent warning headache moments before the explosive headache, the headache persists for hours to days and is usually associated with nausea, vomiting, neck stiffness and possibly a focal neurological deficit and, or depression of the conscious state.

| Treatment of Cough, Exertional and Benign Sex Headache |
| --- |
| The most important aspect of the management of cough, exertional and benign sex headaches is to reassure the patient of their benign nature and to advise them that they will resolve with time. Cough, exertional and benign sex headache may be helped by the introduction of indomethacin 25-100 mg per day, other non-steroidal anti-inflammatory drugs, or a beta-blocker. |

# Ice Cream or Cold Stimulus Headache

Ice-cream headache is now referred to as cold stimulus headache. It occurs when the patient is eating or drinking something very cold such as ice cream and it touches the palate or posterior pharyngeal wall. The patient experiences the onset over seconds of an excruciating, unilateral frontal headache that can be so severe that it may induce profound bradycardia and syncope. This is a common cause of headache in adolescents [32] and is not influenced by eating ice cream more slowly.[33]

# Ice Pick Headache – Primary Stabbing Headache

Ice pick headache, also termed jabs and jolts is now called primary stabbing headache. It a curious entity in which the patient experiences recurrent, brief stabbing pains, often localized to one part of the head, rarely in other parts of the body. The patient describes the pain as lancinating, like a needle, a nail or an ice pick being stabbed into their scalp. The pain lasts seconds only, may occur as a single jab or there may be many stabs within seconds to a minute. The commonest site is the temples. The same site on the opposite side (mirror image) of the head may be similarly affected. Ice pick headaches occur more commonly in patients with migraine. They can occur during or before the migraine but often in isolation.[34] They are benign and do not represent any sinister underlying pathology, reassurance is all that is required.

Ice-pick headache is another of the indomethacin responsive headache syndromes.

## Aseptic or Viral Meningitis

Very rarely, aseptic or viral meningitis may present with the very abrupt onset of severe headache. [16] The associated fever, sweats and the presence of an antecedent upper respiratory tract infection provide clues to the possible diagnosis. A lumbar puncture may be required to differentiate aseptic meningitis from subarachnoid haemorrhage.

# Posture Induced Headache

Severe headache on standing that resolves on lying flat is characteristic of low-pressure headache due to reduced CSF pressure. Low-pressure headache most often occurs after a lumbar puncture but may develop with a CSF leak, the so-called spontaneous low-pressure headache.

## Post Lumbar Puncture Headache

The characteristic and pathognomic feature is a headache that worsens within 15 minutes of standing and resolves within 30 minutes if the patient lies completely flat, [9] particularly if the foot of the bed or the legs are elevated. If the patient lies down on several pillows, the headache will be less severe but not abolished. The headache must resolve to be confident it is a low-pressure headache as all headaches are usually less severe when patients lie down. The headache can be dull or throbbing, frontal, occipital or generalised, worsened by coughing, sneezing, and straining. i.e., non-specific features.

There is often neck discomfort, other associated symptoms include a change in hearing (hyperacusis), nausea, blurred vision, photophobia, horizontal diplopia, occasionally facial numbness, cognitive abnormalities and even coma. All these symptoms resolve when the patient lies completely flat. The headache usually develops within one or two days of the lumbar puncture or epidural, although rare cases occurring 12 days later have been described. [35] The CSF pressure can be measured to confirm the diagnosis. [36] Although it usually resolves spontaneously, there are reports of it persisting for up to 19 months. [37]

Post lumbar puncture headache occurs in as many as 30% of patients when a traditional Quincke needle is employed. [38] This needle has a very sharp tip. The incidence is reduced to as little as 5% with a pencil-point LP needle. It is also less frequent when a smaller gauge needle is used. It occurs in 70% of patients with a 16-19 gauge, 40% with a 20-22 gauge and 12% with a 24-27 gauge. Inserting the bevel parallel rather than at right angles to the fibres of the dura, reinserting the stylet before removing the needle also reduces the risk.[39-40, 176] There is no evidence that bed rest following an LP reduces the incidence of headache. The incidence is also not influenced by whether the lumbar puncture is performed in the sitting or lying position or whether increased fluids are administered. The volume of cerebrospinal fluid (CSF) removed does not increase the incidence of post-lumbar puncture headaches.

> There should be no hesitation in removing copious amounts of CSF for diagnostic purposes.

## Low-Pressure Headache

Low-pressure headache was also referred to as spontaneous intracranial hypotension. The new nomenclature is headache attributed to low CSF pressure. It is identical to the headache seen after a lumbar puncture. This headache relates to a leak of CSF either from the nose following a head injury (rarely a spontaneous leak) or in the majority of patients, the leak is at the level of the spine, particularly the thoracic spine and cervicothoracic junction. [36]

| **Investigation and Treatment of Low Pressure and Post LP Headache** |
|---|
| Subdural fluid collections, pachymeningeal enhancement, pituitary hyperaemia and brain sagging may be visualized on CT scans. Magnetic resonance imaging may be normal, although it may detect pockets of CSF outside the dura. Myelography or CSF isotope studies can often identify the CSF leak [36, 41] but are not necessary to make the diagnosis. Radioisotope cisternography typically shows an absence of activity over the cerebral convexities, even at 24 or 48 hours, and early appearance of activity in the kidneys and urinary bladder. Nasal endoscopy may detect the CSF leak in patients with a fractured base of the skull. Initial treatment is effective in as many as 85% of patients [42] and consists of lying the patient completely flat with the foot of the bed elevated, copious fluids (unproven benefit) and if this fails an epidural blood patch is often effective. [43] Occasionally more than one epidural blood patch may be required, [44] even 19 months after the onset. [37] |

# First Episode of Headache with Gradual Onset

> There is one overarching principle in clinical medicine. DO NOT MISS the treatable or the diagnosis that, if missed, could lead to disastrous consequences.

Cranial arteritis, bacterial meningitis and ethmoid sinusitis are three causes of headache that must not be missed.

## Cranial or Giant Cell Arteritis

Cranial arteritis is also called giant cell arteritis or temporal arteritis as most often the temporal arteries are affected. It is a vasculitis of large and medium-sized arteries. It involves the aorta and its extracranial branches particularly the temporal and occipital arteries.[45] Cranial arteritis is a disorder of the older patient where the mean age is almost 75. [46] It is rare below the age of fifty.[47] It is more common in women, and age-specific incidence rates increase with age. [48] Cranial arteritis is a medical emergency, as a delay in diagnosis may lead to irreversible blindness due to ophthalmic artery occlusion.

Patients present with the insidious onset of severe headache increasing in severity over days or even weeks and often but not invariably associated with one or more of the following:

- scalp tenderness (pain on brushing or washing the hair)
- jaw claudication (pain in the jaw with chewing)

- polymyalgia rheumatica with aches and pains in the shoulder region and often in the proximal legs, occurs in up to 50% of patients.

Occasionally the patient has prominent, tender thrombosed extra-cranial arteries (figure 9.4). Headache is not the only presentation of cranial arteritis. It can present with or be associated with anorexia, weight loss, joint pains, a fever of unknown origin, transient visual obscurations (lasting minutes up to two hours), central retinal artery occlusion or anterior ischaemic optic neuropathy [AION] resulting in unilateral or even bilateral blindness.[49-51] Diplopia (double vision) occurs with ischaemia of the extra-ocular muscles or nerves innervating those muscles. [49]

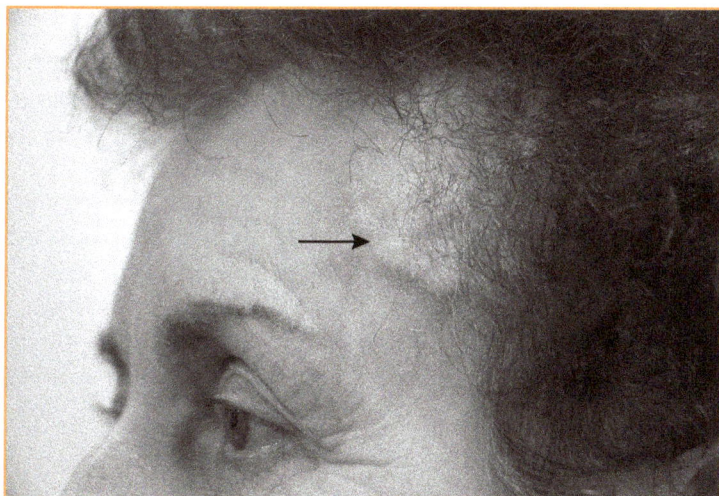

**Figure 9.4** Prominent temporal arteries that are tender and non-pulsatile indicate thrombosis of the vessel.

| Investigation and Treatment of Cranial Giant Cell Arteritis |
| --- |
| The erythrocyte sedimentation rate (ESR) and C-reactive protein (CRP) may be normal initially and repeated testing over the ensuing days and weeks is necessary. Biopsy of the temporal or occipital artery can be diagnostic. The disease process is not contiguous along the vessel, and the biopsy should involve a long segment of the artery; otherwise, the biopsy could be normal. [52] The diagnostic yield is higher with a minimum length of 1 cm. [53] |
| High dose prednisolone is the drug of first choice. The addition of (azathioprine, if methotrexate is not tolerated) lowers the recurrence rate, enables a reduction of the dose of Prednisolone, thus decreasing the risk of serious adverse events with higher dose steroids. [158] |
| Tocilizumab (TCZ), an IL-6 receptor inhibitor is recommended for a maximum of 1 year for refractory and relapsing disease in those who have not received TCZ previously. [159] IL-6 is one of several cytokines that have been implicated in the pathogenesis of cranial arteritis. Other Tumour Necrosis Factor TNFμ inhibitors Abatacept and Ustekinumab are currently being studied in patients with large vessel arteritis.[160-161] |

# Acute Bacterial or Viral Meningitis

Isolated headache, particularly in the absence of fever, is unlikely to be due to meningitis.

In general, patients present with increasingly severe generalised headache developing over several hours rarely days. Headache, fever and neck stiffness occurs in > 90% of patients. [54] Photophobia, nausea and vomiting, a change in mental status, seizures and focal neurological deficits may also occur. Worsening of headache with eye movement is a characteristic feature.

The clinical features of meningitis in its early stages can often be non-specific, yet patients with fulminant meningitis may deteriorate rapidly over hours, particularly meningococcal meningitis. It is important to have a high index of suspicion. Meningococcal meningitis and septicaemia are often associated with a petechial or purpuric rash. [55]
Viral meningitis can be mild such that patients may not present in the early stages.

# Sinusitis

Sinusitis is a rare but commonly over-diagnosed cause of headaches and facial pain. Eighty per cent of patients with either a self or physician diagnosis of sinusitis fulfil the IHS migraine criteria. [101,102] The detection of thickened mucosa in the sinuses with medical imaging is common, but without a fluid level this does not represent acute sinusitis. Frontal and maxillary sinusitis usually present with facial pain and are discussed below. Ethmoid or sphenoid sinusitis presents with severe midline headache behind the nose associated with malaise and low-grade fever. The diagnosis can be challenging if the ostium to the sinus is occluded as there will be no nasal discharge. Tenderness is not present as the ethmoid and sphenoid sinuses are deep within the skull. As the sinusitis progresses, the pain increases over the ethmoidal area; however, the pain can be referred to the medial orbital, eye, and brow. Acute ethmoid sinusitis can progress rapidly, presenting with facial and orbital cellulitis, meningitis or cavernous sinus thrombosis. Although it can have a bacterial, viral, fungal, or allergic aetiology, it is most often bacterial.

# Recurrent Headaches

Most patients with recurrent headaches either have a primary headache syndrome such as migraine and tension-type headache or one of the trigeminal autonomic cephalalgias.

## Migraine

In the 1st two editions of the IHS classification [9,56], migraine was categorised as classical, common or migraine equivalents. In the revised criteria, the classification has changed such that migraine with aura replaced classic migraine, common migraine became migraine without aura, and migraine equivalents was renamed aura without migraine headache. [9]

When the sub-acute onset of headache is accompanied by spreading photopsia (flashing lights), scotomata (patches of visual loss), nausea, vomiting, photophobia, phonophobia and paraesthesia the most likely diagnosis is migraine with aura. However, migraine is not the only cause of such a constellation of symptoms. The simultaneous onset of headache, photopsia, nausea and vomiting can occur with vertebrobasilar ischaemia affecting the occipital lobes. (chapter 10)

It is the progressive evolution of the headache and associated symptoms with the initial symptoms showing signs of either improving or have resolved before the latter symptoms appear or reach their full intensity in terms of severity or distribution that is **pathognomonic** of migraine.

Wolff [57] suggested that the aura resulted from vasoconstriction of the intracranial vessels, and the headache was the consequence of dilatation of the extracranial vessels. The unique changes of cerebral blood flow seen in patients during migraine with aura [58] have been replicated in animal experiments. [59] However, a magnetic resonance imaging study [60] has failed to confirm any changes in cerebral blood flow during nitroglycerin and induced migraine. [61]

Cortical spreading depression of Leäo [62] occurs in migraine. It consists of a slowly propagated wave of depolarization followed by suppression of brain activity. It is heralded by a brief phase of excitation that is immediately followed by prolonged nerve cell depression. [59] Cortical spreading depression (SD) is now widely recognized as the neurophysiological substrate of classical migraine aura and may be involved in migraines without a perceived aura. [63] Cortical spreading depression moves across the cortex at a rate of 3–5 mm/min. This slow spread of cortical depolarization is reflected in the gradual evolution of the associated visual and other focal neurological symptoms associated with migraine. The current theory regarding the pathophysiology is that migraine involves alterations in the sub-cortical aminergic sensory modulatory systems that influence the brain widely. [193]

The more common varieties of migraine in the IHS classification are listed below, with the ICHD 3 names after the hyphen. [9,175]

- Classic – Migraine with typical aura
- Migraine without aura – Migraine without aura
- Migraine without headache, migraine equivalents -Typical aura without headache
- Basilar artery migraine – Migraine with brainstem aura
- Hemiplegic migraine – Hemiplegic migraine
- Status migrainosus – Status migrainosus
- Menstrual migraine – Menstrually-related migraine with aura, Pure menstrual migraine with aura

| Contrarian Point of View[2] |
| --- |
| I have an issue with the ICHD statement that migraine is a unilateral throbbing headache. Over the 45 years I have enjoyed neurology, this has <u>not</u> been my experience. I analysed the headache characteristics in patients with classic migraine (migraine with aura) where most would concur with the diagnosis. In many patients, the headache was constant, not throbbing, and bilateral, not unilateral. I found three characteristic features that seem to occur in virtually all patients. Patients with migraine typically retire to bed without a headache and are either: 1. Awoken in the middle of the night or 2. They awaken at their normal time the following morning with a severe headache. 3. The other characteristic is that the headache increases in severity over a short period, usually minutes up to two hours. |

## Migraine with Aura – Migraine with Typical Aura

Migraine with typical aura is a headache associated with a variable combination of visual, gastrointestinal, and neurological symptoms. Photophobia and phonophobia may occur. Some patients may experience non-specific symptoms such as changes in appetite, drowsiness, yawning and alterations of mood (irritability or depression), anything up to 24 hours before the onset of headache.

An aura occurs in a little over ⅓ of patients, on average lasts 27 minutes, with the headache following within approximately 10 minutes. [64] The pathognemonic feature is that the visual and or neurological symptoms evolve gradually with the initial symptoms disappearing as the latter

---

2  Personal unpublished and unproven observations

either commence or increase in severity. There is a separation in time between each aspect of the aura; the visual, sensory, and other focal neurological symptoms *do not all develop simultaneously.*

## The Aura

### Visual Symptoms

Many visual symptoms can occur during the aura. Photopsia (flashing lights) consist of zigzag or jagged lines, bright spots, or stars. Some patients see walls that resemble a medieval fort, these are referred to as fortification spectra within the fortification spectra, the vision is blurred. Scintillating scotomas are blind spots that flicker and waver between light and dark. A scotoma may occur in the absence of any fortification spectra resulting in patch of loss of vision replaced by greyness or blackness. At times contralateral hemianopia or even total blindness may occur.

### Sensory symptoms

The sensory symptoms consist of tingling or numbness. They commence in one part of the body e.g., the hand, and gradually spread over 10–20 minutes to involve a greater area of the body. Usually, when the sensory symptoms have reached the foot or face, they have either diminished in intensity or are no longer present at the site where they originated. The sensory symptoms persist for up to 20 minutes. They may be ipsilateral or contralateral to the headache. [65] Alterations in speech (dysphasia) and weakness may occur but are much less common.

> Photopsia are not specific to migraine and may occur with posterior vitreous detachment, retinal detachment, or occipital lobe infarction.

## The Headache

The migraine headache is more commonly unilateral and frontal but may be bilateral, occipital, or generalised. The headache begins in the neck in some patients and radiates up to the head. Very rarely, migraine can affect just the face, referred to as lower half headache. Stabbing pains likened to being stabbed by ice pick are common in patients with migraine.[34] They may occur at the time of the migraine and at other times.

The headache increases in severity over minutes to an hour or two (more rapidly than a tension-type headache). A misconception is that migraine headache is throbbing, but this occurs in only 50% of patients. Constant non-throbbing headache is equally as common. The migraine headache is severe, lasting less than four hours in 27%, four to 24 hours in 40%, one to two days in 11% and longer than two days in 22% of patients.[66]

## Migraine Without Aura

The ICHD 3 [175] defines migraine without aura as at least 5 attacks of recurrent moderate to severe unilateral, pulsating headaches lasting 4–72 hours. The headache is either aggravated by or causes avoidance of routine physical activity. It is often, but not invariably, associated with mild nausea and or photophobia and phonophobia. The features that I believe differentiate common migraine from tension-type headaches have been listed above in the contrarian thought box As already stated, many patients do not have a throbbing unilateral headache[3]

---

3  Personal observation

Patients with tension-type headaches or chronic daily headaches typically retire to bed with a headache and awaken the following day with the same headache that fluctuates in severity throughout the day.

It is uncertain whether migraine with aura and migraine without aura are the same disorder as far as treatment is concerned. [67]

## Migraine Without Headache – Typical Aura Without Headache

The term migraine without headache has been replaced by the term typical aura without headache. These are episodes of completely reversible visual and or sensory symptoms with or without speech disturbance developing gradually, lasting less than 60 minutes and without a subsequent headache. [68,69] In essence, these patients experience the symptoms typical of the aura of migraine without subsequently developing a headache. The diagnosis is not difficult when the symptoms have occurred in the past with a migraine headache. When patients have never experienced a migraine, it can be challenging to differentiate such symptoms from transient ischaemic attacks. Once again I stress that the pathognomonic clue that the diagnosis is migraine is that the first symptoms show signs of resolving before subsequent symptoms appear or fully develop. The term fully develop refers to either their intensity or the extent of the area of the body affected. If the neurological symptoms develop simultaneously, or if the initial symptoms are not showing signs of abating as the latter symptoms are developing, then the diagnosis of cerebral ischaemia should be considered.

## Basilar Artery Migraine – Migraine with Brainstem Aura

The term basilar artery migraine has been renamed migraine with brainstem aura. This refers to a migraine headache with aura symptoms originating from the brainstem without motor weakness. To the uninitiated patients with this form of migraine can be terrifying. They present with an altered conscious state, total blindness, visual hallucinations, photopsia, fortification spectra, vertigo, ataxia, perioral and peripheral tingling, or numbness. The symptoms last two to 45 minutes, followed by a severe throbbing headache and vomiting lasting several hours. [70] Basilar artery migraine is more common in young females. Fortunately, the attacks are infrequent.

## Hemiplegic Migraine

Migraine with aura associated with weakness was referred to as hemiplegic migraine. If a first or second-degree relative is affected, it is called familial hemiplegic migraine (FHM). [71] Several types of FHM are identified. [175] A sporadic form is seen in those without a family history. Migraine with aura associated with weakness is extremely rare. This diagnosis should probably left to a neurologist. The unilateral motor symptoms of hemiplegic migraine differ from the more common forms of aura. There is no apparent spread of symptoms, and the duration of motor weakness is much greater than in the other aura types. Patients often have a unilateral weakness for hours to days. [72]

## Menstrual migraine

Menstrual migraine is attacks of migraine without aura in menstruating women occurring exclusively on day 1 (+/- 2 days) of menstruation in at least two out of three menstrual cycles and do not occur when they are not menstruating. Menstrual migraine occurs during or after the time at which oestradiol and progesterone levels fall to their lowest. [73, 74] Some patients experience migraines at other and in these individuals, the menstrual-related migraine may not necessarily have a hormonal basis.

## Retinal Migraine

Retinal migraine [175] is characterized by repeated attacks of monocular visual disturbance, including scintillations, scotomata, or blindness, associated with migraine headache. The diagnostic criteria are:

A Attacks fulfilling criteria for Migraine with aura and B below
B Aura characterized by both of the following:
    **1.** fully reversible, monocular, positive and or negative visual phenomena e.g. scintillations, scotomata or blindness confirmed during an attack by either or both of the following:
      • clinical visual field examination
      • the patient's drawing of a monocular field defect (made after explicit instruction)
    **2.** at least two of the following:
      • spreading gradually over ≥5 minutes
      • symptoms last 5-60 minutes
      • accompanied, or followed within 60 minutes, by headache
C Not better accounted for by another ICHD-3 diagnosis, and other causes of amaurosis fugax have been excluded.

## Vestibular Migraine

Vestibular migraine is not included in the 3rd edition of the IHS Classification of Headache Disorders (ICHD) 2013 beta version [56] nor is it in the main table of the 2018 iteration.[174] There is a different classification in the appendix on the IHS ICHD-3 website that contains the term vestibular migraine. The classification scheme has been modified significantly on this website.[4,5]

| Contrarian Thought |
| --- |
| Both migraine and vertigo are common and may be present in the same individual.<br>My personal observations are that vestibular migraine is rare and frequently over-diagnosed in patients with a previous history of migraine who develop vertigo. I would be more convinced if the vertigo has the pathognomonic feature as with other symptoms of migraine and that is gradual worsening or improvement when other symptoms have either resolved or are lessening in intensity when the vertigo follows them or that the vertigo is improving if it precedes the other symptoms. |

---

4  Accessed 15th May 2021 https://ichd-3.org/appendix/
5  I was unable to find any explanation for the modifications in the appendix.

Diagnostic criteria:

**A** At least five episodes fulfilling criteria C and D

**B** A current or past history of *Migraine without aura* or *Migraine with aura*[i]

**C** Vestibular symptoms[ii] of moderate or severe intensity[iii], lasting between 5 minutes and 72 hours[iv]

**D** At least half of episodes are associated with at least one of the following three migrainous features[v]:

  **1.** headache with at least two of the following four characteristics:

    a) unilateral location

    b) pulsating quality

    c) moderate or severe intensity

    d) aggravation by routine physical activity

  **2.** photophobia and phonophobia

  **3.** visual aura

**E** Not better accounted for by another ICHD-3 diagnosis or by another vestibular disorder[vi].[6]

---

6 **Notes:**

  i  Code also for the underlying migraine diagnosis.

  ii  Vestibular symptoms, as defined by the Bárány Society's Classification of Vestibular Symptoms and qualifying for a diagnosis of A1.6.6 Vestibular migraine, include:

    a) spontaneous vertigo:

      – internal vertigo (a false sensation of self-motion).

      – external vertigo (a false sensation that the visual surround is spinning or flowing).

    b  positional vertigo, occurring after a change of head position.

    c) visually-induced vertigo, triggered by a complex or large moving visual stimulus.

    d) head motion-induced vertigo, occurring during head motion.

    e) head motion-induced dizziness with nausea (dizziness is characterized by a sensation of disturbed spatial orientation; other forms of dizziness are currently not included in the classification of vestibular migraine).

  iii  Vestibular symptoms are rated moderate when they interfere with but do not prevent daily activities and severe when daily activities cannot be continued.

  iv  Duration of episodes is highly variable. About 30% of patients have episodes lasting minutes, 30% have attacks for hours and another 30% have attacks over several days. The remaining 10% have attacks lasting seconds only, which tend to occur repeatedly during head motion, visual stimulation or after changes of head position. In these patients, episode duration is defined as the total period during which short attacks recur. At the other end of the spectrum, there are patients who may take 4 weeks to recover fully from an episode. However, the core episode rarely exceeds 72 hours.

  v  One symptom is sufficient during a single episode. Different symptoms may occur during different episodes. Associated symptoms may occur before, during or after the vestibular symptoms.

  vi  History and physical examinations do not suggest another vestibular disorder, or such a disorder has been considered but ruled out by appropriate investigations or such a disorder is present as a comorbid condition, but episodes can be clearly differentiated. Migraine attacks may be induced by vestibular stimulation. Therefore, the differential diagnosis should include other vestibular disorders complicated by superimposed migraine attacks. NB noted 7 and 8 (labelled here vii and viii to avoid confusion with the footnotes) are missing on the website.

## Principles of Treatment of Migraine

One of the most difficult aspects of treating patients with migraine is that they have not kept accurate records regarding previous therapy. Many patients vaguely recall using a particular drug, often cannot recall the exact name, certainly can't remember what dose they talk, whether it helped or whether it caused side-effects. In the past I advised patient to keep an accurate record, now there are several migraine apps to help patients keep detailed records.[7]

> A major issue in patients with long-standing migraine is their poor record keeping. "I remember a little white tablet but cannot recall the name, how much I took and why I stopped it." I encourage patients to keep a paper or electronic diary, recording the name of the drug, how many times per day they took it, the maximum dose used and the reason for stopping, either lack of efficacy or side effects and what side effects. Many patients are prescribed small doses used for short periods and often stopped for perceived side effects that were probably not due to the medication

The principles of pharmacologic preventive treatment of migraine are:
- use evidence-based treatments when possible and appropriate
- start with a low dose and titrate slowly
- reach a therapeutic dose if possible
- allow for an adequate treatment trial duration
- establish expectations of therapeutic response and adverse events
- maximize adherence [156]
- insist that the patient keep accurate records.

The most appropriate treatment is to identify and eliminate any precipitating factors. Some patients are adamant that their migraine is precipitated by certain foods, particularly in children. [75, 76] The commonest foods include cow's milk, egg, chocolate, oranges, wheat, orange juice, cheese, artificial colourings and preservatives such as benzoic acid and tartrazine found in tinned, packet and junk food. Alcohol seems to be the offending agent in others. Elimination of the offending substance, in theory, should reduce the frequency of migraine. However, a careful study by McQueen et al [77] could not demonstrate any benefit from an elimination diet. Despite this, one encounters patients who are adamant that they had experienced fewer migraine headaches when they eliminated the food they had identified as precipitating their migraine attacks.[8] Treatment begins with a headache and diet diary and the selective avoidance of foods presumed to trigger attacks. [75]

Non-pharmacological treatments are often advocated. Although psychological factors are important migraine triggers, the efficacy of psychological therapy has not been confirmed in controlled trials. Biofeedback-relaxation therapy is effective in some patients. [78] A meta-analysis of acupuncture concluded that there is weak evidence for efficacy. [79] Hypnotherapy is difficult to subject to randomised controlled trials. One unblinded study claimed efficacy.[80] A systematic review of cognitive behavioural therapy concluded there was insufficient evidence to make formal recommendations. [157] Some patients claim that their migraine was helped by a chiropractor or a osteopath performing neck manipulation but there is no objective scientific evidence of benefit.

---

7   The 10 best migraine apps. https://www.medicalnewstoday.com/articles/319508
8   Personal Observation

**The pharmacological treatment of migraine is influenced by:**

1. The frequency and the severity of the attacks.
2. The patient's willingness to accept the potential risk of side effects from drugs
3. Whether vomiting occurs early during the migraine, thus preventing oral therapy. In this latter circumstance, subcutaneous, intravenous, sublingual, intranasal or rectal therapy will need to be employed.

Prophylaxis is indicated if the migraine attacks are frequent. If the migraine attacks are infrequent but very severe and difficult to treat when they occur, many patients will prefer to take prophylactic medication. If the migraines are infrequent, many patients will opt not to expose themselves to the potential risk of side effects of daily drugs. Ultimately the patient decides to choose therapy at the time of the migraine or prophylaxis.

There are many drugs for treating acute migraine and prophylactic therapy.[81] These are likely to change over the ensuing years. As migraine is an unpredictable illness, only the results from randomized controlled trials should decide what therapies are helpful. On the website, links are provided to sites that should contain up-to-date information regarding current recommendations. Currently, recommended therapy for both the individual migraine and prophylaxis is detailed in the appendix of this chapter.

Unfortunately, there is no way of predicting which patient will respond or not respond to a particular therapy. In clinical practice, it is often a matter of trial and error. The principle is to initially use drugs with the least potential side effects and then move to perhaps more potent therapies potentially associated with a greater risk of side effects.

| Treatment of Migraine in Adults |
|---|
| The principles of treatment have been discussed. The appendix contains two tables listing the currently recommended drugs for treating acute attacks (Table 9.2) and for prevention (Table 9.3) of migraine. Only those with level 1 evidence (randomised controlled trials) are included. |
| Krymchantowski has recommended combination therapy to suit the individual patient profile, with the use of analgesics or a non-steroidal anti-inflammatory drug together with a triptan or a gastrokinetic drug. [82] |
| A multicentre, randomized, double-blind, single-dose, placebo-controlled study found that two tablets of 250 mg Acetylsalicylic acid (ASA) + 200 mg Paracetamol + 50 mg Caffeine (Thomapyrin) was statistically more effective than two tablets of 250 mg ASA + 200 mg Paracetamol, two tablets of 500 mg ASA, two tablets of 500 mg Paracetamol, two tablets of 50 mg Caffeine, and placebo in patients who were used to treating their episodic tension-type headache or migraine attacks with non-prescription analgesics. [83] |
| Botulinum toxin type A (BoNTA) is safe, effective, and well-tolerated in reducing the frequency of headache episodes in patients with chronic daily headache,[84, 85] chronic migraine [191] but not acute migraine. [86, 87] Botulinum toxin reduces migraine frequency by only two days per month. [191] and chronic daily headache by seven days per month. [85] |
| A placebo-controlled (sham surgery) study demonstrated that surgical deactivation of peripheral migraine headache trigger sites is an effective alternative treatment for patients who suffer from frequent moderate to severe migraine headaches that are difficult to manage with standard protocols. [88] |
| Since the 1st edition of this book, drugs have been developed that are specifically designed to treat acute attacks as well as prevent migraine as opposed to previous drugs that were used for other purposes but found to be effective in migraine. These drugs are monoclonal antibodies that either target calcitonin gene-related peptide (CGRP) or are CGRP receptor antagonists. At the time of writing these drugs were very expensive and beyond the financial resources of many patients. CGRP is increased in venous blood in patients with a headache due to migraine and cluster headache and normalises after the headache subsides. [see reviews 152,153] |

**Treatment of Menstrual Related Migraine**

Menstrual related migraine does not respond well to the usual prophylactic measures. On the other hand, oestradiol implants or oestradiol gel can render some patients' headache free. [89] These patients do not respond as well to oestradiol implants. Two triptans are useful as prophylaxis, namely frovatriptan 2.5mg BD and naratriptan 1mg BD. [154] Some patients who experienced migraine at menstruation also experienced migraine at other times.

Several drugs, such as non-steroidal anti-inflammatory drugs and the triptans starting two days before the expected onset of menses and continuing for seven days, reduce the severity and duration of the headache but, unlike the oestradiol implants, do not abolish the headaches altogether. naproxen 550mg twice a day [90] and zolmitriptan 2.5 mg oral tablet, 2 or 3 times per day with three doses per day more effective than 2 per day. [91] Sumatriptan 85 mg combined with naproxen sodium 500 mg in a single fixed dose taken within one hour of onset of menstruation has also been shown to be effective but only in a little less than ⅓ of patients. [92] Another alternative is the prostaglandin synthesis inhibitor mefenamic acid at a dose of 500mg 8 hourly commencing at the onset of the headache.[155]

# Curiosities

## Nummular Headache

There is a peculiar primary headache called nummular headache. The pain is highly variable in duration but often chronic. The pain affects a small, circumscribed area of the scalp. It occurs in the absence of any underlying structural lesion. The painful area may be localized in any part of the scalp but is typically in the parietal region. Rarely, nummular headache is bilateral or multifocal, each symptomatic area retaining all the characteristics of nummular headache. Pain intensity is generally mild to moderate but occasionally severe. Superimposed on the background pain, spontaneous or triggered exacerbations may occur. In up to 75% of published cases, the disorder has been chronic (present for longer than three months), but other cases have been described where the duration can be seconds, minutes, hours, or days.

The affected area commonly shows variable combinations of hyperaesthesia, dysaesthesia, paraesthesia, allodynia and/or tenderness.

**The Diagnostic criteria are:**

A Continuous or intermittent head pain fulfilling criterion B
B Felt exclusively in an area of the scalp, with all of the following four characteristics:
   1. sharply contoured
   2. fixed in size and shape
   3. round or elliptical
   4. 1-6 cm in diameter
C Not better accounted for by another ICHD-3 diagnosis[1].

## Hypnic headache

Hypnic headache was previously called alarm clock headache. Hypnic headache consists of frequent, recurrent headache attacks developing only during sleep, awakening the patient from sleep, and lasting up to 4 hours. Hypnic headache is not associated with any other symptoms. Hypnic headache usually begins after age 50 but may occur in younger people. The pain is generally mild to moderate, but severe pain occurs in one-fifth of patients. The pain is bilateral in about two-thirds of cases. Attacks usually last 15 to 180 minutes, occasionally longer. Most cases are persistent, with daily or near-daily headaches, but an episodic subtype (on <15 days/month) may occur.

**Diagnostic criteria:**

A Recurrent headache attacks fulfilling criteria B-E

B Developing only during sleep, causing wakening

C Occurring on ≥10 days/month for >3 months

D Lasting from 15 minutes up to 4 hours after waking

E No cranial autonomic symptoms or restlessness

F Not better accounted for by another ICHD-3 diagnosis[1;2].

Other possible causes of a headache developing during and causing wakening from sleep should be ruled out, with particular attention given to sleep apnoea, nocturnal hypertension, hypoglycaemia and medication overuse. Intracranial disorders must also be excluded. However, the presence of sleep apnoea syndrome does not necessarily exclude the diagnosis of hypnic headache.

| Treatment of Hypnic Headache |
| --- |
| There are no controlled trials. Lithium, caffeine, melatonin, and indomethacin have been effective treatments in several reported cases. |

# External-Compression Headache

External-compression headaches result from sustained compression of pericranial soft tissues. External-compression headaches occur with a tight band around the head without damage to the scalp. The headache can be caused by a hat, a helmet, or goggles worn during swimming or diving.

**Diagnostic criteria:**

A At least two episodes of headache fulfilling criteria B-D

B Brought on by and occurring within 1 hour during sustained external compression of the forehead or scalp

C Maximal at the site of external compression

D Resolving within 1 hour after external compression is relieved

E Not better accounted for by another ICHD-3 diagnosis

# Trigeminal Autonomic Cephalalgias

Cluster headaches, SUNCT Syndrome and the paroxysmal hemicranias belong to a group of disorders that the IHS classifies as trigeminal autonomic cephalalgias. [9,175]

# Cluster Headache

The pain of cluster headache is **strictly unilateral.** It is almost invariably in or around the eye, although it may involve the temple, frontal, or maxillary regions. (Figure 9.5) The pain increases in severity over minutes to an hour or so and is excruciatingly severe. So severe it has been called suicide headache because during the headache patients experience suicidal thoughts.

The headaches last 15-180 minutes and occur every second day or up to eight times per day. There is often reddening and watering of the ipsilateral eye and blockage of the ipsilateral nostril. A transient Horner's syndrome (Figure 4.9, chapter 4) during the headache is virtually pathognomonic. When it does occur in women it is very similar except that women experience more vomiting and other "migrainous symptoms." [93]

The attacks occur in bouts or cluster's thus the name. These may be hours or days apart and there is a curious periodicity often occurring at the same time of the day or night with each subsequent attack and until the cluster resolves. The patient can almost set their clock to the headache. Alcohol can exacerbate the problem and patients voluntarily refrain during the bouts.

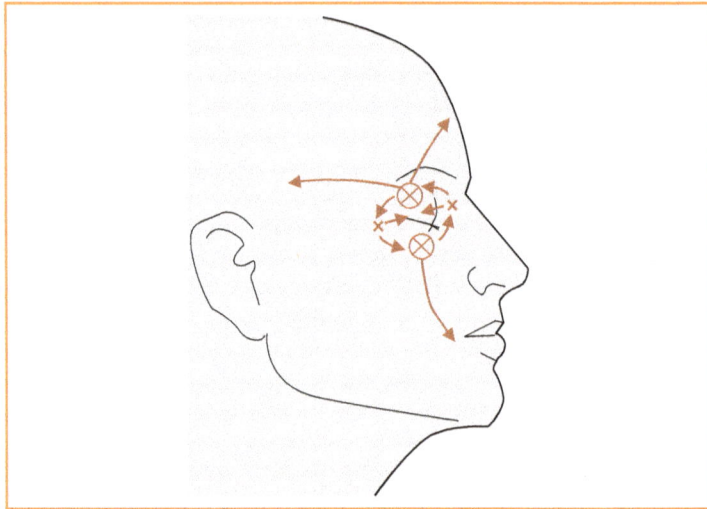

**Figure 9.5** the distribution of pain seen with classic cluster headache. Reproduced from: Headache second edition. Author Neil Hugh Raskin. Publisher Churchill Livingstone, London. figure 6.1 page 230[4]

| Treatment of Cluster Headache [186] |
|---|
| **Acute Attack** |
| 100% Oxygen 12-15l/min via closed face mask 15-20 minutes |
| Sumatriptan (6mg SC,20mg IN), zolmitriptan (2.5mg O or 5-10mg IN) max 10mg/24 hours |
| Dihydroergotamine (1mg SC) |
| Intranasal Lignocaine 4 sprays of 4% into the ipsilateral nostril |
| **Prophylaxis** |
| Verapamil 360-560mg/day (high dose) max 960mg/day |
| Corticosteroids 100mg/day* (O) [187] |
| Lithium Carbonate adjust dose to achieve 0.6-0.8mmol/L |
| Topiramate 100-200mg/day |
| Melatonin(conflicting results) 10mg daily |
| Galcanezumab 300mg at baseline and after 1 month [188] |
| Occipital nerve block/stimulation |
| **Abbreviations:** SC=subcutaneous, IN=intranasal, O=oral |
| *Whilst titrating an increasing dose of verapamil |

# Paroxysmal hemicrania

Paroxysmal hemicrania may either be episodic or chronic and consists of paroxysmal headache attacks where the character and localization of the pain, and the autonomic symptoms (although less severe) are very similar to those observed in cluster headache. However, the attacks are more frequent (by definition more than five per day for half of the time), shorter duration and lack the circadian rhythm seen with cluster headache. One of the diagnostic criteria is the complete abolition of headaches with Indomethacin.

# SUNCT

SUNCT is an acronym for **S**hort-lasting **U**nilateral **N**euralgiform headaches with **C**onjunctival injection and **T**earing. As opposed to cluster headache SUNCT is more common in females. The attacks last between five seconds and four minutes and occur from as few as three times per day to as often as 200 times per day. These headaches are also strictly unilateral and periorbital. They are triggered by touching the periorbital region, talking, or chewing food. The presence of mild conjunctival injection and watering of the ipsilateral eye differentiates the pain from trigeminal neuralgia. The other clue is that triggered pain (pain precipitated by touching a trigger point on the face) shows a refractory period in trigeminal neuralgia but not SUNCT syndrome.

# Tension-Type Headache

Tension-type headache has a variety of other names. Tension headache; muscle contraction headache; stress headache; ordinary headache; essential headache and psychogenic headache. The lifetime prevalence is 30-78%. Tension-type headaches (TTH) consist of mild to moderately severe non-throbbing headaches lasting minutes to days. TTH is not worse with routine physical activity[9], not associated with nausea, phonophobia or photophobia. The most characteristic feature is that the headache fluctuates in severity from hour to hour, day today. It is the main cause of headache that lasts all day every day for months on end. The headache is typically bilateral, although it can be unilateral and is described as a tight sensation around the head or a pressure sensation in the head. Some authorities consider tension-type headache and migraine headache without aura (common migraine) virtually indistinguishable, except that migraine headaches are relatively brief and episodic.[95]

Episodic tension-type headache is common in primary care. [96] Chronic daily headaches are commonly seen in the specialist clinic.[97] Many patients with the clinical features of tension-type headache take issue with the term tension-type, denying that there is tension or stress in their life. Some patients state that they could understand had the headache developed some time ago when there was considerable stress in their life. Others deny any pressure at all. The absence of stress should not preclude a diagnosis of tension-type headache. Similarly, the stress in someone with headaches is only circumstantial evidence that the headaches are tension-type. It is essential to use the diagnostic criteria for tension-type headache and then look for the tension in a patient's life to explain why they have tension-type headache. Lifestyle headaches is a term that most patients are more comfortable to accept. It refers to the fact that they are experiencing a headache because of a lack of balance between their personal, professional and the family

---

9   A Personal observation is that ALL headaches are worse with physical activity.

aspects of their life.[10] I almost invariably see them in patients who have stopped doing things that make their own personal life more enjoyable because of work and family commitments.

| **Treatment of Tension-Type Headache.** |
|---|
| If tension-type headaches are infrequent over the counter medications such as aspirin, paracetamol, ibuprofen or naprosyn are recommended. However, if headaches become more frequent excess use of these medications can create a vicious cycle resulting in medication over-use syndrome. (See below) No drug can cure tension-type headaches. |
| Textbooks advise a multifaceted approach to treating tension-type headaches, employing psychological, physiological and pharmacological therapies. [98] Hypnotherapy, meditation, relaxation therapy, biofeedback and acupuncture have all been advocated. Acupuncture has not been confirmed in randomized controlled trials[79], hypnotherapy resulted in less frequent less prolonged and less intense headaches in a single-blind study. [99] A recent internet-delivered behavioural regimen composed of progressive relaxation, limited biofeedback with autogenic training, and stress management claimed significant benefit compared to symptom monitoring waitlist controls.[100] |
| **Personal Approach** |
| In my experience, most young patients shun pharmacological therapy. Some patients are willing to use short-term pharmacological therapy using the analogy of saving oneself from drowning if the head is above water instead of having no chance if the head is below the water. It is suggested that the patient takes medication for a short time whilst altering their lifestyle[11], regaining a balance between work, family, and self. |

# Chronic Headaches
## Chronic Daily Headache

Chronic daily headache is daily tension-type headaches for six months or more.[12]

Chronic daily headache is defined as a headache on more than 15 days per month or 180 days per year. Approximately 35% to 40% of patients who seek treatment at headache clinics suffer from daily or near-daily headaches. [103] Some 80% of patients with chronic daily headaches have evolved from episodic headaches, predominantly migraine. This is referred to as "transformed migraine." In 20% of patients, the headache is daily from the outset. [104]

Chronic daily headaches may be constant or throbbing, mild, moderate, or severe, and often associated with phonophobia, photophobia, and nausea. Consistently unilateral headaches are seen in only 2% of patients. [105] The headache fluctuates in severity from hour to hour and day to day. Patients retire with a headache and awaken with the headache the following morning.

Excess analgesics or ergotamine overuse (termed medication or analgesic overuse headache**)** and stress are the two leading factors that appear to increase the risk of developing a chronic daily headache. However, in many patients, no obvious reason for their chronic daily headaches can be identified. Episodic migraine often continues once chronic daily headaches develop.

---

10 Personal unpublished and unproven observations. These patients do not have a balance between time for themselves, time for their work and time for their families. Many of these patient's headaches have resolved once they resume the physical or social activity that they had given up because they had become too busy.

11 Personal observation I fixed my own tension headaches within 2 weeks by taking wednesday afternoons off whilst being the only neurologist between Melbourne and Adelaide for 15 years working 12–14-hour days.

12 This term no longer exists in the IHS ICHD-3rd edition, but it is a very real entity in neurological clinics. The revised classification contains two entities, New daily persistent headache (7.1.1-NDPH) and medication-overuse headache (8.2-MOH)

The analgesic overuse syndrome is also referred to as a rebound headache or medication overuse headache (MOH). It is the perpetuation of head pain in chronic headache sufferers caused by frequent and excessive use of immediate relief medications. The IHS [175] diagnostic criteria are:

- Headache present on ≥ 15 days/month in patients with a pre-existing headache disorder
- Regular overuse for >3 months of one or more drugs used for acute and or symptomatic headache treatment.
- Not better accounted for by another ICHD-3 diagnosis

Medications that can cause the medication overuse headache include ergotamine preparations, opiates, triptans and simple analgesics such as aspirin or paracetamol.

---

**Treatment of Chronic Daily Headache**

Spontaneous improvement can occur on discontinuation of the medications causing the problem. Combining a tricyclic antidepressant[13] and cessation of analgesia reduces headache frequency more than cessation of analgesia alone. Kudrow, in his landmark study [107] demonstrated that only 10% resolved if nothing was changed, 30% improved with the addition of a tricyclic antidepressant, 43% when the only course taken was the cessation of analgesia and 70% with a combination of a tricyclic antidepressant and ceasing analgesia. There is no role for the SSRI's or SNRIs. Mirtazapine has similar noradrenergic blocking properties to tricyclic antidepressants. There are case reports claiming benefit, but it has not been subjected to a randomized trial. [182]

There is one study claiming benefit with prednisolone 60 mg/day for 2 days, 40 mg/day for 2 days and 20 mg/day for 2 days, plus ranitidine (to prevent a stomach ulcer) 300 mg/day for 6 days. [183].

Intravenous dihydroergotamine can break the vicious cycle of chronic daily headache, The initial test dose is 0.5mg with a second 0.5mg two hours later. This is followed by 1mg every eight hours for 48-72 hours.[184,185]

Cognitive behaviour therapy and changing lifestyle based on the observation[14] that most of these patients have forgotten they are an individual (as well as being married, a parent or a slave to their work) and there is nothing in their lives that enhances their quality of life.

---

# Headache in Chronic Meningitis

Chronic meningitis is inflammation of the meninges persisting for more than four weeks, associated with a CSF pleocytosis (increased white cell count). [108] In reality, the diagnosis is often delayed, and the average duration of symptoms varies from 17 to 43 months. [109] Chronic meningitis can be infective (cryptococcus, tuberculosis, listeria), non-infective (sarcoidosis, Mollarets, drugs) or malignant. [110] Low-grade fever, headache, and mild neck stiffness may be very subtle. Any one of these features may be absent. Mental status changes, seizures, or focal deficits may evolve over time. [111] The intensity of the headache can slowly worsen, fluctuate, or remain static. The headache is usually bilateral, frontal and retro-orbital. It may be associated with photophobia nausea, vomiting, generalised malaise, and weight loss. The presence of fever suggests an infective aetiology. Although significant weight loss can occur with all causes, it is more common with malignancy. Night sweats, neck stiffness, papilloedema and cranial nerve abnormalities have been described[15]. [112, 113]

---

13 I prefer nortryptiline as it can be broken in half. I start with 12.5mg and increase very slowly to the minimum effective, maximum tolerated dose up to a maximum of 100mg nocte.

14 Personal observation

15 It is one of the causes of a mononeuritis or mononeuritis multiplex. A simple mnenonic to remember the causes of a mononeuritis multiplex is DIAbeTeS M. D for diabetes, I for infections such as leprosy, syphilis, cryptococcus amd mycobacterium, A for arteritis, (forget the bee), T for trauma, S for sarcoid and M for malignancy.

# Idiopathic Intracranial Hypertension

The headache of Idiopathic intracranial hypertension (IIH) is constant or throbbing, worse with coughing or straining (like most headaches) and may mimic chronic tension-type headache. The headache is generalised and of low to moderate severity. At times it can be pulsatile and awaken the patient from sleep. Retro-ocular pain worse with eye movement can occur. [114] Visual obscurations (transient blindness lasting seconds) may occur, especially when straining. Pulsatile tinnitus is not uncommon. Bilateral papilloedema associated with enlargement of the blind spot and normal visual acuity may be the only sign, unless the patient develops cranial nerve palsies, a 6th is the commonest but other cranial nerve palsies can occur. MRI can detect swollen optic nerve sheaths, transverse sinus narrowing and an empty pituitary sella. An LP is required to exclude chronic meningitis and to measure the CSF pressure.

Diagnostic criteria for IIH [192]:
- **A** Papilloedema
- **B** Normal neurological examination (other than 6th nerve palsy)
- **C** Neuroimmaging: normal parent climber (no hydrocephalus, mass, structural lesion or meningeal enhancement). Venous thrombosis excluded in all.
- **D** Normal CSF constituents
- **E** Elevated lumbar puncture pressure ≥25 cm $H_2O$

# When to Worry

The great majority of patients with headaches will have one of the primary headache syndromes. It is often taught that a change in the character or nature of headaches suggests a possible sinister underlying cause but this scenario is very common in patients with migraine who develop chronic daily headache, so-called transformed migraine. The following features should alert the clinician to a possible more significant underlying cause.
- Headache awakening patients from sleep (again very common in migraine)
- Thunderclap onset of headache
- Headaches associated with focal neurological symptoms that accompany or outlast the headache[115]
- Long-lasting headaches (weeks or months)[115], (again common in chronic daily headache)
- Headache with systemic symptoms such as anorexia, weight loss or fever, scalp tenderness and jaw claudication
- New-onset headache in the elderly

# Headache and Brain Tumours

Many patients with headaches fear having a brain tumour (Figure 9.6), fortunately, these are very rare. Although headache is a common symptom of brain tumours, occurring in up to 70% of adults[116] and 60% of children[117] it is the sole manifestation in only 2% of patients. [118] *In primary care, the incidence of a brain tumour with a headache presentation is less than 0.1%.*[11,119] This implies a primary care physician will have to do 1000 imaging procedures on patients with a headache to detect one tumour!

Many of the features of the brain tumour associated headache are non-specific. It is mild to moderately severe, lasting for hours (not all day every day like chronic daily or tension-type headache) developing over weeks or months.[120] Headache awakening the patient from sleep and the presence of instability are the two main clinical features that should alert the clinician to the possibility of a brain tumour.[116, 120] Increasingly severe headache and the development of headache for the first time in elderly patients is another indication of a possible brain tumour.[121]

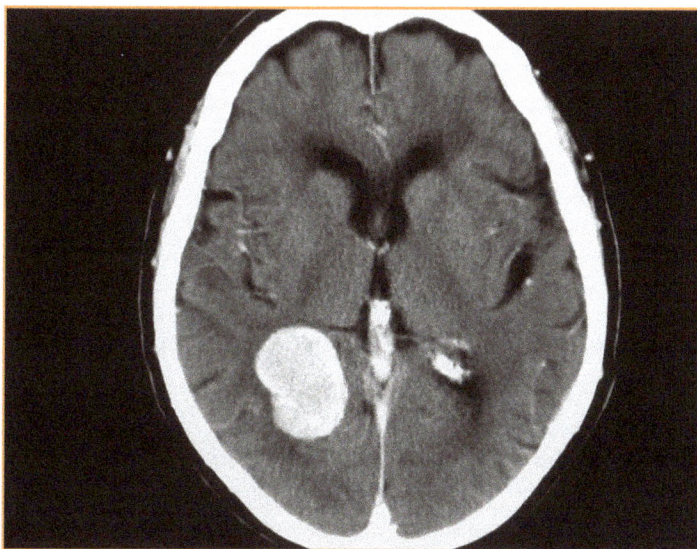

Figure 9.6 A CT scan of the brain demonstrating a large intraventricular meningioma.

# Investigating Headache

The American Academy of Neurology practice guidelines [121] has recommended imaging if:
- the Valsalva manoeuvre worsens the headache
- causes the patient to awaken from sleep
- is a new headache in an older patient
- a progressively worsening headache
- the presence of abnormal neurological findings

Neuroimaging is not warranted for patients with migraine and a normal neurological examination. There should be a lower threshold for neuroimaging in for patients with atypical headache features or patients who do not fulfil the strict definition of migraine.

The American Academy of Neurology guidelines state that there is insufficient evidence to choose between CT scan and MRI scan, nor is there sufficient evidence to indicate whether an enhanced CT scan is better than an unenhanced CT scan when evaluating patients with migraine or other non-acute headaches. [121]

In reality, most patients with headaches are terrified that they have a brain tumour and virtually demand some form of imaging of the brain. Many have had a CT scan well before referral to the neurologist. As opposed to an MRI scan, CT scan exposes young patients to radiation. I avoid CT scans in younger patients

# Facial Pain

There are many causes of facial pain. The more common ones include:
- Trigeminal Neuralgia
- Glossopharyngeal neuralgia
- Pain of Dental Origin
- Sinusitis
- Atypical Facial Pain
- Herpes Zoster Ophthalmicus and post-herpetic neuralgia
- Tolosa-Hunt Syndrome

## Trigeminal Neuralgia

Trigeminal neuralgia consists of brief lancinating pain, abrupt in onset and termination. The pain MUST be within the distribution of the trigeminal nerve. (Figure 1.9 Chapter 1) The pain is most common in the 2nd and 3rd divisions, rarely in the 1st. Although the paroxysms of pain may occur spontaneously, they are often precipitated by trivial stimuli such as washing, shaving, talking, brushing teeth or the wind blowing on the face.

Dental pain and the pain of trigeminal neuralgia are very commonly confused. [122] Both pains are within the distribution of the trigeminal nerve. Dental pain occurs in the distribution of the 2nd or 3rd but not the 1st division of the trigeminal nerve. Both may be precipitated by eating or chewing. **The vital clue** that the problem is trigeminal neuralgia is the presence of a trigger point on the face, an area that, if touched or sometimes even the wind blowing onto the area, will trigger a severe paroxysm of pain. The pain is so severe it makes the patient wince. Hence the term tic douloureux is derived from French, literally meaning a painful tick.

In general, this is a condition of older patients. Compression of the trigeminal nerve in the posterior fossa by an aberrant loop of a vessel is the principal cause. [123] Less commonly, it is symptomatic of another disorder such as a tumour or multiple sclerosis. Younger age, bilateral trigeminal neuralgia, abnormal trigeminal sensation, and corneal reflexes indicate a possible secondary cause. [12]

## Glossopharyngeal Neuralgia

The pain of Glossopharyngeal neuralgia is severe transient (seconds only) stabbing pain experienced in the ear, tonsillar fossa, base of the tongue or beneath the angle of the jaw. It is commonly provoked by coughing, swallowing, or talking. In between the spasms of pain, there may be a dull discomfort. In some patients, the pain is predominantly in the ear. In others, it is in the pharynx. The pain is beyond the glossopharyngeal nerve distribution, reflecting involvement in the auricular and pharyngeal branches of the vagus nerve.[127] Occasionally the pain is so severe that it results in transient asystole (no cardiac electrical activity).[128]

| Treatment of Trigeminal and Glossopharyngeal Neuralgia |
| --- |
| Carbamazepine or Oxcarbazepine are the drugs of choice for trigeminal and glossopharyngeal neuralgia. Baclofen and lamotrigine are alternatives.[12] If medical therapy fails, posterior fossa micro-vascular decompression is the treatment of choice.[123] In patients unable to undergo intracranial surgery, a percutaneous rhizotomy of the trigeminal ganglion is useful.[12] |

# Pain of Dental Origin

The pain of dental origin is very difficult to diagnose, particularly when due to a deep root abscess where the dentist often cannot see anything wrong with the tooth. The pain is a constant aching sensation, often fluctuating in severity at times very distressing. **The vital clue** is that pain of dental origin can be precipitated by contact of hot (and to a lesser extent cold) fluids on the affected tooth. [124]

A practical bedside test is to put ice blocks in a glass of water and ask the patient to swirl the ice-cold water around on the suspected side of the mouth. Warn the patient that this may cause a very severe pain attack. Start with the lower jaw and then the upper jaw. This may help localise the offending tooth. On occasions, pain is referred to the cheek when the problem is in the lower jaw.

---

Facial pain confined to the distribution of the 2nd or 3rd divisions of the trigeminal nerve is most likely trigeminal neuralgia or dental pain. A trigger spot on the face is pathognomonic for trigeminal neuralgia. Pain of dental origin may be triggered by drinking hot and less commonly cold fluids.

---

# Sinusitis

Acute sinusitis frequently follows an upper respiratory tract infection. Ipsilateral facial pain over the region of the infected sinus, associated with fever and purulent rhinorrhoea. [125] Clinical signs and symptoms most helpful in the diagnosis of maxillary and frontal sinusitis are the presence of a purulent nasal discharge, cough, purulent secretions observed on nasal examination and tenderness over the sinus. [126] A word of warning, many patients, have asymptomatic thickening of the mucosa of their maxillary and, to a lesser extent, frontal sinuses. In this setting, a diagnosis of sinusitis should be avoided in the absence of symptoms to suggest infection and no fluid level in the sinus on imaging.

# Persistent Idiopathic Facial Pain

Persistent idiopathic facial pain was previously referred to as atypical facial pain. Idiopathic facial pain consists of persistent facial pain that does not have the features of the cranial neuralgias and cannot be attributable to any other cause, i.e. it does not fit a recognized pattern.

The pain is deep, poorly localized, although most commonly in the region of the nasolabial fold or chin, present most of the day almost every day. Occasionally, the condition follows surgery or trauma in the trigeminal nerve distribution.[129] There are no abnormal neurological signs and no cause found despite detailed investigation. The aetiology of this condition is unclear; some authorities suggest depression plays a significant role although this is controversial. Very rarely patients presenting with facial pain will have a nasopharyngeal carcinoma.

---

**Treatment of Persistent Idiopathic Facial Pain**

Tricyclic antidepressants, such as amitryptiline, imipramine or nortriptyline are the treatment of choice for persistent idiopathic facial pain. [97, 130, 131] One should commence with the lowest possible dose and increase very, very slowly to the minimum effective or maximum tolerated dose. Often this is 75-100mg nocte.

---

# Post-Herpetic Neuralgia

Facial pain, usually burning in nature, in the distribution of the first division of the trigeminal nerve may precede by several days the onset of the characteristic rash of herpes zoster. Once the rash, consisting of blisters, appears the diagnosis is straightforward. Post-herpetic neuralgia may develop in as many as 50% of patients (more common in the elderly) where pain may persist for months or even years after the rash has resolved. The pain is stabbing or burning in nature, touching the skin lightly evokes pain, referred to as hyperaesthesia.

| Treatment of Herpes Zoster and Post Herpetic Neuralgia |
|---|
| Herpes Zoster vaccine reduces the incidence of herpes zoster and postherpetic neuralgia [132]. It is recommended for all persons aged ≥ 60 years if there are no contraindications. This includes persons who report a previous episode of zoster or who have a chronic medical condition.[133] |
| Treatment with Antiviral therapy [134] and a small dose of a tricyclic antidepressant such as amitryptiline 25mg once herpes zoster develops will lead to a more rapid reduction in the severity of the pain and the incidence of postherpetic neuralgia. [135] |
| Corticosteroids have been claimed to reduce the incidence of post-hepatic neuralgia in small unblinded, controlled trials. [136, 137] A Cochrane review concluded that there is insufficient evidence to justify their use. [138] Tricyclic antidepressants, such as amitryptiline, imipramine or nortriptyline are the treatment of choice for post-herpetic neuralgia. [97, 130, 131] |

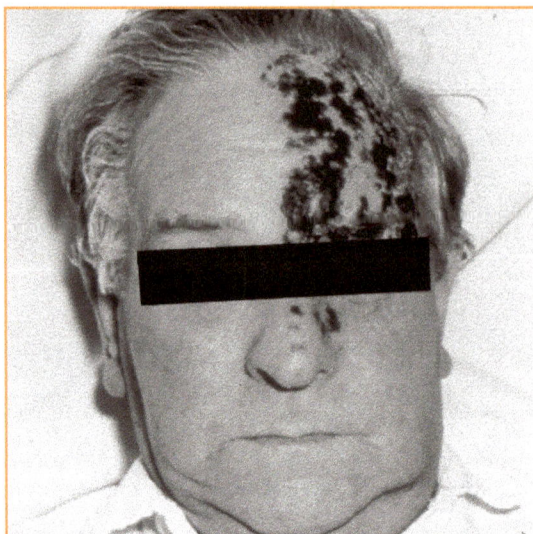

**Figure 9.7** Severe Herpes Zoster Ophthalmicus

# Tolosa-Hunt Syndrome

Tolosa–Hunt syndrome is a rare disorder due to a granulomatous inflammatory process of the cavernous sinus and or superior orbital fissure. Tolosa–Hunt syndrome is characterized by episodic orbital and periorbital pain with paralysis of the 3rd, 4th, or 6th cranial nerves developing within two weeks of the onset of pain. Occasionally the 1st division of the 5th cranial nerve may be affected. Tolosa–Hunt syndrome can remit spontaneously over days to weeks but may relapse. Many conditions that can produce a painful ophthalmoplegia that need to be excluded.

These include Graves' disease, Wegener's granulomatosis, sarcoidosis, diabetes, cavernous sinus thrombosis, aneurysm, and lymphoma. There is an excellent discussion in the review by Lutt et al. [139]

The IHS diagnostic criteria are:

- One or more episodes of unilateral orbital pain persisting for weeks if untreated
- Paresis of one or more of the third, fourth and or sixth cranial nerves and or demonstration of granulomas by MRI or biopsy
- Paresis coincides with the onset of pain or follows it within two weeks
- Pain and paresis resolve within 72 hours when treated adequately with corticosteroids
- Other causes have been excluded by appropriate investigations

---

**Investigation and Treatment of Tolosa-Hunt Syndrome**

An MRI scan is abnormal in more than 90% of patients. It reveals a convex enlargement of the symptomatic cavernous sinus by an abnormal tissue isointense with the grey matter on short repetition time (TR) and echo time (TE) images and iso-hypointense on long TR/TE images. This abnormal tissue enhances markedly after contrast injection. [140] The mass may extend into the superior orbital fissure. [141] The MRI scan may remain abnormal following the resolution of symptoms.

High dose corticosteroids are the treatment of choice and are more likely to induce resolution and avoid recurrence than lower dose regimes. Pain but not the neurological signs usually subside rapidly, often within 72 hours. It has been recommended that this rapid response can be diagnostic criterium. However, a response to treatment DOES NOT confirm the diagnosis. Many of the other conditions causing painful ophthalmoplegia also respond to corticosteroids, probably not as promptly.

---

# References

1   *Dorland's Pocket Medical Dictionary*. 21st ed. 1968, Philadelphia, London, Toronto: W.B.Saunders Company.

2   Selby, G., *Migraine and its Varients*. 1983, NSW: ADIS Health Science Press. 153.

3   Headache. *Handbook of Clinical Neurology*, ed. P.J. Vinken, G.W. Bruyn, and H.L. Klawans. 1986, Amsterdam. 556.

4   Raskin, N.H., *Headache*. Edition: 2, illustrated, revised ed. 1988: Churchill Livingstone. 396.

5   Lance, J.W. and P.J. Goadsby, *Mechnism and Management of Headache*. 7th ed. 2004: Butterworth-Heinemann.

6   Olesen, J., et al., *The Headaches*. 1169 ed. 2005: Lippincott Williams & Wilkins.

7   You, J.J., et al., Indications for and results of outpatient computed tomography and magnetic resonance imaging in Ontario. *Can Assoc Radiol J*, 2008. 59(3): p. 135-43.

8   Jacob, J., Mechanisms of fever occurring in migraine. *Adv Neurol,* 1982. **33**: p. 127-33.

9   Classification and diagnostic criteria for headache disorders, cranial neuralgias and facial pain. Headache Classification Committee of the International Headache Society. *Cephalalgia* 1988; 8 Suppl 7: 1-96.

10  Evans, R.W., Diagnostic testing for the evaluation of headaches. *Neurol Clin,* 1996. 14(1): p. 1-26.

11  Rasmussen, B.K. and J. Olesen, Symptomatic and nonsymptomatic headaches in a general population. *Neurology*, 1992. 42(6): p. 1225-31.

12  Gronseth, G., et al., Practice parameter: the diagnostic evaluation and treatment of trigeminal neuralgia (an evidence-based review): report of the Quality Standards Subcommittee of the American Academy of Neurology and the European Federation of Neurological Societies. *Neurology*, 2008. 71(15): p. 1183-90.

13  Young, W.B. and T.D. Rozen, Bilateral cluster headache: case report and a theory of (failed) contralateral suppression. *Cephalalgia*, 1999. 19(3): p. 188-90.

14  Leone, M., A. Rigamonti, and G. Bussone, Cluster headache sine headache: two new cases in one family. *Cephalalgia*, 2002. 22(1): p. 12-4.

15  Rozen, T.D., Atypical presentations of cluster headache. *Cephalalgia*, 2002. 22(9): p. 725-9.

16  Landtblom, A.M., et al., Sudden onset headache: a prospective study of features, incidence and causes. *Cephalalgia*, 2002. 22(5): p. 354-60.

17  Morgenstern, L.B., et al., Worst headache and subarachnoid hemorrhage: prospective, modern computed tomography and spinal fluid analysis. *Ann Emerg Med*, 1998. 32(3 Pt 1): p. 297-304.

18  Bo, S.H., et al., Acute headache: a prospective diagnostic work-up of patients admitted to a general hospital. *Eur J Neurol*, 2008. 15(12): p. 1293-9.

19  Seet, C.M., Clinical presentation of patients with subarachnoid haemorrhage at a local emergency department. *Singapore Med J*, 1999. 40(6): p. 383-5.

20  Verweij, R.D., E.F. Wijdicks, and J. van Gijn, Warning headache in aneurysmal subarachnoid hemorrhage. A case-control study. *Arch Neurol*, 1988. 45(9): p. 1019-20.

21  Jakobsson, K.E., et al., Warning leak and management outcome in aneurysmal subarachnoid hemorrhage. *J Neurosurg*, 1996. 85(6): p. 995-9.

22  Markus, H.S., A prospective follow up of thunderclap headache mimicking subarachnoid haemorrhage. *J Neurol Neurosurg Psychiatry*, 1991. 54(12): p. 1117-8.

23  Wijdicks, E.F., H. Kerkhoff, and J. van Gijn, Long-term follow-up of 71 patients with thunderclap headache mimicking subarachnoid haemorrhage. *Lancet*, 1988. 2(8602): p. 68-70.

24  Qureshi, A.I., et al., Spontaneous intracerebral hemorrhage. *N Engl J Med*, 2001. 344(19): p. 1450-60.

25  Symonds, C., Cough headache. *Brain*, 1956. 79(4): p. 557-68.

26  Pascual, J., et al., Cough, exertional, and sexual headaches: an analysis of 72 benign and symptomatic cases. *Neurology*, 1996. 46(6): p. 1520-4.

27  Diamond, S. and J.L. Medina, Prolonged benign exertional headache: clinical characteristics and response to indomethacin. *Adv Neurol*, 1982. 33: p. 145-9.

28  Mathew, N.T., Indomethacin responsive headache syndromes. *Headache*, 1981. 21(4): p. 147-50.

29  Rooke, E.D., Benign exertional headache. *Med Clin North Am*, 1968. 52(4): p. 801-8

30  Kriz, K., [Coitus as a factor in the pathogenesis of neurologic complications]. *Cesk Neurol*, 1970. 33(3): p. 162-7.

31  Lance, J.W., Headaches occurring during sexual intercourse. *Proc Aust Assoc Neurol*, 1974. 11: p. 57-60.

32  Fuh, J.L., et al., Ice-cream headache--a large survey of 8359 adolescents. *Cephalalgia*, 2003. 23(10): p. 977-81.

33  Kaczorowski, M. and J. Kaczorowski, Ice cream evoked headaches (ICE-H) study: randomised trial of accelerated versus cautious ice cream eating regimen. *BMJ*, 2002. 325(7378): p. 1445-6.

34  Raskin, N.H. and R.K. Schwartz, Icepick-like pain. *Neurology*, 1980. 30(2): p. 203-5.

35  Reamy, B.V., Post-epidural headache: how late can it occur? *J Am Board Fam Med*, 2009. 22(2): p. 202-5.

36  Mokri, B., Spontaneous intracranial hypotension. *Curr Neurol Neurosci Rep*, 2001. 1(2): p. 109-17.

37  Wilton, N.C., J.H. Globerson, and A.M. de Rosayro, Epidural blood patch for postdural puncture headache: it's never too late. *Anesth Analg*, 1986. 65(8): p. 895-6.

38  Thoennissen, J., et al., Does bed rest after cervical or lumbar puncture prevent headache? A systematic review and meta-analysis. *Cmaj*, 2001. 165(10): p. 1311-6.

39  Evans, R.W., et al., Assessment: prevention of post-lumbar puncture headaches: report of the therapeutics and technology assessment subcommittee of the American Academy of Neurology. *Neurology*, 2000. 55(7): p. 909-14.

40  Armon, C. and R.W. Evans, Addendum to assessment: Prevention of post-lumbar puncture headaches: report of the Therapeutics and Technology Assessment Subcommittee of the American Academy of Neurology. *Neurology*, 2005. 65(4): p. 510-2.

41　Moriyama, E., et al., Quantitative analysis of radioisotope cisternography in the diagnosis of intracranial hypotension. *J Neurosurg*, 2004. 101(3): p. 421-6.

42　Turnbull, D.K. and D.B. Shepherd, Post-dural puncture headache: pathogenesis, prevention and treatment. B*r J Anaesth*, 2003. 91(5): p. 718-29.

43　van Kooten, F., et al., Epidural blood patch in post-dural puncture headache: a randomised, observer-blind, controlled clinical trial. *J Neurol Neurosurg Psychiatry*, 2008. 79(5): p. 553-8.

44　Ho, K.Y. and T.J. Gan, Management of persistent post-dural puncture headache after repeated epidural blood patch. *Acta Anaesthesiol Scand*, 2007. 51(5): p. 633-6.

45　Schwedt, T.J., D.W. Dodick, and R.J. Caselli, Giant cell arteritis. *Curr Pain Headache Rep*, 2006. 10(6): p. 415-20.

46　Salvarani, C., et al., Reappraisal of the epidemiology of giant cell arteritis in Olmsted County, Minnesota, over a fifty-year period. *Arthritis Rheum*, 2004. 51(2): p. 264-8.

47　Pipinos, II, et al., Giant-cell temporal arteritis in a 17-year-old male. *J Vasc Surg*, 2006. 43(5): p. 1053-5.

48　Salvarani, C., et al., The incidence of giant cell arteritis in Olmsted County, Minnesota: apparent fluctuations in a cyclic pattern. *Ann Intern Med*, 1995. 123(3): p. 192-4.

49　Danesh-Meyer, H.V. and P.J. Savino, Giant cell arteritis. *Curr Opin Ophthalmol*, 2007. 18(6): p. 443-9.

50.　Tal, S., V. Guller, and A. Gurevich, Fever of unknown origin in older adults. *Clin Geriatr Med*, 2007. 23(3): p. 649-68, viii.

51　Schmidt, D., Ocular ischemia syndrome - a malignant course of giant cell arteritis. *Eur J Med Re*s, 2005. 10(6): p. 233-42.

52　Tehrani, R., et al., Giant cell arteritis. *Semin Ophthalmol*, 2008. 23(2): p. 99-110.

53　Taylor-Gjevre, R., et al., Temporal artery biopsy for giant cell arteritis. *J Rheumatol*, 2005. 32(7): p. 1279-82.

54　Roos, K.L., Acute bacterial meningitis. *Semin Neurol*, 2000. 20(3): p. 293-306.

55　Rosenstein, N.E., et al., Meningococcal disease. *N Engl J Med*, 2001. 344(18): p. 1378-88.

56　The International Classification of Headache Disorders, 3rd edition (beta version). *Cephalalgia* 2013; 33(9): 629-808.

57　Wolff, H., *Headache and other head pain*. 2nd ed. 1963, New York: Oxford University Press.

58　Olesen, J., B. Larsen, and M. Lauritzen, Focal hyperemia followed by spreading oligemia and impaired activation of rCBF in classic migraine. *Ann Neurol*, 1981. 9(4): p. 344-52.

59　Lauritzen, M., Pathophysiology of the migraine aura. The spreading depression theory. *Brain*, 1994. 117 ( Pt 1): p. 199-210.

60　VanDenBrink, A.M., D.J. Duncker, and P.R. Saxena, Migraine headache is not associated with cerebral or meningeal vasodilatation--a 3T magnetic resonance angiography study. *Brain*, 2009. 132(Pt 6): p. e112; author reply e113.

61　Schoonman, G.G., et al., Migraine headache is not associated with cerebral or meningeal vasodilatation--a 3T magnetic resonance angiography study. *Brain*, 2008. 131(Pt 8): p. 2192-200.

62　Leao, A.A.P., Spreading depression of activity in cerebral cortex. *J Neurophysiol*. 1944. 7: p. 359-90.

63　Ayata, C., Spreading depression: from serendipity to targeted therapy in migraine prophylaxis. *Cephalalgia*, 2009. 29(10): p. 1095-114.

64　Kelman, L., The aura: a tertiary care study of 952 migraine patients. *Cephalalgia*, 2004. 24(9): p. 728-34.

65　Jensen, K., et al., Classic migraine. A prospective reporting of symptoms. *Acta Neurol Scand*, 1986. 73: p. 359-362.

66　Selby, G. and J.W. Lance, Observations on 500 cases of migraine and allied vascular headache. J *Neurol Neurosurg Psychiatry*, 1960. 23: p. 23-32.

67　Welch, K.M., Drug therapy of migraine. *N Engl J Med*, 1993. 329(20): p. 1476-83.

68　Fisher, C.M., Late-life migraine accompaniments as a cause of unexplained transient ischemic attacks. *Can J Neurol Sci*, 1980. 7(1): p. 9-17.

69    Kunkel, R.S., Acephalgic migraine. *Headache*, 1986. 26(4): p. 198-201.

70    Bickerstaff, E.R., The basilar artery and the migraine epilepsy syndrome. *Proc R Soc Med*, 1962. 55: p. 167-9.

71    Glista, G.G., J.F. Mellinger, and E.D. Rooke, Familial hemiplegic migraine. *Mayo Clin Proc*, 1975. 50(6): p. 307-11.

72    Foroozan, R. and F.M. Cutrer, Transient neurologic dysfunction in migraine. *Neurol Clin*, 2009. 27(2): p. 361-78.

73    Somerville, B.W., The role of progesterone in menstrual migraine. *Neurology*, 1971. 21(8): p. 853-9.

74    Somerville, B.W., The role of estradiol withdrawal in the etiology of menstrual migraine. *Neurology*, 1972. 22(4): p. 355-65.

75    Millichap, J.G. and M.M. Yee, The diet factor in pediatric and adolescent migraine. *Pediatr Neurol*, 2003. 28(1): p. 9-15.

76    Egger, J., et al., Is migraine food allergy? A double-blind controlled trial of oligoantigenic diet treatment. *Lancet*, 1983. 2(8355): p. 865-9.

77    McQueen, J., et al., *A controlled trial of dietary modification in migraine in New advances in headache research*, F.C. Rose, Editor. 1989, Smith-Gordon: London. p. 235-242.

78    Holroyd, K.A. and D.B. Penzien, Pharmacological versus non-pharmacological prophylaxis of recurrent migraine headache: a meta-analytic review of clinical trials. *Pain*, 1990. 42(1): p. 1-13.

79    Melchart, D., et al., Acupuncture for recurrent headaches: a systematic review of randomized controlled trials. *Cephalalgia*, 1999. 19(9): p. 779-86; discussion 765.

80    Anderson, J.A., M.A. Basker, and R. Dalton, Migraine and hypnotherapy. *Int J Clin Exp Hypn*, 1975. 23(1): p. 48-58.

81    Goadsby, P.J., Advances in the pharmacotherapy of migraine. How knowledge of pathophysiology is guiding drug development. *Drugs R D*, 1999. 2(6): p. 361-74.

82    Krymchantowski, A.V., Acute treatment of migraine. Breaking the paradigm of monotherapy. *BMC Neurol*, 2004. 4: p. 4.

83    Diener, H.C., Medication overuse is more than just taking too much. *Cephalalgia*, 2005. 25(7): p. 481.

84    Silberstein, S.D., et al., Botulinum toxin type A for the prophylactic treatment of chronic daily headache: a randomized, double-blind, placebo-controlled trial. *Mayo Clin Proc*, 2005. 80(9): p. 1126-37.

85    Mathew, N.T., et al., Botulinum toxin type A (BOTOX) for the prophylactic treatment of chronic daily headache: a randomized, double-blind, placebo-controlled trial. *Headache*, 2005. 45(4): p. 293-307.

86    Aurora, S.K., et al., Botulinum toxin type a prophylactic treatment of episodic migraine: a randomized, double-blind, placebo-controlled exploratory study. *Headache*, 2007. 47(4): p. 486-99.

87    Relja, M., et al., A multicentre, double-blind, randomized, placebo-controlled, parallel group study of multiple treatments of botulinum toxin type A (BoNTA) for the prophylaxis of episodic migraine headaches. *Cephalalgia*, 2007. 27(6): p. 492-503.

88    Guyuron, B., et al., A placebo-controlled surgical trial of the treatment of migraine headaches. *Plast Reconstr Surg*, 2009. 124(2): p. 461-8.

89    Magos, A.L., K.J. Zilkha, and J.W. Studd, Treatment of menstrual migraine by oestradiol implants. *J Neurol Neurosurg Psychiatry*, 1983. 46(11): p. 1044-6.

90    Sances, G., et al., Naproxen sodium in menstrual migraine prophylaxis: a double-blind placebo controlled study. *Headache*, 1990. 30(11): p. 705-9.

91    Tuchman, M.M., et al., Oral zolmitriptan in the short-term prevention of menstrual migraine: a randomized, placebo-controlled study. *CNS Drugs*, 2008. 22(10): p. 877-86.

92    Mannix, L.K., et al., Combination treatment for menstrual migraine and dysmenorrhea using sumatriptan-naproxen: two randomized controlled trials. *Obstet Gynecol*, 2009. 114(1): p. 106-13.

93    Rozen, T.D., et al., Cluster headache in women: clinical characteristics and comparison with cluster headache in men. *J Neurol Neurosurg Psychiatry*, 2001. 70(5): p. 613-7.

94   May, A., et al., EFNS guidelines on the treatment of cluster headache and other trigeminal-autonomic cephalalgias. *Eur J Neurol*, 2006. 13(10): p. 1066-77.

95   Zeigler, A.K. and R.t. Hassanein, *Migraine muscle contraction headache dichotomy studied by statistical analysis of headache symptoms., in Advances in migraine research and therapy*, F.C. Rose, Editor. 1995, Raven Press: New York. p. 7-11.

96   Rasmussen, B.K., et al., Epidemiology of headache in a general population--a prevalence study. *J Clin Epidemiol*, 1991. 44(11): p. 1147-57.

97   Lance, J.W. and D.A. Curran, Treatment of Chronic Tension Headache. *Lancet*, 1964. 1(7345): p. 1236-9.

98   Lance, J.W. and P.J. Goadsby, *Mechanisms and Management of Headache*. 7th ed. 2005: Elsevier, Butterworth, Heinemann.

99   Melis, P.M., et al., Treatment of chronic tension-type headache with hypnotherapy: a single-blind time controlled study. *Headache*, 1991. 31(10): p. 686-9.

100  Devineni, T. and E.B. Blanchard, A randomized controlled trial of an internet-based treatment for chronic headache. *Behav Res Ther,* 2005. 43(3): p. 277-92.

101  Blau, J.N., A note on migraine and the nose. *Headache*, 1988. 28(7): p. 495.

102  Schreiber, C.P., et al., Prevalence of migraine in patients with a history of self-reported or physician-diagnosed "sinus" headache. *Arch Intern Med*, 2004. 164(16): p. 1769-72.

103  Mathew, N.T., U. Reuveni, and F. Perez, Transformed or evolutive migraine. *Headache*, 1987. 27(2): p. 102-6.

104  Mathew, N.T., Transformed migraine, analgesic rebound, and other chronic daily headaches. *Neurol Clin*, 1997. 15(1): p. 167-186.

105  Solomon, S., R.B. Lipton, and L.C. Newman, Clinical features of chronic daily headache. *Headache*, 1992. 32(7): p. 325-9.

106  Silberstein, S.D., et al., The International Classification of Headache Disorders, 2nd Edition (ICHD-II)--revision of criteria for 8.2 Medication-overuse headache. *Cephalalgia*, 2005. 25(6): p. 460-5.

107  Kudrow, L., Paradoxical effects of frequent analgesic use. *Adv Neurol*, 1982. 33: p. 335-41.

108  Ellner, J.J. and J.E. Bennett, *Chronic meningitis Medicine (Baltimore)*, 1976. 55(5): p. 341-69.

109  Smith, J.E. and A.J. Aksamit, Jr., Outcome of chronic idiopathic meningitis. *Mayo Clin Proc*, 1994. 69(6): p. 548-56.

110  Coyle, P.K., Overview of acute and chronic meningitis. *Neurol Clin*, 1999. 17(4): p. 691-710.

111. Helbok, R., et al., Chronic meningitis. J *Neurol*, 2009. 256(2): p. 168-75.

112. Anderson, N.E. and E.W. Willoughby, Chronic meningitis without predisposing illness--a review of 83 cases. *Q J Med*, 1987. 63(240): p. 283-95.

113. Ginsberg, L. and D. Kidd, Chronic and recurrent meningitis. *Pract Neurol*, 2008. 8(6): p. 348-61.

114. Wall, M., The headache profile of idiopathic intracranial hypertension. *Cephalalgia*, 1990. 10(6): p. 331-5.

115. Schoenen, J. and P.S. Sandor, Headache with focal neurological signs or symptoms: a complicated differential diagnosis. *Lancet Neurol*, 2004. 3(4): p. 237-45.

116. Suwanwela, N., K. Phanthumchinda, and S. Kaoropthum, Headache in brain tumor: a cross-sectional study. H*eadache*, 1994. 34(7): p. 435-8.

117. The epidemiology of headache among children with brain tumor. Headache in children with brain tumors. The Childhood Brain Tumor Consortium. *J Neurooncol*, 1991. 10(1): p. 31-46.

118. Schankin, C.J., et al., Characteristics of brain tumour-associated headache. *Cephalalgia*, 2007. 27(8): p. 904-11.

119. Hamilton, W. and D. Kernick, Clinical features of primary brain tumours: a case-control study using electronic primary care records. *Br J Gen Pract*, 2007. 57(542): p. 695-9.

120. Pfund, Z., et al., Headache in intracranial tumors. *Cephalalgia*, 1999. 19(9): p. 787-90; discussion 765.

121 American Academy of Neurology. *Report of the Quality Standards Sub-Committee of the American Academy of Neurology*. The utility of neuroimaging in the evaluation of headache in patients with normal neurological examinations. 2008 [cited (accessed 17 April 2009).]; Available from: www.aan.com/professionals/practice/pdfs/gl0088.pdf

121 Tew, J.M.J. and H. van Loveren, *Percutaneous rhizotomy in the treatment of intractable facial pain (trigeminal, glossopharyngeal, and vagal nerves), in Operative Neurosurgical Techniques: Indications, Methods, and Results*. ed 2, H.H. Schmidek and W.H. Sweet, Editors. 1998, Orlando: Grune & Stratton. p. 1111-1123.

123 Jannetta, P.J., Arterial compression of the trigeminal nerve at the pons in patients with trigeminal neuralgia. *J Neurosurg*, 1967. 26(1): p. Suppl:159-62.

124 Heir, G.M., Facial pain of dental origin--a review for physicians. *Headache*, 1987. 27(10): p. 540-7.

125 Evans, K.L., Recognition and management of sinusitis. *Drugs*, 1998. 56(1): p. 59-71.

126 Diaz, I. and D.M. Bamberger, Acute sinusitis. *Semin Respir Infect*, 1995. 10(1): p. 14-20.

127 Rushton, J.G., J.C. Stevens, and R.H. Miller, Glossopharyngeal (vagoglossopharyngeal) neuralgia: a study of 217 cases. *Arch Neurol*, 1981. 38(4): p. 201-5.

128 Bruyn, G.W., Glossopharyngeal neuralgia, in Handbook of clinical neurology. *Headache*, P.J. Vincken, Bruyn, G.W. & Klawans, H.L., Editor. 1986, Elsevier: Amsterdam. p. 487-494.

129 Siccoli, M.M., C.L. Bassetti, and P.S. Sandor, Facial pain: clinical differential diagnosis. *Lancet Neurol*, 2006. 5(3): p. 257-67.

130 Lascelles, R.G., Atypical facial pain and depression. *Br J Psychiatry*, 1966. 112(488): p. 651-9.

131 Feinmann, C., M. Harris, and R. Cawley, Psychogenic facial pain: presentation and treatment. *Br Med J* (Clin Res Ed), 1984. 288(6415): p. 436-8.

132 Oxman, M.N., et al., A vaccine to prevent herpes zoster and postherpetic neuralgia in older adults. *N Engl J Med*, 2005. 352(22): p. 2271-84.

133 Harpaz, R., I.R. Ortega-Sanchez, and J.F. Seward, Prevention of herpes zoster: recommendations of the Advisory Committee on Immunization Practices (ACIP). *MMWR Recomm Rep*, 2008. 57(RR-5): p. 1-30; quiz CE2-4.

134 Wood, M.J., et al., Oral acyclovir therapy accelerates pain resolution in patients with herpes zoster: a meta-analysis of placebo-controlled trials. *Clin Infect Dis*, 1996. 22(2): p. 341-7.

135 Bowsher, D., The effects of pre-emptive treatment of postherpetic neuralgia with amitriptyline: a randomized, double-blind, placebo-controlled trial. *J Pain Symptom Manage*, 1997. 13(6): p. 327-31.

136 Eaglstein, W.H., R. Katz, and J.A. Brown, The effects of early corticosteroid therapy on the skin eruption and pain of herpes zoster. *Jama*, 1970. 211(10): p. 1681-3.

137 Keczkes, K. and A.M. Basheer, Do corticosteroids prevent post-herpetic neuralgia? *Br J Dermatol*, 1980. 102(5): p. 551-5.

138 He, L., et al., Corticosteroids for preventing postherpetic neuralgia. *Cochrane Database Syst Rev*, 2008(1): p. CD005582.

139 Lutt, J.R., et al., Orbital inflammatory disease. *Semin Arthritis Rheum*, 2008. 37(4): p. 207-22.

140 Pascual, J., et al., Tolosa-Hunt syndrome: focus on MRI diagnosis. *Cephalalgia*, 1999. 19 Suppl 25: p. 36-8.

141 Kline, L.B. and W.F. Hoyt, The Tolosa-Hunt syndrome. *J Neurol Neurosurg Psychiatry*, 2001. 71(5): p. 577-82.

142 Schoenen, J., J. Jacquy, and M. Lenaerts, Effectiveness of high-dose riboflavin in migraine prophylaxis. A randomized controlled trial. *Neurology*, 1998. 50(2): p. 466-70.

143 MacLennan, S.C., et al., High-dose riboflavin for migraine prophylaxis in children: a double-blind, randomized, placebo-controlled trial. *J Child Neurol*, 2008. 23(11): p. 1300-4.

144 Dodick, D.W., et al., Topiramate versus amitriptyline in migraine prevention: a 26-week, multicenter, randomized, double-blind, double-dummy, parallel-group noninferiority trial in adult migraineurs. *Clin Ther*, 2009. 31(3): p. 542-59.

145 Louis, P. and E.L. Spierings, Comparison of flunarizine (Sibelium) and pizotifen (Sandomigran) in migraine treatment: a double-blind study. *Cephalalgia*, 1982. 2(4): p. 197-203.

146 Pryse-Phillips, W.E., et al., Guidelines for the diagnosis and management of migraine in clinical practice. *Canadian Headache Society. Cmaj*, 1997. 156(9): p. 1273-87.

147 Evers, S., et al., EFNS guideline on the drug treatment of migraine - report of an EFNS task force. *Eur J Neurol*, 2006. 13(6): p. 560-72.

148 Geraud, G., A. Compagnon, and A. Rossi, Zolmitriptan versus a combination of acetylsalicylic acid and metoclopramide in the acute oral treatment of migraine: a double-blind, randomised, three-attack study. *Eur Neurol*, 2002. 47(2): p. 88-98.

149 Sorge, F. and E. Marano, Flunarizine v. placebo in childhood migraine. A double-blind study. *Cephalalgia*, 1985. 5 Suppl 2: p. 145-8.

150 Diener, H.C., et al., Efficacy, tolerability and safety of oral eletriptan and ergotamine plus caffeine (Cafergot) in the acute treatment of migraine: a multicentre, randomised, double-blind, placebo-controlled comparison. *Eur Neurol*, 2002. 47(2): p. 99-107.

151 Ferrari, M.D., et al., Oral triptans (serotonin 5-HT(1B/1D) agonis*ts) in acute migraine treatment: a meta-analysis of 53 trials. Lancet*, 2001. 358(9294): p. 1668-75.

152 Charles A, Pozo-Rosich P. Targeting calcitonin gene-related peptide: a new era in migraine therapy. *Lancet* 2019; 394(10210): 1765-74.

153 Ashina M, Vasudeva R, Jin L, et al. Onset of Efficacy Following Oral Treatment With Lasmiditan for the Acute Treatment of Migraine: Integrated Results From 2 Randomized Double-Blind Placebo-Controlled Phase 3 Clinical Studies. *Headache* 2019; 59(10): 1788-801.

154 MacGregor EA. Prevention and treatment of menstrual migraine. Drugs 2010; 70(14): 1799-818.

155 Al-Waili NS. Treatment of menstrual migraine with prostaglandin synthesis inhibitor mefenamic acid: double-blind study with placebo. *Eur J Med Res* 2000; 5(4): 176-82.

156 American Headache S. The American Headache Society Position Statement On Integrating New Migraine Treatments Into Clinical Practice. *Headache: The Journal of Head and Face Pain* 2019; 59(1): 1-18.

157 Harris P, Loveman E, Clegg A, Easton S, Berry N. Systematic review of cognitive behavioural therapy for the management of headaches and migraines in adults. *British Journal of Pain* 2015; 9(4): 213-24.

158 Ness T, Bley TA, Schmidt WA, Lamprecht P. The diagnosis and treatment of giant cell arteritis. *Dtsch Arztebl Int* 2013; 110(21): 376-85; quiz 86.

159 Coath F, Gillbert K, Griffiths B, et al. Giant cell arteritis: new concepts, treatments and the unmet need that remains. *Rheumatology* 2018; 58(7): 1123-5.

160 Frohman L, Wong ABC, Matheos K, Leon-Alvarado LG, Danesh-Meyer HV. New developments in giant cell arteritis. *Survey of Ophthalmology* 2016; 61(4): 400-21.

161 Guevara M, Kollipara CS. Recent Advances in Giant Cell Arteritis. *Current Rheumatology Reports* 2018; 20(5): 25.

162 Schoenen J, Jacquy J, Lenaerts M. Effectiveness of high-dose riboflavin in migraine prophylaxis. A randomized controlled trial. *Neurology* 1998;50(2):466–470.

163 MacLennan SC, et al. High-dose riboflavin for migraine prophylaxis in children: A double-blind, randomized, placebo-controlled trial. *J Child Neurol* 2008;23(11):1300–1304.

164 Dodick DW, et al. Topiramate versus amitriptyline in migraine prevention: A 26-week, multicenter, randomized, double-blind, double-dummy, parallel-group noninferiority trial in adult migraineurs. *Clin Ther* 2009;31(3):542–559.

165 Louis P, Spierings EL. Comparison of flunarizine (Sibelium) and pizotifen (Sandomigran) in migraine treatment: A double-blind study. *Cephalalgia* 1982;2(4):197–203.

166 Pryse-Phillips WE, et al. Guidelines for the diagnosis and management of migraine in clinical practice. Canadian Headache Society. *CMAJ* 1997;156(9):1273–1287.

167 Evers S, et al. EFNS guideline on the drug treatment of migraine – report of an EFNS task force. *Eur J Neurol* 2006;13(6):560–572.

168 Geraud G, Compagnon A, Rossi A. Zolmitriptan versus a combination of acetylsalicylic acid and metoclopramide in the acute oral treatment of migraine: A double-blind, randomised, three-attack study. *Eur Neurol* 2002;47(2):88–98.

169 Sorge F, Marano E. Flunarizine v. placebo in childhood migraine. A double-blind study. *Cephalalgia* 1985;5(Suppl 2):145–148.

170 Diener HC, et al. Efficacy, tolerability and safety of oral eletriptan and ergotamine plus caffeine (Cafergot) in the acute treatment of migraine: A multicentre, randomised, double-blind, placebo-controlled comparison. *Eur Neurol* 2002;47(2):99–107.

171 Ferrari MD, et al. Oral triptans (serotonin 5-HT(1B/1D) agonists) in acute migraine treatment: A meta-analysis of 53 trials. *Lancet* 2001;358(9294):1668–1675.

172 Ashina M, Vasudeva R, Jin L, et al. Onset of Efficacy Following Oral Treatment With Lasmiditan for the Acute Treatment of Migraine: Integrated Results From 2 Randomized Double-Blind Placebo-Controlled Phase 3 Clinical Studies. *Headache* 2019; 59(10): 1788-801.

173 Charles A, Pozo-Rosich P. Targeting calcitonin gene-related peptide: a new era in migraine therapy. *Lancet* 2019; 394(10210): 1765-74.

174 American Headache Society. The American Headache Society Position Statement on Integrating New Migraine Treatments into Clinical Practice. *Headache: The Journal of Head and Face Pain* 2019; 59(1): 1-18.

175 Headache Classification Committee of the International Headache Society (IHS) The International Classification of Headache Disorders, 3rd edition. *Cephalalgia* 2018; 38(1): 1-211.

176 Ahmed SV, Jayawarna C, Jude E. Post lumbar puncture headache: diagnosis and management. *Postgrad Med J* 2006; 82(973): 713-6.

177 Ailani J, Burch RC, Robbins MS, Society tBoDotAH. The American Headache Society Consensus Statement: Update on integrating new migraine treatments into clinical practice. *Headache: The Journal of Head and Face Pain*; n/a(n/a).

178 Dodick DW, Turkel CC, DeGryse RE, et al. OnabotulinumtoxinA for treatment of chronic migraine: pooled results from the double-blind, randomized, placebo-controlled phases of the PREEMPT clinical program. *Headache* 2010; 50(6): 921-36.

179 Lipton RB, Nye BL, Hirman J, Aurora SK, Shrewsbury SB. Treatment consistency across multiple migraine attacks: Results from the phase 3 open-label STOP 301 study. *Headache* 2021; 61(Abstract P-183): 148.

180 Croop R, Madonia J, Conway CM, al. e. Intranasal zavegepant is effective and well tolerated for the acute treatment of migraine: A phase 2/3 dose-ranging clinical trial. *Headache 2021;61(S1):104-105*; 61: 1-4-105.

181 Kuruvilla DE, Starling AJ, Tepper SJ, Mann JI, Johnson M. A phase 3 randomized, double-blind, sham-controlled trial of e-TNS for the acute treatment of migraine (TEAM) *Headache* 2021; 61(Abstract IOR-02).

182 Bendtsen L, Jensen R. Mirtazapine is effective in the prophylactic treatment of chronic tension-type headache. *Neurology* 2004; 62(10): 1706-11.

183 Krymchantowski AV, Barbosa JS. Prednisone as initial treatment of analgesic-induced daily headache. *Cephalalgia* 2000; 20(2): 107-13.

184 Raskin NH. Repetitive intravenous dihydroergotamine as therapy for intractable migraine. *Neurology* 1986; 36(7): 995-7.

185 Ford RG, Ford KT. Continuous intravenous dihydroergotamine in the treatment of intractable headache. *Headache* 1997; 37(3): 129-36.

186 Hoffmann J, May A. Diagnosis, pathophysiology, and management of cluster headache. *Lancet Neurol* 2018; 17(1): 75-83.

187 Obermann M, Nägel S, Ose C, et al. Safety and efficacy of prednisone versus placebo in short-term prevention of episodic cluster headache: a multicentre, double-blind, randomised controlled trial. *Lancet Neurol* 2021; 20(1): 29-37.

188 Goadsby PJ, Dodick DW, Leone M, et al. Trial of Galcanezumab in Prevention of Episodic Cluster Headache. *N Engl J Med* 2019; 381(2): 132-41.

189 Caliskan, E., et al. (2016). "Can we evaluate cranial aneurysms on conventional brain magnetic resonance imaging?" *Journal of neurosciences in rural practice* 7(1): 83-86.

190 Gates, P. C., et al. (1986). "Primary intraventricular hemorrhage in adults." *Stroke* 17: 872-877.

191 Herd, C. P., et al. (2019). "Cochrane systematic review and meta-analysis of botulinum toxin for the prevention of migraine." *BMJ Open* 9(7): e027953.

192 Mollan, S. P., et al. (2018). "Evaluation and management of adult idiopathic intracranial hypertension." *Pract Neurol* 18(6): 485-488.

193 Goadsby, P. J., Holland, P. R., Martins-Oliveira, M., Hoffmann, J., Schankin, C. and Akerman, S. Pathophysiology of Migraine: A Disorder of Sensory Processing, *Physiol Rev* 2017; 97 (2):553-622

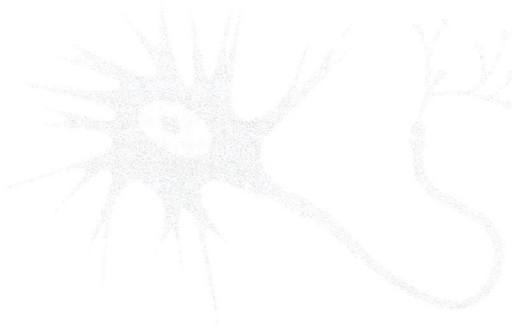

# Cerebrovascular Disease

Cerebrovascular disease (CVD) is one of the commonest problems encountered in clinical neurology. Hippocrates (460–375 BCE) is credited with introducing the concept of apoplexy (derived from the Greek word for seizure, *apoplēxia, in the sense of being struck down)* to describe patients with stroke. He also noted that 'it is difficult to cure a mild case of apoplexy and impossible to cure a severe case'. Until recently, this essentially was the case. Thus the focus should be on **primary and secondary prevention**.

Although the management of cerebrovascular disease, particularly acute ischaemic stroke, has changed dramatically since the 1st edition of this book, the basic principles remain the same. This chapter will discuss these principles and secondary prevention of stroke. Appendix E deals with epidemiology and primary stroke prevention, whilst Appendix F discusses thrombolysis and clot retrieval.

## Minor Stroke or TIA: Does it Matter?

In the past, symptoms of cerebral ischaemia that last less than 24 hours were labelled a **transient ischaemic attack** (TIA), whilst symptoms that last more than 24 hours were designated a stroke. [1] However, **cerebral infarction** (CI) can be detected on diffusion-weighted magnetic resonance imaging (dwMRI) in as many as one-third of patients with symptoms lasting less than 24 hours. [2,3] This has led some authorities to recommend a change in the definition of TIA to "any neurological dysfunction caused by focal brain, spinal cord, or retinal ischemia, without acute infarction". [5, 6] An MRI detected acute infarct predicts both a short and long-term increased risk of stroke. [4, 153] This implies that all patients with TIA undergo a dwMRI scan within seven days. Both impractical and impossible outside major institutions. Although it may indicate the subsequent risk of stroke, it does not appear to influence the acute management of TIA.

There are essentially two types of patients with cerebral ischaemia:
- those with minor symptoms that may or may not resolve within a defined period and thus are candidates for secondary prevention.
- Those with a severe and disabling neurological deficit, where the horse has already bolted the stable door!

In the former group, prompt assessment and appropriate treatment provide an opportunity to prevent severe stroke. [7] The risk of stroke after TIA or minor stroke is similar (Table 10.1), once again suggesting that the separation between TIA and minor stroke is arbitrary and of little clinical value. Thus, all patients with minor symptoms of cerebral ischaemia, regardless of how long the symptoms last, should be treated as a matter of urgency.

| Presenting Symptom | Subsequent risk of stroke | | |
| --- | --- | --- | --- |
| | 7 days | 1 month | 3 months |
| TIA | 8%<br>(2.3% to 13.7%) | 11.5%<br>(4.8% to 18.2%) | 17.3%<br>(9.3% to 25.3%) |
| Minor stroke | 11.5%<br>(4.8% to 11.2%) | 15.0%<br>(7.5% to 22.5%) | 18.5%<br>(10.3% to 26.7%) |

**Table 10.1** The subsequent risk of stroke after TIA and minor stroke (95% confidence intervals in brackets). [11]

All patients with minor cerebral ischaemia should be evaluated as a matter of urgency.
Recurrent stereotyped TIAs indicate a tight stenosis that could be either a large artery or a very small perforating vessel.

Forty per cent of patients who subsequently suffer a stroke after a TIA will do so within the first seven days; in 17%, the TIA will be on the day of the stroke, while in 9%, it will be on the day prior. [8] Unfortunately, many patients ignore minor symptoms and do not seek urgent medical advice. The opportunity to prevent stroke is lost. The subsequent risk of early stroke after minor cerebral ischaemia is greatest with severe carotid stenosis and patients with repeated or crescendo TIAs, the so-called 'capsular warning syndrome'. [9, 10]

The basic principles of management of most patients with CVD are simple (Figure 10.1). At times, however, they can be complex. Some patients have more than one potential underlying pathological cause. [12] Patients can present with a cerebral infarct one time and an intracerebral haemorrhage another time. [13,14] The symptoms and signs of a small intracerebral haemorrhage can be identical to a cerebral infarct of a similar size in the same area. Many patients have coexistent medical problems that make the choice of subsequent therapy difficult.

This chapter will discuss the general principles of diagnosis, investigation, and management of the more common manifestations of CVD. It is far from comprehensive. For more detail, the reader can consult one of the many excellent books on the subject. [15–20] Many websites also help the clinician keep abreast of the latest developments.[1]

As treatment is currently largely disease-specific and different diseases affect different regions, accurate localisation of the problem within the cerebral hemispheres, brainstem or cerebellum is essential. It would, at this point, be helpful to review chapters 1 and 4 before reading further.

---

1 http://www.cochrane.org/reviews/en/topics/93_reviews.html,
http://www.strokeassociation.org/presenter.jhtml?identifier=1200037, http://www.strokecenter.org/).

# Principles of Management

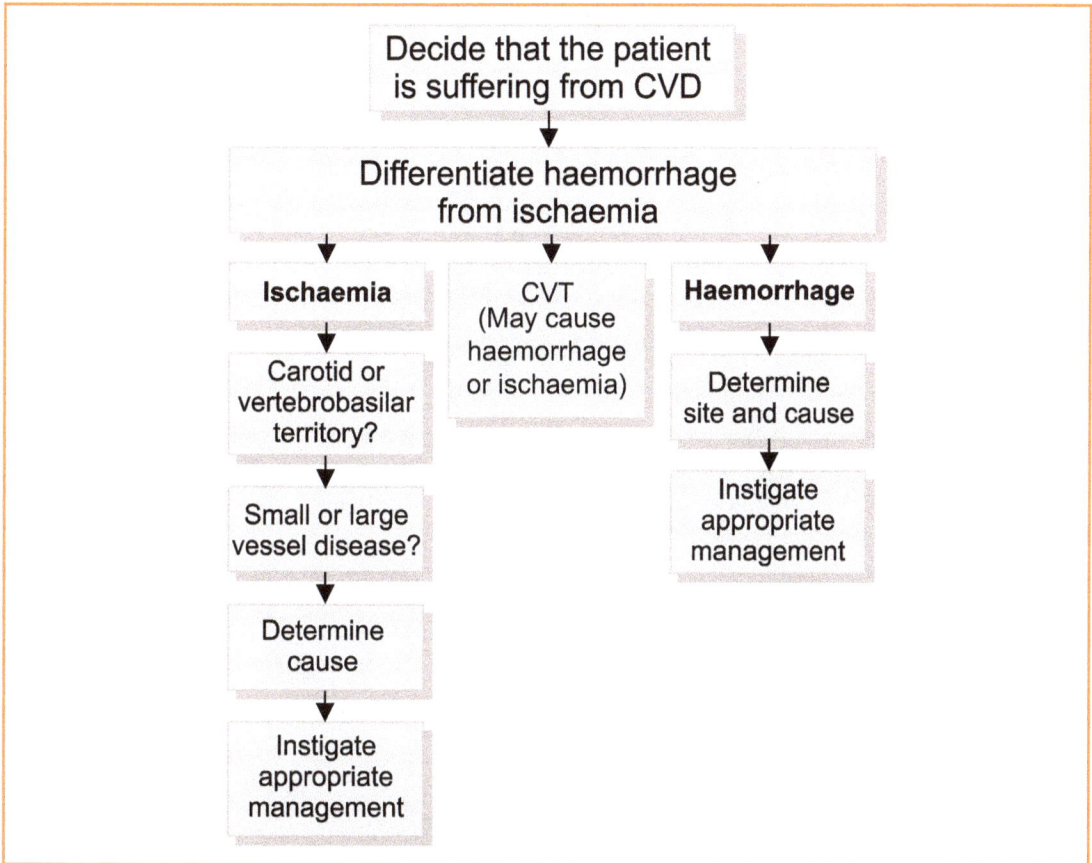

**Figure 10.1** Principles of managing patients with cerebral vascular disease (CVD). CVT=cerebral vein thrombosis

Carotid territory refers to cerebral ischaemia in the distribution of the main artery at the front of the neck: the carotid and its branches, the anterior and middle cerebral arteries. Vertebrobasilar territory refers to the arteries at the back of the neck. The two vertebral arteries merging to form the basilar artery. The posterior inferior cerebellar arteries arise from the vertebral artery. The anterior inferior cerebellar, the superior cerebellar, the posterior cerebral, and the small paramedian perforating arteries originate from the basilar. (Figure 10.2)

Computerised tomography (CT) scans, MRI scans, duplex carotid ultrasound, and echocardiography (transthoracic and trans-oesophageal) have revolutionised CVD management. They can, in most instances, readily establish if a patient has CVD, differentiate between haemorrhage and infarction, localise the exact site of the lesion, determine if it is a lacunar infarct and most likely establish the aetiology. The difficulty is that not everybody has access to such facilities. The tests are not always positive in patients suspected of having CVD (particularly in patients with transient symptoms). Asymptomatic cerebral infarction [21] and asymptomatic carotid stenosis are not uncommon. Therefore, a careful history and, if there are abnormal neurological signs, a detailed neurological examination is essential in managing CVD patients.

# Deciding the Problem is CVD

Cerebral vascular disease should be suspected when a patient presents with the sudden or subacute onset of a focal neurological deficit *associated with loss of function*. The neurological deficit is usually of sudden onset within minutes, if not quicker, particularly with an embolic source from the heart or atherosclerotic vascular disease in the major extracranial vessels. Other modes of onset include stepwise stuttering (related to thrombosis rather than embolism) or fluctuating deficit. [22, 23]

The more *common presentations* with the area of the brain and the blood vessels affected (Figure 102, 10.3A and B) include:

**Vertebrobasilar territory ischaemia** (VBI)

- Ataxia, nausea and vomiting with or without vertigo: cerebellar infarction, posterior inferior, anterior inferior and superior cerebellar arteries, or cerebellar haemorrhage.
- Dysphagia, dysarthria, and ataxia: lateral medullary syndrome, vertebral or posterior inferior cerebellar artery (almost always on an ischaemic basis).
- Pure motor hemiparesis affecting arm and leg: paramedian pontine syndrome, paramedian perforating vessels (almost always on an ischaemic basis).
- Horizontal diplopia looking to one side: unilateral internuclear ophthalmoplegia, small perforating arteries deep within the brainstem (almost always on an ischaemic basis)
- Hemianopia: occipital infarction, posterior cerebral artery (almost always on an ischaemic basis).

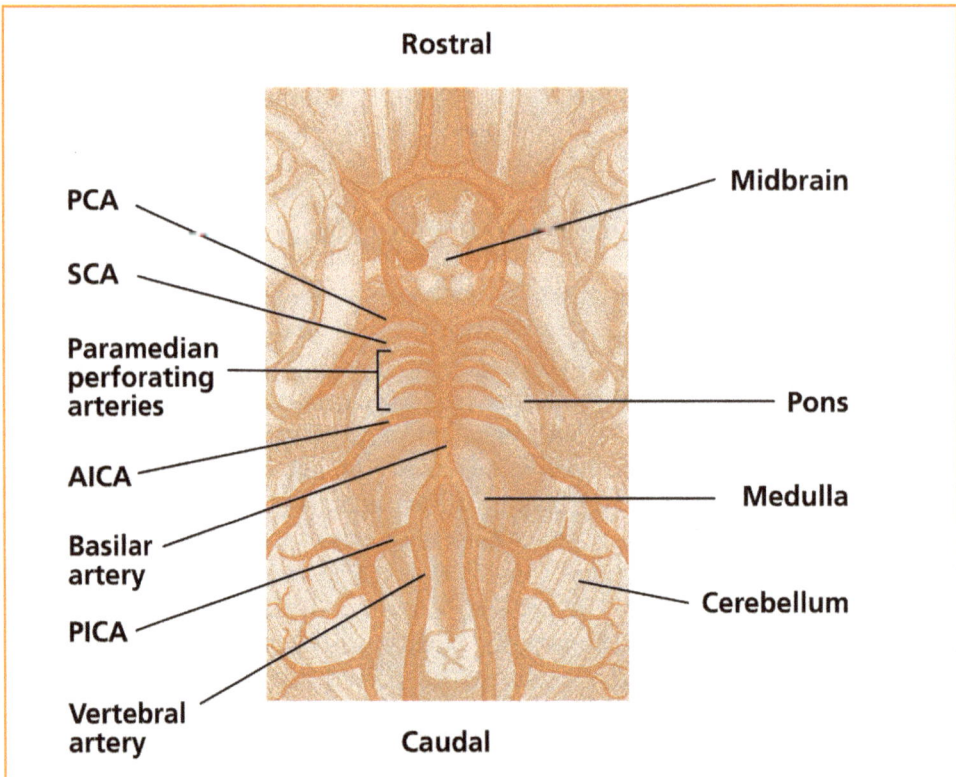

**Figure 10.2** The circle of Willis and the vertebrobasilar blood vessels. Abbreviations: PCA:Posterior cerebral artery, SCA:Superior cerebellar artery, AICA:Anterior inferior cerebellar artery, PICA:Posterior inferior cerebellar artery. Illustration Sandra Coventry

236

**Carotid territory ischaemia** (Figure 10.3 A and B)

- Amaurosis fugax, transient or permanent monocular visual loss: retina ischaemia, ipsilateral internal carotid artery (almost always on an ischaemic basis)
- Non-fluent dysphasia and right-sided hemiparesis: dominant hemisphere frontal lobe, left middle cerebral artery (almost always on an ischaemic basis)
- Fluent dysphasia with or without a hemianopia: dominant parietal or temporal lobe, left middle cerebral artery
- Left-sided weakness and neglect, with or without hemianopia: non-dominant parietal lobe, right middle cerebral artery
- Pure motor hemiparesis affecting the face, arm, and leg equally: lacunar infarct in the internal capsule deep within the cerebral hemisphere, small perforating artery

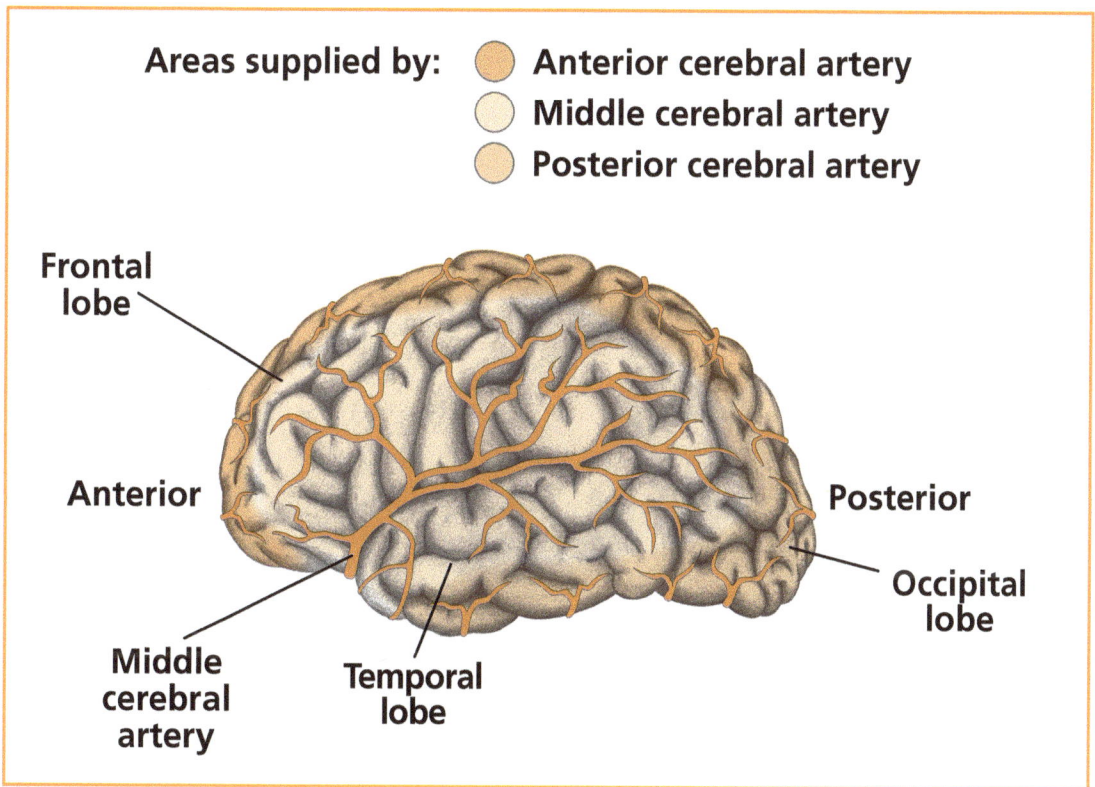

**Figure 10.3A** Cerebral hemispheres, lateral aspect showing area supplied by the middle cerebral artery. Illustration Sandra Coventry

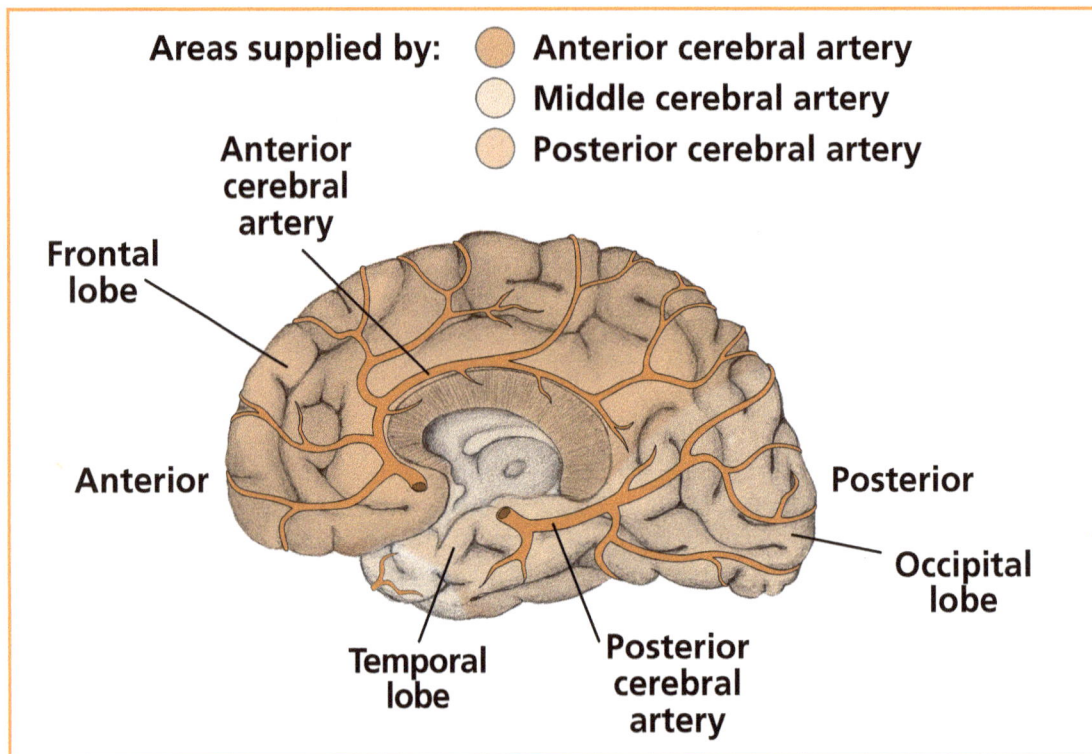

Areas supplied by:
- ● **Anterior cerebral artery**
- ○ **Middle cerebral artery**
- ○ **Posterior cerebral artery**

Anterior cerebral artery

Frontal lobe

Anterior

Posterior

Occipital lobe

Temporal lobe

Posterior cerebral artery

**Figure 10.3B** Cerebral hemispheres, medial aspect showing areas supplied by the anterior and posterior cerebral arteries. Illustration Sandra Coventry

There should be an increased level of suspicion in older patients when one or more risk factors or other manifestations of atherosclerotic vascular disease in the coronary or peripheral arteries are present. Remember, however, that this is prior probability, i.e. it increases the likelihood that it is CVD, but patients with risk factors can have problems unrelated to CVD.

The longer the deficit takes to develop the less one can be certain that the problem is CVD.

# Imaging in Cerebrovascular Disease

CT scanning of the brain is often normal in the first 6 hours and sometimes up to 24 hours after cerebral infarction. MRI can detect ischaemic changes as early as 1.5 hours after onset. Thus it can be abnormal in patients with TIA's. [24] Diffusion-weighted MRI (dwMRI; Figure 10.4) has a sensitivity of > 90–95% for detecting early (within the first 6 hours after onset) ischaemic changes as opposed to a CT scan with a sensitivity of only 70–75%. [1, 25] Both CT and MRI can miss very small lacunar infarcts, although MRI is more sensitive than CT. CT perfusion is discussed in appendix F.

> 🔑
>
> A normal dwMRI does not exclude cerebral ischaemia: when performed in the first few hours for small lacunar infarcts in the brainstem or deep hemisphere. [1]

> 🔑
>
> It is important to remember that CVD can occur: at any age, even in childhood in patients without risk factors for stroke with symptoms that do not always develop suddenly.

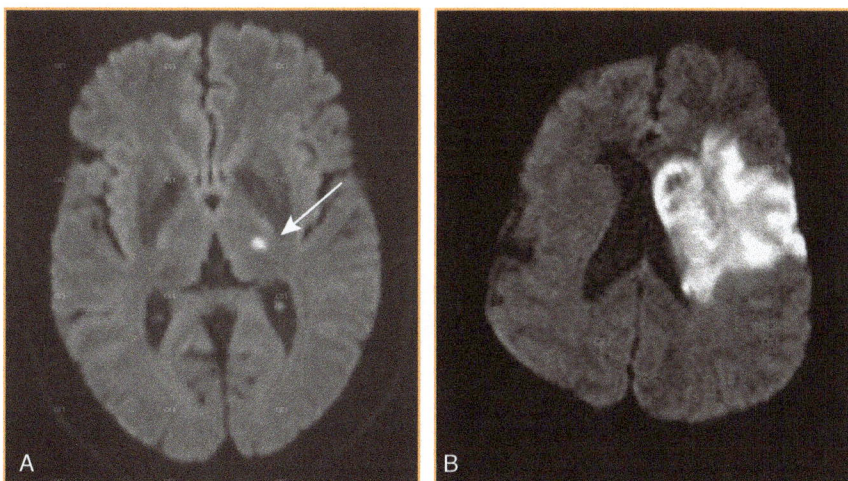

Figure 10.4 DwMRI showing **A** lacunar infarct and **B** large artery middle cerebral artery distribution infarction

DwMRI should be performed within the first week after onset as the changes are transient. The presence of dwMRI abnormalities helps to differentiate long-standing old 'asymptomatic' ischaemic changes from acute cerebral infarct.

# Differentiating Haemorrhage from Infarction
## More in Keeping with Haemorrhage

- *Early depression of the conscious state and vomiting.* Although these two clinical features can occur in brainstem infarction or haemorrhage, both can also reflect a rapid increase in intracranial pressure and should raise the suspicion of intracerebral haemorrhage within the hemisphere.
- *Headache* in a patient with a pure motor hemiparesis is more suggestive of haemorrhage. [28]
- Neither vomiting nor early depression of the conscious state occurs with a small haematoma mimicking a lacune. However, more than 80% of patients with pure motor hemiparesis or pure sensory loss affecting the face, arm and leg equally will have a lacunar infarct. Only a tiny percentage are secondary to intracerebral haemorrhage. [29, 30]

# More in Keeping with Ischaemia

- *Antecedent transient ischaemic attack(s)* with the same symptoms before the stroke would indicate ischaemia rather than haemorrhage. For example, repeated stereotyped episodes of weakness affecting the face, arm, and leg are typical of the capsular warning syndrome, invariably due to lacunar or striatocapsular infarction. [10, 31]
- *The neurological deficit gradually spreads* from one part of the body to the rest. For example, if it initially involves the arm and then spreads to the face and the leg, it is more likely to be ischaemic in origin.
- *Spontaneous improvement within the first few hours* favours ischaemia rather than haemorrhage.

# Haemorrhagic Stroke

Intracranial haemorrhage occurs in the extradural, subdural, subarachnoid spaces, intracerebral or intraventricular. (Figure 10.5) Each bleeding site is associated with a different symptom complex and result from different causes.

# Extradural Haematoma

Extradural haematoma (EDH) occurs with a severe head injury. It is almost invariably associated with a fractured skull and middle meningeal artery rupture. It is rarely confused with a stroke.

The patient may be unconscious from the start or deteriorate within minutes to hours with severe headache, vomiting, hemiparesis and subsequent coma. Treatment is urgent surgical evacuation.

# Subdural Haematoma

Acute subdural haematoma (SDH) resulting from rupture of the veins that cross the subdural space is rarely confused with cerebral ischaemia.

An acute subdural haematoma usually results from trauma to the head. On the other hand, almost half of patients with chronic subdural hematomas will not have a history of head trauma. In older people, the trauma can seem trivial such as striking one's head on the corner of a cupboard. There is an increased risk of chronic subdural haematoma in patients on anticoagulants.

In younger patients, subdural haematomas present with headache, nausea, confusion and hemiparesis. If acute, the conscious state can be depressed. In the elderly, hemiparesis is not always a feature. [26] The combination of a reduced conscious state, a dilated pupil (related to a 3rd nerve palsy) and a contralateral hemiparesis indicates life-threatening transtentorial herniation and is a surgical emergency. Occasionally, chronic subdural haematomas are bilateral and may present with an apraxic gait similar to the gait disturbance with frontal lobe pathology. (See Chapter 5)

Acute and large chronic subdural haematomas require surgical evacuation, but some chronic subdural haematomas resolve with conservative treatment. Hyperventilation, mannitol, hypertonic saline, inducing coma and partial craniectomy are used to reduce raised intracranial pressure.

# Subarachnoid Haemorrhage

Subarachnoid haemorrhage (SAH) is most often (85%) related to a ruptured berry aneurysm (a small out-pouching that looks like a berry at the point of bifurcation of an intracranial artery). Less often, it is associated with: an arteriovenous malformation (a congenital disorder of blood vessels in the brain, brainstem or spinal cord consisting of a complex, tangled web of abnormal arteries and veins connected by one or more fistulas [abnormal communications]); a non-aneurysmal perimesencephalic haemorrhage [32] where the bleeding is centred anterior to the midbrain or pons, with or without extension of blood around the brainstem, into the suprasellar cistern or the proximal Sylvian fissures; or it may be traumatic in origin. [33]

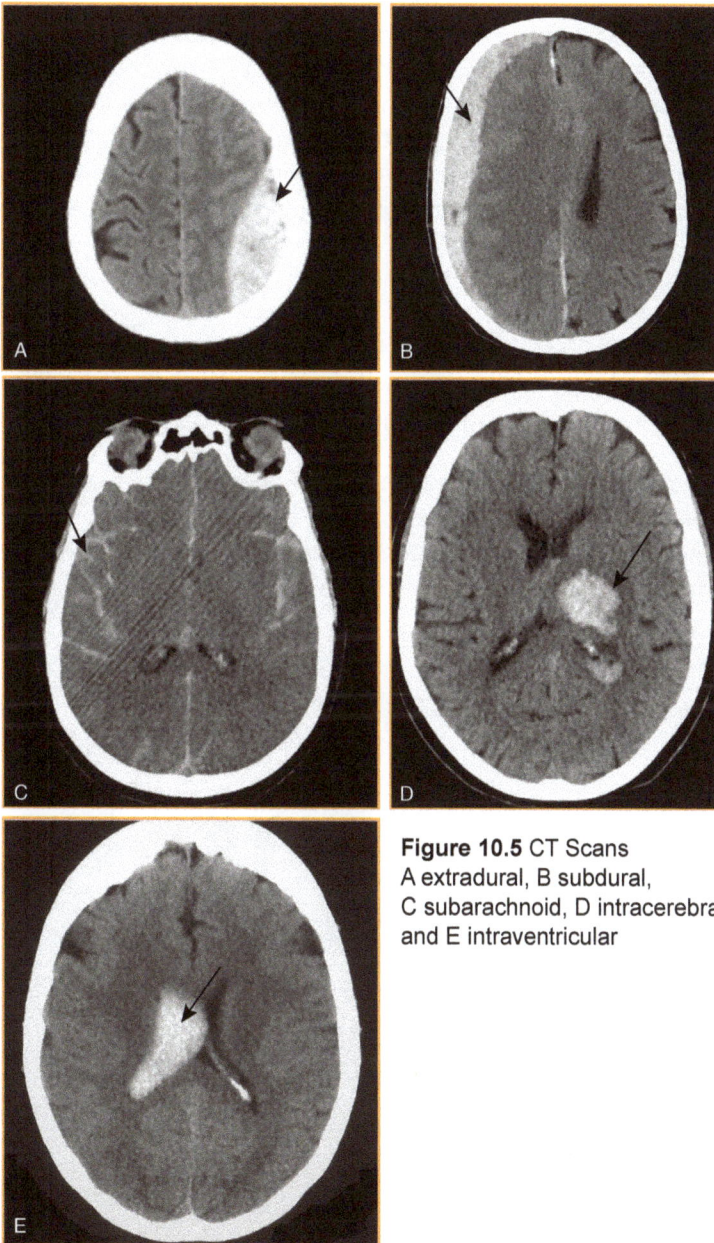

**Figure 10.5** CT Scans
A extradural, B subdural,
C subarachnoid, D intracerebral
and E intraventricular

Subarachnoid haemorrhage (SAH) presents in most patients with the sudden onset of a very severe headache, nausea and vomiting with or without depression of the conscious state. Although SAH is discussed under the heading of CVD, it rarely is confused with a stroke. Occasional patients will have a focal neurological deficit if bleeding also occurs in the brain.

# Intracerebral Haemorrhage

Traditional teaching has been that the leading cause of intracerebral haemorrhage is rupture of a Charcot–Bouchard aneurysm. This aneurysm was said to form on tiny intracerebral vessels in the setting of long-standing hypertension. [34] However, the existence of these aneurysms has been questioned. [154] The haemorrhages occur in characteristic sites, as shown in Figures 10.6 A and B.

Putaminal and basal ganglia haemorrhages are most often seen in patients with hypertension. Lobar haemorrhage is secondary to cerebral amyloid angiopathy(CAA). CAA is also referred to as congophilic angiopathy or cerebrovascular amyloidosis. CAA is the deposition of amyloid protein in the walls of the small blood vessels, with resulting fragility of the wall and tendency to rupture. Anticoagulants and less often vascular malformations or rarely aneurysms may cause lobar haemorrhage.

Classically seen with hypertension, cerebellar haemorrhage is a not uncommon site in patients with anticoagulant-related haemorrhage.

# Intraventricular Haemorrhage

Intraventricular haemorrhage is usually secondary to rupture into the ventricles from an intracerebral haemorrhage. Primary intraventricular bleeding is infrequent and presents with a depressed conscious state or headache and vomiting with or without confusion. Focal neurological signs are absent. [35]

**Figure 10.6 A** sites of intracerebral haemorrhage in the cerebral hemispheres (reproduced with permission HJM Barnett)

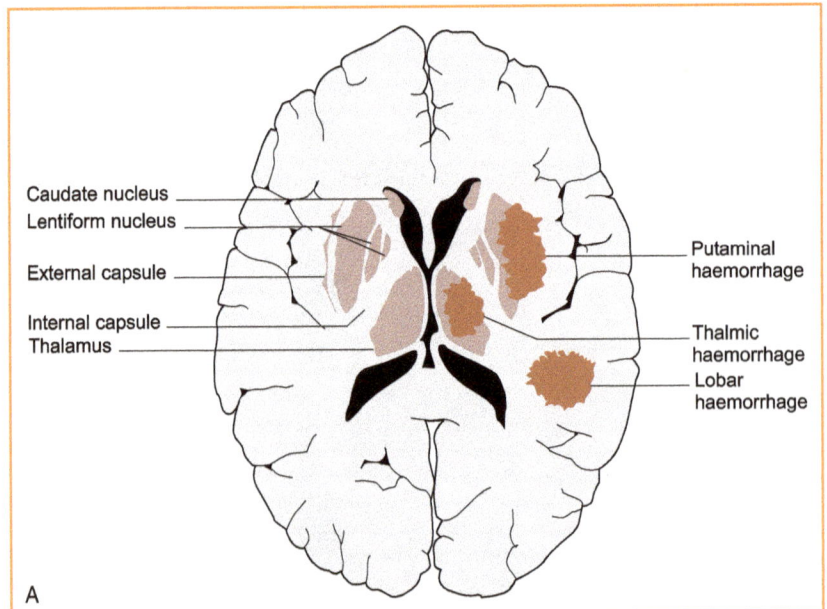

Caudate nucleus
Lentiform nucleus
External capsule
Internal capsule
Thalamus
Putaminal haemorrhage
Thalmic haemorrhage
Lobar haemorrhage

A

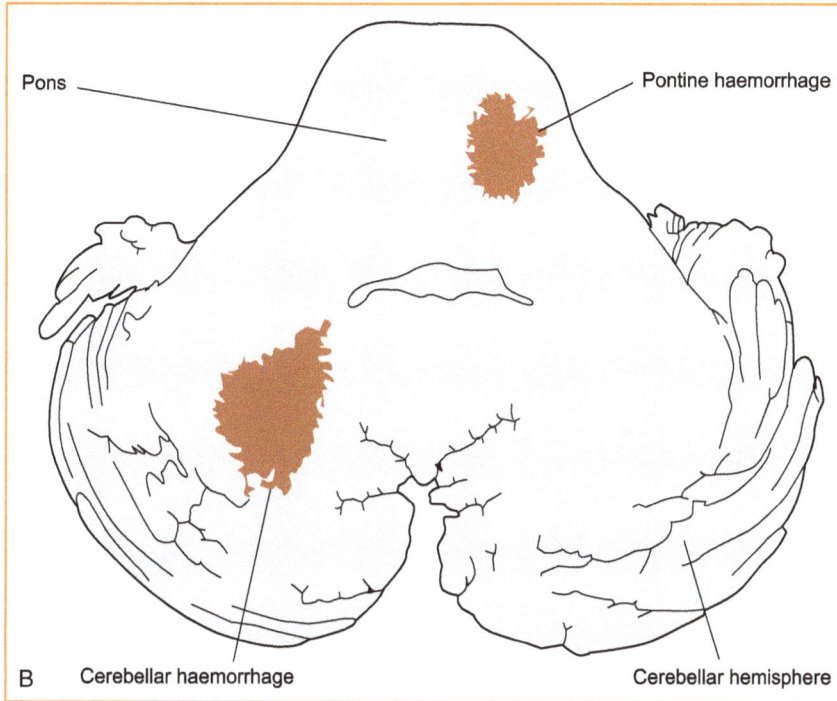

**Figure 10.6 B** sites of intracerebral haemorrhage in cerebellum and brainstem (reproduced with permission HJM Barnett)

---

**Management of Intracranial Haemorrhage**

- **Extradural and acute subdural haematomas.** Surgical evacuation.
- **Chronic subdural haematomas.** Can be treated conservatively, although many will require surgical evacuation.
- **Subarachnoid haemorrhage.** Transfer as a matter of urgency to a neurosurgical unit with expertise in the management of SAH. Endovascular intervention using a variety of coils, stents and other unproven devices has supplanted direct clipping of aneurysms. [37, 201] Early intervention prevents re-bleeding. Nimodipine is used to treat cerebral vasospasm. [202]
- **Intracerebral haemorrhage** (ICH) [38] If the ICH is small, it can be managed conservatively. Treatment of larger ICH's consists of ventilatory support, blood pressure control, reversal of any preexisting coagulopathy, intracranial pressure monitoring, osmotherapy, fever control, seizure prophylaxis, treatment of hyperglycaemia and nutritional supplementation. [39] Despite these measures there is some doubt that mortality is reduced. [40] The only study of mannitol failed to show any benefit at 3 months. [41] The role of surgery is clearly established [42] with cerebellar haemorrhages, but the role of surgery in hemisphere haemorrhages is less well defined. The two randomized trials, STITCH and STITCH II found no clinical benefit for early surgical evacuation of intraparenchymal hematoma in patients with spontaneous supratentorial hemorrhage when compared with best medical management plus delayed surgery if necessary. However, the results of the STITCH trials may not be generalizable, because of the high rates of patient crossover from medical management to the surgical group. [203,204]

# Ischaemic Cerebrovascular Disease

Ischaemic stroke accounts for the great majority of patients with CVD. When managing a patient with ischaemic stroke, one needs to consider whether the ischaemia relates to arterial or, much less likely, venous disease. In patients with arterial related cerebral ischaemia, it is necessary to differentiate between small and large vessel disease. Small vessel disease is due to the occlusion of small perforating vessels. Stroke in the area supplied by large arteries is most likely to be embolic in origin either from the heart, the arch of the aorta or the large arteries in the neck (Figures 10.7 and 10.8).

## Is it a large artery, small vessel, or cerebral venous disease?

Differentiating between a stroke due to a large artery versus small vessel disease can sometimes be challenging. Access to diffusion-weighted MRI in the first week after stroke enables differentiation between large and small vessel ischaemia. Small vessel disease is referred to as lacunar syndrome. The lacune is where there is occlusion of the tiny vessels, usually due to lipohyalinosis. Occlusion of slightly larger feeding vessels is due to atheromatous or embolic occlusion at the origin of the penetrating vessel. [36] Although many lacunar syndromes have been described, the advent of sophisticated imaging has revealed that large artery territory infarcts can mimic many of the clinical features of these syndromes.

The most helpful lacunar syndromes are pure motor hemiparesis and pure sensory loss affecting the contralateral face, arm and leg equally. These point to infarction in the deep hemisphere, in particular, the internal capsule and less likely the paramedian brainstem, although in this situation, the face may not be affected if the infarct is below the mid pons.

The third helpful lacunar syndrome is the unilateral internuclear ophthalmoplegia (INO). INO occurs with infarction of the ipsilateral median longitudinal fasciculus. INO results from ostial atheroma occlusion of a small perforating branches of the P2 segment of the posterior cerebral artery. There may be associated significant basilar artery atheroma.

The value of the lacunar syndromes is that they usually identify patients with small vessel disease. Other lacunar syndromes are less predictive of small vessel disease. Syndromes such as ataxic hemiparesis (also referred to as crural paresis and homolateral ataxia), dysarthria, clumsy hand syndrome and sensorimotor stroke can occasionally be seen in large artery ischaemia. The advent of CT and MRI has allowed the detection of many more 'atypical lacunar syndromes' infarcts and highlighted that the clinical features could be very varied. [43]

The risk factors associated with small vessel disease are virtually identical to those associated with large vessel disease. However, lacunar infarcts are more common in patients with long-standing hypertension and diabetes. It is not uncommon for patients with a lacunar infarct to have multiple potential causes for ischaemia, such as an ipsilateral internal carotid artery stenosis or a cardiac source for embolism. [12]

Dysphasia, visual field disturbances and the cortical sensory signs all indicate involvement of the cortex and, therefore, are related to large artery disease. An epileptic seizure associated with the stroke would also indicate cortical involvement and large artery disease.

# If it is Large Artery Cerebral Ischaemia, what is the Vascular Territory?

The reason for differentiating between carotid territory versus vertebrobasilar territory ischaemia is the differences in therapeutic options.

At times it can be challenging to differentiate between anterior and posterior circulation ischaemia. As discussed in Chapter 2, many neurological symptoms and signs are non-specific in terms of their ability to localise a problem to a particular part of the nervous system. In contrast, others accurately identify the part of the nervous system affected. Hemiparesis affecting the arm and leg with or without the ipsilateral facial weakness; unilateral sensory abnormalities affecting the primary sensory modalities of pain, temperature, vibration and proprioception; and dysarthria are non-specific symptoms with poor localising value. They indicate the lesion is in the CNS above the level of the uppermost symptoms and or signs. For example, if the face, arm and leg are affected by weakness or altered sensation, the problem is above the 7th nerve nucleus and the 5th nerve nucleus, respectively, in the pons, but we cannot localise the exact site of the lesion. A hemiparesis affecting the arm and a leg in the absence of any other signs can occur with lesions in the contralateral brainstem or hemisphere.

## Carotid Territory Ischaemia

Visual field defects and dysphasia, together with the parietal cortical signs discussed in Chapter 5, would indicate the involvement of the cerebral hemispheres.

## Vertebrobasilar Territory Ischaemia

The presence of bilateral weakness or sensory disturbance, diplopia or vertigo associated with weakness or sensory disturbance indicates that the problem is in the brainstem. Nausea, vomiting and an inability to stand are not pathognomonic for CVD. When these symptoms are due to CVD, it almost invariably points to cerebellar infarction or haemorrhage.

---

Symptoms of cerebral ischaemia in two different vascular territories within a short time indicate that the likely source is proximal, either the heart or the arch of the aorta.

---

# If it is Large Artery Cerebral Ischaemia, what is the Underlying Pathology?

Cerebral ischaemia results from multiple potential sources, some extremely rare. Figures 10.7 and 10.8 show the more common causes from the heart, arch of the aorta and the major extracranial and intracranial vessels. It is helpful to consider these two diagrams when dealing with a patient with CVD and always ask where the embolic material has arisen?

*The commonest causes of large artery cerebral ischaemia are:*

- Embolism from the heart in patients with atrial fibrillation, less commonly thrombus within the left ventricle in the setting of myocardial infarction or a cardiomyopathy
- Atheroma or thrombus from the arch of the aorta or the major extracranial vessels secondary to atherosclerotic vascular disease.
- Cerebral infarction related to infective or marantic endocarditis is extremely rare.

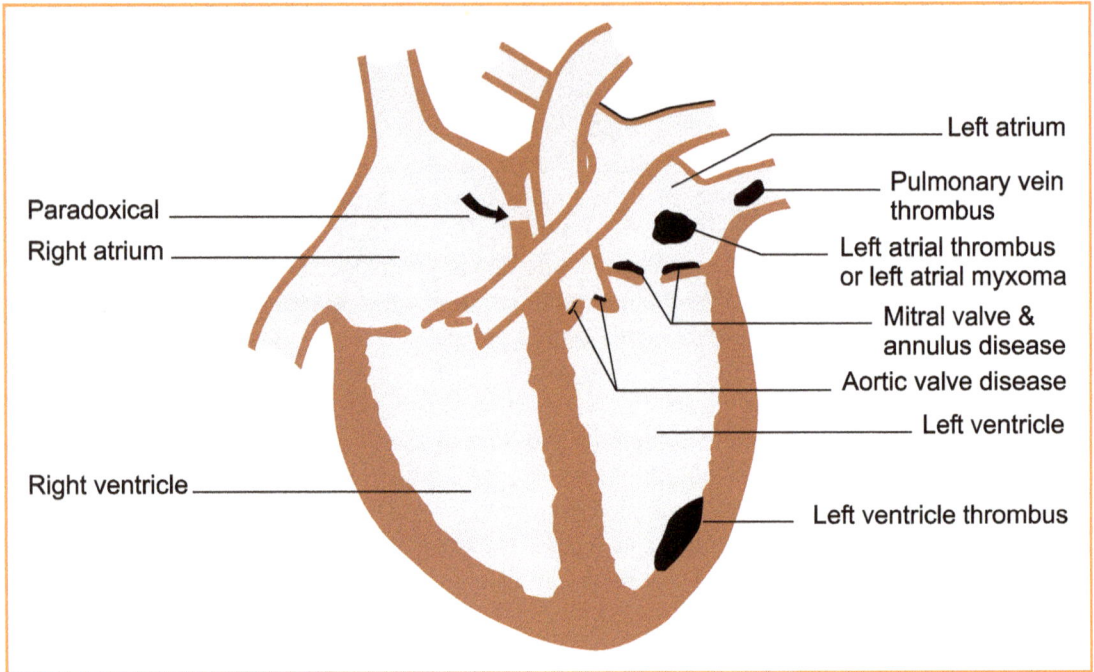

Figure 10.7 The heart and sources of emboli Reproduced with permission from *Stroke: Pathophysiology, Diagnosis and Management*, edited by HJM Barnett et al., 1986, Churchill Livingstone, Figure 54.2, p 1088 [44]

In many patients with cerebral ischaemia, particularly younger patients, current investigations cannot elucidate the cause in as many as 30–40%. [48] This is referred to as cryptogenic stroke. In some patients with 'cryptogenic stroke,' atrial fibrillation is subsequently detected. [40]

| Contrarian Thought |
| --- |
| Knowing that arteriosclerosis commences in-utero, increases in severity with advancing age, and that superimposed atherosclerotic vascular disease begins in childhood leads one to suspect that the cause of cryptogenic stroke relates to atherosclerotic vascular disease, not severe enough to be detected by current imaging techniques. |

# The Cerebral Circulation

Two common carotid arteries bifurcate in the neck into the internal and external carotid arteries. The anterior and middle cerebral arteries arise from the internal carotid. Two vertebral arteries join intracranially to form the basilar artery. Major branches arise from the vertebral and basilar arteries to supply the lateral brainstem and cerebellum. These include the posterior inferior cerebellar artery (PICA), usually arises from the vertebral, the anterior inferior cerebellar artery (AICA), the superior cerebellar artery (SCA) and the posterior cerebral arteries (PCA) that supply the occipital lobes (all branches of the basilar). (Figure 10.8)

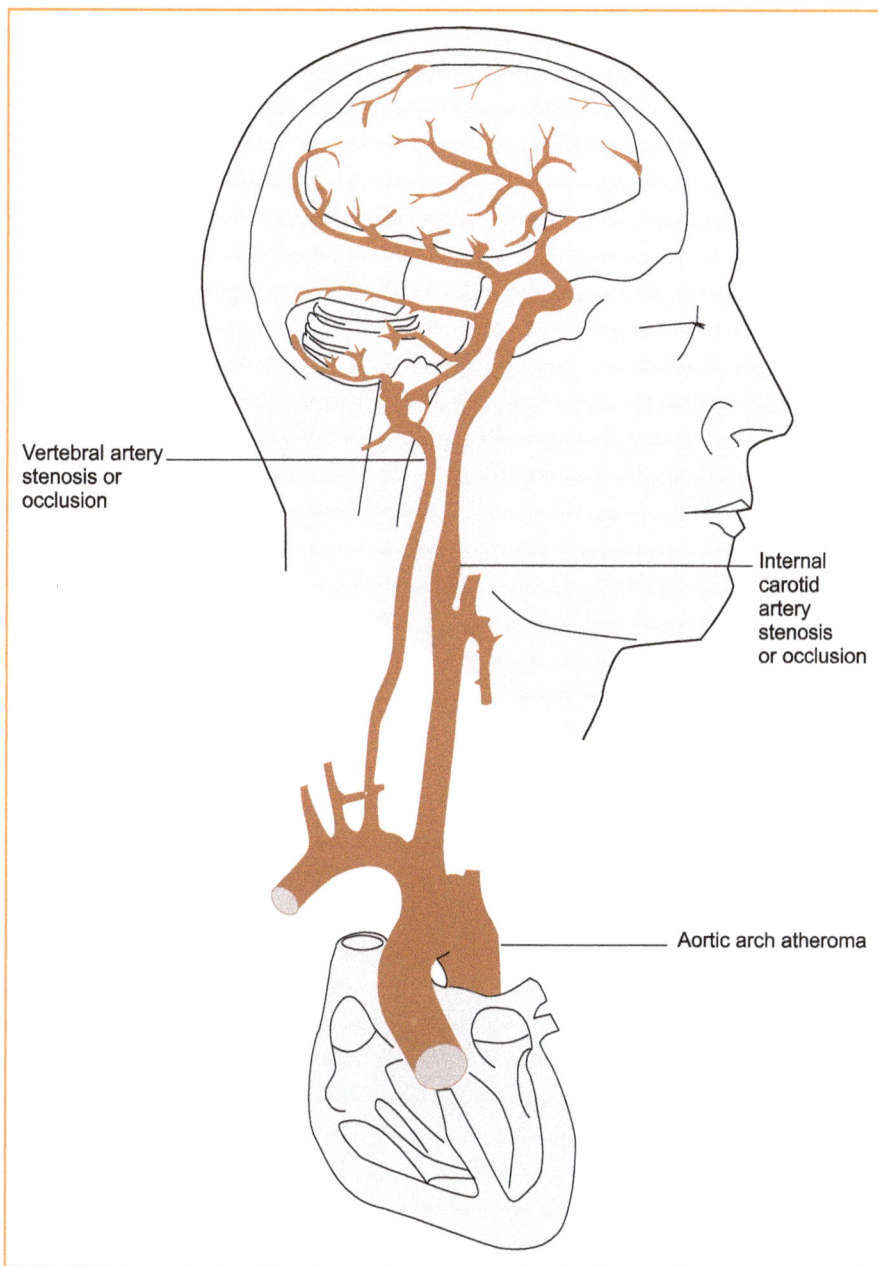

**Figure 10.8** The heart, major vessels, and intracranial vessels. Reproduced with the permission of H.J.M. Barnett.

# Cerebral Vein Thrombosis

Cerebral vein thrombosis is very rare. Blood drains via the cortical veins into the superior sagittal sinus (SSS) of the venous system. The SSS merges with the straight sinus (SS) to form the torcular herephili that then drains into the internal jugular veins via the lateral sinuses (Figure 10.9).

247

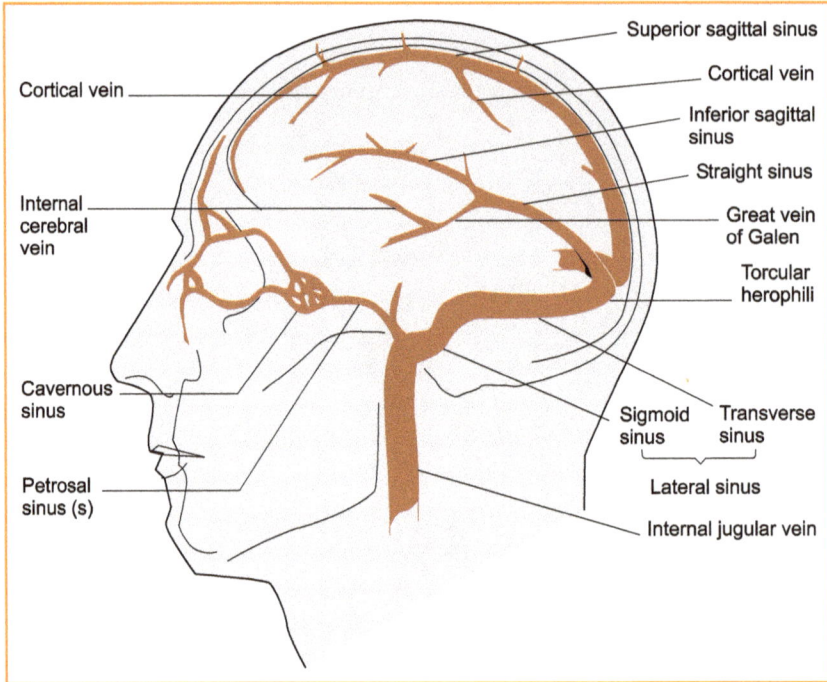

**Figure 10.9** Cerebral venous system Reproduced with permission from 'Cardiogenic stroke' by PC Gates, HJM Barnett, MD Silver, in Stroke: Pathophysiology, Diagnosis and Management, edited by HJM Barnett et al., 1986, Churchill Livingstone, Figure 35.1, p 732 [44]

The resultant clinical syndrome depends on what part of the venous system is affected. [44]

- **Lateral sinus:** usually results in intracranial hypertension, resembling idiopathic intracranial hypertension(IIH) with raised intracranial pressure causing headache and papilloedema.
- **Superior sagittal sinus** thrombosis may also result in intracranial hypertension. It more commonly causes severe headache, focal or generalised convulsions, and a focal neurological deficit, predominantly hemiparesis due to associated cortical vein thrombosis.
- **Cavernous sinus thrombosis** presents with unilateral periorbital pain, impaired ocular movements, proptosis (protruding eye) and chemosis (conjunctival oedema and erythema).
- **Deep venous system** thrombosis (the straight sinus and its tributaries) is very rare. It presents with headache, vomiting, fever and a depressed conscious state.

# Three Stroke Syndromes not to miss

There are three-stroke syndromes that, if missed, can result in a severe adverse outcome. These include cerebellar haemorrhage or infarction, severe symptomatic carotid stenosis and basilar artery stenosis.

## Cerebellar Haemorrhage or Infarction

Patients with cerebellar haemorrhage or infarction are at significant risk of brain stem compression and secondary hydrocephalus (dilatation of the 3rd and lateral ventricles) due to swelling of the cerebellar hemisphere. Prompt neurosurgical intervention can be lifesaving.

Patients present in a variety of ways. The commonest is an inability to walk associated with severe nausea and vomiting with or without vertigo and headache. In some patients, the vomiting is so intense that it results in a Mallory–Weiss tear of the oesophagus, causing haematemesis. In patients with posterior inferior cerebellar artery territory infarcts, a triad of vertigo, headache and gait imbalance predominates at stroke onset. In patients with superior cerebellar artery infarcts, gait disturbance dominates at onset; vertigo and headache are significantly less common. [50] There will be cranial nerve involvement if the infarct also involves the lateral brainstem. For example, with a posterior inferior cerebellar artery territory, infarct, there is often an associated lateral medullary syndrome.

*Note*: Lateral medullary syndrome also occurs with vertebral artery disease. [51]

# Symptomatic Severe Carotid Stenosis

Symptomatic carotid stenosis of greater than 70% is associated with a 26% risk of stroke in the ensuing 18 months. [52, 53] There is a significant risk of recurrent ischaemia in the first week after the initial symptoms; thus, *assessment and treatment should NOT be delayed.* The risk of stroke *prior to endarterectomy* in the OXVASC subpopulation (where there was a significant delay in performing endarterectomy with only 43% of patients with ≥ 50% stenosis undergoing endarterectomy by 12 weeks) was 21% (95% CI: 8 to 34%) at two weeks and 32% (95% CI: 17 to 47%) at 12 weeks. Half the strokes were disabling or fatal. [54] Contralateral carotid occlusion increases the risk of early recurrence. [55]

Patients with carotid stenosis may present with a severe stroke without warning; however, a number will have an antecedent TIA that provides an opportunity to intervene and prevent the stroke. Carotid stenosis should be suspected in patients who present with transient monocular blindness (amaurosis fugax) or ipsilateral hemisphere ischaemia. The presence of a carotid bruit increases the likelihood of severe carotid stenosis. Focal involvement of one limb or dysphasia with symptoms lasting longer than 1 hour are more likely to indicate the presence of severe carotid stenosis than a lacunar syndrome. [56–58] Carotid stenosis is more common in patients with diabetes, smokers [59] and if there is coexistent coronary artery or peripheral vascular disease.

# Basilar Artery Stenosis

The prognosis of untreated basilar artery thrombosis is abysmal. Although basilar artery occlusion may be the initial presenting symptom, two-thirds of these patients experience in the weeks to months before the thrombosis a flurry of episodes of transient cerebral ischaemia that become more frequent just before occlusion. [60] Tetraparesis is rare and occurs more frequently when the basilar artery syndrome is related to embolism rather than stenosis with superimposed thrombosis. Patients can present with any combination of symptoms reflecting brainstem involvement, including a depressed conscious state, weakness, sensory abnormalities, vertigo, nausea and vomiting, and diplopia. [60]

Once again, vertigo with diplopia and bilateral symptoms indicate involvement of the brainstem. It is important to remember that not all patients with severe basilar artery stenosis will have symptoms that indicate a brainstem problem. Repeated brief stereotyped TIAs should alert the clinician to the possibility of a tight stenosis and prompt urgent investigations.

# Three Rare Causes of Stroke
## Extracranial Arterial Dissection

Dissection of the carotid and vertebral arteries is one of the more common causes of stroke in young patients. In 50% of patients, there will be no history of head or neck trauma; it can occur even during coughing or sneezing. This author has seen patients who developed arterial dissection by simply turning their heads quickly to one side. Carotid artery dissection is more common than vertebral artery dissection

Essentially there are two presentations:
1. isolated Horner's syndrome with ipsilateral pain in the head, face or neck with internal carotid artery occlusion and negligible risk of cerebral ischaemia [61]
2. focal cerebral ischaemia.

Although an infarct may be the presenting event, it is more common for patients to have transient cerebral ischaemia some days or weeks after the onset of the headache. The headache is of sudden onset, often severe affecting the neck, ear, face, temple or forehead. In more than 90% of cases, it is ipsilateral to the dissection. If the dissection extends intracranially (more common with vertebral artery dissection), rupture of the artery may occur, resulting in SAH. Vertebral artery dissection may very rarely extend into the basilar artery. Recanalisation occurs in most patients, and the risk of recurrent events is negligible but not zero. This low risk of recurrent symptoms has led to considerable debate regarding the most appropriate treatment. There is no information from randomised controlled trials to guide therapy. This author has seen several cases of recurrent cerebral ischaemia, often when therapy was suboptimal. In these cases, the ischaemia was in a more distal vessel than the initial ischaemic symptoms. For example, in patients with occipital lobe infarction when the initial presenting problem was lateral brainstem ischaemia. Ischaemia in a different vascular territory supports the hypothesis that thromboembolism is the cause of recurrent ischaemia. It also endorses the use of anticoagulants. [135]

---

**Management of Arterial Dissection**

Arterial dissection can be detected on imaging studies such as MRI, MR angiography with fat saturation or CT angiography if MRI is not available. The sensitivity of duplex carotid ultrasound in the internal carotid artery (80–96%) and the vertebral arteries (70–86%) is not high enough to exclude extracranial arterial dissection. [62]

There are no adequate randomized trials to guide treatment. The risk of recurrent events is with the initial presentation, and the long-term risk of recurrence is negligible.

- For patients with ischaemic stroke or TIA and extracranial arterial dissection, either heparin followed by a short course of warfarin [135] or NOAC's [205] is recommended by most clinicians.
- In patients with ischaemic stroke and extracranial arterial dissection, the European Stroke Organisation guidelines(ESO) [208] recommend IV thrombolysis within 4.5 hours or mechanical thrombectomy for large vessel occlusion in the anterior circulation. Endovascular or surgical intervention is recommended in patients with intracranial arterial dissection and subarachnoid haemorrhage. The ESO recommends either antiplatelet therapy or anticoagulation in the acute phase, as there is no evidence favouring one or the other.
- Some clinicians keep patients on lifelong antiplatelet therapy despite the low risk of recurrence.
  In the very rare patient who has recurrent ischaemia, despite adequate antithrombotic therapy and in the absence of any scientific proof of efficacy, some authorities would recommend endovascular stenting [63] or direct surgical intervention, despite the fact that surgery is associated with a high complication rate of stroke and death (10–12%). [64]

# Patent Foramen Ovale

Patent foramen ovale (PFO) is present in up to 27% of the general population, and in 2% of the population it is associated with an atrial septal aneurysm (ASA). An ASA is bulging of the atrial wall into the left atrium by as little as 1.2 up to 15 mm. It can occur in the absence of a PFO. The overall rate of recurrent stroke is 0.61-1.25 per 100 patient years. [128] The presence of an ASA or large right-to-left shunt increases the risk of stroke. In a large French study [46], the risk of recurrent cerebral ischaemia was 2.3% with PFO alone and 15.2% if there was also an ASA. Other studies have failed to confirm the increased risk with an ASA. [65] A patent foramen ovale (PFO) is associated with an increased risk of stroke, particularly in young adults. [45, 46] Thrombus has been visualised traversing the patent foramen ovale. [47] However, coexistent deep venous thrombosis (DVT) is detected in as few as 5% of patients.

| Management of Cerebral Ischaemia with PFO |
| --- |
| Current American Heart Association/American Stroke Association guidelines recommend antiplatelet therapy in patients with an ischaemic stroke or TIA associated with a PFO. Warfarin is recommended for high-risk patients, those who have other indications for oral anticoagulation. This includes those with an underlying hypercoagulable state or evidence of venous thrombosis. When the 1st edition was published, there was insufficient data to recommend PFO closure in patients with a first stroke. [66] Subsequently, several randomised controlled trials have established a role for PFO closure in high-risk patients. These include those with a large right to left shunt (>30 microbubbles within three cardiac cycles after opacification of the right atrium) or with an ASA. [129-133] The RRR over 3.2 years after closure was an impressive 77%, the ARR was 4.02% (1.25% per year) and the NNT is 24.9. [131] |

# Antiphospholipid Antibody Syndrome

Antiphospholipid syndrome (APS) is an autoimmune disorder where blood clots occur within arteries, veins, and small blood vessels. Antiphospholipid (APL) antibodies were first described in 1906. [67] They are a heterogeneous group of autoantibodies directed against phospholipid-binding proteins. They consist of the lupus anticoagulants (LA), anticardiolipin antibodies (aCL) and anti-Beta-2-glycoprotein-I antibody (aβ2GPI). LA prolong phospholipid-dependent coagulation assays. aCL target a molecular congener of cardiolipin and aβ2GPI in combination with C-reactive protein and thrombomodulin regulate the complement and coagulation systems, both up and down.

The presence of the lupus anticoagulant increases the risk of stroke 40-fold. [152] Patients who are LA negative but with persistently positive aCL antibodies are also at increased risk. [150] The diagnostic criteria for the Antiphospholipid Antibody Syndrome remain controversial. [150] The minimum is one clinical manifestation (e.g. stroke, TIA) with positive tests for circulating antiphospholipid antibodies, including lupus anticoagulant, anticardiolipin and anti-Beta-2-glycoprotein-1 antibody (aβ2GPI) IgG or IgM at medium-high values, detected at least twice 12 weeks apart. The presence of anti-β2-glycoprotein-1 also increases the risk for venous and arterial thrombosis. However, aPL test results need to be interpreted cautiously. Not every person who has a positive aPL test result necessarily has APS or a clinically relevant aPL positivity.

APS is the presence of these antibodies in patients with arterial or venous thrombosis. The association between APL antibodies and stroke is strongest for young adults less than 50 years of age. [68] Recurrent thrombotic events are common despite treatment. [69] APL antibodies should be tested in all young patients, particularly if there is a combination of arterial and venous thrombosis. Recurrent cerebral ischaemia is common, and the risk of stroke is greatest with higher IgG anticardiolipin titres. [70]

---

**Management of the Antiphospholipid Antibody Syndrome**

Low dose Aspirin (75-100mg/day) is recommended for primary prevention in high-risk patients who are APL positive. [151] Lim et al. [71] recommended moderate-intensity aspirin in patients with first ischaemic stroke. Current guidelines recommend high-intensity Warfarin (PT INR 3.0-4.0), low dose Aspirin (75-100mg/day), with moderate intensity Warfarin (PT INR 20-3.0). At the time of writing, there is insufficient evidence to support the use of novel or direct anticoagulants (DOAC or) in APS. [155] The clinical relevance of transient or low titre APL antibodies remains uncertain.

---

# Management of Ischaemic CVD

The principles of management are discussed below. However, treatment will evolve rapidly. The reader should seek up-to-date information and guidelines from the American Heart Association stroke website and other websites dedicated to cerebral vascular disease[2].

Essentially, managing patients with cerebral ischaemia involves treating the initial episode and secondary prevention through risk factor modification and cause-specific therapy adapted to the individual patient based on their coexistent medical conditions, concurrent medications, and social circumstances.

Many patients with CVD have multiple medical problems such as hypertension, diabetes, peptic ulcer, chronic obstructive airways, coronary artery or peripheral vascular disease that will influence the choice of therapy. They are often taking a large number of medications that may either contraindicate the introduction of new drugs or result in adverse drug interactions. The presence or absence of a supportive family has a significant impact on management, as does the type of work that the patient is involved with and, of course, whether their house is suitable for someone who may have a residual neurological deficit resulting in some incapacity.

Initial management depends on whether the patient presents with a minor episode of cerebral ischaemia such as a TIA or minor stroke or with a severe stroke.

## Management of Acute Ischaemic Stroke

The American Heart Association Stroke Council has issued extensive guidelines for all aspects of the early management of patients with ischaemic stroke[3]. [140,142,143]

The general principles are discussed in this chapter. Thrombolysis and clot retrieval are discussed in appendix F.

Patients should be prioritised in the emergency department, preferably by a stroke team using organised protocols primarily to establish that the patient is suffering from cerebral ischaemia.

The severity of the stroke should be assessed using the National Institute of Health Stroke Severity Scale (NIHSS) and the modified Rankin Score (mRS Score). [145]

CT scans should be graded using the Alberta Stroke Program Early CT Score. [146-148]

---

2   The American Heart Association http://www.americanheart.org/presenter.jhtml?identifier=3004586

    The Cochrane collaboration http://www.cochrane.org/reviews/en/topics/93_reviews.html

    The stroke trials registry http://www.strokecenter.org/trials/

3   AHA website, https://www.ahajournals.org/

# Initial urgent bedside clinical assessment

- The pulse, looking for atrial fibrillation, the temperature that if elevated may indicate sepsis and respiratory rate if elevated, may indicate pneumonia.
- The blood pressure should be measured (checking for the very rare case of hypertensive encephalopathy with a diastolic pressure > 120 mm Hg and determining if the blood pressure needs to be reduced to administer thrombolysis).
- The heart should be auscultated to check for a cardiac murmur that may indicate infective endocarditis, a rare cause of stroke in < 1% of cases per year.
- An urgent ECG should be performed (to detect atrial fibrillation (AF) or the asymptomatic myocardial infarct, the latter, particularly in patients with diabetes).

# Immediate Investigations

## Imaging

- A CT scan may be the only modality available in many places. It can rule out intracranial haemorrhage and other pathology such as tumours that may mimic a stroke. It may not detect all instances of cerebral ischaemia. MRI, if available, can detect ischaemic changes after 1½ hours duration, and diffusion-weighted MRI can differentiate recent from old stroke if undertaken within two weeks of the event. Both CT and MRI perfusion studies can assess the viable ischaemic penumbra to help select patients suitable for thrombolysis. Either CT or MR angiography can demonstrate the presence of large vessel occlusion suitable for endovascular clot retrieval. [116,149] This is discussed in appendix F.

## Blood Tests

- Complete (or full) blood examination, platelet count, C-reactive protein (CRP) and ESR should be requested in all patients. Anaemia and an elevated CRP or ESR suggest possible endocarditis. An altered platelet count may indicate rarer pathological processes such as thrombotic thombocytopaenic purpura (TTP) or essential thrombocytosis.
- There are two reasons to measure the blood glucose; firstly, if raised, it can detect asymptomatic diabetes and secondly, hypoglycaemia may present with a focal deficit mimicking a stroke.
- Serum electrolytes and renal function tests, as many patients are on diuretics that may cause hyponatraemia or hypokalaemia, and impaired renal function will influence the choice of antihypertensive medication.
- Prothrombin time/international normalised ratio (PT INR), particularly necessary in patients on warfarin.
- An elevated activated partial thromboplastin time (APTT) suggests possible lupus anticoagulant syndrome, particularly in young patients.
- Reduced oxygen saturation occurs with aspiration pneumonia and in heavy smokers with chronic obstructive airways disease.

# Subsequent Investigations

## Assessing the Internal Carotid Artery

The modality of choice for non-invasive carotid artery assessment depends mainly on the clinical indications for imaging and the skills available in individual centres. Digital subtraction angiography was the gold standard imaging technique used in the North American Symptomatic Carotid Endarterectomy Trial. Until recently, 3-D carotid duplex ultrasonography (DUS) has been the modality of choice and will continue to be, in some places, the technique of choice due to the inability to access CTA and MRA. The sensitivity and specificity of duplex ultrasound, CTA and MRA are shown in table 10.2. [73] DUS has limitations; it can miss severe carotid stenosis and cannot assess the arch of the aorta or the intracranial circulation. Both CTA and MRA can accurately assess the severity of the stenosis at the carotid bifurcation and provide images of the aortic arch and intracranial circulation. CTA and MRA are not suitable for all patients because of contraindications. CTA has a sensitivity and specificity for detecting carotid occlusion of 97% and 99%, respectively. [115,156] The advantage of MRI is that it is non-invasive.

| | Sensitivity (95% CI) | Specificity (95% CI) |
|---|---|---|
| Duplex Ultrasound | 86 (84-89) | 87 (84-90) |
| CTA | 85 (79-89) | 93 (89-96) |
| Contrast enhanced MRA | 94 (88-97) | 93 (89-96) |

Table 10.2 The sensitivity and specificity of duplex carotid ultrasound, CTA, and MRI to detect>70% ICA Stenosis. [115]

A screening test should be performed within the first 24 hours in patients with suspected large artery carotid territory ischaemia with a mild deficit to detect carotid stenosis > 50%. The reason is the high risk of early recurrent ischaemia in patients with severe ICA stenosis. It can be delayed and performed as an outpatient in patients with lacunar ischaemia and vertebrobasilar ischaemia.

# Looking for a Cardiac Source of Embolism

A more proximal source should be considered in patients with large artery territory ischaemia with normal arterial vessels to the area of ischaemia or when a patient experiences two episodes of ischaemia in two different vascular territories within a short period of time (hours to weeks), occasionally this can be to the spleen or lower limbs. This involves monitoring cardiac rhythm to detect AF and ultrasonography of the heart to look for potential sources of embolism.

## Cardiac monitoring

Cardiac monitoring is usually undertaken on all in-patients presenting with cerebral ischaemia. More prolonged monitoring for AF should be considered in patients with ischaemia in the territory of one of the major vessels without any disease in that vessel to account for the symptoms. [49] AF is more likely to be present in patients ≥ 62 years of age, with an NIHSS ≥ 8, extensive cortical ischaemia without extracranial large artery stenosis and a dilated left atrium as detected on transthoracic echocardiogram. [76] It is appropriate to monitor patients with large artery territory ischaemia with normal arteries to that territory for several days whilst there are other reasons for them to be an inpatient. Subsequently, patients can be monitored with holter monitoring, loop recorders or smartwatches. Prolonged monitoring is recommended in patients with a suspected cardiac source for embolism with no explanation on transthoracic (TTE) or transoesophageal echocardiography (TOE/TEE).

Smartwatches can detect suspected AF that can be confirmed by wearing an ECG patch for 7 days, [157, 206] although signal quality is an issue. [158] ECG skin patches have detected AF in a little over 5% of high risk (age ≥55 years with ≥2 of the following risk factors: coronary disease, heart failure, hypertension, diabetes, sleep apnea) patients. [159] Implantable loop recorders detect AF in more patients with stroke the longer they are monitored. [160,161] Using a loop recorder AF was detected in 19.1% of patients with cryptogenic stroke after a median follow-up of 10.7 months. [162] Currently, the routine use of loop recorders is not recommended by the European Heart Rhythm Association. [163] They question the cost-effectiveness and clinical utility. They also pointed out the lack of a temporal relationship between the AF and the occurrence of stroke. [165]

Prolonged monitoring for AF is not recommended in patients with a contraindication to anticoagulation, lacunar infarct and those with a significant ipsilateral carotid stenosis. [74]

| Contrarian thought |
| --- |
| The risk of stroke with isolated AF is very low. Most severe ischaemic strokes are secondary to thrombus, not platelet embolism. The $CHA_2DS_2$-Vasc score reflects the risk factors in ALL patients with stroke, not only those with AF. Most studies of anticoagulation in non-AF patients have included low-risk patients and have not shown a benefit. I suspect a study of anticoagulation in patients without AF and a high $CHA_2DS_2$-Vasc score would demonstrate benefit. |

### Echocardiography

Transthoracic echocardiography (TTE) can detect enlargement of the left atrium and abnormalities of the left ventricle. A TTE bubble study (saline with tiny air bubbles injected into the vein) can detect a PFO, assess the severity of the right to left shunt but not the presence of an atrial septal aneurysm (ASA). Transoesophageal[4] (TOE) is more sensitive at detecting PFO, infective endocarditis vegetations and aortic arch atheroma. TOE is more invasive and may cause an oesophageal rupture in elderly patients. At this point in time there is no consensus on who should have structural imaging of the heart, with some advocating all patients and others recommending a more restricted use. One could argue against a TOE as there is no convincing evidence regarding the treatment of aortic arch atheroma. Cardiomyopathy or dyskinetic anterior left ventricular wall, both indications for the use of anticoagulation, can be detected with TTE. TOE should be performed in suspected infective endocarditis and to identify appropriate patients for PFO closure (< 55 years of age with PFO, large right to left shunt and an associated atrial septal aneurysm). [166]

# General Supportive Care and Treatment of Acute Complications

Guidelines continue to be updated and modified, and once again, it is important to consult current guidelines. [140,141]
- *Airway support and ventilator assistance* are recommended for patients with decreased consciousness or who have bulbar dysfunction causing compromise of the airway.

---

4   In the USA the spelling is TEE, tranesophageal echocardiography

- Patients can lie flat or sit up at 30 degrees. [167]
- Hypoxic patients with stroke should receive *supplemental oxygen*.
- Patients should be *screened for dysphagia* and placed nil orally if they fail the screening test.
- The *management of arterial hypertension* remains controversial. It needs to be less than 185/110 mmHg if thrombolysis is contemplated. Blood pressure typically decreases spontaneously during the acute phase of ischemic stroke, starting within 90 minutes after the onset of symptoms. Elevated blood pressure should be lowered slowly with labetalol and or nicardipine, [143] aiming to reduce it by 15% in the first 24 hours. [141]
- Hyperglycaemia and hypoglycaemia should be treated.
- *Prevention of DVT* with prompt initiation of subcutaneous anticoagulation in all patients.
- *Fever should prompt a septic workup.* Sources of fever should be treated, and antipyretic medications should be administered to lower temperature in febrile patients.
- The patient's *chest and IV sites should be examined daily* as chest infections, aspiration pneumonia (even in patients who are nil orally and who have nasogastric tubes inserted) and IV site infections or thrombosis occur in the first few days after stroke. Frequent changing of the IV is ideal but challenging in patients with poor venous access.
- *Urinary tract infections are common complications* of patients with ischaemic stroke and require prompt attention.
- *Seizures,* either focal or generalised, may occur in a small percentage of patients with cortical cerebral ischaemia, usually within the first 24 hours.
- *Myocardial ischaemia* is seen in the occasional patient.
- *Pulmonary embolism* may occur despite prophylactic anticoagulants.

## Dysphagia screen

Many patients with stroke develop dysphagia that predisposes them to aspiration pneumonia. The dysphagia is often transient but may persist for days to weeks, and patients will require nasogastric feeding. In some patients, swallowing does not recover, and these patients require long-term feeding with a percutaneous endoscopic gastrostomy (PEG) tube. Although controversial, [77, 168] the risk of aspiration may be reduced with dysphagia screening. [78] A dysphagia screen is undertaken on all patients. If the patient fails the screen, they should be placed nil orally until a speech therapist undertakes a formal assessment of swallowing as soon as possible[5]. As dysphagia is often temporary, it is not unreasonable to defer insertion of a nasogastric tube until it is clear that improvement is not occurring.

## Intravenous therapy

Intravenous therapy is often required in the first 24–48 hours in patients who fail a dysphagia screen. Normal saline should be used, not 5% glucose, as the latter enters the intracellular space and will exacerbate cerebral oedema.

---

5 The Barwon Health Stroke unit has a speech therapist 7 day per week to ensure all patients are assessed for dysphagia. The Barwon Health Dysphagia Screen is shown in Appendix G.

# Antiplatelet agents

The International Stroke Trial (IST) [88] and the Chinese Acute Stroke Trial (CAST) [89] have both demonstrated a non-significant trend towards a better outcome with antiplatelet agents. A combined analysis of both trials showed a statistically significant benefit in reducing the incidence of recurrent stroke with aspirin given in the first 24–48 hours of acute stroke. In patients undergoing thrombolysis, aspirin should be withheld for 24 hours. The recommended dose of aspirin is 160–300mg. [90] In patients with minor ischemic stroke or high-risk TIA, those who received dual antiplatelet therapy with a combination of clopidogrel and aspirin had a lower risk of major ischemic events but a higher risk of major bleeding at 90 days than those who received aspirin alone. [164] The recommended duration of dual antiplatelet therapy varies. Both the Australian Stroke foundation and the European Stroke Organisation [210] recommend only three weeks[6], The AHA/ASA do not specify an exact duration but indicate that the risk outweighs the benefit beyond 90 days [194]. Triple platelet therapy in a trial of aspirin, clopidogrel and dipyridamole versus clopidogrel alone or aspirin and dipyridamole was associated with a significantly increased risk of significant bleeding. [165]

# Anticoagulants

Apart from prophylaxis for DVT, anticoagulants are not recommended in acute completed (maximum deficit already present at time patient presents) ischaemic stroke. [91]

# Urgent Management of Minor Ischaemic Stroke

One of the most challenging aspects of caring for CVD patients is managing minor ischaemic stroke and TIA. Many patients do not recognise that minor neurological symptoms may represent a warning of a more severe stroke and do not seek medical attention. In other patients, the interval between the initial symptom and the subsequent severe cerebral infarct is brief and therefore, the time to intervene is limited. It is sometimes impossible to be certain clinically whether the symptoms represent cerebral ischaemia and thus prompt emergency investigations or whether it is a less urgent problem when investigations could wait. Finally, having decided the patient has cerebral ischaemia, the question arises as to whether one can access the urgent imaging required as an out-patient[7]. All these questions are not readily answered.

Patients with suspected minor cerebral ischaemia should be assessed as a matter of urgency. The urgent bedside assessment involves palpating the pulse, measuring the blood pressure, respiratory rate and temperature. An urgent ECG (to detect AF and clinically silent myocardial infarction), CT of the brain (to exclude haemorrhage and other stroke mimics) and, if carotid territory ischaemia, imaging the carotid bifurcation to check for severe carotid stenosis should be undertaken. If there is uncertainty about whether it is carotid territory, then err on the safe side and obtain urgent imaging because missing a severe symptomatic internal carotid stenosis is potentially disastrous. The earliest risk of recurrence is in patients with large artery atherosclerotic vascular disease, accounting for more than one-third of recurrent cerebral ischaemia within the

---

6  https://app.magicapp.org/#/guideline/5781

7  It is not uncommon in Australia for patients to be admitted to hospital in order to obtain the necessary urgent investigations.

first seven days. [92] Ideally carotid arteries should be imaged on the same day as half of all recurrent strokes during the seven days after a TIA occur in the first 24 hours. [92]

A vexed question is whether to admit the patient to a hospital. Although therapy can be administered on an outpatient basis, some argue that in the high-risk group, admission to the hospital provides an excellent opportunity for the urgent detection of subsequent cerebral infarction and prompt administration of thrombolytic therapy and clot retrieval. The reality is that most hospitals do not have the resources to admit all patients, nor do they have clot retrieval.

In recent years the ABCD3-I score has been developed that takes into account the imaging-based diagnosis of TIA. [189-192] ABCD3-I is an expanded version of the ABCD2 score. (Table 10.3) It has been suggested that the ABCD2 score can identify patients with a greater likelihood of early recurrence of cerebral ischaemia. Patients with a score ≥ 4 should be admitted to the hospital for urgent assessment. [93] An ABCD2 score <4 can be investigated as outpatients.

| ABCD2 Score (Maximum score 7) | Points |
|---|---|
| Age ≥ 60 years | 1 |
| Blood pressure ≥ 140/90 mmHg | 1 |
| Unilateral weakness | 2 |
| Speech impairment without weakness | 1 |
| Duration of event ≥ 60 min | 2 |
| Duration of event = 10–59 min | 1 |
| Diabetes | 1 |
| ABCD3-I (Maximum score 13 i.e. 7 from ABCD2 +6) | |
| ≥ 2 TIA's within seven days | 2 |
| Ipsilateral ≥50% ICA stenosis | 2 |
| Acute DWI hyperintensity on MRI | 2 |

Table 10.3 The ABCD2 and ABCD3-I scores for prediction of early and 90-day stroke risk [93] [8]

In the SOS-TIA registry of 1,176 patients, an ABCD2 score < 4 would have missed 20% of patients requiring urgent treatment for carotid stenosis > 50%, intracranial stenosis, AF, and other major cardiac causes of embolism. [94] The authors in the SOS-TIA study advocated a carotid ultrasound or CT angiogram of the carotid arteries and ECG as part of the emergency assessment. Patients with recurrent TIAs and patients with severe carotid stenosis should be admitted for evaluation and with a view to urgent endarterectomy. A prospective Norwegian TIA study [193] found that neither score predicted the short term, 90 day or one-year risk of stroke.

Severe symptomatic extracranial ICA stenosis is the one entity that can cause severe stroke that is preventable. The carotid bifurcation should be assessed urgently within 24 hours, preferably immediately in all patients with carotid territory TIA or minor stroke. In patients with posterior circulation TIA or minor stroke, assessing the ICA's for asymptomatic stenosis can be deferred.

---

8   ABCD3-I/ABCD2 toolkit https://neurotoolkit.com/abcd3-i/

# Secondary Prevention

The same principles apply in secondary as they do in primary prevention (Appendix E). Risk factor modification includes treatment of hypertension, atrial fibrillation, asymptomatic carotid stenosis, hyperlipidaemia, diabetes, obesity and cessation of smoking.

In the last decade, the recommendations regarding the optimal level for blood pressure have undergone enormous and controversial changes. [169,170] Before the 2017 guidelines, the target blood pressure was <140/90. The new 2018 ESC/TSH, Canadian, Korean, Japan, and Latin America hypertension guidelines have maintained this target unless the patient is at high risk. The ACC/IHA 2017 guidelines have recommended treatment if the blood pressure exceeds 130/80. This would mean that nearly 50% of the population will require treatment for hypertension! To complicate matters even further, it is recognised that measuring blood pressure using a sphygmomanometer and a stethoscope can be inaccurate. Many individuals suffer from white coat hypertension, i.e. the blood pressure goes up when they attend a doctor. Electronic digital measuring devices and home blood pressure monitoring should be used to confirm the presence of hypertension. [171] In clinical practice, many patients with hypertension are elderly and cannot tolerate blood pressure reduction to the recommended levels in the current guidelines. A realistic approach is to reduce the blood pressure as close as possible to 120/80 provided there are no side effects from treatment.

This remainder of this section discusses antiplatelet therapy, anticoagulation, carotid endarterectomy and carotid stenting.

# Antiplatelet Therapy

All patients with noncardioembolic cerebral ischaemia should receive antiplatelet therapy, unless contraindicated. There is considerable debate about the actual dose. The early trials studied 1200 mg/day. [95, 96] The addition of dipyridamole to aspirin was shown to be superior to aspirin alone. [97, 98] Clopidogrel was shown to be equivalent to aspirin + dipyridamole. [99]

| Current AHA/ASA Council recommendations [194] include: |
| --- |
| Patients with noncardioembolic ischemic stroke or TIA, aspirin 50 to 325 mg daily, clopidogrel 75 mg, or the combination of aspirin 25 mg and extended-release dipyridamole 200 mg twice daily |
| Patients with recent minor (NIHSS score ≤3) noncardioembolic ischemic stroke or high-risk TIA (ABCD2 score ≥4), dual antiplatelet therapy (aspirin plus clopidogrel) should be initiated early (ideally within 12–24 hours of symptom onset and at least within 7 days of onset) and continued for 21 to 90 days, followed by single antiplatelet therapy. |

Long-term combination therapy with aspirin and clopidogrel is not recommended because of an increased risk of bleeding. [101, 172] Clopidogrel-related bleeding cannot be reversed. Many patients are unable to tolerate dipyridamole because of headaches. The headache may resolve if the drug is introduced at a small dose and increased gradually, and the patient can persevere for a few days to weeks despite the headache. [102]

There is an increased risk of intracranial haemorrhage complicating head trauma with clopidogrel, not seen with aspirin. [103]

Although warfarin is often prescribed in patients with recurrent events on antiplatelet therapy, it is no more beneficial than aspirin in patients with atherosclerotic vascular disease. [104]

# Endarterectomy for Symptomatic Carotid Stenosis

The North American Symptomatic Carotid Endarterectomy Trial (NASCET) [105] and the European Carotid Surgery Trial (ECST) [106] both demonstrated significant benefit (absolute risk reduction of 17% and 14%, respectively) of carotid endarterectomy in patients with a 70% or more *symptomatic* stenosis of the internal carotid artery. The benefit for patients with symptomatic 50—69% stenosis was modest. The absolute risk reduction was only 1%. [107]

| The European Society of Vascular Surgeons (ESVS) published guidelines recommend [108]: |
| --- |
| carotid endarterectomy (CEA) in symptomatic patients with > 50% stenosis if the perioperative stroke/death rate is < 6%, preferably within two weeks of the patient's last symptoms aspirin at a dose of 75—325 mg daily, and statins are given before, during and following CEA. |

The reported complications rates of endarterectomy vary enormously from one institution to another. Hard to believe figures as low as 0% to as high as 21%. [109, 110] An acceptable complication rate for patients with symptomatic stenosis is < 6%.

| |
| --- |
| The results of treatment (in this case, endarterectomy) in the literature are irrelevant. The only relevant complication rate is that of the surgeon operating on your patient! |

# Carotid Artery Stenting
## Symptomatic extracranial internal carotid stenosis

The ESVS guidelines [108] recommend carotid artery stenting (CAS) in patients at high risk for CEA. CAS should be performed in high-volume centres with documented low perioperative stroke and death rates, and using dual antiplatelet treatment with aspirin and clopidogrel.

A 2021 Cochrane review concluded that in patients with symptomatic extracranial internal carotid artery stenosis, CAS compared to CEA is associated with a higher risk of stroke or death within 30 days of treatment and stated that CEA is still the procedure of choice. [111]

## Intracranial stenosis

Although intracranial stenting appears to be feasible, a 2009 review concluded that the widespread application of intracranial stenting outside the setting of randomised trials and in inexperienced centres was not justified. [86] Both the SAMMPRIS [112] and VISSIT [113] trials demonstrated an increased peri-procedural risk compared to aggressive medical therapy. Even though the FDA has approved the wingspan stent[9] AHA guidelines state that stenting for intracranial stenosis is investigational and of unknown utility. [207] The guidelines also advise against extracranial to intracranial bypass surgery and recommend aspirin 50-325mg/day, treatment of blood pressure and hypercholesterolaemia.

---

9   In patients 22-80 years of age who had intracranial arterial stenosis of 70-99% with two or more strokes despite medical treatment with the most recent stroke more than eight days before the procedure,

# Ischaemic stroke or TIA related to cardiac disease

The most recent guidelines were updated in 2021 [194}

## Atrial Fibrillation

The recommendations applying to both persistent and paroxysmal (intermittent) AF have changed significantly since the 1st edition and will almost certainly change in the future. Thus it is essential to consult up to date guidelines.

| AHA/ASA guidelines [194] recommend for patients with AF and an elevated $CHA_2DS_2$-VASc score: |
| --- |
| ≥2 in men and ≥3 in women, oral anticoagulation, with one of the following warfarin, dabigatran, rivaroxaban, apixaban or edoxaban. [124] |
| • DOACs such as dabigatran, rivaroxaban, apixaban, and edoxaban over warfarin in DOAC-eligible patients with AF. |
| • Warfarin in patients with AF associated with moderate-to-severe mitral stenosis. (Target INR, 2.5; range, 2.0–3.0) Warfarin requires weekly checks of the international normalisation ratio (INR) during initiation and monthly after that. |
| • Patients who are unable to take oral anticoagulants, aspirin 325 mg/day. |

In patients where anticoagulation is contraindicated and in those who have had life-threatening bleeding, the European Stroke Consortium (ESC) recommends left atrial appendage (LAA) occlusion initially combined with dual antiplatelet therapy using aspirin and clopidogrel. [173] The guidelines issued by the American Heart Association, American College of Cardiology (ACC) and the Heart Rhythm Society, on the other hand, restrict LAA occlusion to those undergoing cardiac surgery. [124]

The US Preventive Services Task Force (USPSTF) states that there is insufficient evidence to justify screening asymptomatic individuals for AF. [209] In the LOOP study [198], only 20% of patients with AF who suffered a stroke were in AF at the time of the event.[10]

## Acute Myocardial Infarction (MI) with Left Ventricular (LV) Mural Thrombus

The incidence of LV thrombus has decreased to as few as 7 per 10,000 patients [174] since the introduction of percutaneous coronary intervention (PCI).

| AMI with left ventricular thrombus |
| --- |
| • Oral anticoagulation aiming for a PT INR of 2.0–3.0. The duration of therapy has never been clearly defined. The ACC recommends three months [175], the ESC 6 months [176], whilst the ACC/AHA do not state the duration of therapy.[177] More extended periods of anticoagulation is recommended if there is persisting wall motion abnormality and or LV thrombus is detected on repeat contrast echocardiography. [178] The DOAC's have not been subjected to randomised trials but have been used in a small number of patients with "presumed efficacy". [179] |
| • Aspirin should be used concurrently for ischaemic coronary artery disease during oral anticoagulant therapy in doses up to 162 mg/day. |

---

10 Personal Communication Jesper Hastrup Svensen

# Dilated Cardiomyopathy

Anticoagulation was recommended in patients with an ejection fraction of <35%, where the embolism rate is approximately 4%. However, whilst the WATCH [180] and WARCEF [181] trials confirmed a slight advantage over aspirin, the bleeding complications outweighed the benefits. [182] Anticoagulation is recommended in patients with dilated cardiomyopathy only if associated with atrial fibrillation, prosthetic heart valves, known mural thrombus or previous thromboembolism. Low dose aspirin was beneficial in the SAVE [183] and SOLVD studies. [184]

| Dilated Cardiomyopathy with AF |
| --- |
| • Warfarin (INR, 2.0–3.0) with associated AF<br>• Low dose aspirin isolated dilated cardiomyopathy without AF |

# Valvular Heart Disease

The AHA and ACC guidelines[11] have been updated twice [137,138] since the 1st edition, again emphasizing the importance of regularly checking for updated guidelines. Anticoagulation is indicated in patients with AF and a $CHA_2DS_2$-VASc score of 2 or greater in the setting of native aortic valve disease, tricuspid valve disease, or mitral regurgitation. Isolated (no AF) mitral regurgitation, aortic and tricuspid valve disease are not an indication for anticoagulation.

| Rheumatic mitral stenosis |
| --- |
| • Whether or not AF is present, long-term warfarin therapy with a target INR of 2.5 (range, 2.0–3.0).<br>• Add aspirin if recurrent emboli on warfarin.<br>• The role of DOAC's has not been established. [139] |
| **Mitral valve prolapse** |
| • Antiplatelet therapy is not recommended in patients with MVP in the absence of cerebral ischaemia.<br>• Mitral annular calcification<br>• Antiplatelet therapy. |
| **Prosthetic heart valves** |
| Modern mechanical prosthetic heart valves.<br>• Warfarin with an INR target of 3.0 (range, 2.5–3.5)<br>• Plus aspirin 75–100 mg/day<br>DOACs should not be used in patients with mechanical prosthetic heart valves |

# Embolic Stroke of Undetermined Cause

Embolic Stroke of Undetermined Cause (ESUC) aka cryptogenic stroke accounts for 30% to 40% of ischemic stroke. [195] Two trials of anticoagulation in patients with cryptogenic stroke failed to show any benefit from rivaroxaban [196] or dabigatran [197] over aspirin. Unfortunately, these two studies did not look at just patients with high $CHADS_2$ or $CHA_2DS_2$-VASc scores.

---

11  https://www.acc.org/guidelines/hubs/valvular-heart-disease

# Management of Patients with Anticoagulation-Associated Intracranial Haemorrhage

The general principles of management that apply to the management of intracerebral haemorrhage unrelated to anticoagulation should be followed. [185] There is little scientific evidence in the literature to guide management of this situation. Temporary interruption of anticoagulation therapy seems safe for patients with intracranial haemorrhage and mechanical heart valves without previous evidence of systemic embolisation. Discontinuation for 1–2 weeks should be sufficient to observe the evolution of a parenchymal haematoma, clip or coil a ruptured aneurysm, or evacuate an acute subdural haematoma. Others have argued for a 6-month cessation of anticoagulation. Some would recommend heparin during the period of warfarin withdrawal. [117-119]

The most sensible approach would appear to be to reverse the anticoagulant immediately. Warfarin is reversed with either vitamin K or fresh frozen plasma and withhold anticoagulation for at least 10-14 days. This approach does not reverse DOAC's. Currently, the only specific reversal agent for dabigatran, idarucizumab, is widely available, while andexanet alfa, which reverses factor Xa inhibitors, was only approved in the United States in May 2018. Ciraparantag, designed to reverse all DOACs and other anticoagulants, is being investigated in clinical trials. [186]

The decision to resume anticoagulation after 3–4 weeks would depend on the underlying risk for thromboembolism. Two trials, one of apixaban the other of warfarin or a NOAC, failed to answer whether it is safe to resume anticoagulation. [199,200] Current recommendations state that patients be monitored more carefully, and the PT INR be kept at the lower end of the therapeutic range. [66] (*Note*: If the intracranial haemorrhage is SAH related to rupture of an aneurysm, the anticoagulation should not be resumed until the aneurysm is secured.) In patients with artificial heart valves, the risk of recurrent embolism is so high that anticoagulation must be recommenced, and, in patients with AF and a high $CHA_2DS_2$-VASc score, the benefits would outweigh the risks. Anticoagulation can be safely resumed in selected patients with intracerebral haemorrhage. The optimal timing of anticoagulation resumption after ICH is still unknown. [187]

The European Stroke Initiative recommends restarting warfarin after 10 to 14 days in patients with a strong indication for anticoagulation, such as a history of embolic stroke with atrial fibrillation. [188] Anticoagulation should be considered in patients with a high $CHA_2DS_2$-VASc score. The presence of cerebral amyloid angiopathy, microbleeds on gradient-echo magnetic resonance imaging or anticipated difficulty controlling the international normalised ratio argue against resumption. Many clinicians start subcutaneous heparinoids in low doses 24 to 72 hours after ICH to prevent deep vein thrombosis. [188]

As already discussed, the use of the left atrial appendage occlusion device can be considered in patients with atrial fibrillation if resumption of anticoagulation would represent a significant risk of recurrent intracerebral haemorrhage.

# References

1   *Ad hoc* committee established by the Advisory Council for the National Institute of Neurological and Communicative Disorders and Stroke, National Institutes of Health. A classification and outline of cerebrovascular diseases. II. *Stroke* 1975;6(5):564–616.

2   Brazzelli M, Chappell FM, Miranda H, et al. Diffusion-weighted imaging and diagnosis of transient ischemic attack. *Ann Neurol* 2014; **75**(1): 67-76.

3   Kidwell CS, et al. Diffusion MRI in patients with transient ischemic attacks. *Stroke* 1999;30(6):1174–1180.

4   Purroy F, et al. Higher risk of further vascular events among transient ischemic attack patients with diffusion-weighted imaging acute ischemic lesions. *Stroke* 2004;35(10):2313–2319.

5   Easton JD, et al. Definition and evaluation of transient ischemic attack: A scientific statement for healthcare professionals from the American Heart Association/American Stroke Association Stroke Council; Council on Cardiovascular Surgery and Anesthesia; Council on Cardiovascular Radiology and Intervention; Council on Cardiovascular Nursing; and the Interdisciplinary Council on Peripheral Vascular Disease. The American Academy of Neurology affirms the value of this statement as an educational tool for neurologists. *Stroke* 2009;40(6):2276–2293.

6   Albers GW, et al. Transient ischemic attack — proposal for a new definition. *N Engl J Med* 2002;347(21):1713–1716.

7   Rothwell PM, et al. Effect of urgent treatment of transient ischaemic attack and minor stroke on early recurrent stroke (EXPRESS study): A prospective population-based sequential comparison. *Lancet* 2007;370(9596):1432–1442.

8   Rothwell PM, Warlow CP. Timing of TIAs preceding stroke: Time window for prevention is very short. *Neurology* 2005;64(5):817–820.

9   Lovett JK, Coull AJ, Rothwell PM. Early risk of recurrence by subtype of ischemic stroke in population-based incidence studies. *Neurology* 2004;62(4):569–573.

10  Rothrock JF, et al. 'Crescendo' transient ischemic attacks: Clinical and angiographic correlations. *Neurology* 1988;38(2):198–201.

11  Coull AJ, Lovett JK, Rothwell PM. Population based study of early risk of stroke after transient ischaemic attack or minor stroke. Implications for public education and organisation of services. *BMJ* 2004;328(7435):326.

12  Moncayo J, et al. Coexisting causes of ischemic stroke. *Arch Neurol* 2000;57(8):1139–1144.

13  Wang HC, et al. Risk factors for acute symptomatic cerebral infarctions after spontaneous supratentorial intra-cerebral hemorrhage. *J Neurol* 2009;256(8):1281–1287.

14  Ariesen MJ, et al. Predictors of risk of intracerebral haemorrhage in patients with a history of TIA or minor ischaemic stroke. *J Neurol Neurosurg Psychiatry* 2006;77(1):92–94.

15  Caplan LR. *Posterior circulation disease: Clinical findings, diagnosis, and management.* ;vol 1Boston: Blackwell Science; 1996.

16  Vinken PJ, Bruyn GW, Klawans HL (eds). Vascular diseases: Handbook of clinical neurology, vol. 53–55. Elsevier Science Publishers; 1988.

17  Bogousslavsky J, Caplan LR. *Uncommon causes of stroke.* Cambridge: Cambridge University Press; 2001.

18  Bogousslavsky J, Caplan LR. *Stroke syndromes.* 2nd edn Cambridge: Cambridge University Press; 2001.

19  Barnett HJM, et al. *Stroke, pathophysiology, diagnosis and management.* 3rd edn New York: Churchill Livingstone; 1998.

20  Warlow CP, et al. *Stroke: A practical guide to management.* Oxford: Blackwell Science; 2001.

21  Kempster PA, Gerraty RP, Gates PC. Asymptomatic cerebral infarction in patients with chronic atrial fibrillation. *Stroke* 1988;19(8):955–957.

22  Bogousslavsky J, Van Melle G, Regli F. The Lausanne Stroke Registry: Analysis of 1,000 consecutive patients with first stroke. *Stroke* 1988;19(9):1083–1092.

23   Mohr JP, et al. The Harvard Cooperative Stroke Registry: A prospective registry. *Neurology* 1978;28(8):754–762.

24   Kucinski T, et al. Correlation of apparent diffusion coefficient and computed tomography density in acute ischemic stroke. *Stroke* 2002;33(7):1786–1791.

25   Saur D, et al. Sensitivity and interrater agreement of CT and diffusion-weighted MR imaging in hyperacute stroke. *AJNR Am J Neuroradiol* 2003;24(5):878–885.

26   Patrick D, Gates PC. Chronic subdural haematoma in the elderly. *Age Ageing* 1984;13(6):367–369.

27   Mori E, Tabuchi M, Yamadori A. Lacunar syndrome due to intracerebral hemorrhage. *Stroke* 1985;16(3):454–459.

28   Arboix A, et al. Haemorrhagic pure motor stroke. *Eur J Neurol* 2007;14(2):219–223.

29   Arboix A, et al. Clinical study of 99 patients with pure sensory stroke. *J Neurol* 2005;252(2):156–162.

30   Arboix A, et al. Clinical study of 222 patients with pure motor stroke. *J Neurol Neurosurg Psychiatry* 2001;71(2):239–242.

31   Donnan GA, et al. The capsular warning syndrome: Pathogenesis and clinical features. *Neurology* 1993;43(5):957–962.

32   Schwartz TH, Solomon RA. Perimesencephalic nonaneurysmal subarachnoid hemorrhage: Review of the literature. *Neurosurgery* 1996;39(3):433–440:discussion 440.

33   van Gijn J, Rinkel GJ. Subarachnoid haemorrhage: Diagnosis, causes and management. *Brain* 2001;124(Pt 2):249–278.

34   Sutherland GR, Auer RN. Primary intracerebral hemorrhage. *J Clin Neurosci* 2006;13(5):511–517.

35   Gates PC, et al. Primary intraventricular hemorrhage in adults. *Stroke* 1986;17:872–877.

36   Fisher CM. Lacunar strokes and infarcts: A review. *Neurology* 1982;32(8):871–876.

37   Derdeyn CP, et al. The International Subarachnoid Aneurysm Trial (ISAT): A position statement from the Executive Committee of the American Society of Interventional and Therapeutic Neuroradiology and the American Society of Neuroradiology. *Am J Neuroradiol* 2003;24(7):1404–1408.

38   Broderick J, et al. Guidelines for the management of spontaneous intracerebral hemorrhage in adults: 2007 update: A guideline from the American Heart Association/American Stroke Association Stroke Council, High Blood Pressure Research Council, and the Quality of Care and Outcomes in Research Interdisciplinary Working Group. *Stroke* 2007;38(6):2001–2023.

39   Rincon F, Mayer SA. Clinical review: Critical care management of spontaneous intracerebral hemorrhage. *Crit Care* 2008;12(6):237.

40   Qureshi AI, Mendelow AD, Hanley DF. Intracerebral haemorrhage. *Lancet* 2009;373(9675):1632–1644.

41   Misra UK, et al. Mannitol in intracerebral hemorrhage: A randomised controlled study. *J Neurol Sci* 2005;234:41–45.

42   Elijovich L, Patel PV, Hemphill 3rd JC. Intracerebral hemorrhage. *Semin Neurol* 2008;28(5):657–667.

43   Arboix A, et al. Clinical study of 39 patients with atypical lacunar syndrome. *J Neurol Neurosurg Psychiatry* 2006;77(3):381–384.

44   Gates PC, Barnett HJM, Silver MD. Cardiogenic Stroke. *Stroke: pathophysiology, diagnosis and management*. New York: Churchill Livingstone; 1986. p. 1085–1110.

45   Lechat P, et al. Prevalence of patent foramen ovale in patients with stroke. *N Engl J Med* 1988;318(18):1148–1152.

46   Mas JL, et al. Recurrent cerebrovascular events associated with patent foramen ovale, atrial septal aneurysm, or both. *N Engl J Med* 2001;345(24):1740–1746.

47   Srivastava TN, Payment MF. Images in clinical medicine: Paradoxical embolism—thrombus in transit through a patent foramen ovale. *N Engl J Med* 1997;337(10):681.

48   Guercini F, et al. Cryptogenic stroke: Time to determine aetiology. *J Thromb Haemost* 2008;6(4):549–554.

49   Elijovich L, et al. Intermittent atrial fibrillation may account for a large proportion of otherwise cryptogenic stroke: A study of 30-day cardiac event monitors. *J Stroke Cerebrovasc Dis* 2009;18(3):185–189.

50    Kase CS, et al. Cerebellar infarction. Clinical and anatomic observations in 66 cases. *Stroke* 1993;24(1):76–83.

51    Kim JS. Pure lateral medullary infarction: Clinical-radiological correlation of 130 acute, consecutive patients. *Brain* 2003;126(Pt 8):1864–1872.

52    European Carotid Surgery Trialists' Collaborative Group. MRC European Carotid Surgery Trial: Interim results for symptomatic patients with severe (70–99%) or with mild (0–29%) carotid stenosis. *Lancet* 1991;337(8752):1235–1243.

53    North American Symptomatic Carotid Endarterectomy Trial Collaborators. Beneficial effect of carotid endarterectomy in symptomatic patients with high-grade carotid stenosis. *N Engl J Med* 1991;325(7):445–453.

54    Fairhead JF, Mehta Z, Rothwell PM. Population-based study of delays in carotid imaging and surgery and the risk of recurrent stroke. *Neurology* 2005;65(3):371–375.

55    Kastrup A, et al. Risk factors for early recurrent cerebral ischemia before treatment of symptomatic carotid stenosis. *Stroke* 2006;37(12):3032–3034.

56    Harrison MJ, Marshall J. Indications for angiography and surgery in carotid artery disease. *BMJ* 1975;1(5958):616–618.

57    Harrison MJ, Marshall J, Thomas DJ. Relevance of duration of transient ischaemic attacks in carotid territory. *BMJ* 1978;1(6127):1578–1579.

58    Harrison MJ, Iansek R, Marshall J. Clinical identification of TIAs due to carotid stenosis. *Stroke* 1986;17(3):391–392.

59    Mast H, et al. Cigarette smoking as a determinant of high-grade carotid artery stenosis in Hispanic, black, and white patients with stroke or transient ischemic attack. *Stroke* 1998;29(5):908–912.

60    Voetsch B, et al. Basilar artery occlusive disease in the New England Medical Center Posterior Circulation Registry. *Arch Neurol* 2004;61(4):496–504.

61    West TE, Davies RJ, Kelly RE. Horner's syndrome and headache due to carotid artery disease. *BMJ* 1976;1(6013):818–820.

62    Nebelsieck J, et al. Sensitivity of neurovascular ultrasound for the detection of spontaneous cervical artery dissection. *J Clin Neurosci* 2009;16(1):79–82.

63    Malek AM, et al. Endovascular management of extracranial carotid artery dissection achieved using stent angioplasty. *Am J Neuroradiol* 2000;21(7):1280–1292.

64    Muller BT, et al. Surgical treatment of 50 carotid dissections: Indications and results. *J Vasc Surg* 2000;31(5):980–988.

65    Homma S, et al. Effect of medical treatment in stroke patients with patent foramen ovale: Patent foramen ovale in Cryptogenic Stroke Study. *Circulation* 2002;105(22):2625–2631.

66    Sacco RL, et al. Guidelines for prevention of stroke in patients with ischemic stroke or transient ischemic attack: A statement for healthcare professionals from the American Heart Association/American Stroke Association Council on Stroke: Co-sponsored by the Council on Cardiovascular Radiology and Intervention: The American Academy of Neurology affirms the value of this guideline. *Circulation* 2006;113(10):e409–e449.

67    Wassermann A, Neisser A, Bruck C. Eine serodiagnostische Reaction bei Syphilis [German]. *Dtsch Med Wochenschr* 1906;32:745–746.

68    The Antiphospholipid Antibodies in Stroke Study (APASS) Group. Anticardiolipin antibodies are an independent risk factor for first ischemic stroke. *Neurology* 1993;43(10):2069–2073.

69    Cervera R, et al. Morbidity and mortality in the antiphospholipid syndrome during a 5-year period: A multicentre prospective study of 1000 patients. *Ann Rheum Dis* 2009;68(9):1428–1432.

70    Levine SR, et al. Recurrent stroke and thrombo-occlusive events in the antiphospholipid syndrome. *Ann Neurol* 1995;38(1):119–124.

71    Lim W, Crowther MA, Eikelboom JW. Management of antiphospholipid antibody syndrome: A systematic review. *JAMA* 2006;295(9):1050–1057.

72  Adams Jr. HP, et al. Guidelines for the early management of adults with ischemic stroke: A guideline from the American Heart Association/American Stroke Association Stroke Council, Clinical Cardiology Council, Cardiovascular Radiology and Intervention Council, and the Atherosclerotic Peripheral Vascular Disease and Quality of Care Outcomes in Research Interdisciplinary Working Groups: The American Academy of Neurology affirms the value of this guideline as an educational tool for neurologists. *Stroke* 2007;38(5):1655–1711.

73  Jahromi AS, et al. Sensitivity and specificity of color duplex ultrasound measurement in the estimation of internal carotid artery stenosis: A systematic review and meta-analysis. *J Vasc Surg* 2005;41(6):962–972.

74  Morris JG, Duffis EJ, Fisher M. Cardiac workup of ischemic stroke: Can we improve our diagnostic yield?. *Stroke* 2009;40(8):2893–2898.

75  Vivanco Hidalgo RM, et al. Cardiac monitoring in stroke units: Importance of diagnosing atrial fibrillation in acute ischemic stroke. *Rev Esp Cardiol* 2009;62(5):564–567.

76  Suissa L, et al. Score for the targeting of atrial fibrillation (STAF): A new approach to the detection of atrial fibrillation in the secondary prevention of ischemic stroke. *Stroke* 2009;40(8):2866–2868.

77  Perry L, Hamilton S, Williams J. Formal dysphagia screening protocols prevent pneumonia. *Stroke* 2006;37(3):765.

78  Hinchey JA, et al. Formal dysphagia screening protocols prevent pneumonia. *Stroke* 2005;36(9):1972–1976.

79  The National Institute of Neurological Disorders and Stroke rt-PA Stroke Study Group. Tissue plasminogen activator for acute ischemic stroke. *N Engl J Med* 1995;333(24):1581–1587.

80  Clark WM, et al. Recombinant tissue-type plasminogen activator (Alteplase) for ischemic stroke 3 to 5 hours after symptom onset. The ATLANTIS Study: A randomised controlled trial. Alteplase Thrombolysis for Acute Noninterventional Therapy in Ischemic Stroke. *JAMA* 1999;282(21):2019–2026.

81  Del Zoppo GJ, et al. Expansion of the time window for treatment of acute ischemic stroke with intravenous tissue plasminogen activator: A Science Advisory from the American Heart Association/American Stroke Association. *Stroke* 2009;40(8):2945–2948.

82  Hacke W, et al. Thrombolysis with alteplase 3 to 4.5 hours after acute ischemic stroke. *N Engl J Med* 2008;359(13):1317–1329.

83  Wahlgren N, et al. Thrombolysis with alteplase for acute ischaemic stroke in the Safe Implementation of Thrombolysis in Stroke-Monitoring Study (SITS-MOST): An observational study. *Lancet* 2007;369(9558):275–282.

84  Smith WS, et al. Safety and efficacy of mechanical embolectomy in acute ischemic stroke: Results of the MERCI trial. *Stroke* 2005;36(7):1432–1438.

85  Smith WS, et al. Mechanical thrombectomy for acute ischemic stroke: Final results of the Multi MERCI trial. *Stroke* 2008;39(4):1205–1212.

86  Groschel K, et al. A systematic review on outcome after stenting for intracranial atherosclerosis. *Stroke* 2009;40(5):e340–e347.

87  IMS II Trial Investigators. The Interventional Management of Stroke (IMS) II Study. *Stroke* 2007;38(7):2127–2135.

88  International Stroke Trial Collaborative Group. The International Stroke Trial (IST): A randomised trial of aspirin, subcutaneous heparin, both, or neither among 19435 patients with acute ischaemic stroke. *Lancet* 1997;349(9065):1569–1581.

89  CAST (Chinese Acute Stroke Trial) Collaborative Group. CAST: Randomised placebo-controlled trial of early aspirin use in 20,000 patients with acute ischaemic stroke. *Lancet* 1997;349(9066):1641–1649.

90  Sandercock PA, et al. Antiplatelet therapy for acute ischaemic stroke. *Cochrane Database Syst Rev* 2008(3):CD000029.

91  Gubitz G, Sandercock P, Counsell C. Anticoagulants for acute ischaemic stroke. *Cochrane Database Syst Rev* 2004(3):CD000024.

92  Chandratheva A, et al. Population-based study of risk and predictors of stroke in the first few hours after a TIA. *Neurology* 2009;72(22):1941–1947.

93 Johnston SC, et al. Validation and refinement of scores to predict very early stroke risk after transient ischaemic attack. *Lancet* 2007;369(9558):283–292.

94 Amarenco P, et al. Does ABCD2 score below 4 allow more time to evaluate patients with a transient ischemic attack?. *Stroke* 2009;40(9):3091–3095.

95 Bousser MG, et al. "AICLA" controlled trial of aspirin and dipyridamole in the secondary prevention of athero-thrombotic cerebral ischemia. *Stroke* 1983;14(1):5–14.

96 The Canadian Cooperative Study Group. A randomised trial of aspirin and sulfinpyrazone in threatened stroke. *N Engl J Med* 1978;299(2):53–59.

97 Diener HC, et al. European Stroke Prevention Study. 2: Dipyridamole and acetylsalicylic acid in the secondary prevention of stroke. *J Neurol Sci* 1996;143(1–2):1–13.

98 The ESPS Group. The European Stroke Prevention Study (ESPS). Principal end-points. *Lancet* 1987;2(8572):1351–1354.

99 Diener HC, et al. Effects of aspirin plus extended-release dipyridamole versus clopidogrel and telmisartan on disability and cognitive function after recurrent stroke in patients with ischaemic stroke in the Prevention Regimen for Effectively Avoiding Second Strokes (PRoFESS) trial: A double-blind, active and placebo-controlled study. *Lancet Neurol* 2008;7(10):875–884.

100 CAPRIE Steering Committee. A randomised, blinded, trial of clopidogrel versus aspirin in patients at risk of ischaemic events (CAPRIE). *Lancet* 1996;348(9038):1329–1339.

101 Diener HC, et al. Aspirin and clopidogrel compared with clopidogrel alone after recent ischaemic stroke or transient ischaemic attack in high-risk patients (MATCH): Randomised, double-blind, placebo-controlled trial. *Lancet* 2004;364(9431):331–337.

102 Theis JG, Deichsel G, Marshall S. Rapid development of tolerance to dipyridamole-associated headaches. *Br J Clin Pharmacol* 1999;48(5):750–755.

103 Wong DK, Lurie F, Wong LL. The effects of clopidogrel on elderly traumatic brain injured patients. *J Trauma* 2008;65(6):1303–1308.

104 Sacco RL, et al. Comparison of warfarin versus aspirin for the prevention of recurrent stroke or death: Subgroup analyses from the Warfarin-Aspirin Recurrent Stroke Study. *Cerebrovasc Dis* 2006;22(1):4–12.

105 North American Symptomatic Carotid Endarterectomy Trial Collaborators. Beneficial effect of carotid endarterectomy in symptomatic patients with high-grade carotid stenosis. *N Engl J Med* 1991;325(7):445–453.

106 European Carotid Surgery Trialists' Collaborative Group. MRC European Carotid Surgery Trial: Iinterim results for symptomatic patients with severe (70–99%) or with mild (0–29%) carotid stenosis. *Lancet* 1991;337(8752):1235–1243.

107 Chaturvedi S, et al. Carotid endarterectomy – an evidence-based review: Report of the Therapeutics and Technology Assessment Subcommittee of the American Academy of Neurology. *Neurology* 2005;65(6):794–801.

108 Liapis CD, et al. ESVS guidelines. Invasive treatment for carotid stenosis: Indications, techniques. *Eur J Vasc Endovasc Surg* 2009;37(4 Suppl):1–19.

109 Fode NC, et al. Multicenter retrospective review of results and complications of carotid endarterectomy in 1981. *Stroke* 1986;17(3):370–376.

110 Brott T, Thalinger K. The practice of carotid endarterectomy in a large metropolitan area. *Stroke* 1984;15(6):950–955.

111 Müller MD, Lyrer PA, Brown MM, Bonati LH. Carotid Artery Stenting Versus Endarterectomy for Treatment of Carotid Artery Stenosis. *Stroke* 2021; 52(1): e3-e5.

112 Chimowitz MI, Lynn MJ, Derdeyn CP, et al. Stenting versus aggressive medical therapy for intracranial arterial stenosis. *N Engl J Med* 2011; 365(11): 993-1003.

113 Zaidat OO, Fitzsimmons BF, Woodward BK, et al. Effect of a balloon-expandable intracranial stent vs medical therapy on risk of stroke in patients with symptomatic intracranial stenosis: the VISSIT randomized clinical trial. *Jama* 2015; 313(12): 1240-8.

114  Wacher K, et al. Carotid endarterectomy deemed safer than stenting. *World Neurology* 2010;25(1):15.

115  Saxena A, Ng EYK, Lim ST. Imaging modalities to diagnose carotid artery stenosis: progress and prospect. *Biomed Eng Online* 2019; 18(1): 66.

116  Demeestere J, Wouters A, Christensen S, Lemmens R, Lansberg MG. Review of Perfusion Imaging in Acute Ischemic Stroke. *Stroke* 2020; 51(3): 1017-24.206

117  Wijdicks EF, et al. The dilemma of discontinuation of anticoagulation therapy for patients with intracranial hemorrhage and mechanical heart valves. *Neurosurgery* 1998;42(4):769–773.

118  Ananthasubramaniam K, et al. How safely and for how long can warfarin therapy be withheld in prosthetic heart valve patients hospitalised with a major hemorrhage?. *Chest* 2001;119(2):478–484.

19   Bertram M, et al. Managing the therapeutic dilemma: Patients with spontaneous intracerebral hemorrhage and urgent need for anticoagulation. *J Neurol* 2000;247(3):209–214.

120  Lip GY, Nieuwlaat R, Pisters R, Lane DA, Crijns HJ. Refining clinical risk stratification for predicting stroke and thromboembolism in atrial fibrillation using a novel risk factor-based approach: the euro heart survey on atrial fibrillation. *Chest* 2010; 137(2): 263-72.

121  Friberg L, Rosenqvist M, Lip GY. Evaluation of risk stratification schemes for ischaemic stroke and bleeding in 182 678 patients with atrial fibrillation: the Swedish Atrial Fibrillation cohort study. *Eur Heart J* 2012; 33(12): 1500-10.

122  Patel P, Pandya J, Goldberg M. NOACs vs. Warfarin for Stroke Prevention in Nonvalvular Atrial Fibrillation. *Cureus* 2017; 9(6): e1395.

123  Salazar CA, del Aguila D, Cordova EG. Direct thrombin inhibitors versus vitamin K antagonists for preventing cerebral or systemic embolism in people with non-valvular atrial fibrillation. *Cochrane Database of Systematic Reviews* 2014; (3).

124  January CT, Wann LS, Calkins H, et al. 2019 AHA/ACC/HRS Focused Update of the 2014 AHA/ACC/HRS Guideline for the Management of Patients with Atrial Fibrillation: A Report of the American College of Cardiology/American Heart Association Task Force on Clinical Practice Guidelines and the Heart Rhythm Society in Collaboration with the Society of Thoracic Surgeons. *Circulation* 2019; 140(2): e125-e51.

125  Pisters R, Lane DA, Nieuwlaat R, de Vos CB, Crijns HJ, Lip GY. A novel user-friendly score (HAS-BLED) to assess 1-year risk of major bleeding in patients with atrial fibrillation: the Euro Heart Survey. *Chest* 2010; 138(5): 1093-100.

126  Lip GY, Nieuwlaat R, Pisters R, Lane DA, Crijns HJ. Refining clinical risk stratification for predicting stroke and thromboembolism in atrial fibrillation using a novel risk factor-based approach: the euro heart survey on atrial fibrillation. *Chest* 2010; 137(2): 263-72.

127  Udayachalerm S, Rattanasiri S, Angkananard T, Attia J, Sansanayudh N, Thakkinstian A. The Reversal of Bleeding Caused by New Oral Anticoagulants (NOACs): A Systematic Review and Meta-Analysis. *Clin Appl Thromb Hemost* 2018; 24(9_suppl): 117s-26s.

128  Farb A, Ibrahim NG, Zuckerman BD. Patent Foramen Ovale after Cryptogenic Stroke — Assessing the Evidence for Closure. *New England Journal of Medicine* 2017; 377(11): 1006-9.

129  Saver JL, Carroll JD, Thaler DE, et al. Long-Term Outcomes of Patent Foramen Ovale Closure or Medical Therapy after Stroke. *New England Journal of Medicine* 2017; **377**(11): 1022-32.

130  Mas J-L, Derumeaux G, Guillon B, et al. Patent Foramen Ovale Closure or Anticoagulation vs. Antiplatelets after Stroke. *New England Journal of Medicine* 2017; 377(11): 1011-21.

131  Sondergaard L, Kasner SE, Rhodes JF, et al. Patent Foramen Ovale Closure or Antiplatelet Therapy for Cryptogenic Stroke. *N Engl J Med* 2017; 377(11): 1033-42.

132  Meier B, Kalesan B, Mattle HP, et al. Percutaneous Closure of Patent Foramen Ovale in Cryptogenic Embolism. *New England Journal of Medicine* 2013; 368(12): 1083-91.

133  Mas JL, Derumeaux G, Guillon B, et al. Patent Foramen Ovale Closure or Anticoagulation vs. Antiplatelets after Stroke. *N Engl J Med* 2017; 377(11): 1011-21.

134  Crisostomo RA, Garcia MM, Tong DC. Detection of Diffusion-Weighted MRI Abnormalities in Patients with Transient Ischemic Attack. *Stroke* 2003; **34**(4): 932-7.

135 Caplan LR. Dissections of brain-supplying arteries. *Nat Clin Pract Neurol* 2008; 4(1): 34-42.

136 Khan F, Tritschler T, Kimpton M, et al. Long-Term Risk for Major Bleeding During Extended Oral Anticoagulant Therapy for First Unprovoked Venous Thromboembolism : A Systematic Review and Meta-analysis. *Ann Intern Med* 2021; 174(10):1420-1429

137 Nishimura RA, Otto CM, Bonow RO, et al. 2014 AHA/ACC guideline for the management of patients with valvular heart disease: a report of the American College of Cardiology/American Heart Association Task Force on Practice Guidelines. *J Thorac Cardiovasc Surg* 2014; 148(1): e1-e132.

138 Nishimura RA, Otto CM, Bonow RO, et al. 2017 AHA/ACC Focused Update of the 2014 AHA/ACC Guideline for the Management of Patients with Valvular Heart Disease: A Report of the American College of Cardiology/American Heart Association Task Force on Clinical Practice Guidelines. *J Am Coll Cardiol* 2017; 70(2): 252-89.

139 Owens RE, Kabra R, Oliphant CS. Direct oral anticoagulant use in nonvalvular atrial fibrillation with valvular heart disease: a systematic review. *Clin Cardiol* 2017; 40(6): 407-12.

140 Powers WJ, Derdeyn CP, Biller J, et al. 2015 American Heart Association/American Stroke Association Focused Update of the 2013 Guidelines for the Early Management of Patients with Acute Ischemic Stroke Regarding Endovascular Treatment: A Guideline for Healthcare Professionals from the American Heart Association/American Stroke Association. *Stroke* 2015; 46(10): 3020-35.

141 Powers WJ, Rabinstein AA, Ackerson T, et al. 2018 Guidelines for the Early Management of Patients with Acute Ischemic Stroke: A Guideline for Healthcare Professionals from the American Heart Association/American Stroke Association. *Stroke* 2018; 49(3): e46-e110.

142 Powers WJ, Rabinstein AA, Ackerson T, et al. Guidelines for the Early Management of Patients with Acute Ischemic Stroke: 2019 Update to the 2018 Guidelines for the Early Management of Acute Ischemic Stroke: A Guideline for Healthcare Professionals from the American Heart Association/ American Stroke Association. *Stroke* 2019; 50(12): e344-e418.

143 Turc G, Bhogal P, Fischer U, et al. European Stroke Organisation (ESO) - European Society for Minimally Invasive Neurological Therapy (ESMINT) Guidelines on Mechanical Thrombectomy in Acute Ischemic Stroke. *Journal of NeuroInterventional Surgery* 2019: neurintsurg-2018-014569.

144 Jauch EC, Saver JL, Adams HP, Jr., et al. Guidelines for the early management of patients with acute ischemic stroke: a guideline for healthcare professionals from the American Heart Association/ American Stroke Association. *Stroke* 2013; 44(3): 870-947.

145 Quinn TJ, Dawson J, Walters MR, Lees KR. Functional outcome measures in contemporary stroke trials. *Int J Stroke* 2009; 4(3): 200-5.

146 Pexman JH, Barber PA, Hill MD, et al. Use of the Alberta Stroke Program Early CT Score (ASPECTS) for assessing CT scans in patients with acute stroke. *AJNR Am J Neuroradiol* 2001; 22(8): 1534-42.

147 Barber PA, Demchuk AM, Zhang J, Buchan AM. Validity and reliability of a quantitative computed tomography score in predicting outcome of hyperacute stroke before thrombolytic therapy. ASPECTS Study Group. Alberta Stroke Programme Early CT Score. *Lancet* 2000; 355(9216): 1670-4.

148 Nagel S, Sinha D, Day D, et al. e-ASPECTS software is non-inferior to neuroradiologists in applying the ASPECT score to computed tomography scans of acute ischemic stroke patients. *Int J Stroke* 2017; 12(6): 615-22.

149 Christensen AF, Christensen H. Editorial: Imaging in Acute Stroke—New Options and State of the Art. *Frontiers in Neurology* 2018; 8(736).

150 Ruiz-Irastorza G, Crowther M, Branch W, Khamashta MA. Antiphospholipid syndrome. *Lancet* 2010; 376(9751): 1498-509.

151 Ruiz-Irastorza G, Cuadrado MJ, Ruiz-Arruza I, et al. Evidence-based recommendations for the prevention and long-term management of thrombosis in antiphospholipid antibody-positive patients: report of a task force at the 13th International Congress on antiphospholipid antibodies. *Lupus* 2011; 20(2): 206-18.

152 Urbanus RT, Siegerink B, Roest M, Rosendaal FR, de Groot PG, Algra A. Antiphospholipid antibodies and risk of myocardial infarction and ischaemic stroke in young women in the RATIO study: a case-control study. *Lancet Neurol* 2009; 8(11): 998-1005.

153 Hurford R, Li L, Lovett N, et al. Prognostic value of "tissue-based" definitions of TIA and minor stroke. *Neurology* 2019; 92(21): e2455.

154 Challa VR, Moody DM, Bell MA. The Charcot-Bouchard aneurysm controversy: impact of a new histologic technique. *J Neuropathol Exp Neurol* 1992; 51(3): 264-71.

155 Andrade D, Cervera R, Cohen H, et al. 15th International Congress on Antiphospholipid Antibodies Task Force on Antiphospholipid Syndrome Treatment Trends Report. In: Erkan D, Lockshin MD, eds. Antiphospholipid Syndrome: Current Research Highlights and Clinical Insights. Cham: Springer International Publishing; 2017: 317-38.

156 Yang CW, Carr JC, Futterer SF, et al. Contrast-Enhanced MR Angiography of the Carotid and Vertebrobasilar Circulations. *American Journal of Neuroradiology* 2005; 26(8): 2095.

157 Perez MV, Mahaffey KW, Hedlin H, et al. Large-Scale Assessment of a Smartwatch to Identify Atrial Fibrillation. *New England Journal of Medicine* 2019; 381(20): 1909-17.

158 Dörr M, Nohturfft V, Brasier N, et al. The WATCH AF Trial: SmartWATCHes for Detection of Atrial Fibrillation. *JACC: Clinical Electrophysiology* 2019; 5(2): 199-208.

159 Turakhia MP, Ullal AJ, Hoang DD, et al. Feasibility of Extended Ambulatory Electrocardiogram Monitoring to Identify Silent Atrial Fibrillation in High-risk Patients: The Screening Study for Undiagnosed Atrial Fibrillation (STUDY-AF). *Clinical cardiology* 2015; 38(5): 285-92.

160 Tsivgoulis G, Katsanos AH, Kohrmann M, et al. Duration of Implantable Cardiac Monitoring and Detection of Atrial Fibrillation in Ischemic Stroke Patients: A Systematic Review and Meta-Analysis. *J Stroke* 2019; 21(3): 302-11.

161 Hindricks G, Pokushalov E, Urban L, et al. Performance of a New Leadless Implantable Cardiac Monitor in Detecting and Quantifying Atrial Fibrillation Results of the XPECT Trial. *Circulation: Arrhythmia and Electrophysiology* 2010; 3(2): 141-7.

162 Bettin M, Dechering D, Kochhauser S, et al. Extended ECG monitoring with an implantable loop recorder in patients with cryptogenic stroke: time schedule, reasons for explantation and incidental findings (results from the TRACK-AF trial). *Clin Res Cardiol* 2019; 108(3): 309-14.

163 Gorenek BC, Bax J, Boriani G, et al. Device-detected subclinical atrial tachyarrhythmias: definition, implications, and management-an European Heart Rhythm Association (EHRA) consensus document, endorsed by Heart Rhythm Society (HRS), Asia Pacific Heart Rhythm Society (APHRS) and Sociedad Latinoamericana de Estimulacion Cardiaca y Electrofisiologia (SOLEACE). *Europace* 2017; 19(9): 1556-78.

164 Johnston SC, Easton JD, Farrant M, et al. Clopidogrel and Aspirin in Acute Ischemic Stroke and High-Risk TIA. *New England Journal of Medicine* 2018; 379(3): 215-25.

165 Bath PM, Woodhouse LJ, Appleton JP, et al. Antiplatelet therapy with aspirin, clopidogrel, and dipyridamole versus clopidogrel alone or aspirin and dipyridamole in patients with acute cerebral ischaemia (TARDIS): a randomised, open-label, phase 3 superiority trial. *Lancet* 2018; 391(10123): 850-9.

166 Mas J-L, Derumeaux G, Guillon B, et al. Patent Foramen Ovale Closure or Anticoagulation vs. Antiplatelets after Stroke. *New England Journal of Medicine* 2017; 377(11): 1011-21.

167 Anderson CS, Arima H, Lavados P, et al. Cluster-Randomized, Crossover Trial of Head Positioning in Acute Stroke. *N Engl J Med* 2017; 376(25): 2437-47.

168 Smith EE, Kent DM, Bulsara KR, et al. Effect of Dysphagia Screening Strategies on Clinical Outcomes After Stroke: A Systematic Review for the 2018 Guidelines for the Early Management of Patients with Acute Ischemic Stroke. *Stroke* 2018; 49(3): e123-e8.

169 Whelton PK, Carey RM, Aronow WS, et al. 2017 ACC/AHA/AAPA/ABC/ACPM/AGS/APhA/ASH/ASPC/NMA/PCNA Guideline for the Prevention, Detection, Evaluation, and Management of High Blood Pressure in Adults: Executive Summary. *A Report of the American College of Cardiology/American Heart Association Task Force on Clinical Practice Guidelines* 2018; 71(19): 2199-269.

170 Ihm SH, Bakris G, Sakuma I, Sohn IS, Koh KK. Controversies in the 2017 ACC/AHA Hypertension Guidelines: Who Can Be Eligible for Treatments Under the New Guidelines?- An Asian Perspective. *Circ J* 2019; 83(3): 504-10.

171 Cloutier L, Daskalopoulou SS, Padwal RS, et al. A New Algorithm for the Diagnosis of Hypertension in Canada. *Can J Cardiol* 2015; 31(5): 620-30.

172 Johnston SC, Easton JD, Farrant M, et al. Clopidogrel and Aspirin in Acute Ischemic Stroke and High-Risk TIA. *N Engl J Med* 2018; 379(3): 215-25.

173 Kirchhof P, Benussi S, Kotecha D, et al. 2016 ESC Guidelines for the management of atrial fibrillation developed in collaboration with EACTS. *Eur Heart J* 2016; 37(38): 2893-962.

174 Lee JM, Park JJ, Jung HW, et al. Left ventricular thrombus and subsequent thromboembolism, comparison of anticoagulation, surgical removal, and antiplatelet agents. *J Atheroscler Thromb* 2013; 20(1): 73-93.

175 Guyatt GH, Akl EA, Crowther M, Gutterman DD, Schuunemann HJ. Executive summary: Antithrombotic Therapy and Prevention of Thrombosis, 9th ed: American College of Chest Physicians Evidence-Based Clinical Practice Guidelines. *Chest* 2012; 141(2 Suppl): 7s-47s.

176 Steg PG, James SK, Atar D, et al. ESC Guidelines for the management of acute myocardial infarction in patients presenting with ST-segment elevation. *Eur Heart J* 2012; 33(20): 2569-619.

177 O'Gara PT, Kushner FG, Ascheim DD, et al. 2013 ACCF/AHA guideline for the management of ST-elevation myocardial infarction: a report of the American College of Cardiology Foundation/American Heart Association Task Force on Practice Guidelines. *J Am Coll Cardiol* 2013; 61(4): e78-e140.

178 Habash F, Vallurupalli S. Challenges in management of left ventricular thrombus. *Ther Adv Cardiovasc Dis* 2017; 11(8): 203-13.

179 Kajy M, Shokr M, Ramappa P. Use of Direct Oral Anticoagulants in the Treatment of Left Ventricular Thrombus: Systematic Review of Current Literature. *Am J Ther* 2019.

180 Massie BM, Collins JF, Ammon SE, et al. Randomized trial of warfarin, aspirin, and clopidogrel in patients with chronic heart failure: the Warfarin and Antiplatelet Therapy in Chronic Heart Failure (WATCH) trial. *Circulation* 2009; 119(12): 1616-24.

181 Homma S, Thompson JL, Sanford AR, et al. Benefit of warfarin compared with aspirin in patients with heart failure in sinus rhythm: a subgroup analysis of WARCEF, a randomized controlled trial. *Circulation Heart failure* 2013; 6(5): 988-97.

182 Mischie AN, Chioncel V, Droc I, Sinescu C. Anticoagulation in patients with dilated cardiomyopathy, low ejection fraction, and sinus rhythm: back to the drawing board. *Cardiovasc Ther* 2013; 31(5): 298-302.

183 Dries DL, Rosenberg YD, Waclawiw MA, Domanski MJ. Ejection fraction and risk of thromboembolic events in patients with systolic dysfunction and sinus rhythm: evidence for gender differences in the studies of left ventricular dysfunction trials. *J Am Coll Cardiol* 1997; 29(5): 1074-80.

184 Loh E, Sutton MS, Wun CC, et al. Ventricular dysfunction and the risk of stroke after myocardial infarction. *N Engl J Med* 1997; 336(4): 251-7.

185 Cordonnier C, Demchuk A, Ziai W, Anderson CS. Intracerebral haemorrhage: current approaches to acute management. *The Lancet* 2018; 392(10154): 1257-68.

186 Crowther M, Cuker A. How can we reverse bleeding in patients on direct oral anticoagulants? *Kardiol Pol* 2019; 77(1): 3-11.

187 Li Y-G, Lip GYH. Anticoagulation Resumption After Intracerebral Hemorrhage. *Current atherosclerosis reports* 2018; 20(7): 32.

188 Steiner T, Kaste M, Forsting M, et al. Recommendations for the management of intracranial haemorrhage – part I: spontaneous intracerebral haemorrhage. The European Stroke Initiative Writing Committee and the Writing Committee for the EUSI Executive Committee. *Cerebrovasc Dis* 2006; 22(4): 294-316.

189 Merwick A, Albers GW, Amarenco P, et al. Addition of brain and carotid imaging to the ABCD² score to identify patients at early risk of stroke after transient ischaemic attack: a multicentre observational study. *Lancet Neurol* 2010; 9(11): 1060-9

190 Song B, Fang H, Zhao L, et al. Validation of the ABCD3-I score to predict stroke risk after transient ischemic attack. *Stroke* 2013; 44(5): 1244-8.

191 Knoflach M, Lang W, Seyfang L, et al. Predictive value of ABCD2 and ABCD3-I scores in TIA and minor stroke in the stroke unit setting. *Neurology* 2016; 87(9): 861-9.

192 Kiyohara T, Kamouchi M, Kumai Y, et al. ABCD3 and ABCD3-I scores are superior to ABCD2 score in the prediction of short- and long-term risks of stroke after transient ischemic attack. *Stroke* 2014; 45(2): 418-25.

193 Ildstad F, Ellekjær H, Wethal T, Lydersen S, Fjærtoft H, Indredavik B. ABCD3-I and ABCD2 Scores in a TIA Population with Low Stroke Risk. *Stroke Res Treat* 2021; 2021: 8845898.

194 Kleindorfer DO, Towfighi A, Chaturvedi S, et al. 2021 Guideline for the Prevention of Stroke in Patients with Stroke and Transient Ischemic Attack: A Guideline from the American Heart Association/American Stroke Association. *Stroke* 2021; 52(70): e364-e467.

195 Yaghi S, Bernstein RA, Passman R, Okin PM, Furie KL. Cryptogenic Stroke. *Circulation Research* 2017; 120(3): 527-40.

196 Hart RG, Sharma M, Mundl H, et al. Rivaroxaban for Stroke Prevention after Embolic Stroke of Undetermined Source. *N Engl J Med* 2018; 378(23): 2191-201.

197 Diener H-C, Sacco RL, Easton JD, et al. Dabigatran for Prevention of Stroke after Embolic Stroke of Undetermined Source. *New England Journal of Medicine* 2019; 380(20): 1906-17.

198 Svendsen JH, Diederichsen SZ, Højberg S, et al. Implantable loop recorder detection of atrial fibrillation to prevent stroke (The LOOP Study): a randomised controlled trial. *The Lancet*.

199 Schreuder F, Van Nieuwenhuizen K, Hofmeijer J, Kerkhoff H, al. e, Investigators TA-AT. APACHE-AF: Apixaban versus antiplatelet drugs or no antithrombotic drugs after anticoagulation-associated intracerebral haemorrhage in patients with atrial fibrillation. A randomised, open-label phase II clinical trial. European Stroke Organisation Conference (ESOC) 2021. Virtual: ESOC; 2021.

200 Al-Shahi Salman R, Keerie C, Stephen J, et al. Effects of oral anticoagulation for atrial fibrillation after spontaneous intracranial haemorrhage in the UK: a randomised, open-label, assessor-masked, pilot-phase, non-inferiority trial. *The Lancet Neurology* 2021; 20(10): 842-53.

201 Molyneux A. International Subarachnoid Aneurysm Trial (ISAT) of neurosurgical clipping versus endovascular coiling in 2143 patients with ruptured intracranial aneurysms: a randomised trial. *The Lancet* 2002; 360(9342): 1267-74.

202 Allen GS, Ahn HS, Preziosi TJ, et al. Cerebral Arterial Spasm – A Controlled Trial of Nimodipine in Patients with Subarachnoid Hemorrhage. *New England Journal of Medicine* 1983; 308(11): 619-24.

203 Mendelow AD, Gregson BA, Fernandes HM, et al. Early surgery versus initial conservative treatment in patients with spontaneous supratentorial intracerebral haematomas in the International Surgical Trial in Intracerebral Haemorrhage (STICH): a randomised trial. *Lancet* 2005; 365(9457): 387-97.

204 Mendelow AD, Gregson BA, Rowan EN, Murray GD, Gholkar A, Mitchell PM. Early surgery versus initial conservative treatment in patients with spontaneous supratentorial lobar intracerebral haematomas (STICH II): a randomised trial. *Lancet* 2013; 382(9890): 397-408.

205 Caprio FZ, Bernstein RA, Alberts MJ, et al. Efficacy and safety of novel oral anticoagulants in patients with cervical artery dissections. *Cerebrovasc Dis* 2014; 38(4): 247-53.

206 Seshadri DR, Bittel B, Browsky D, et al. Accuracy of Apple Watch for Detection of Atrial Fibrillation. *Circulation* 2020; 141(8): 702-3.

207 Kernan WN, Ovbiagele B, Black HR, et al. Guidelines for the Prevention of Stroke in Patients with Stroke and Transient Ischemic Attack. *Stroke* 2014; 45(7): 2160-236.

208 Debette S, Mazighi M, Bijlenga P, et al. ESO guideline for the management of extracranial and intracranial artery dissection. *European Stroke Journal* 2021; 6(3): XXXIX-LXXXVIII.

209 US Preventive services Task Force UPST. Screening for Atrial Fibrillation: US Preventive Services Task Force Recommendation Statement. *JAMA* 2022; 327(4): 360-7.

210 Dawson, J., et al. (2021). "European Stroke Organisation expedited recommendation for the use of short-term dual antiplatelet therapy early after minor stroke and high-risk TIA." *Eur Stroke J* 6(2): Clxxxvii-cxci.

# chapter 10 Cerebrovascular Disease

# Common Neck, Arm and Upper Back Problems

Neck and arm pain and sensory disturbance with or without weakness in the arm are widespread complaints. This chapter will discuss the more frequently encountered peripheral nervous system (lower motor neuron)[1] problems and the non-neurological conditions seen in everyday clinical practice and will detail those features that help differentiate one problem from another. The chapter is divided into three sections reflecting the regions of complaints most often seen in clinical practice:

1. the neck
2. the shoulder and upper arm
3. the forearm and hand.

A few rare conditions will be discussed because a delay in diagnosis may result in long-term disability. These are suprascapular nerve entrapment, thoracic outlet syndrome, radial tunnel syndrome (posterior interosseous nerve entrapment) and complex regional pain syndrome.

There are *only four neurological symptoms* that can develop in a limb:

1. pain
2. weakness (with or without wasting)
3. altered sensation
4. incoordination.

When a patient presents complaining of problems in the arm, the critical thing to establish is whether the symptoms relate to a non-neurological or a neurological problem and if the latter, whether it is a peripheral ('lower motor neuron') or central ('upper motor neuron') problem. Remember, the peripheral nervous system in the upper limb consists of the anterior horn cell in the spinal cord, the motor and sensory nerve roots, brachial plexus, peripheral nerves, neuromuscular junctions, and muscle. A central nervous system problem is anything above the level of the anterior horn cell, i.e. in the spinal cord, brainstem, deep cerebral hemisphere, and cortex (Figure 1.1). The pattern of weakness, sensory disturbance, and reflexes will help determine whether the problem is in the central or peripheral nervous. It is also essential to establish whether the symptoms are intermittent or persistent as different conditions present with paroxysmal whilst others present with persistent symptoms. Pain in the arm is only occasionally related to the nervous system but, when it is, it almost invariably indicates a problem in the peripheral nervous system as central causes of pain are infrequent.

---

1   see chapters 1 and three for a discussion of upper versus a lower motor neuron problem.

> Most patients with pain in the arm have a non-neurological problem.
> Although there are rare central nervous system causes of pain, the great majority of patients with neurological symptoms in the arm associated with pain will have a problem in the peripheral nervous system.

Symptoms arising from peripheral nerve lesions can occur as a result of three mechanisms:

- Direct trauma, in which case the neurological symptoms +/- signs will be present from the moment of trauma
- Compression of the nerve (referred to as entrapment syndrome), where the symptoms will be persistent and, as the degree of compression worsens, the severity of the symptoms (in terms of intensity and the extent of involvement of the muscles or area of sensation supplied by the particular nerve or nerve root) will increase
- Irritation of nerves without persistent weakness or sensory loss is seen with entrapment syndromes. The symptoms are initially intermittent and often provoked by certain activities; after repeated and prolonged irritation, damage may result in persistent weakness and or sensory loss.

# Neck Pain

Although pain in the neck is common, symptoms arising in the neck are often poorly localised, and a precise diagnosis is not always possible.

## Acute Spasm of the Neck Muscles

One of the more common causes of neck pain is an acute spasm of the neck muscles. The exact cause of the spasm is uncertain, but it appears to be related to bad posture. Patients often awake with severe neck pain, with the neck twisted to one side and pain aggravated by attempts to turn the head.

The most common form is *torticollis*, often referred to as a '*wry neck*'. It is a self-limiting condition, resolving within days. More severe and disabling but rare forms of congenital and acquired spasmodic torticollis occur [1] but are beyond the scope of this book.

## Non-Specific Neck Pain

Many patients present with *non-specific neck pain* in the centre and or to the side of the neck that is constant but fluctuating in severity and present most days. The pain is usually bilateral, often associated with stiffness in the neck, and is aggravated by neck movement. In many patients, it is over the trapezius muscle. There are no associated neurological symptoms in the limbs and no sensory symptoms in the neck to suggest the pain is of nerve root origin. Occasionally, the pain radiates to the base of the skull. The trapezius and sternocleidomastoid muscles are often tense and tender to palpate, but the relationship of this finding to the neck discomfort is not clear.

The aetiology of this entity is uncertain. However, it is not uncommon in patients with psychological problems such as anxiety or depression. [2]

# Whiplash

Another common cause of neck pain is whiplash, often the result of motor vehicle collisions with sudden flexion and extension of the neck. Again, various symptoms develop, and not all patients experience all symptoms.

- Within hours, less commonly a few days after a whiplash injury, the patient complains of neck pain and stiffness, with or without a decreased range of neck motion. Tenderness on palpation of the neck muscles and even the spinal processes is common. The pain may radiate into the shoulders or down the spine to the thoracic region.
- Headache frequently occurs together with insomnia, complaints of poor memory and difficulty concentrating. [3]
- A small percentage of patients will develop non-specific and diffuse arm pain with or without subjective weakness and or sensory symptoms in the arm that are clearly beyond the distribution of a single nerve or nerve root and are thus not related to nerve root compression. In addition, unlike cervical nerve root compression, the pain and neurological symptoms in the arm are often aggravated by movement of both the arm and the neck, whilst the pain of nerve root compression may be aggravated by movement of the neck but not the arm.
- Imaging is invariably normal, although the asymptomatic degenerative disease commonly present in older patients is often incorrectly invoked to cause the symptoms.
- The duration of symptoms varies from a few weeks to months or even years (the late whiplash syndrome, a controversial entity. [4]) Pain settles within weeks in 90–95% of patients.
- The aetiology of whiplash is unknown. Curiously, it is not seen in Lithuania, with little awareness of the syndrome and no accident compensation scheme. [5, 6]

# Cervical Spondylosis

Cervical spondylosis or degenerative changes in the cervical spine is very common. It is often asymptomatic, particularly in the elderly. Although neck pain aggravated by neck movement may occur, the neck pain may not be due to spondylosis. *Therefore,* other possible causes should be considered. Cervical spondylosis is more likely to be symptomatic if neck pain is associated with pain radiating into the shoulder or arm, with or without weakness and or sensory symptoms in the nerve root distribution. Thus, it is crucial to ascertain the arm pain and sensory symptom distribution.

---

**Management of Whiplash**

This section discusses the management of minor neck injuries that result from whiplash, not the initial assessment of patients with trauma in whom cervical spine injuries could be present. The Canadian C-spine rule [8] is a decision-making tool to determine when medical imaging should be undertaken.

Imaging is not justified in patients with mild symptoms or under 65 years of age. [3] Plain X-rays, CT, or MRI scans rarely demonstrate any abnormality, even in more severe cases. Therefore, most patients with mild pain can be reassured and advised to lead a normal life without restrictions. [3]

With more severe pain, a period of abstinence from intense training and sporting activities is recommended. Simple analgesia or a non-steroidal anti-inflammatory drug (NSAID) can be prescribed. It is essential to advise patients with severe pain that recovery is very likely but may take months. In these cases, lifestyle, including work, is often restricted.

The role of physical therapy is controversial. However, the Bone and Joint Decade 2000–2010 Task Force on Neck Pain and its Associated Disorders concluded that 'best evidence suggests that treatments involving manual therapy and exercise are more effective than alternative strategies for patients with neck pain. [9]

Management of cervical nerve root compression is discussed in the section' Pain with or without focal neurological symptoms in the shoulder and upper arm'.

---

## Cervical Radiculopathy

Cervical radiculopathy arising from the 3rd and 4th cervical nerve roots is rare. Compression of the 3rd cervical nerve root causes unilateral pain in the suboccipital region, extending to the back of the ear and in the dorsal or lateral aspect of the neck. C4 radiculopathy results in unilateral pain that may radiate to the posterior neck, trapezius region, and anterior chest but does not radiate into the upper extremity. [7] Neither is associated with any weakness, but sensory symptoms in the C3 or C4 nerve root distribution can occur. When radiculopathy is associated with spinal cord compression, there will be an upper motor neuron pattern of weakness usually in all four but may just affect the lower limbs. There may be sensory symptoms with a sensory level with loss of sensation below the site of compression.

# Problems Around the Shoulder and Upper Arm

This section discusses common neurological and non-neurological conditions affecting the shoulder and upper arm that can result in pain with or without focal neurological symptoms and focal neurological symptoms in the absence of pain.

## Pain with or without Focal Neurological Symptoms in the Shoulder and Upper Arm

Several neurological and non-neurological conditions can cause pain in and around the shoulder. These include:
- nerve root compression of the 4th, 5th, and 6th cervical nerve roots
- brachial neuritis
- suprascapular nerve entrapment syndrome
- arthritis of the shoulder joint
- adhesive capsulitis
- bursitis
- rotator cuff pathology

Pain in the shoulder and upper arm most often relates to diseases of the joints, ligaments, or bones. The pain occurs in the absence of neurological symptoms and is aggravated by movement of the shoulder joint. There may be localised tenderness at the site of the pain. The presence of joint swelling and or tenderness is another clue that the pain is not of neurological origin.

Figure 11.1 lists the common causes of pain in the shoulder region.

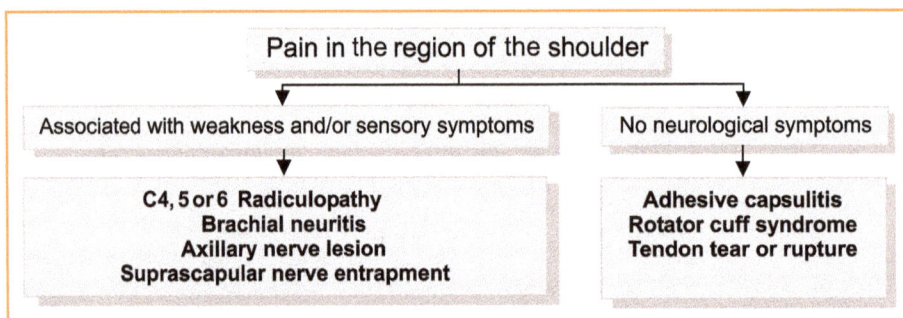

**Figure 11.1** Painful conditions affecting the shoulder region

# Neurological Causes

## Radicular Pain

Radicular pain will be in the area supplied by the nerve root and may be aggravated by moving the neck. If weakness and or sensory disturbance occur it will be in the nerve root distribution. However, pain may occur in the absence of or precede neurological symptoms by days or even weeks. Although radicular pain may affect the upper (C4–C5) arm, it is more common in the lower (C6–8) arm.

Shoulder pain not influenced by movement of the shoulder suggests a possible C5 nerve root problem. If numbness develops, it is along the mid-portion of the top of the shoulder and extends laterally to the upper arm but not into the forearm. There may be a weakness of the supraspinatus, infraspinatus, and deltoid.[7]

## Brachial Neuritis or Neuralgic Amyotrophy

Brachial neuritis or neuralgic amyotrophy are terms used to describe a syndrome of severe pain and weakness affecting the brachial plexus. Brachial neuritis can be hereditary (familial) or probable immune-mediated. The diagnosis should be suspected when severe shoulder pain aggravated by shoulder movement is associated with weakness and sensory disturbance in the arm. [10] There is no 'gold standard' diagnostic test for brachial neuritis.

---

Ascertain whether the arm pain is aggravated by movement of the arm, suggesting local pathology in the arm, or aggravated by movement of the neck, indicating possible referred pain from nerve root compression.
- Pain occurring simultaneously with neurological symptoms is of neurological origin. Arm pain may or may not be neurological in origin in the absence of neurological symptoms.
- If testing the strength of muscles around a joint evokes marked pain, this may cause the patient not to exert a full effort and give the incorrect impression that there may be a weakness when the pain actually limits the effort.

---

# Symptoms

The classic symptoms begin with the subacute onset over weeks of increasingly severe constant unilateral pain predominantly in the shoulder girdle; less commonly, the pain may come on rapidly. Rarely, bilateral cases occur, but one side is usually affected for up to 2 days before the other side is involved. [11] This constant pain persists on average for approximately 3–4 weeks but may last as little as a few days or up to 60 days or more. Movement-evoked severe stabbing pain can persist for months in many patients. In a small proportion of cases, the pain can radiate from the shoulder to the arm, the cervical spine or neck down into the arm, the scapular or dorsal region to the chest wall and or arm or be confined to a lower plexus distribution (e.g. medial arm and or hand, axilla).

The shoulder pain is aggravated by the movement of the shoulder, not the neck. Associated weakness and sensory disturbance in the arm indicates a neurological cause for the pain. Although local heat to the shoulder region occasionally relieves the pain, this is non-specific. As well as the brachial plexus, individual nerves, such as the suprascapular, axillary, musculocutaneous, long thoracic, and radial nerves, can be affected. [11]

Progressive weakness develops over days. It may commence within 24 hours or up to 4 weeks after the onset of the pain. [11] Although any part of the plexus can be involved, the upper brachial plexus is more commonly affected in males. In contrast, the middle and lower brachial plexus is more widely affected in females. Wasting may occur with prolonged symptoms. Recovery can take months or even years. Sensory involvement is common and sensory symptoms can be diffuse and non-localising.

Recurrent attacks occur in a little over a quarter of patients. Familial cases termed hereditary neuralgic amyotrophy (HNA), have been described. In North America, 55% of HNA patients have an abnormality of the SEPT9 gene.[67] Only 5% of European cases have a SEPT9 mutation. Hereditary neuropathy with pressure palsy is a distinct disorder more commonly affecting individual nerve palsies. It can mimic neuralgic amyotrophy and is related to a defect in the peripheral myelin protein 22. [12]

## Axillary Nerve Lesion

Axillary nerve lesions are usually related to traumatic dislocation of the shoulder joint due to either a sporting injury or a tonic-clonic seizure. Less commonly, they occur with a fracture of the neck of the humerus or following shoulder surgery. As with all single nerve (mononeuritis) lesions, some are idiopathic (unknown cause).

### Symptoms

Difficulty or inability to the lift arm. There may be a patch of numbness over the lower end of the deltoid.

### Examination

Weakness of shoulder abduction due to the weakness of the deltoid muscle. (Figure 11.2) Remember, the supraspinatus muscle is responsible for the initial 30° of abduction. There may be a small patch of numbness over the lower aspect of the deltoid. When the lesion relates to dislocation, there is often pain in the shoulder aggravated by movement of the shoulder. Usually, the presence of pain and weakness with a history of trauma to the shoulder is a strong pointer to the diagnosis. The prognosis for recovery is variable. [13]

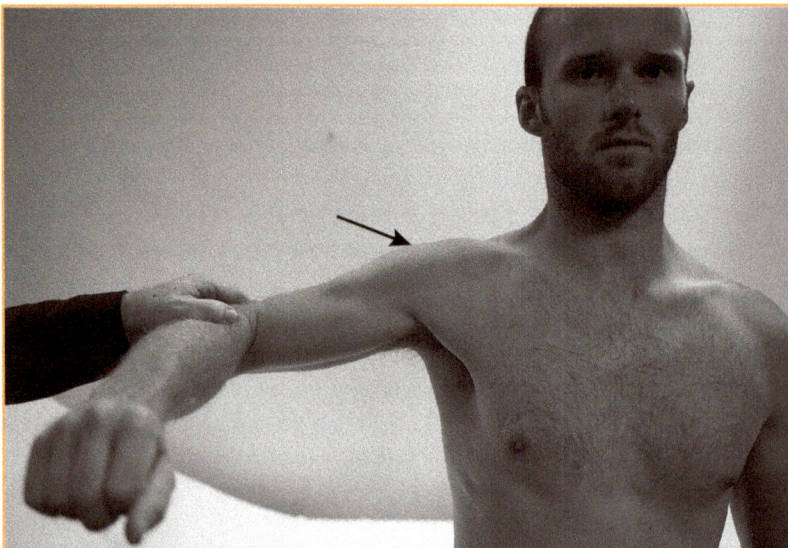

**Figure 11.2** Testing the deltoid muscle (the arrow points to the deltoid muscle, supplied by the axillary Nerve

## Suprascapular Nerve Entrapment

The suprascapular Nerve arises from the junction of the 5th and 6th cervical nerve roots. It runs an oblique course across the supraspinatus fossa, relatively fixed on its floor and tethered underneath the transverse scapular ligament. It passes through the scapular notch and supplies the supraspinatus and infraspinatus muscles. Suprascapular nerve entrapment syndrome is local compression by the suprascapular ligament. It may also be idiopathic in origin or due to rarer causes. [14] Although very rare, it is a diagnosis where it is more likely to resolve with prompt treatment.

## Symptoms

The pain is deep and diffuse, localised to the posterior and lateral aspects of the shoulder and may radiate into the arm, neck, or upper anterior chest wall. Certain scapular motions may be painful, causing the patient to restrict shoulder movement. Adduction of the arm across the body tenses the nerve and may increase the pain. Occasionally, the patient may complain of burning, aching, or crushing pain.

## Examination

Weakness is confined to the supraspinatus and infraspinatus muscles. Remember, pain may give the appearance of weakness with the patient unable to exert a full effort. The clue that the weakness relates to pain from the shoulder joint and not a suprascapular nerve entrapment is that the deltoid and subscapularis muscles will also "appear weak". Severe suprascapular nerve entrapment results in atrophy and weakness of the supraspinatus and infraspinatus muscles (Figure 11.3).

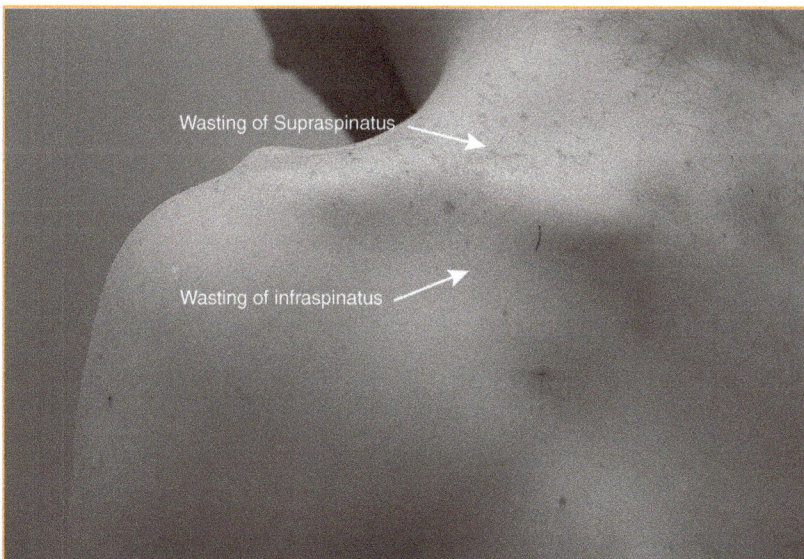

**Figure 11.3** Suprascapular nerve entrapment with marked wasting of the supraspinatus and infraspinatus muscles

**Treatment of Suprascapular Nerve Entrapment**

Confirmation of the diagnosis depends on the nerve conduction studies (NCS) and electromyography (EMG). Some authorities [15] argue that a normal EMG does not exclude the diagnosis. Others [16] state that an abnormal EMG is essential in confirming the diagnosis. A prolonged latency from stimulation at Erb's point to either the supraspinatus or infraspinatus muscle is diagnostic. Treatment is surgical decompression. [14]

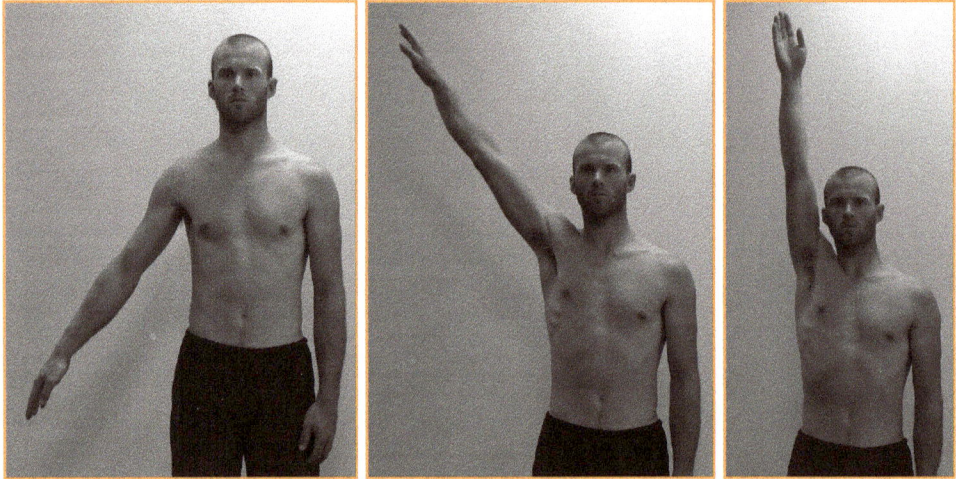

**Figure 11.4** Testing of a painful arc and the impingement test. Pain is experienced between 60° and 120° of abduction.

# Non-Neurological Causes of Shoulder Pain

The following section may seem out of place, but neurologists are often asked to see patients with pain of non-neurological origin. This section assists in differentiating neurological and non-neurological causes of pain.

Pain radiating below the elbow to the hand is unrelated to shoulder pathology. Ascertain whether the arm pain is aggravated by:
• movement of the arm, suggesting local pathology in the arm
• movement of the neck, indicating possible referred pain from nerve root compression.

## Adhesive Capsulitis

Adhesive capsulitis or 'frozen shoulder' causes pain and stiffness in the shoulder. As a result, there is a restricted range of movement at the shoulder joint. It is more common in patients over the age of 40. A full range of movement of the shoulder joint is incompatible with the diagnosis. X-rays are normal. The aetiology is unclear. It is a common complication of the inability to move the shoulder joint in patients with paralysis of the upper limb.

# Rotator Cuff Impingement Syndrome

The Rotator cuff impingement syndrome is the commonest non-neurological cause of pain affecting the shoulder joint. The rotator cuff consists of the four tendons of the teres minor, subscapularis, infraspinatus, and supraspinatus muscles. The rotator cuff is compressed against the acromion, causing bursitis, tendinitis, and eventually a rotator cuff tear. Partial or complete tears or inflammation (tendinitis, tendinosis, calcific tendinitis) associated with rotator cuff injury occur in the region where these tendon-muscle complexes attach to the humerus. [17]

# Symptoms

Symptoms are pain, initially after and then during activity. The pain is relieved by rest. Patients over 40 are more susceptible to rotator cuff tendinosis. The most prominent complaint is pain with overhead use or athletic activities. Night pain and an inability to lie on that side are common. [17] Although the pain may radiate into the arm and the neck, it is aggravated by movement of the shoulder and not the neck. Pain in the shoulder between 60° and 120° of abduction is typical of a rotator cuff problem called painful arc syndrome (Figure 11.4).

---

**Management of Rotator Cuff Syndrome**

Plain X-rays can be helpful to diagnose calcific tendinitis, acromial spur, humeral head cysts or superior migration of the humeral head, but in most cases are typically normal. Arthrography, ultrasound, CT, and MRI are the definitive tests in diagnosing rotator cuff injury. Arthrography and ultrasound of the shoulder can help determine whether or not there is a full-thickness tear in the rotator cuff. An MRI can detect a full or partial tear, chronic tendinosis, or other cause of shoulder pain. [18]

- Physiotherapy is superior to NSAIDs alone. [19] Physical therapy with stretching exercises will improve most patients, but the pain may take several months to subside. [20]
- Subacromial corticosteroid injections are recommended for non-responders [21]; however, these injections are difficult to give, and the needle is not always placed accurately. [22] In addition, corticosteroid injections may increase the subsequent risk of tendon rupture. Repeated injections are associated with a higher failure rate for surgical repair of ruptured tendons. [23] Corticosteroid injection is the preferred and definitive treatment for trochanteric bursitis. [24]
- Non-surgical management is the initial treatment for all patients. Subacromial decompression has been recommended for the impingement syndrome but has not been shown in randomised trials to be more beneficial than physical therapy. [25, 26] Surgical repair of rotator cuff tears can result in less pain and increased strength and movement; recovery can take up to 6 months. [27, 68]
- Hydrodilatation for frozen shoulder is no better than manipulation. [69] It provides more rapid relief of symptoms than intra-articular or subacromial injection of corticosteroids. However, at six months, the results were identical. [70] Hydrodilatation is less effective than arthroscopic capsular release. [71]

---

# Painless weakness affecting the shoulder region and upper arm

The two most common conditions that cause painless weakness around the shoulder and upper arm are nerve root compression and winging of the scapula. Less commonly, an axillary nerve palsy can result in painless weakness of the deltoid muscle.

# Cervical Nerve Root Compression

Cervical nerve root compression more commonly affects the lower cervical nerve roots (C7–T1). Compression of the C5 or C6 nerve root and an upper cord brachial plexus problem [28] can cause painless weakness in the shoulder and upper arm region. [29, 30] The weakness will affect the C5 and C6 innervated muscles around the shoulder, i.e. supraspinatus, infraspinatus, subscapularis, deltoid, biceps, and brachialis. Brachioradialis will also be weak with C6 radiculopathy. More commonly, cervical radiculopathy is associated with pain radiating into the upper arm. Figure 11.5 demonstrates how to test supraspinatus, infraspinatus, and subscapularis.

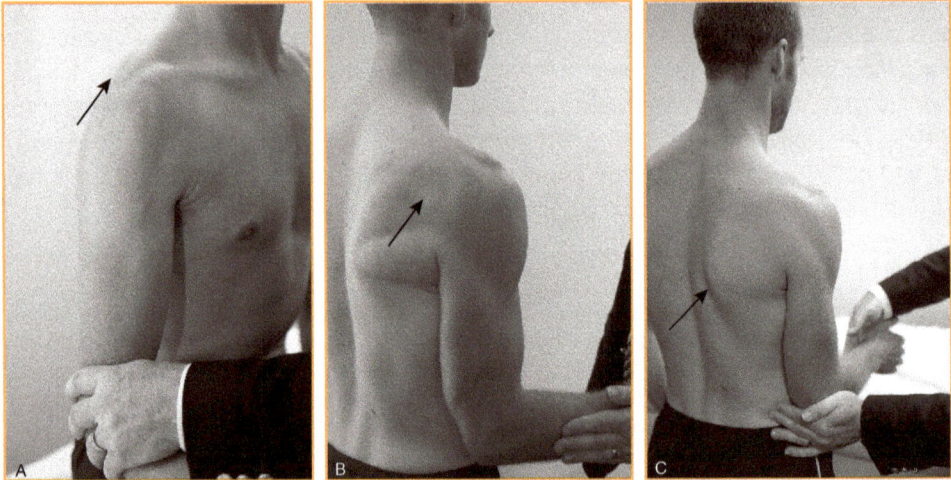

Figure 11.5 A Method of testing the supraspinatus. As the arm is abducted 20–30° away from the chest wall, the examiner pushes on the elbow, trying to force the arm back against the chest wall. B Method of testing the infraspinatus. The elbow is kept next to the chest wall; the semi-flexed forearm is externally rotated against resistance. C Method of testing the subscapularis. The arm is bent at a right angle at the elbow, and the forearm is semi-pronated. The elbow is kept against the chest wall. The patient is asked to rotate the forearm towards the body. The examiner tries to prevent this by pushing the forearm in the opposite direction.

# Winging of the Scapula

Most patients with winging of the scapula due to a mononeuritis of the long thoracic nerve to the serratus anterior muscle are unaware of the problem until someone points out that their shoulder blade protrudes (Figure 11.6). Occasional patients notice difficulty reaching high places with the affected arm with or without mild shoulder pain. [31] There is no treatment and whilst most patients recover spontaneously, this may take up to 2 years and occasional cases never recover.

# Examination

To test the serratus anterior muscle, have the patient's arm horizontal to the floor and pushing against the examiner's hand, or alternatively, as shown in figure 11.6, ask the patient to push against the wall, whilst the examiner looks to see if the scapula comes off the chest wall, indicating weakness of the serratus anterior muscle.

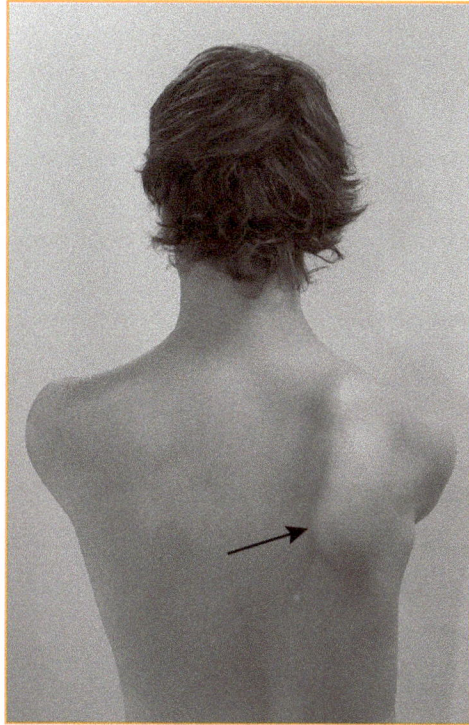

**Figure 11.6** Winging of the scapula due to weakness of the Serratus Anterior muscle

## Painless numbness affecting the shoulder and upper arm

Sensation over the lower aspect of the neck, shoulder and upper arm is from the 3rd to 5th cervical nerve roots. As degenerative disease predominantly affects the lower part of the cervical spine (C6, C7, C8 and T1), it is uncommon to see an isolated sensory loss in the distribution of the C3-C5 nerve roots. However, the sensory loss will be in a dermatome pattern if it does occur, as shown in Figures 1.12 and 1.13 (chapter one).

# Problems in the Forearms and Hands

## Numbness in the hand, forearm, or both

The commonest problems are carpal tunnel syndrome (CTS) at the wrist and an ulnar nerve lesion at the elbow (tardy ulnar palsy). Median nerve lesions can be confused with C6 radiculopathy as both supply sensation to the lateral aspect of the hand. An ulnar nerve lesion may be confused with a C8–T1 radiculopathy or a lower cord brachial plexus lesion as they all supply sensation to the medial aspect of the hand and forearm.

Figure 11.7 lists the clinical features of some of the problems affecting the forearms and hands. It separates them into those that cause paroxysmal and those that cause persistent symptoms. Occasionally the pain is absent, and the patient presents with the other clinical features after an injury, such as isolated coldness or altered sweating. [54]

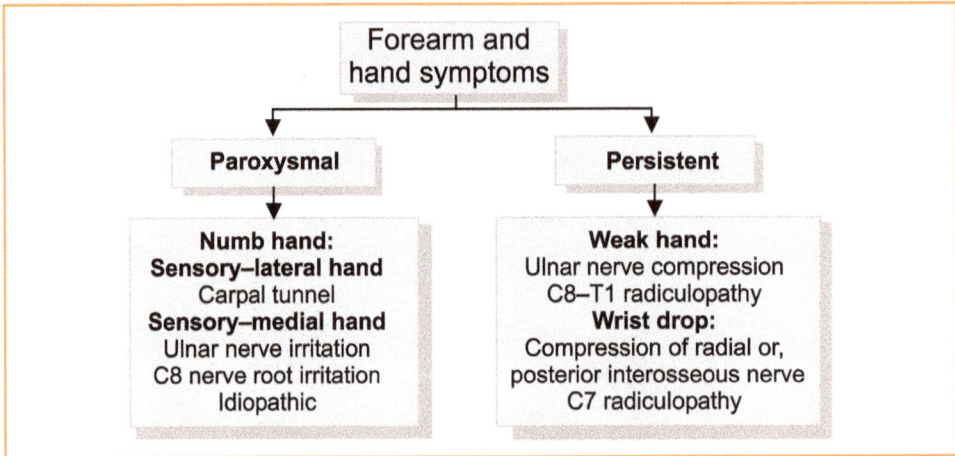

Figure 11.7 The essential diagnostic clues in patients with symptoms in the forearms and hands

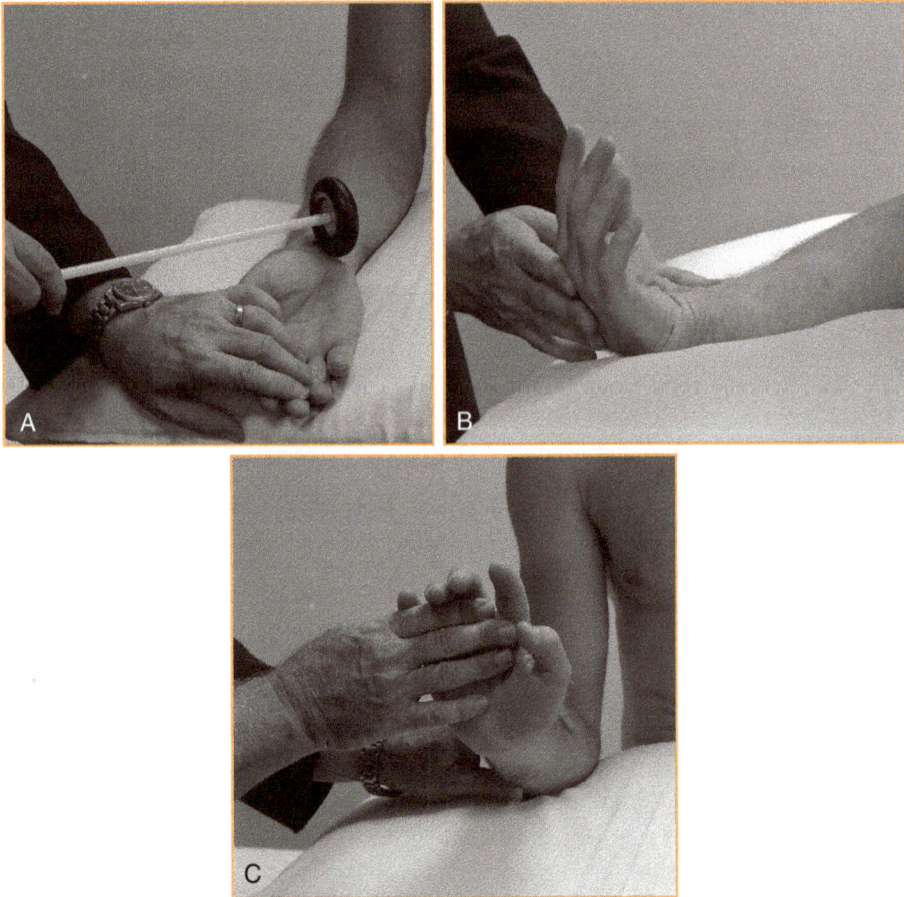

Figure 11.8 A Tinel's sign. The median nerve is tapped using the tendon hammer several times from several centimeters above the wrist and across the wrist for 2–3 cm. B, C Phalen's sign. The classic description is that the wrist is flexed (B) for up to 60 seconds and, if positive, the patient will experience transient altered sensation in the fingers and hand within the distribution of the median nerve. Some patients do not experience paraesthesia in the hands with wrist flexion but may with wrist extension (C).

# Carpal Tunnel Syndrome

Carpal tunnel syndrome is probably the most common neurological condition encountered in clinical practice. The annual incidence is approximately 3–4 per 1000 patients. It is more common during pregnancy and may resolve spontaneously after delivery. It is also more common in patients who gain excessive weight and may resolve with weight loss. If it is bilateral, it is essential to exclude hypothyroidism. There is a high incidence of CTS in patients with diabetes, although it is rarely the presenting symptom of that diagnosis.

## Symptoms

Carpal tunnel syndrome presents in two ways.

1. In most patients, the symptoms are due to irritation and compression of the median nerve at the wrist by the flexor retinaculum of the carpal tunnel. Patients experience intermittent paraesthesia (numbness, pins and needles or tingling) or dysaesthesia (an unpleasant sensation). The sensory branches of the median nerve innervate the lateral 3½ digits; however, many patients find it difficult to localise the sensory symptoms and often describe sensory disturbance well beyond the lateral 3½ digits. [32] The duration of altered sensation varies from a few minutes up to 30 minutes or rarely longer.

2. A different presentation is seen in older patients. They often present with either persistent altered sensation within the median nerve distribution on the hand or marked wasting of the thenar eminence (the muscles at the base of the thumb), with little in the way of the intermittent nocturnal sensory symptoms that occur with irritation of the nerve.

The characteristic and almost pathognomonic (diagnostic for a particular disease) complaint is waking in the middle of the night or in the morning with altered sensation in one or more often both hands that is relieved by shaking, moving, or hanging the arm and hand out of the side of the bed. Other activities that may precipitate the symptoms include driving, knitting, reading, mowing the lawn, or using hand tools.

> Little else other than CTS causes paroxysmal, nocturnal bilateral sensory symptoms.

Some patients complain of pain in the hand that may even extend up the arm even as far as the shoulder. [33] It is reasonable to accept that the pain may be related to CTS if the pain occurs only when the patient has simultaneous sensory symptoms. On the other hand, if the patient experiences pain with no sensory symptoms, this pain is very unlikely due to CTS and will not resolve with surgery for carpal tunnel syndrome. A common complaint is that the pain did not respond to carpal tunnel surgery. This is because the pain was not related to the median nerve compression, and the patient had two conditions, e.g. arthritis or occupational overuse syndrome. Patients should be advised that this pain may not be due to CTS and therefore may not resolve with appropriate treatment of CTS. This may explain the high failure rate seen in some studies. [44] The presence of pain, swelling and tenderness is not typical of CTS and suggests an alternative diagnosis.

## Examination

In young patients, weakness and sensory loss are absent. However, they may have a positive Tinel's or Phalen's sign (Figure 11.8). Tinel's sign is the precipitation of fleeting pain or sensory symptoms radiating into the palm and fingers when the median nerve is tapped at the wrist. Phalen's sign [35] is the presence of altered sensation in some or all lateral 3½ digits precipitated by forced flexion or extension of the wrist. The wrist may need to be bent for up to 60 seconds.

The sensitivity and specificity of the clinical examination for the diagnosis of carpal tunnel syndrome is 84% and 72%, respectively. The sensitivity and specificity of Tinel's sign were 60% and 67%, respectively, and of Phalen's sign were 75% and 47%, respectively. [36]

The electrophysiological diagnosis of carpal tunnel syndrome is discussed in Appendix H, 'Nerve conduction studies and electromyography'. C6 radiculopathy can cause an altered sensation on the lateral aspect of the forearm and hand. Figure 11.9 list the features that help differentiate a carpal tunnel from C6 radiculopathy.

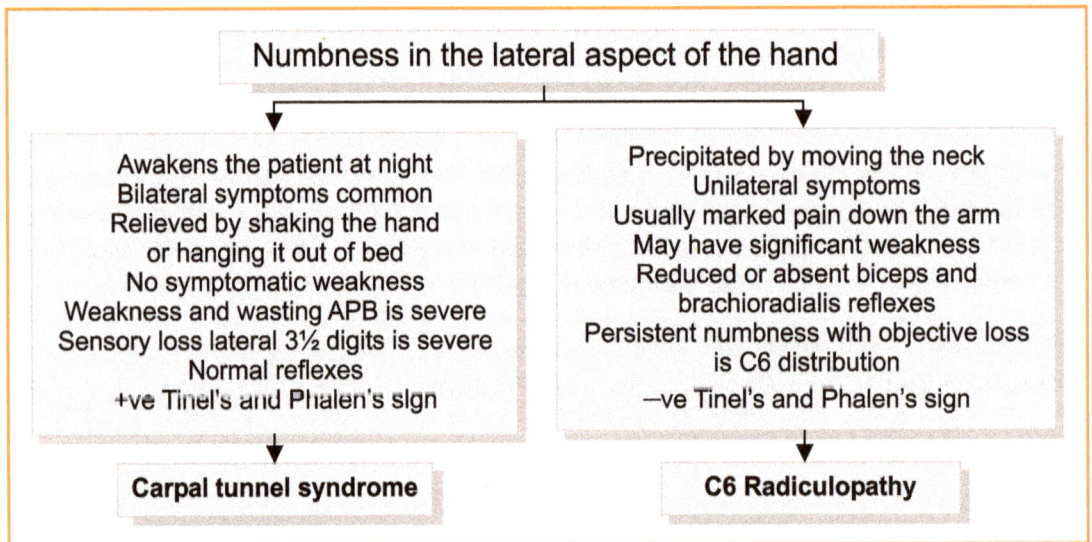

Numbness in the lateral aspect of the hand

Awakens the patient at night
Bilateral symptoms common
Relieved by shaking the hand
or hanging it out of bed
No symptomatic weakness
Weakness and wasting APB is severe
Sensory loss lateral 3½ digits is severe
Normal reflexes
+ve Tinel's and Phalen's sign

**Carpal tunnel syndrome**

Precipitated by moving the neck
Unilateral symptoms
Usually marked pain down the arm
May have significant weakness
Reduced or absent biceps and
brachioradialis reflexes
Persistent numbness with objective loss
is C6 distribution
−ve Tinel's and Phalen's sign

**C6 Radiculopathy**

Figure 11.9 The clinical features of carpal tunnel syndrome versus C6 radiculopathy

## Pronator Syndrome

The pronator syndrome is compression of the median nerve at the elbow between the two heads of the pronator teres muscle. Sensory symptoms are identical to carpal tunnel, but patients complain of a vague pain in the volar forearm and weakness because the flexor pollicus longus (Figure 11.17) and the median innervated portion of flexor digitorum profundus muscles are weak (Figure 11.10). As a result, patients cannot make a pincer grip with their thumb and index finger.

Abnormalities consistent with CTS diagnosis demonstrated on nerve conduction studies (NCS) do not imply that some or all of the patient's symptoms are related.

Asymptomatic median nerve compression detected by NCS is not uncommon.
Normal NCS does not exclude a mild CTS.

### Therapeutic Options for Treating Carpal Tunnel Syndrome

A conservative is appropriate if the symptoms are not severe, the patient tolerates them, and the nerve conduction studies are normal or reveal very mild abnormalities. Symptoms may resolve, particularly after pregnancy or with weight loss.

Splinting the wrists at night can provide symptomatic benefit. [37] However, in a randomised controlled trial, surgery was better than splinting. [38]

Corticosteroid injection into the wrist is beneficial in some patients, although the long-term benefit is unproven. [39] Repeat injections (8 weeks after the first) are of no value. [40] In an open randomised study, surgical carpal tunnel release was more cost-effective and resulted in a better symptomatic and neurophysiological outcome than corticosteroid injections. [41,42]

Surgery provides long-term benefits and is recommended in patients with more severe symptoms, regardless of the severity of the NCS abnormalities. Nocturnal or daytime paraesthesia resolve entirely in more than 90% of patients. [41] Surgery is also recommended in patients with severe NCS abnormalities regardless of the severity of the symptoms. The results of surgery in elderly patients who present with permanent wasting and sensory disturbance with no sensory response on NCS are less favourable. [43] Based on a retrospective questionnaire, some authors concluded that surgical carpal tunnel decompression has a significant failure rate. [44] In the questionnaire, patients stated whether they were better, unchanged, or worse after surgery. NCS can predict the response to surgery, with patients who have mid-range severity abnormalities having better results than those with either very severe or no abnormality. [44] In research studies, the response to surgery was assessed using the Global Symptom Score (GSS). This scoring system rates symptoms on a scale of 0 (no symptoms) to 10 (severe) in five categories: pain, numbness, paraesthesia, weakness/clumsiness, and nocturnal awakening. The sum of the scores in each category is the GSS. [45]

## Ulnar Nerve Lesions

Ulnar nerve lesions at the elbow are usually *unilateral,* bilateral cases are rare. Intermittent symptoms occur when the patient leans their elbow on a desk or the arm of a chair. Isolated sensory symptoms may occur or can precede weakness for months or even years. The more common presentation is the gradual onset of numbness and or pins and needles affecting the medial 1½ digits and the medial aspect of the hand on both the palmar and dorsal surfaces. Pins and needles or numbness are the initial symptom in most patients. Weakness results with ongoing compression, eventually wasting of the hypothenar eminence (base of the 4th and 5th digits), the interossei, medial two lumbricals (the small muscles between the metacarpal bones of the hand) and the 1st dorsal interosseous (the muscle between the thumb and index finger) occurs. An ulnar nerve lesion at the elbow is called a 'tardy ulnar palsy'. Compression of the ulnar nerve at the wrist level will affect the deep branch of the ulnar nerve and will not produce any sensory disturbance.

```
┌─────────────────────────────────────────────────────────────────┐
│         ┌───────────────────────────────────────────┐           │
│         │ Numbness medial "2 digits" and weakness in hand │      │
│         └───────────────────────────────────────────┘           │
│                                                                   │
│   ┌──────────────────────────┐   ┌──────────────────────────┐   │
│   │   Little or no pain       │   │         Pain*            │   │
│   │ Numbness medial 1½ digits │   │  Numbness medial 2 digits │   │
│   │   Weak long flexors of    │   │   Weak long flexors of    │   │
│   │      medial 2 digits      │   │      medial 4 digits      │   │
│   └──────────────────────────┘   └──────────────────────────┘   │
│                                                                   │
│   ┌──────────────────────────┐   ┌──────────────────────────┐   │
│   │   Ulnar nerve at elbow    │   │    C8-T1 Radiculopathy    │   │
│   └──────────────────────────┘   └──────────────────────────┘   │
│                                                                   │
│                                   ┌──────────────────────────┐   │
│                                   │    Horner's syndrome      │   │
│                                   │ Consider apical lung malignancy │
│                                   └──────────────────────────┘   │
└─────────────────────────────────────────────────────────────────┘
```

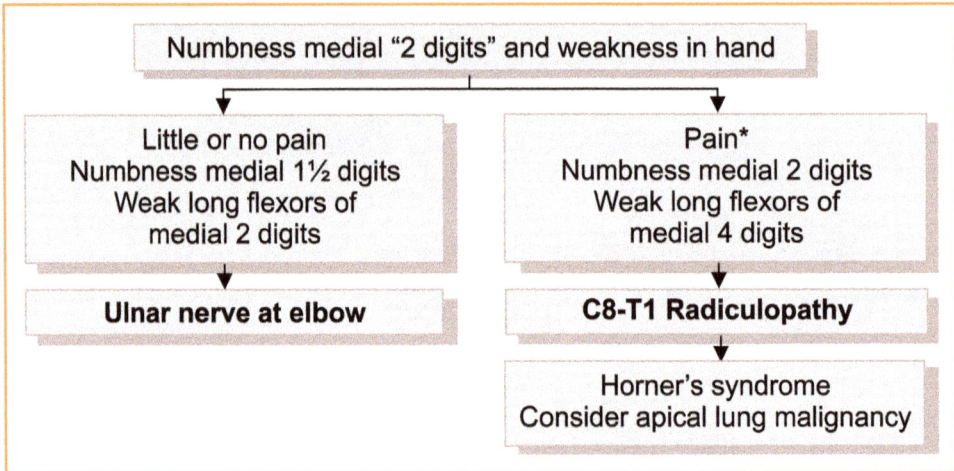

**Figure 11.10** Differentiating the two causes of numbness on the medial aspect of the hand

## Idiopathic Sensory Disturbance

Many patients complain of intermittent paraesthesia, with variable intensity and distribution predominantly affecting the medial aspect of the forearm and hand. The paraesthesia is never associated with any weakness or objective loss of sensation and, despite extensive investigations, no cause is detected. The cause of this problem is unclear. It can mimic the symptoms of an ulnar nerve lesion, a lower cord brachial plexus problem or a C8–T1 radiculopathy.

## Weakness with or without numbness in hand and forearm

The commonest condition affecting the hand is CTS. Symptomatic weakness is not a feature of CTS as only the abductor pollicus brevis muscle is involved. Although patients may notice wasting of the thenar eminence they are not aware of weakness. Ulnar nerve lesions at the elbow and C8–T1 radiculopathy have almost identical symptoms but the signs are different. Figure 11.10 lists the features that differentiate these two entities. Weakness of the extensor muscles of the wrist and hand can result from radial nerve lesions or C7 radiculopathy; subtle differences lead to the correct diagnosis (see the 5*3*5. rule below).

## Anterior Interosseous Nerve Entrapment

Compression of the anterior interosseous nerve between the two heads of pronator teres produces weakness of the flexor pollicus longus (Figure 11.17) and the lateral half of the flexor digitorum profundus (Figure 11.11). There is a weakness of flexion of the distal phalanx of the thumb and lateral two digits.[72] The patient cannot make a pincer grip similar to entrapment of the median nerve in the pronator syndrome. However, there are no sensory symptoms or signs.

## Ulnar Nerve Lesions

Occasionally, patients with compression of the ulnar nerve at the elbow will present with progressive weakness in the hand with little sensory disturbance. Another cause for isolated weakness is compression of or injury to the deep branch of the ulnar nerve at the wrist. There is a variable weakness of the abductor digiti minimi (Figure 11.16-abduction of the little finger) and more severe weakness of the small interosseous muscles (abduction and adduction of the digits), the 3rd and 4th lumbricals (flexion of the metacarpophalangeal joints) and the 1st dorsal interosseous muscle.

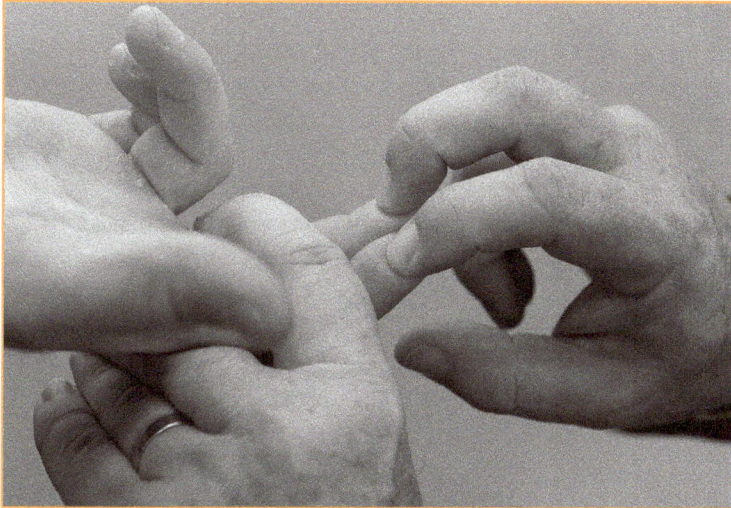

**Figure 11.11** Testing the long flexors of the lateral two digits. The examiner's other hand is used to prevent the patient from flexing the fingers at the proximal interphalangeal joint by flexor digitorum superficialis that is supplied by the median nerve.

## Ulnar Nerve Lesion at the Elbow versus C8–T1 Radiculopathy

Both conditions can present with a gradual onset of weakness of the hand associated with altered sensation affecting the medial two digits and the medial aspect of the forearm. However, with ulnar nerve lesions the numbness is mainly confined to the fingers and hand with a small amount of numbness on the underside of the forearm. The hand weakness is usually more marked with radiculopathy as more muscles that grip objects are affected. In neither will there be any change in the reflexes. Figure 11.9 lists the differences between these two entities. Figures 11.11 and 11.12 show how to test the long flexors of the distal phalanges of the medial four digits. The lower cord of the brachial plexus may very rarely be affected, e.g. with a tumour in the apex of the lung, and if the sympathetic ganglion is involved an ipsilateral Horner's syndrome will occur.

## Examination

Careful examination of *the pattern of weakness will differentiate these two entities*. Both will cause weakness of finger abduction (abductor digit minimi, the interossei and lumbricals) and the 1st dorsal interosseous whilst an ulnar nerve lesion at the elbow causes selective weakness of flexion of the distal phalanges of the medial two digits due to involvement of the flexor digitorum profundus muscle. On the other hand, a C8–T1 radiculopathy or lower cord brachial plexus lesion will cause weakness of flexion of the distal phalanges of all four medial digits.

To test these muscles the fingers are prevented from flexing at the proximal interphalangeal joint. The examiner asks the patient to bend the tips of their fingers while the examiner attempts to straighten them. The lateral two (Figure 11.10) are supplied by the median nerve, the medial two (Figure 11.12) by the ulnar nerve.

291

# Thoracic Outlet Syndrome

The reason for discussing thoracic outlet syndrome (TOS) [48] is that non-neurologists frequently suspect it in patients with paraesthesia, affecting the medial aspect of the forearm and hand. Especially in the absence of an ulnar nerve lesion. [49] Thoracic outlet syndrome is a controversial entity. It can occur in children and young adults. [50, 51] There are three types: arterial, venous, and neurogenic. Neurogenic is more common than vascular (arterial and venous) TOS, but both are very rare. It relates to brachial plexus compression, usually from scarred scalene muscles secondary to neck trauma. Compression can also occur with a cervical rib; however, the absence of a cervical rib on X-ray does not exclude the diagnosis as compression may be due to a fibrous band that is the continuation of the cervical rib.

The most frequent neurological symptom is aching pain in the side or back of the neck extending across the shoulder and down the arm. Tingling and numbness are common in the forearm and hand in the ulnar (C8–T1) distribution. Paraesthesia in the medial forearm and hand is a common complaint (90%), with the 5th finger involved four times as often as the thumb. One clue to the diagnosis is the precipitation of the paraesthesia with overhead activity or carrying heavy objects. [52] Objective sensory loss is uncommon, and muscle weakness and wasting are late signs; once they develop, the prognosis for recovery is poor. Sensory signs can occur without weakness and vice versa.

There is no reliable laboratory diagnostic test to confirm or exclude the diagnosis. The presence of a cervical rib is not proof, as this is a common incidental finding in asymptomatic individuals.

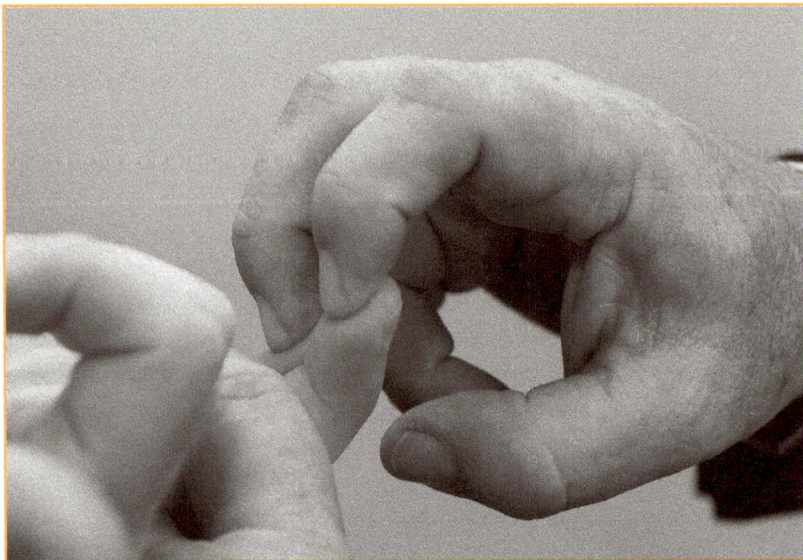

**Figure 11.12** Testing the long flexors of the medial two digits. The examiner's other hand prevents the flexor digitorum superficialis, supplied by the median nerve, from flexing the fingers at the proximal interphalangeal joint.

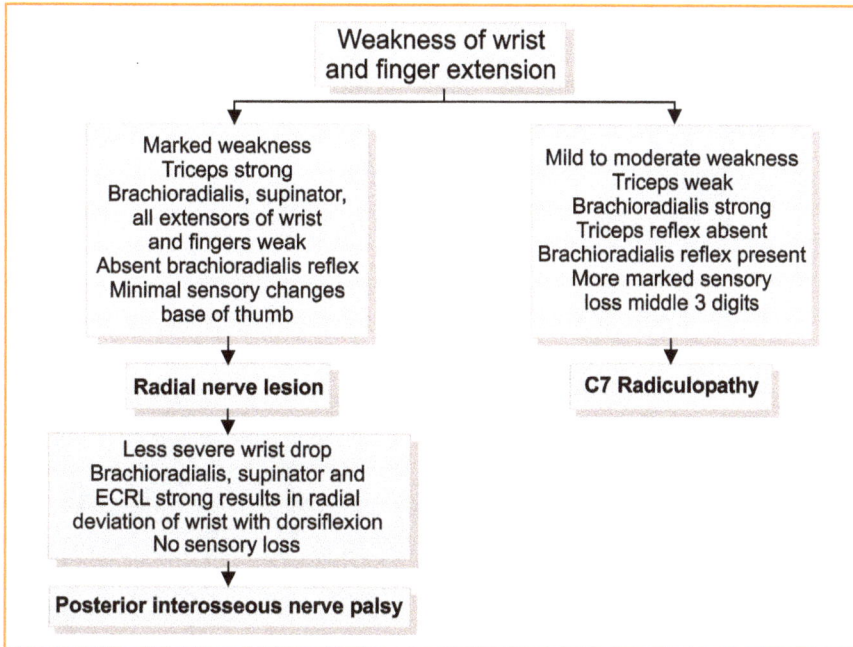

**Figure 11.13** Differentiating between a C7 radiculopathy and a radial nerve lesion

# Radial Nerve Palsy (Saturday night palsy)

The term 'Saturday night palsy' refers to the intoxicated patient who falls asleep in the chair and awakens with a wrist drop due to radial nerve compression in the radial groove of the humerus in the upper arm. The typical story is a patient awakening with a painless wrist drop with an inability to extend the wrist and fingers occasionally associated with mild sensory loss at the base of the first and second digits on the dorsal surface (Figure 1.14, chapter one).

Classical teaching has recommended a conservative approach with a wrist splint while the patient makes a complete recovery within days to weeks. *However, alternative pathology should be considered in patients with radial nerve palsy who have not 'slept on their arm'.* In two cases, the author has seen alternate pathology. In the first, a fibrous band caused progressive weakness over several weeks, and surgery led to a complete resolution. In the second, the radial nerve weakness was of sudden onset during the day and was due to torsion of the nerve. A delayed diagnosis resulted in a poor outcome despite surgery.

## Symptoms

- There is a weakness of supinator, brachioradialis and the extensors of the wrist, fingers, and thumb.
- The apparent weakness of the small muscles of the hand is due to the wrist drop. However, strength in the adductor and abductor muscles of the fingers is normal when tested with the hand flat on a hard surface eliminating the wrist drop (Figure 11.14).
- The triceps reflex is preserved.
- The brachioradialis reflex is reduced or absent.
- The degree of weakness of wrist and finger extension is severe, resulting in the wrist drop.

# Radial Nerve Palsy versus a C7 Radiculopathy

Patients with C7 radiculopathy may also present with wrist and finger extension weakness. However, it is less severe and usually associated with radicular arm pain. Figure 11.13 lists the differences between C7 radiculopathy and a radial nerve lesion. Figure 11.14 shows how to examine the three muscles around the elbow (biceps, brachioradialis and triceps) to determine if it is a radial nerve palsy and figure 11.15 shows how to test finger abduction when finger and wrist extension are weak.

## Radial Tunnel Syndrome, Posterior Interosseous Nerve Entrapment

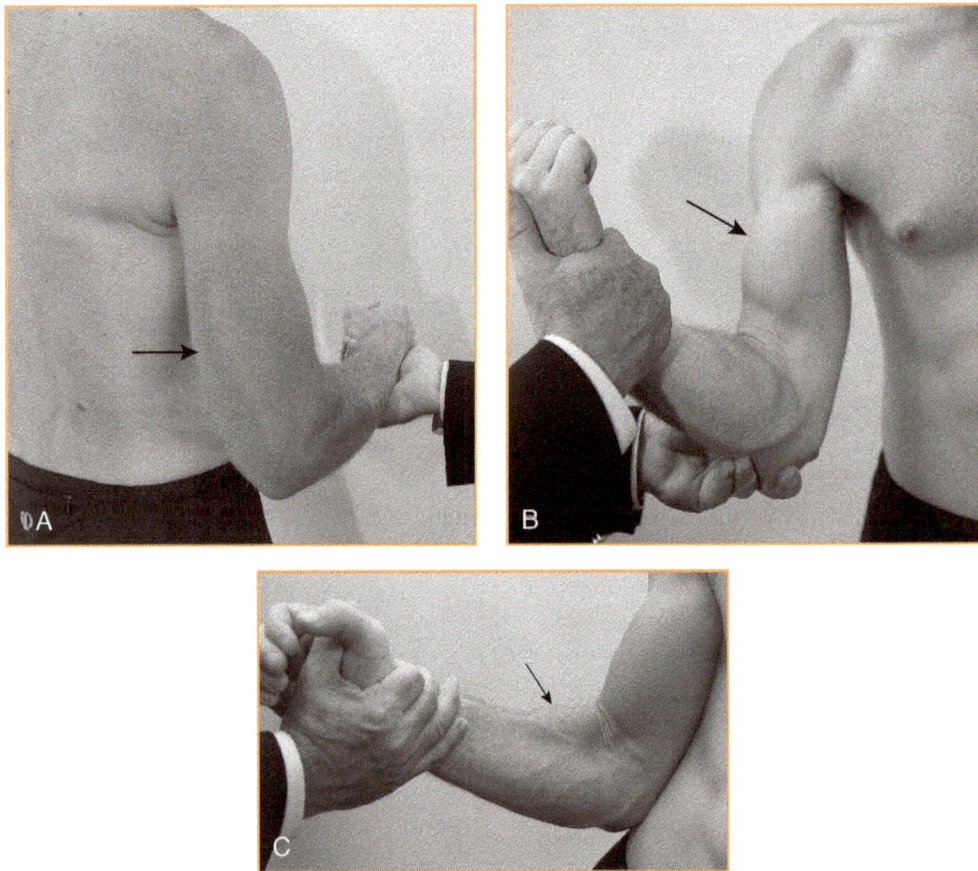

**Figure 11.14** Method of testing the 3 muscles around the elbow: **A** triceps. Ask the patient to extend the elbow from 90° of flexion. It is essential NOT to fully bend the elbow when testing the triceps as this will produce a false positive weakness of elbow extension. B the biceps (arrow). The forearm is fully supinated, and the patient bends the elbow. **C** brachioradialis. The arm is semi-pronated and flexed at the elbow, and the patient bends the arm at the elbow

Radial tunnel syndrome is an infrequent cause of weakness affecting the extensor muscles of the wrist and hand. Once again, a delay in recognition is more likely to result in a poor outcome with treatment. The posterior interosseous nerve is compressed in an aponeurotic (deep fascia attached to muscle) cleft in the supinator muscle.

The pain of radial tunnel syndrome is similar to the pain of lateral epicondylitis. It is located 3—4 cm distal to the lateral epicondyle on the dorsal aspect of the forearm. With more prolonged compression, progressive weakness and wasting of the extensor muscles occurs (excluding the extensor carpi radialis, a muscle that deviates the wrist laterally with extension) in the absence of any sensory symptoms.

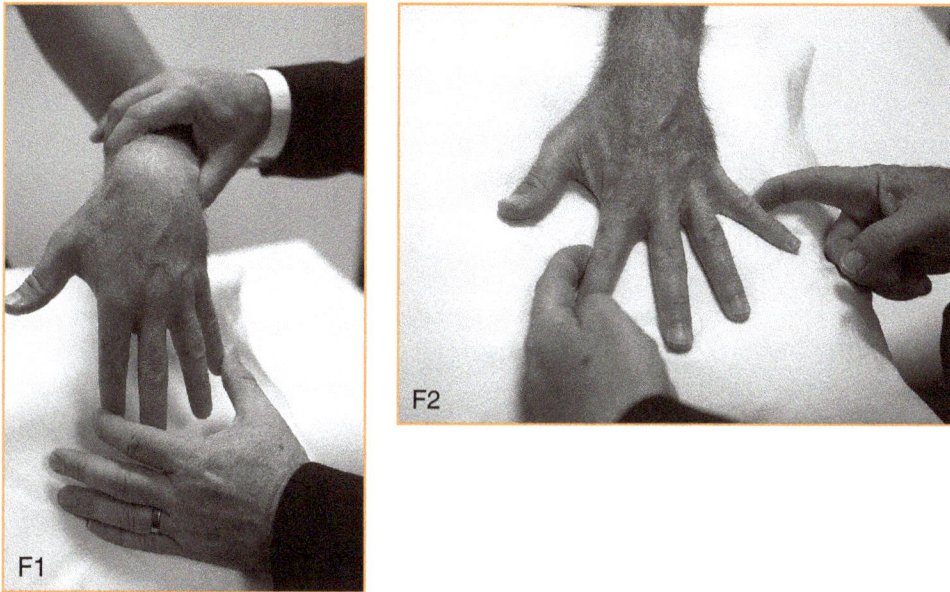

**Figure 11.15** Method of testing finger abduction and adduction in the presence of wrist drop **F1** can give a false impression that the ulnar innervated muscles that abduct and adduct the fingers are weak. F2 Ask the patient to place the palm on a firm surface so that the fingers rest firmly on the surface and then test adduction and abduction The strength will be normal with a radial nerve lesion and weak with an ulnar nerve lesion.

# Pain in the forearm

Forearm pain is more often due to lateral epicondylitis (tennis elbow), tenosynovitis or occupational overuse syndrome. If the pain is of neurological origin, it is likely due to a C6, C7 or C8 radiculopathy. Although the ulnar and radial nerves innervate the muscles and skin of the forearm, lesions of these nerves rarely, if ever, cause pain.

## Lateral and Medial Epicondylitis

Lateral epicondylitis is also referred to as tennis elbow. It occurs not only in tennis players. It produces pain and tenderness over the lateral aspect of the elbow. The pain radiates into the dorsal aspect of the proximal forearm extensor muscles and is exacerbated by clenching the fist, e.g., lifting heavy objects. There is no sensory disturbance or weakness, although the pain may limit the patient's ability to exert a total effort, mimicking weakness. An overuse injury affects the muscles (extensor radialis brevis) and tendons attached to the lateral epicondyle of the distal humerus.

A similar condition affects the medial epicondyle. Golfers elbow is the layperson's term for medial epicondylitis. Once again it is not confined to golfers. There is pain down the medial aspect of the forearm to the wrist. There are no sensory symptoms, and the only "weakness" is pain induced inability to exert a full effort.

| Treatment of Lateral and Medial Epicondylitis |
|---|
| There is little consensus on the treatment for lateral epicondylitis (conservative or operative). Rest, counterforce supportive forearm bracing and non-steroidal anti-inflammatory drugs (NSAIDs) often provide relief of symptoms. Wrist splinting is sometimes used, but the efficacy is uncertain. In many patients, the problem eventually resolves spontaneously. |

# Occupational Overuse Syndrome

Repetition strain injury (RSI) or occupational overuse syndrome (OOS) is a controversial entity. The term encompasses a range of conditions characterised by discomfort or persistent pain in muscles, tendons, and other soft tissues with or without physical manifestations. OOS is caused or aggravated by repetitive movement, sustained constrained postures or forceful movements. This condition occurs among workers performing tasks involving either repetitive and or forceful movements of the limb. For example, it is common amongst keyboard operators and machinists.

Pain is the predominant symptom and is diffuse, occurring in the hand, wrist, forearm, elbow, shoulder, scapular region, and neck, clearly beyond any single nerve or nerve root distribution. There is also diffuse tenderness of muscles, joints, and ligaments in the forearm and, less commonly, the upper arm. [53]

The aetiology is uncertain and treatment limited.

# Tendinosis or Tenosynovitis

The term tendinosis does not imply an inflammatory aetiology. Tendonitis and tenosynovitis denote inflammation of the tendon sheath. There is pain aggravated by movement of the tendon, with swelling and crepitus on palpation of the affected tendons or tendon sheath. The most commonly affected tendons are the dorsal extensors of the wrist. Pain occurs in the absence of any sensory disturbance or actual weakness, although once again the pain can be severe enough to prevent the patient from exerting a full effort with the complaint of weakness.

| |
|---|
| Pain can limit the ability to exert a full effort giving the false impression of weakness |

# Forearm Pain Related to Cervical Radiculopathy

Forearm pain can occur with C6, C7 and C8 radiculopathies.

## Relationship between symptoms and nerve root involvement

Sensory symptoms, if present, will be in the distribution of the nerve roots (Figures 1.12 and 1.13,chapter one).

The particular nerve root involved will influence the distribution of the pain.
- Forearm pain along the lateral border (radial side) indicates a C6 lesion.
- Pain involving the whole arm radiating into the 3rd digit suggests C7 (as the C7 nerve root supplies the periosteum of bone)
- Pain on the medial (ulnar side) indicates C8 nerve root pathology.
- Suprascapular pain (C5 or C6), interscapular pain (C7 or C8) or scapular pain (C8).

Cervical radiculopathy may be acute or chronic:
- Acute cervical radiculopathy with significant pain is more common in younger patients. It usually results from a tear in the annulus fibrosis and subsequent prolapse of the nucleus pulposus (the jelly-like substance in the middle of the spinal disc) or the disc itself.
- Subacute radiculopathy occurs in patients with preexisting cervical spondylosis. These patients experience occasional neck pain and develop insidious symptoms, affecting a single or multiple nerve roots.
- Chronic nerve root compression occurs spontaneously or when acute or subacute radiculopathies fail to respond to treatment. The gradual onset of wasting and weakness of the small muscles of the hand and forearm, sometimes associated with fasciculations, is seen in the elderly, leading to the suspicion of motor neuron disease.

Radicular pain may be precipitated or exacerbated by activities that stretch the involved nerve root, such as coughing, sneezing, valsalva and specific cervical movements or positions. It is NOT influenced by movement of the arm. C7 nerve root compression is the commonest and C6 is the second most common nerve root affected. Rarely, radiculopathy can result from benign neural tumours such as a neurofibroma or meningioma, Malignancy affecting the cervical vertebrae is very rare, although extradural malignancy can cause nerve root compression.

Although not present in all patients, the clue to the diagnosis is that the arm pain is NOT influenced by moving the arm. Instead, it may be exacerbated by turning the neck in some but not in all directions.

It is important to remember that the first seven cervical nerve roots emerge above the corresponding vertebra and the 8th below the 7th cervical vertebrae. Thus, C6 nerve root compression will occur between the 5th and 6th cervical vertebrae.

## Confirming the Diagnosis of Cervical Nerve Root Compression

- A plain X-ray of the cervical spine with anteroposterior, lateral, and oblique views will often demonstrate disc space narrowing or degenerative changes. Therefore, it is *essential to request oblique views* to see the foramen through which the nerve roots emerge. Plain x-rays do not confirm nerve root compression.
- If the pain does not settle with conservative (non-surgical) treatment an MRI scan of the cervical spine can usually identify the underlying pathology.
- A CT scan (i.e. without myelography) of the cervical spine provides good detail of the actual bony anatomy, but very poor visualization of soft tissues and nerves. Only occasionally does it identify the underlying pathology causing nerve root compression. Thus a CT scan is not recommended for cervical radiculopathy.
- When the main complaint is arm pain, surgery almost invariably relieves the pain. However, the weakness and sensory loss may take some months to resolve and in some cases, it never resolves.

| Principles of Management for Cervical Nerve Root Compression |
| --- |
| Treatment is determined by the patient's ability to tolerate pain. Therefore, motor, and sensory symptoms in isolation are not indications for surgery, as one cannot guarantee the resolution of such symptoms. |
| There are some [77] that would recommend surgery if the patient develops progressive weakness in the distribution of a compressed nerve root. This is controversial as there is no evidence to support this approach. |
| Some patients who have little tolerance for pain request surgery as soon as possible. If patients can tolerate the pain, it often resolves within 4–6 weeks. |
| If moving the neck aggravates the pain, a collar that immobilises the neck can provide symptomatic benefit until the pain resolves. |
| Analgesics and fluoroscopically guided transforaminal placement of corticosteroids close to the disc–nerve root interface and near the dorsal root ganglia are beneficial. [54] |
| Despite the lack of scientific evidence of benefit, some patients appear to settle with oral corticosteroids (50 mg per day of prednisolone for ten days). Some relapse when the steroids are withdrawn. [3] |
| The pain improves more rapidly with surgery. However, at one year, there is no difference between surgery and conservative management. [55] A Cochrane review concluded there was insufficient evidence to indicate whether surgery or conservative management was the optimal treatment. [56] |

# Complex Regional Pain Syndrome

Although rare, complex regional pain syndrome <u>must not be missed</u>. The consequences of a delay in diagnosis are often severe and prolonged problems. Symptoms can recur once or many times, months or even years later.

Complex regional pain syndrome was first described in the 16th century by Ambrose Paré. [75] Various terms describe this entity, including causalgia, shoulder–hand syndrome, reflex sympathetic dystrophy and Sudeck's atrophy. The current nomenclature refers to complex regional pain syndrome (CRPS) types I and II. The difference between types I and II is the presence of a nerve lesion in type II with the latter termed causalgia [Greek: kausos(heat) + algos (pain)]. Causalgia is a burning pain in the area supplied by the injured nerve. The pain is evoked by innocuous skin stimulation (allodynia) with an abnormally exaggerated response to a painful stimulus (hyperpathia). It is usually in the hand or foot after partial injury of a nerve or one of its major branches. Pain is more severe in type II.

| The Budapest criteria for CRPS. [76] |
| --- |
| A. **They should report continuing pain disproportionate to the inciting event.** |
| B. **They should report at least one symptom in three of the four following categories:** |
|    1. Sensory: Reports of hyperalgesia and/or allodynia, |
|    2. Vasomotor: Reports of temperature asymmetry and/or skin colour changes and/or skin colour asymmetry, |
|    3. Sudomotor/oedema: Reports of oedema and/or sweating changes and/or sweating asymmetry, |
|    4. Motor/trophic: Reports of decreased range of motion and/or motor dysfunction (weakness, tremor, dystonia) and/or trophic changes (hair, skin, nails). |
| C. **Additionally, they must display at least one sign at the time of evaluation in two or more of the following categories:** |
|    1. Sensory: Evidence of hyperalgesia (to pinprick) and/or allodynia (to light touch or deep somatic pressure), |
|    2. Vasomotor: Evidence of temperature asymmetry and/or skin colour changes and/or asymmetry, |
|    3. Sudomotor/oedema: Oedema and/or sweating changes and/or sweating asymmetry, |
|    4. Motor/trophic: Evidence of decreased range of motion and/or motor dysfunction (weakness, tremor, dystonia) and/or trophic changes (hair, skin, nails). |
| D. **Finally, there is no other diagnosis that better explains the signs and symptoms.** |

## Clinical features

CRPS may develop after a trivial injury and sometimes complicates minor surgery, e.g., carpal tunnel. The essential clinical features include:

- *persistent pain* developing within days to weeks after the injury or surgery.
- In type I, the pain is not confined to the distribution of a single nerve or nerve root
- initially increased temperature, then fluctuating between a sense of increased heat or coldness and subsequently persistent coldness
- swelling in the region of the pain
- changes in the colour of the skin, often described as mottled
- less frequently, excessive, or reduced sweating. [59]

---

**Management of Complex Regional Pain Syndrome**

Numerous treatments exist for CRPS type 1 with little evidence to support them. [60, 61] These include:
- corticosteroids[2] [62] in the form of oral prednisolone 40 mg/day for 14 days, followed by 10 mg/week taper.
- intravenous guanethidine. [63, 64]
- chemical and surgical sympathectomy. A Cochrane review concluded that there was no evidence of benefit. [61]
- Spinal cord stimulation.
- Dorsal root ganglion stimulation.

A randomised comparative trial of dorsal root ganglion stimulation compared to spinal cord stimulation found a 50% reduction in pain in 82% and 55%, respectively. [73]

  Some have argued that, with so little to offer therapeutically, it is not on an empirical basis unreasonable to treat with one or two sympatholytic procedures. [58] Drug treatment is based, not unreasonably, on experience gained in treating neuropathic pain in general. Drugs such as opioids, gabapentin and tricyclic antidepressants are recommended but have not yet been shown in randomised controlled trials to be effective in CRPS. Bisphosphonates, including pamidronate, clodronate and alendronate, have been advocated by some authorities. [65] Phenoxybenzamine (intravenous [66] and oral [67]) has also been reported to result in resolution of early CPRS type I. (It is essential to warn men of the side effect of retrograde ejaculation.)

---

# The 5*3*5 Rule for Examining the Upper Limb

This chapter has discussed how to examine the muscles of the upper limb and the various conditions that affect the upper limb. It is challenging, if not impossible, for the non-neurologist to remember the underlying neuroanatomy of each muscle. The 5*3*5 rule enables a non-neurologist to diagnose virtually every nerve and nerve root problem causing weakness in the upper limb without knowing the neuroanatomy. Essentially the rule consists of examining 5 muscles around the shoulder (Figure 11.18) , 3 muscles around the elbow (Figure 1.19) and 5 muscles around the wrist and hand (Figure 1.20). Establish which muscles are weak and then consult the tables below to determine the cause of the weakness.

  Figure 11.16 shows the remaining muscles that have not been described thus far in this chapter that need to be tested with the 5*3*5 rule.

---

2  Despite the lack of evidence the author has seen patients who have improved with steroids and gaunethidine.

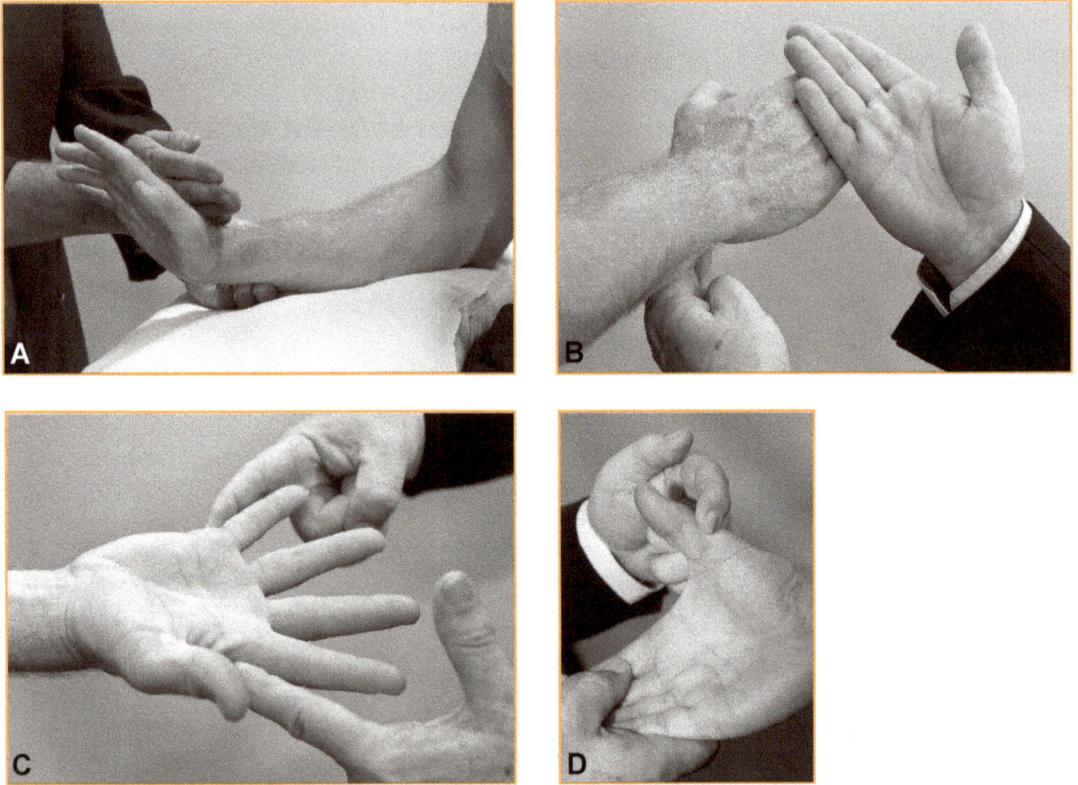

**Figure 11.16 A.** Extension of the wrist and fingers muscles of the wrist. **B.**The patient extends the wrist whilst the examiner places the back of their hand over the back of the patient's hand. Both exert a full effort. When testing finger extension the examiner places their 5th digit over the knuckles (MCP joints) of the patient. This places the patients MCP joints under the examiners 2nd digit, both exert a full effort and if the strength is normal the fingers will remain extended. This technique reduces the possibility of producing a "false +ve weakness" that can occur using other methods such as pushing down on the extended fingers with the ulnar border of the hand. **C.** shows how to test finger abduction, note the examiner is pushing on the base not the tip of the fingers. **D.** shows how to test abduction of the thumb, note the examiner is pushing on the base not the tip of the thumb.

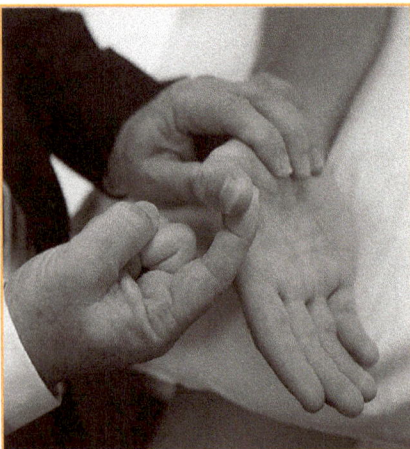

**Figure 11.17** Testing flexor pollicus longus that flexes the distal phalanx of the thumb

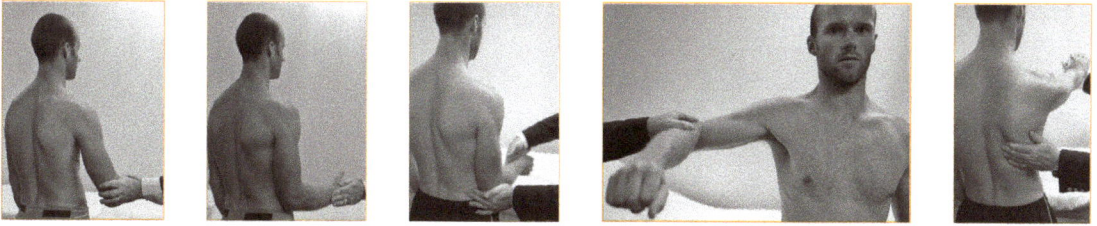

**Figure 11.18** The 5 muscles around the shoulder

| Muscle Number Action | Condition | | | | | |
|---|---|---|---|---|---|---|
| | **Axillary nerve** | **C5 Radiculopathy** | **C6 Radiculopathy** | **Suprascapular nerve** | **Winging of Scapula** | **Upper motor neurone weakness** |
| **S1** Abduction 1st 30 degrees Fig 11.5 A | No | Yes | Yes | Yes | No | No |
| **S2** External rotation Fig 11.5 B | No | Yes | Yes | Yes | No | No |
| **S3** Internal rotation Fig 11.5 C | No | Yes | Yes | No | No | No |
| **S4** Abduction 90 degrees Fig 11.2 | Yes | Yes | Yes | No | No | Yes (2nd muscle to become weak) |
| **S5** Arm extended pushing against resistence Fig 11.6 | No | No | No | No | Yes | |
| **E1** Elbow Flexion (palm supinated) Fig 11.14 B | No | Yes | Yes | No | No | No |
| **E3** Elbow Extension Fig 11.14 C | No | No | No | No | No | 3rd muscle to become weak |

**Table 1:** The five muscles around the shoulder plus the two at the elbow to differentiate peripheral nerve lesions as listed. NB the differentiation between a C5 and C6 radiculopathy is not possible with this technique. However, it will point to a C5 or C6 radiculopathy as the cause, and imaging can elucidate the exact site. **S**=shoulder, **E**=elbow and **W**=wrist. To differentiate a C5 from C6 radiculopathy, examine the rhomboids (C5) and supinator (C6). They are not illustrated in this book.

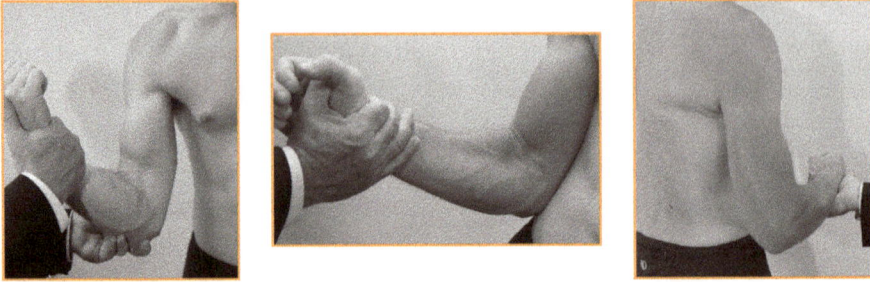

Figure 11.19 The 3 muscles around the elbow

| Muscle No. Muscle Name Action | C6 Radiculopathy | C7 Radiculopathy | Musculocutaneous nerve | Radial nerve | Upper Motor Neurone Weakness |
|---|---|---|---|---|---|
| **E1** Biceps, Elbow flexion-supinated Fig 11.14 | **Yes** | No | **Yes** | No | No |
| **E2** Elbow Flexion semi-supinated Fig 11.14 | **Yes** | No | No | **Yes** | No |
| **E3** Elbow Extension Fig 11.14 | No | **Yes** | No | Yes/No* | **Yes** 3rd muscle to become weak |
| **W1** Wrist & Finger Extension Fig 11.16 | No | **Yes** | No | **Yes** | **Yes** Only if finger extension is weak |
| **W2** Finger Abduction Fig 11.16 | No | No | No | Yes** | **Yes** 1st muscle to become weak |

**Table 2:** The three muscles around the elbow and the 2 of the five muscles in the wrist and hand involved in a radial nerve lesion, as well as an upper motor neuron weakness *Weakness of triceps, is seen with the extremely rare proximal radial nerve lesion due to fracture of the humerus or direct trauma[3]. [74] **E**=elbow and **W**=wrist ** Finger abduction appears weak if tested with the wrist and fingers dangling but is strong if the hand is placed flat on a hard surface.

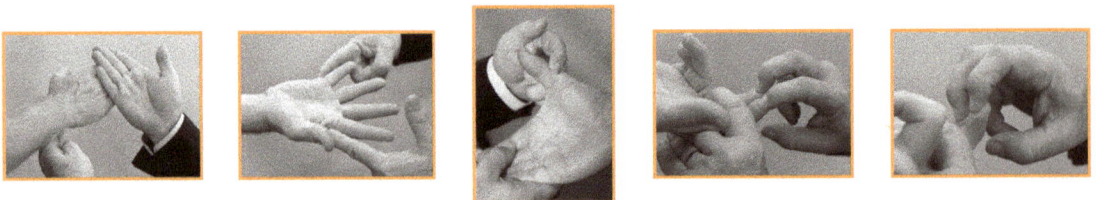

Figure 1.20 The 5 muscles around the wrist and hand. Nb wrist and finger extension are shown separately but are both "muscle 1 in the table)

---

3    In 40 years of clinical practice this author has never encountered a case.

| Muscle No. Muscle Action | Median nerve at Wrist | Median nerve at Elbow | Ulnar nerve at Wrist | Ulnar nerve at Elbow | C8-T1 Radiculopathy | Upper Motor Neurone Weakness |
|---|---|---|---|---|---|---|
| **W1** Wrist & Finger Extension Fig 11.16 | No | No | No | No | No | **Yes** (1st of 2 muscles to become weak) |
| **W2** Finger Abduction Fig 11.16 | No | No | **Yes** | **Yes** | **Yes** | **Yes** (2nd of 2 muscles to become weak) |
| **W3** Abduction of thumb Fig 11.16 | **Yes** | **Yes** | No | No | No | No |
| **W4** Long flexors digits 2 & 3 Fig 11.11 | No | **Yes** | No | No | **Yes** | No |
| **W5** Long flexors digits 4 & 5 Fig 11.12 | No | No | No | **Yes** | **Yes** | No |

**Table 3:** The five muscles around the hand. The flexor digitorum profundus muscle innervates the long flexors of the four fingers (not the thumb). The median nerve innervates the lateral half of this muscle, whilst the ulnar nerve innervates the medial half. Thus, the lateral portion flexes the distal phalanges of the 2nd and 3rd digits (muscle 4), whilst the medial portion flexes the distal phalanges of the 4th and 5th digits (muscle 5). **W**=wrist

# References

1   Dauer WT, et al. Current concepts on the clinical features, aetiology, and management of idiopathic cervical dystonia. *Brain* 1998;121(Pt 4):547–560.

2   Linton SJ. A review of psychological risk factors in back and neck pain. *Spine* 2000;25(9):1148–1156.

3   Jansen GB, et al. Whiplash injuries: Diagnosis and early management. The Swedish Society of Medicine and the Whiplash Commission Medical Task Force. *Eur Spine J* 2008;17(Suppl 3):S355–S417.

4   Radanov BP, Sturzenegger M, Di Stefano G. Long-term outcome after whiplash injury: A 2-year follow-up considering features of injury mechanism and somatic, radiologic, and psychosocial findings. *Medicine (Baltimore)* 1995;74(5):281–297.

5   Obelieniene D, et al. Pain after whiplash: A prospective controlled inception cohort study. *J Neurol Neurosurg Psychiatry* 1999;66(3):279–283.

6   Schrader H, et al. Natural evolution of late whiplash syndrome outside the medicolegal context. *Lancet* 1996;347(9010):1207–1211.

7   Harrop JS, et al. Neurological manifestations of cervical spondylosis: An overview of signs, symptoms, and pathophysiology. *Neurosurgery* 2007;60(Supp1 1):S14–S20.

8   Stiell IG, et al. The Canadian C-spine rule versus the NEXUS low-risk criteria in patients with trauma. *N Engl J Med* 2003;349(26):2510–2518.

9   Hurwitz EL, et al. Treatment of neck pain: Noninvasive interventions. Results of the Bone and Joint Decade 2000–2010 Task Force on Neck Pain and Its Associated Disorders. *J Manipulative Physiol Ther* 2009;32(2 Suppl):S141–S175.

10  van Alfen N, van Engelen BG. The clinical spectrum of neuralgic amyotrophy in 246 cases. *Brain* 2006;129(2):438–450.

11  Cruz-Martinez A, Barrio M, Arpa J. Neuralgic amyotrophy: Variable expression in 40 patients. *J Periph Nerv Syst* 2002;7(3):198–204.

12  Chance PF. Inherited focal, episodic neuropathies: Hereditary neuropathy with liability to pressure palsies and hereditary neuralgic amyotrophy. *Neuromol Med* 2006;8(1–2):159–174.

13  Perlmutter GS. Axillary nerve injury. *Clin Orthop Relat Res* 1999;368:28–36.

14  Post M. Diagnosis and treatment of suprascapular nerve entrapment. *Clin Orthop Relat Res* 1999;368:92–100.

15  Zoltan JD. Injury to the suprascapular nerve associated with anterior dislocation of the shoulder: Case report and review of the literature. *J Trauma* 1979;19(3):203–206.

16  Solheim LF, Roaas A. Compression of the suprascapular nerve after fracture of the scapular notch. *Acta Orthop Scand* 1978;49(4):338–340.

17  Rodgers JA, Crosby LA. Rotator cuff disorders. *Am Fam Physician* 1996;54(1):127–134.

18  Lewis JS. Rotator cuff tendinopathy/subacromial impingement syndrome: Is it time for a new method of assessment?. *Br J Sports Med* 2009;43(4):259–264.

19  Pajareya K, et al. Effectiveness of physical therapy for patients with adhesive capsulitis: A randomised controlled trial. *J Med Assoc Thai* 2004;87(5):473–480.

20  Hawkins RH, Dunlop R. Nonoperative treatment of rotator cuff tears. *Clin Orthop Relat Res* 1995;321:178–188.

21  Blair B, et al. Efficacy of injections of corticosteroids for subacromial impingement syndrome. *J Bone Joint Surg Am* 1996;78(11):1685–1689.

22  Yamakado K. The targeting accuracy of subacromial injection to the shoulder: An arthrographic evaluation. *Arthroscopy* 2002;18(8):887–891.

23  Watson M. Major ruptures of the rotator cuff: The results of surgical repair in 89 patients. *J Bone Joint Surg Br* 1985;67(4):618–624.

24  Stephens MB, Beutler AI, O'Connor FG. Musculoskeletal injections: A review of the evidence. *Am Fam Physician* 2008;78(8):971–976.

25  Haahr JP, Andersen JH. Exercises may be as efficient as subacromial decompression in patients with subacromial stage II impingement: 4–8-years' follow-up in a prospective, randomised study. *Scand J Rheumatol* 2006;35(3):224–228.

26  Gartsman GM, O'Connor PD. Arthroscopic rotator cuff repair with and without arthroscopic subacromial decompression: A prospective, randomised study of one-year outcomes. *J Shoulder Elbow Surg* 2004;13(4):424–426.

27  Codsi MJ. The painful shoulder: When to inject and when to refer. *Cleve Clin J Med* 2007;74(7):473–474:477–478, 480–482.

28  Schott GD. A chronic and painless form of idiopathic brachial plexus neuropathy. *J Neurol Neurosurg Psychiatry* 1983;46(6):555–557.

29  Shimizu S, et al. Radiculopathy at the C5/6 intervertebral foramen resulting in isolated atrophy of the deltoid. An aberrant innervation complicating diagnosis. Report of two cases. *Eur Spine J* 2008;17(Suppl 2): S338–S341.

30  Yoss RE, et al. Significance of symptoms and signs in localisation of involved root in cervical disk protrusion. *Neurology* 1957;7(10):673–683.

31  Wiater JM, Flatow EL. Long thoracic nerve injury. *Clin Orthop Relat Res* 1999;368:17–27.

32  Caliandro P. et al. Distribution of paresthesias in carpal tunnel syndrome reflects the degree of nerve damage at wrist. *Clin Neurophysiol* 2006;117(1):228–231.

33   Bland JD. Treatment of carpal tunnel syndrome. *Muscle Nerve* 2007;36(2):167–171.

34   Tinel J. *Presse Medicale* 1915;47:388.

35   Phalen GS. The birth of a syndrome or carpal tunnel revisited. *J Hand Surg Am* 1981;6(2):109–110.

36   Katz JN, et al. The carpal tunnel syndrome: Diagnostic utility of the history and physical examination findings. *Ann Intern Med* 1990;112(5):321–327.

37   O'Connor D, Marshall S, Massy-Westropp N. Non-surgical treatment (other than steroid injection) for carpal tunnel syndrome. *Cochrane Database Syst Rev* 2003(1): CD003219.

38   Gerritsen AA, et al. Splinting vs surgery in the treatment of carpal tunnel syndrome: A randomised controlled trial. *JAMA* 2002;288(10):1245–1251.

39   Marshall S, Tardif G, Ashworth N. Local corticosteroid injection for carpal tunnel syndrome. *Cochrane Database Syst Rev* 2007(2): CD001554.

40   Wong SM, et al. Single vs two steroid injections for carpal tunnel syndrome: A randomised clinical trial. *Int J Clin Pract* 2005;59(12):1417–1421.

41   Hui AC, et al. A randomised controlled trial of surgery vs steroid injection for carpal tunnel syndrome. *Neurology* 2005;64(12):2074–2078.

42   Korthals-de Bos IB et al. Surgery is more cost-effective than splinting for carpal tunnel syndrome in the Netherlands: Results of an economic evaluation alongside a randomised controlled trial. *BMC Musculoskelet Disord* 2006;7:86.

43   Iida J, et al. Carpal tunnel syndrome: Electrophysiological grading and surgical results by minimum incision open carpal tunnel release. *Neurol Med Chir (Tokyo)* 2008;48(12):554–559.

44   Bland JD. Do nerve conduction studies predict the outcome of carpal tunnel decompression?. *Muscle Nerve* 2001;24(7):935–940.

45   Herskovitz S, Berger AR, Lipton RB. Low-dose, short-term oral prednisone in the treatment of carpal tunnel syndrome. *Neurology* 1995;45(10):1923–1925.

46   Weber RA, Rude MJ. Clinical outcomes of carpal tunnel release in patients 65 and older. *J Hand Surg Am* 2005;30(1):75–80.

47   Leit ME, Weiser RW, Tomaino MM. Patient-reported outcome after carpal tunnel release for advanced disease: A prospective and longitudinal assessment in patients older than age 70. *J Hand Surg Am* 2004;29(3):379–383.

48   Peet RM, et al. Thoracic-outlet syndrome: Evaluation of a therapeutic exercise program. *Proc Staff Meet Mayo Clin* 1956;31(9):281–287.

49   Sanders RJ, Hammond SL, Rao NM. Diagnosis of thoracic outlet syndrome. *J Vasc Surg* 2007;46(3):601–604.

50   Maru S, et al. Thoracic outlet syndrome in children and young adults. *Eur J Vasc Endovasc Surg* 2009;38(5):560–564.

51   Gunther T, et al. Late outcome of surgical treatment of the non-specific neurogenic thoracic outlet syndrome. *Neurol Res* 2009:[vol]:[pages].

52   Leffert RD, Perlmutter GS. Thoracic outlet syndrome: Results of 282 transaxillary first rib resections. *Clin Orthop Relat Res* 1999;368:66–79.

53   Dennett X, Fry HJ. Overuse syndrome: A muscle biopsy study. *Lancet* 1988;1(8591):905–908.

54   Slipman CW, Chow DW. Therapeutic spinal corticosteroid injections for the management of radiculopathies. *Phys Med Rehabil Clin N Am* 2002;13(3):697–711.

55   Persson LC, Lilja A. Pain, coping, emotional state, and physical function in patients with chronic radicular neck pain. A comparison between patients treated with surgery, physiotherapy, or neck collar — a blinded, prospective randomised study. *Disabil Rehabil* 2001;23(8):325–335.

56   Fouyas IP, Statham PF, Sandercock PA. Cochrane review on the role of surgery in cervical spondylotic radiculomyelopathy. *Spine (Phila Pa 1976)* 2002;27(7):736–747.

57  Stanton-Hicks M, et al. Reflex sympathetic dystrophy: Changing concepts and taxonomy. *Pain* 1995;63(1):127–133.

58  Schott GD. Complex? Regional? Pain? Syndrome?. *Pract Neurol* 2007;7(3):145–157.

59  Veldman PH, et al. Signs and symptoms of reflex sympathetic dystrophy: Prospective study of 829 patients. *Lancet* 1993;342(8878):1012–1016.

60  Cepeda MS, Carr DB, Lau J. Local anesthetic sympathetic blockade for complex regional pain syndrome. *Cochrane Database Syst Rev* 2005(4): CD004598.

61  Mailis A, Furlan A. Sympathectomy for neuropathic pain. *Cochrane Database Syst Rev* 2003(2): CD002918.

62  Christensen K, Jensen EM, Noer I. The reflex dystrophy syndrome response to treatment with systemic corticosteroids. *Acta Chir Scand* 1982;148(8):653–655.

63  Hannington-Kiff JG. Intravenous regional sympathetic block with guanethidine. *Lancet* 1974;1(7865):1019–1020.

64  Bonelli S, et al. Regional intravenous guanethidine vs stellate ganglion block in reflex sympathetic dystrophies: A randomised trial. *Pain* 1983;16(3):297–307.

65  Robinson JN, Sandom J, Chapman PT. Efficacy of pamidronate in complex regional pain syndrome type I. *Pain Med* 2004;5(3):276–280.

66  Malik VK, et al. Intravenous regional phenoxybenzamine in the treatment of reflex sympathetic dystrophy. *Anesthesiology* 1998;88(3):823–827.

67  Inchiosa Jr. MA, Kizelshteyn G. Treatment of complex regional pain syndrome type I with oral phenoxybenzamine: Rationale and case reports. *Pain Pract* 2008;8(2):125–132.

68  Serin HM, Yılmaz S, Kanmaz S, et al. A rare cause of brachial plexopathy: hereditary neuralgic amyotrophy. *Turk Pediatri Ars* 2019; 54(3): 189-91.

68  Cederqvist S, Flinkkilä T, Sormaala M, et al. Non-surgical and surgical treatments for rotator cuff disease: a pragmatic randomised clinical trial with 2-year follow-up after initial rehabilitation. *Annals of the Rheumatic Diseases* 2021; **80**(6): 796.

69  Quraishi NA, Johnston P, Bayer J, Crowe M, Chakrabarti AJ. Thawing the frozen shoulder. *The Journal of Bone and Joint Surgery British volume* 2007; 89-B(9): 1197-200.

70  Yoon JP, Chung SW, Kim J-E, et al. Intra-articular injection, subacromial injection, and hydrodilatation for primary frozen shoulder: a randomized clinical trial. *Journal of Shoulder and Elbow Surgery* 2016; 25(3): 376-83.

71  Gallacher S, Beazley JC, Evans J, et al. A randomized controlled trial of arthroscopic capsular release versus hydrodilatation in the treatment of primary frozen shoulder. *Journal of Shoulder and Elbow Surgery* 2018; 27(8): 1401-6.

72  Rodner CM, Tinsley BA, O'Malley MP. Pronator syndrome and anterior interosseous nerve syndrome. *J Am Acad Orthop Surg* 2013; 21(5): 268-75.

73  Deer TR, Levy RM, Kramer J, et al. Dorsal root ganglion stimulation yielded higher treatment success rate for complex regional pain syndrome and causalgia at 3 and 12 months: a randomized comparative trial. *Pain* 2017; 158(4): 669-81.

74  Düz, B., et al. (2010). "Analysis of proximal radial nerve injury in the arm." *Neurol India* 58(2): 230-234.

75  Feliu, M. H. and C. L. Edwards (2010). "Psychologic factors in the development of complex regional pain syndrome: history, myth, and evidence." *Clin J Pain* 26(3): 258-263.

76  Shim, H., et al. (2019). "Complex regional pain syndrome: a narrative review for the practising clinician." *Br J Anaesth* 123(2): e424-e433.

77  Decker, R. C. (2011). "Surgical treatment and outcomes of cervical radiculopathy." *Phys Med Rehabil Clin N Am* 22(1): 179-191.

# Back Pain and Common Leg Problems with or without Difficulty Walking

Patients experience difficulty walking due to pain in their legs. The commonest cause of leg pain is arthritis of the joints in the lower limbs. In the absence of pain, altered strength (which may be due to a lower motor or upper motor neuron problem) or sensation (particularly proprioception) in the lower limbs and impaired balance resulting from either a cerebellar disturbance or vestibular problems may cause difficulty walking. In addition, difficulty walking can occur with Parkinson's syndrome and an apraxic gait due to frontal lobe problems.

Back pain is discussed as it is a common complaint seen by neurologists. After a brief discussion of back pain, there is a description of the clinical features of the various neurological disorders affecting the peripheral nervous system and the non-neurological conditions in the upper and lower leg and foot that may or may not result in difficulty walking. Akathisia, erythromelalgia, painful legs and moving toes and are also discussed.

Difficulty walking related to central nervous system problems is discussed in Chapter 13.

# Back Pain

Almost everyone at some stage in their lives will experience an episode of low back pain. A search of the internet using Entrez PubMed yields more than 80,000 articles. Google scholar more than four million and Google more than 1.6 trillion articles!

> The single most important thing is to ascertain is whether the pain is in the lumbar or thoracic region as the underlying causes are very different.

## Essential facts about back pain

Most *low back (lumbar) pain* is non-specific and relates to soft tissue problems or degenerative disease affecting the lumbosacral spine. If there is nerve root compression (sciatica), the most likely causes are osteoarthritis or lumbar disc protrusion.

307

On the other hand, thoracic back pain is often more sinister. Patients who subsequently develop malignant cord compression experience thoracic back pain for days or weeks before the neurological symptoms. Pain related to osteoporotic vertebral fractures is common in the thoracic region. Rarely, thoracic back pain may be the presenting symptom of a ruptured aortic aneurysm.

Pain from facet joints and the sacroiliac joints may respond to radiofrequency ablation,[109] thus a discussion of these entities would seem reasonable. Essentially it is difficult to distinguish facet joint problems from other causes of low back pain. Degenerative changes include joint space narrowing, sclerosis, subchondral sclerosis and erosions, cartilage thinning, calcification of the joint capsule, hypertrophy of articular processes and of the ligamentum flavum causing impingement of the foramina and osteophytes. However, similar abnormalities can be seen in asymptomatic individuals. Imaging guided controlled blocks with local anaesthetics plus or minus steroids are the only reliable tool in the diagnosis of facet joint pain as a cause of low back pain. If there is complete short-term relief of pain this suggests the pain may be originating in the facet joints and consideration of radiofrequency ablation of the nerves innervating the facet joints. [109]

No pathognomonic clinical history, physical examination finding, or imaging study exists that aids clinicians in making a reliable diagnosis. of sacroiliac joint (SIJ) pain [110] However, imaging combined with clinical provocative tests might help to identify patients for further investigation. Although provocative physical examination tests have not received reliable consensus, if three or more provocative tests (FABER, gapping test/distraction, compression test/approximation test, thigh thrust test/femoral shear test, Gaenslen test/pelvic torsion test and the sacral thrust test/sacral base spring test) are positive, pursuing a diagnostic SIJ injection is considered reasonable[1]. [110]

Routine imaging early on in the course of low back pain is of no benefit. [1] However, with thoracic back pain, an MRI scan can detect spinal metastases in patients with normal plain X-rays or CT scans. [2] A nuclear bone scan can also detect metastases in the vertebral column before cord compression, however, MRI is superior. [3]

In most patients with low back pain, symptoms resolve with exercises and the passage of time, without the need for surgical intervention.

---

**Treatment of Chronic Low Back Pain**

Chronic low back pain can be challenging to treat. Although there is limited evidence for the efficacy of aquatic exercises [8], this author[2] had seen numerous patients where back pain improved with regular swimming, at least three times per week and 20 minutes at a time.

Physical therapy and non-steroidal anti-inflammatory drugs (NSAIDs) are the cornerstones of non-surgical treatment. [4] Superficial heat is the only therapy with reasonable evidence of efficacy. Bed rest often advocated for acute low back pain with continuing ordinary activity may lead to a more rapid recovery. [5] There is conflicting evidence of the efficacy for spinal manipulation in low back pain. [6, 7] Massage and acupuncture are better than no treatment but have not been compared to conventional treatment. Radiofrequency ablation/ denervation of the medial branches innervating the joints has been shown in several trials to be effective for back pain related to facet and sacroiliac joints, whilst the evidence is mixed for discogenic disease. [108]

*Note:* A randomised controlled study detected higher ambulation rates in patients with malignant spinal cord compression given high-dose dexamethasone before radiotherapy than radiotherapy alone. (81% v 63% at three months, respectively; P = 0.046).

---

1  The paper by Thawrani et al [110] has an algorithm to aid in the management of SIJ pain and the details on how to perform each of the provocative tests.

2  Personal Observation

# Problems in the Upper Leg

## Painless numbness

## Meralgia Paraesthetica

Meralgia paraesthetica is very common, particularly in patients who are overweight. It is essentially about the only cause of numbness in the thigh or upper leg because compression of the sensory nerve roots in the upper lumbar (L2–3) spine is very rare. This condition is due to compression of the lateral cutaneous nerve of the thigh beneath the inguinal ligament just medial to the anterior superior iliac spine. Pressure over this point is often associated with tenderness.

### Symptoms

- Symptoms may be intermittent although subsequently many patients often develop a permanently altered sensation.
- Symptoms vary from a mildly altered sensation over the anterolateral aspect of the thigh, often only noticed when the patient touches the thigh or clothes brush up against the thigh. Some patients develop a marked alteration in sensation with persistent numbness within the distribution of the lateral cutaneous nerve of the thigh but not always involving the entire extent. The distribution of the pain is not that of a nerve root.
- Others complain of pain; some experience dysaesthesia which is an unpleasant sensation when the skin is touched lightly.
- The presence of weakness or an altered knee reflex excludes the diagnosis.
- The condition may be unilateral or bilateral.

### Examination

The most straightforward test is to stroke the skin over the lateral aspect of the thigh. If there is an altered sensation, test light touch from where you find an abnormal sensation in all four directions, thus mapping out the exact pattern and sensory loss. I draw on the leg to then show the patient the illustration shown in figure 12.1 Another diagnostic test is to inject local anaesthetic in the region of the lateral cutaneous nerve beneath the inguinal ligament; a quick resolution of symptoms is considered diagnostic. [9]

| Management of Meralgia Paraesthetica |
| --- |
| Once the benign nature of the condition is explained, the great majority of patients do not request any specific treatment. In many patients, the problem may resolve spontaneously. [9] Patients with pain or dysaesthesia may respond to a corticosteroid injection and, if that fails, decompression of the nerve or avulsion of the nerve (neurectomy). [10] This latter procedure will replace dysaesthesia with permanent numbness. Regardless of the treatment chosen, most patients remain free of symptoms following treatment. [9, 11] |

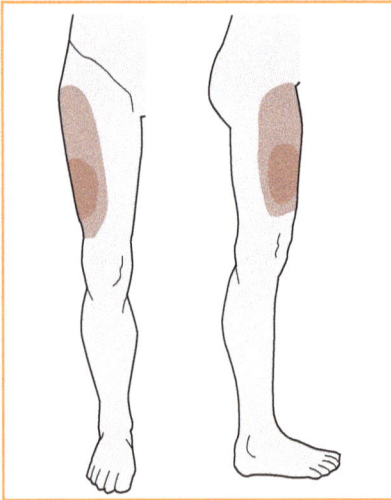

Figure 12.1 The area of sensation supplied by the lateral cutaneous nerve of the thigh Reproduced from Aids to the Examination of the Peripheral Nervous System. 4th edn, Brain, 2000, WB Saunders, Figure 78. p 50.

# Pain and Weakness in the Upper Leg

## Diabetic Amyotrophy/Femoral Amyotrophy/Lumbosacral Neuritis

The clinical features of lumbosacral neuritis, femoral amyotrophy and diabetic amyotrophy are virtually identical.

### Symptoms

- Increasingly severe pain in the buttocks, hips and thighs developing over hours to days is the initial presenting symptom. It is most often unilateral, but as in brachial neuritis, the contralateral side may be affected, usually within 1–2 weeks.
- The pain is followed by severe weakness and subsequently marked wasting of the quadriceps muscles. Paraesthesia in the anterior aspect of the thigh and, at times, the shin may also occur. The weakness can be so severe to render the patient unable to walk.
- Sensory symptoms are usually minimal.
- Weight loss is not uncommon. [12]

### Examination

The examination reveals weakness of hip flexion and knee extension with an absent knee-jerk. Although it may occur at any age, lumbosacral neuritis is more common in the middle-aged to elderly. [13] The aetiology of these conditions is uncertain but thought to be an inflammatory vasculitis. [12, 14]

| Management of Diabetic Amyotrophy/Femoral Amyotrophy/Lumbosacral Neuritis |
|---|
| Although the condition may resolve spontaneously, it may take many months or years. Immunomodulatory therapy, including corticosteroids or even cytotoxic drugs, may shorten the duration of the illness. In several case reports, intravenous immunoglobulin has led to a more rapid improvement. [15, 16] This includes diabetic amyotrophy.[80] |
| At this point, there are no randomised controlled trials to guide therapy, but significant disability persists for months or years in the absence of specific treatment. [86] |

> In both lumbosacral neuritis and polymyalgia rheumatica there is constant pain. The worsening of pain with movement of the hips is seen only in polymyalgia and the presence of severe weakness and sensory disturbance occurs only in lumbosacral neuritis.

## Polymyalgia Rheumatica

Polymyalgia rheumatica occurs in middle-aged to elderly patients.

## Symptoms

Aching and stiffness predominantly affecting the shoulders, but in 50–70% of cases may also affect the hips. [17] The condition is believed to be related to synovitis of the proximal joints and extra-articular synovial structures. The pain is constant day and night, as opposed to osteoarthritis of the hips, where the pain mainly occurs on weight-bearing. It often radiates to the knee and is exacerbated by movement of the proximal leg. Although initially, it may be unilateral, almost invariably, patients develop bilateral symptoms.

A low-grade fever, fatigue and anorexia may occur in as many as 40% of patients, and the presence of high spiking fevers should alert the clinician to the possibility of associated giant-cell arteritis affecting the aorta and major branches. Cranial arteritis causes headaches, scalp tenderness and jaw claudication. (Chapter 9, 'Headache and facial pain', for further discussion).

## Examination

The examination reveals restricted active and passive movement of the hips in the absence of any joint swelling.

| Management of Polymyalgia Rheumatica |
|---|
| The erythrocyte sedimentation rate is usually raised, although it may be normal in the early stages. It is often necessary to repeat the ESR 1-2 weeks later. Corticosteroids are the treatment of choice. Doses of 10–20 mg/day almost invariably leads to a rapid resolution of the aching and stiffness within days. This fast response to low dose corticosteroids is considered diagnostic. |
| Occasional patients may require higher doses for more extended periods. [17] If the patient fails to respond to prednisolone within one week, the diagnosis should be questioned. |
| Early cessation of steroids may lead to a relapse, and treatment with low-dose steroids should continue for 1–2 years. [18] Methotrexate has been shown in a randomised controlled trial to be an effective steroid-sparing agent. |

## Drug-Induced Muscle Pain and or Weakness

Many pharmaceutical agents, including lipid-lowering agents, NSAIDs, antineoplastic drugs and even over-the-counter essential amino acids, such as L-tryptophan, can result in myalgia or even myositis, causing muscle pain, cramps, swelling, tenderness, and weakness. [19, 20] This list is almost certain to enlarge with the advent of new therapeutic agents.

In any patient presenting with myalgia or muscle weakness, every drug that they are taking should be checked to see if they cause myalgia or myositis. Some drugs produce a pure muscle disorder; others are associated with neuropathy. The pharmacy department of the public hospital is a handy resource, as is the patient's pharmacist.

# Weakness in the upper leg

## Inflammatory Muscle Diseases

The classification of inflammatory muscle diseases (IMD, also referred to as idiopathic inflammatory myopathies) has changed [81] with the availability to test for myositis specific and associated antibodies. The traditional view that IMD was a disease confined to muscles is no longer the case. Inflammation frequently affects other organs, including the skin, joints, lungs, gastrointestinal tract, and heart. The current subgroups of IMD include polymyositis, dermatomyositis, inclusion body myositis (IBM), immune-mediated necrotising myopathy(IMNM), and overlap myositis, including antisynthetase syndrome. IMD is rare, and most general practitioners are unlikely to encounter one or two cases during their working careers. Several excellent reviews [82-84] and the Myositis Support and Understanding Association founded in 2015 by Jerry Williams are reliable sources of up-to-date information[3].

Patients present with the insidious onset of proximal weakness in the arms and legs in the absence of sensory disturbance. The weakness is bilateral but may be asymmetrical. Pain in the muscles occurs in approximately 50% of cases but is rarely severe. Dysphagia, neck weakness and impaired respiratory function may occur. [21] Inclusion body myositis (IBM) has finger flexor or quadriceps weakness, endomysial inflammation, and invasion of non-necrotic muscle fibres and rimmed vacuoles in their muscles. The knee reflex is often absent in IBM, whereas, in polymyositis and dermatomyositis, the reflexes are preserved. Dermatomyositis is associated with skin rashes such as the heliotrope erythema over joints (Gottron sign) and papules over joints (Gottron papules). Gottron sign and Gottron papules occur over areas that experience stretching, including the metacarpophalangeal, proximal interphalangeal and distal interphalangeal joints, knees, and elbows[4]. These skin rashes can occur in the absence of any muscle weakness, an entity called amyopathic dermatomyositis. Dermatomyositis is associated with a six-fold increase in malignancy. [85-86] Immune-mediated necrotising myopathy is associated with necrotic muscle fibres, often with little if any inflammatory cell infiltrate. Antisynthetase syndrome is characterised by the presence of myositis, interstitial lung disease, mechanic's hand (roughening and cracking of the skin of the tips and sides of the fingers), arthritis and Raynaud phenomenon (some features might predominate) together with an antisynthetase antibody. [84]

---

3   https://understandingmyositis.org/ The Myositis Support and Understanding Association is a volunteer group with medical and scientific advisers on the board. It took Jerry Williams several years for the diagnosis of dermatomyositis to be established.

4   Images of the skin manifestations are in the paper by Lundberg, de Vesser and Werth. [84]

| Management of Myositis |
|---|
| The creatinine kinase (CK) level is elevated, usually less than < 100 times normal. A normal CK does not exclude the diagnosis with dermatomyositis, thyrotoxic myositis, statin-induced myositis, Parvovirus B19 myositis and in some cases of polymyositis. |

The nerve conduction studies (NCS) should be normal, but electromyography may demonstrate a typical myopathic pattern associated with fibrillation potentials and positive sharp waves indicating an inflammatory muscle disorder together with small amplitude polyphasic potentials (BSAPP's) when the patient is as asked to contract the muscle and with a full recruitment pattern with submaximal effort.

Magnetic resonance imaging(MRI), contrast-enhanced ultrasound and positron emission tomography may demonstrate abnormalities in muscles in some patients with inflammatory myositis to identify the optimal site for a muscle biopsy. [22] A whole-body MRI is recommended, although caution is needed as oedema is non-specific. The sensitivity and specificity of imaging in IMD has not been established. Currently available myositis-specific autoantibodies are present in 50% of patients. They support the diagnosis and aid in the classification and subclassification of IIM's.

Muscle biopsies with histopathological and immunohistochemical evaluation are still crucial in many cases to rule out other causes of myopathy. [84] If immune-mediated necrotising myopathy related to statins is suspected, anti-HMGCR antibodies should be ordered as they are not part of the panel of the myositis specific antibody panel.

| Treatment |
|---|

Corticosteroids are the cornerstone of treatment [83] despite the lack of any randomised controlled trials. [23] High dose steroids are associated with significant side effects. In rapidly progressive disease IV methylprednisolone 1000mg daily for 3 days is recommended. In others, 1mg/kg (up to 100mg) for 3-4 weeks gradually decreasing after that if the patient has responded, changing to alternate day therapy. Response is defined as increased strength not feeling better nor a decreased CK.

If strength has not improved the corticosteroids should be rapidly decreased so that other immunomodulatory drugs can be commenced. These include azathioprine, methotrexate, cyclosporine, and mycophenolate mofetil. Cyclophosphamide or tacrolimus are recommended when interstitial lung disease is present.

Intravenous immunoglobulin (IVIG), 2mg/kg in divided doses for 2-5 days is recommended in non-responders and is of proven value in dermatomyositis. [87]

In those who do not respond to steroids and IVIG, rituximab (an anti-CD20 antibody), at a dose of 2 g (divided into two infusions 2 weeks apart) seems effective in some patients with dermatomyositis, polymyositis, or necrotising autoimmune myositis, particularly in patients with anti-Jo-1, anti- Mi-2, or anti-SRP antibodies.

If symptoms are mild, it is not unreasonable to cease the statin and observe as remission can occur. Immune-mediated necrotising myositis requires intensive immunosuppressive therapy. Initial treatment with corticosteroids 1mg/kg/day should be combined with methotrexate, azathioprine or mycophenolate. If no response after 8-12 weeks IVIG or rituximab is recommended. Triple therapy including IVIG ,may be required.

Tumour necrosis factor inhibitors (infliximab, adalimumab, and etanercept) are ineffective and may worsen or trigger disease. [88] Apart from exercise there is no specific treatment for inclusion body myositis at the time of writing this text. Glucocorticoids, methotrexate, cyclosporine, azathioprine, IVIG and mycophenolate are ineffective. [83]

# Muscle Weakness due to Endocrine Dysfunction

Hyperthyroidism, hypothyroidism, and Addison's disease may all present with muscle weakness. Usually, there are associated manifestations that to point to the underlying endocrine disorder. Hyperthyroidism may cause periodic paralysis [24] or rhabdomyolysis [25], and hypothyroidism may present with muscle hypertrophy. [26] The weakness will resolve with correction of the endocrine disturbance.

## Peripheral Neuropathy

Acute (AIDP) and chronic (CIDP) inflammatory demyelinating peripheral neuropathy, the immune mediated neuropathies and IgG- or IgA-related peripheral neuropathies can cause significant proximal weakness in the lower limbs. However, this rarely occurs in isolation. These patients usually present with generalised weakness affecting the proximal and distal muscles in all four limbs, neck weakness with or without respiratory muscle weakness. Peripheral neuropathy is discussed in more detail later in this chapter.

# Lower Legs and Feet Problems
## Unpleasant sensations in the feet

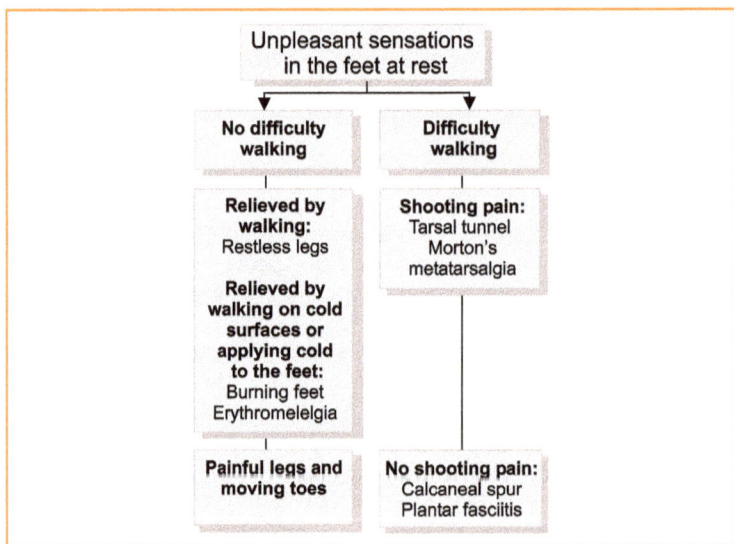

**Figure 12.2** Suggested approach to evaluating unpleasant sensations in the feet.

Unpleasant sensations in the lower legs at rest are common. When the symptoms are improved by walking, the likely diagnosis is restless legs syndrome (RLS), burning feet or painful legs and moving toes. Unpleasant sensations worse with weight-bearing indicate local foot pathology. Figure 12.2 shows an approach to patients with discomfort or unpleasant sensation in their feet. Erythromelalgia and painful legs moving toes are extremely rare.

The pain is worse with weight-bearing in non-neurological causes of pain in the feet. These include osteoarthritis in the ankle or joints of the feet, a calcaneal spur, metatarsalgia affecting the metatarsal bones under the balls of the foot and plantar fasciitis. The neurological causes of pain in the feet that can cause difficulty walking include Morton's neuroma and tarsal tunnel syndrome. Although the pain is worse with weight-bearing, subtle differences exist, such as the nature of the pain and altered sensation that occurs with the neurological causes to help differentiate the various entities. These will be discussed.

# Unpleasant Sensations at Rest that do not Cause Difficulty Walking

Restless legs syndrome (RLS) and burning feet are the two common conditions that cause unpleasant sensations in the feet and lower legs. They do not interfere with walking; in fact, the symptoms improve with walking with RLS and walking on a cold surface with burning feet.

## Restless legs syndrome

Restless legs syndrome [27–31] affects 5-10% of the population. It was first described by Thomas Willis in 1685. Karl Ekbom named it restless legs syndrome in 1945. [103] However, many patients complain that most doctors do not seem to be aware of the entity or know much about it. A more appropriate term is restless limbs syndrome because it can also affect the upper limbs in more severe cases, and, rarely, symptoms may be confined to the upper limbs.

The essential features of RLS are:
- Patients develop symptoms when they are not moving for prolonged periods, such as sitting at the dinner table, on an aeroplane, in a lecture or movie.
- Symptoms are particularly severe in bed at night.
- Patients find it very difficult to describe the nature of the symptoms except to say that they are unpleasant.[5]
- There is an irresistible urge to move the legs
- Patients cannot keep their limbs still because of this unpleasant sensation deep inside the limb, not over the surface or affecting the skin.
- The pain is in the feet, shins, calves, and often seems to cross joints not in the distribution of a single nerve, nerve root or in the pattern of peripheral neuropathy.
- Symptoms persist on and off for hours until patients are forced to move their legs.
- Although the symptoms can be either confined to or are more severe in one leg, both legs are usually affected.
- Patients invariably pace the floor at night to obtain relief, but, unlike burning feet syndrome, they do not need to walk on cold surfaces, and the symptoms are not relieved by moving the feet to where the sheets are colder.
- There are no symptoms during the day unless the patient sits down.
- Sleep is disturbed whether the patient is sleeping at night or during the day.
- The neurological examination of the affected limbs should be normal unless associated with peripheral neuropathy. In this setting, one may find absent ankle reflexes, weakness of dorsiflexion of the toes and feet and possible peripheral sensory loss affecting the distal aspect of the feet circumferentially up from the tip of the toes.

| International RLS Study Group (IRLSG) diagnostic criteria |
| --- |
| a. Desire to move the extremities usually associated with discomfort or disagreeable sensations in the extremities. |
| b. Motor Restlessness-patients move to relieve the discomfort, for example walking, or to provide a counter-stimulus to relieve the discomfort, for example, rubbing the legs. |
| c. Symptoms are worse at rest with at least temporary relief by activity. |
| d. Symptoms are worse later in the day or at night. |

---

5   One patient described it as one leg boxing the other all night. Others described aching, gnawing sensations.

The condition can occur at any age, although most patients will have experienced their first symptom before 30. It affects women more than men. The symptoms are more marked in the presence of renal failure, iron deficiency and pregnancy. Periodic limb movements (see below) occur in 80-90% of patients with RLS.

Conditions that may be confused with restless leg syndrome include peripheral vascular disease (PVD), *periodic limb movements, akathisia* and a curious entity called *painful legs and moving toes.*

| Management of Restless Legs Syndrome |
| --- |
| The **aetiology** of RLS is unclear, although there is a genetic factor with autosomal dominant and autosomal recessive inheritance. However, genome-wide association studies account for only a tiny proportion of the genetically determined susceptibility to RLS. No monogenic cause has been found. [31] Low levels of iron in the brain possibly related to impaired transport across the blood-brain barrier has been found, even in those with normal serum iron. [104] Neurotransmitter dysfunction, in particular, the dopaminergic system is thought to play a role but the mechanism is unknown.<br><br>As it is inherited as an autosomal dominant condition, a family history of RLS can be present in up to 90% of patients. Patients may not be aware of the specific name but can recall their parents or grandparents pacing the floor at night. Other patients will initially say that there is no other family member affected but, when sent away to enquire, discover one or more relatives who have the condition. In many but not all patients, involuntary jerking of the limbs referred to as myoclonus may occur. RLS symptoms increase in severity with increasing age and duration of the disease. |

| Treatment |
| --- |
| Exclude iron deficiency and renal failure. Prescribe iron supplements if iron deficiency is found. Abstinence from alcohol, caffeine, nicotine, and drugs that may exacerbate the problem is advocated. [32] Some patients can minimise their symptoms by either exercising just before retiring to bed or running several kilometres during the day. In most patients, such exercise is not practical, and drug therapy is necessary. [30]<br><br>Dopamine agonists such as Ropinirole, Rotigotine and Pramipexole are of proven efficacy and have been the recommended drugs of choice. [30, 33,35,36] Unfortunately, they can also cause impulse control disorders, such as compulsive gambling and daytime sleepiness. It is now realised that they cause augmentation of symptoms and should be avoided if possible.<br><br>The alpha$_2$delta ligands, Gabapentin and pregabalin are now regarded as first line options. Gabapentin enacarbil is an extended-release form. There is moderate evidence of efficacy.[31]<br><br>Other medications include benzodiazepines such as clonazepam [34], rotigotine transdermal patches [37], in severe cases opiates such as oxycodone [38] and in very severe cases methadone.[6] [39]<br><br>Antihistamine's, anti-nausea drugs, antidepressants, serotonergic reuptake inhibitors, neuroleptics, β blockers, some anticonvulsants, and lithium should be avoided as they can exacerbate symptoms of RLS. [89]<br><br>A small, short, randomised trial of dipyridamole demonstrated benefit with a reduction in the IRLSG severity scale. [102] |

# Periodic Limb Movements (PLM)

Periodic limb movement (PLM) share a similar pathophysiology and often respond to the same treatment as RLS. They are also one of the parasomnias and are diagnosed by polysomnography (sleep study). PLM is the repetitive movements of the legs, bilateral, simultaneous but not always symmetrical. The diagnostic criteria are at least four leg movements in a 90-s period and the severity is rated by the number of movements per hour with > 50 being severe. Contractions should be more than 0.5 seconds and less than 5 seconds. The feet and toes curl upwards. In the rare instances when the arms are involved, there is repetitive flexion of the elbows. [105]

---

6   Personal observations: In several patients with very severe restless leg syndrome methadone has provided significant benefit, although tachyphylaxis has occurred requiring increased doses. Methadone is approved by the Australian pharmaceutical benefits scheme on an authority prescription for the treatment of severe restless legs.

## Peripheral Vascular Disease (PVD)

The characteristic feature of PVD is exercise-induced leg pain relieved by rest, but occasionally it can cause pain at rest. The symptoms are confined to the lower limbs, and upper limb symptoms would exclude this diagnosis. The pain is in the feet and calves; very rarely, buttock pain can occur due to the involvement of the internal iliac artery. The peripheral pulses will be challenging to palpate with PVD.

## Akathisia

Akathisia consists of a distressing inner sense of restlessness with a desire to move not just the limbs but the entire body. Patients will rock back and forwards whilst standing or sitting, keep shifting their weight, shuffling, crossing and uncrossing legs, et cetera. It is seen in patients who have been exposed to dopamine antagonists. Whereas the unpleasant sensations associated with RLS are alleviated by walking or moving the limbs, patients with akathisia cannot obtain relief with movement.

| Treatment of Akathisia |
|---|
| Akathisia is drug-induced, particularly soon after commencing antipsychotic medications. It also occurs when antipsychotics are ceased, or the dose is reduced. [90] Early recognition is essential and either reducing the dose or discontinuing the antipsychotic altogether. Another strategy is to change to a newer antipsychotic medication with a perceived lower risk of akathisia, such as risperidone, clozapine, or olanzapine. Propranolol is the drug of choice to try and suppress akathisia. [20] |

## Painful Legs and Moving Toes

Painful legs and moving toes may develop in the setting of spinal cord and cauda equina trauma, lumbar root lesions, injuries to bony or soft tissues of the feet and peripheral neuropathy. It is not familial, is not thought to be related to RLS, and no cause can be established in most patients. [40]

It consists of the continuous or semi-continuous involuntary writhing movements of the toes associated with pain in the affected extremity. [41] Symptoms may begin on one side and become bilateral; movements may be momentarily suppressed by voluntary action or exacerbated by changing posture. [40] Pain preceding the movements was most commonly burning in nature. Movements consist of flexion/extension, abduction/adduction and fanning or clawing of toes/fingers and sometimes the foot or hand. [42] Surface electromyography (EMG) showed abnormalities suggestive of both chorea and dystonia. The movements are partially suppressible and diminished but still apparent during light sleep.

| Treatment of Painful legs and Moving Toes |
|---|
| Spontaneous resolution is rare. GABAergic agents such as pregabalin and gabapentin are most effective in controlling pain and movements. [42] |

## Burning feet syndrome

Patients with burning feet syndrome complain of an unpleasant burning sensation involving mainly the soles of the feet and occasionally the dorsal aspect of the feet and the legs below the knees that predominantly occurs in bed at night. They prefer to remove the bed covers and move their feet to where the sheets are colder or walk on cold surfaces for relief.

In some patients, burning feet occurs in the setting of a distal sensory peripheral neuropathy related to diabetes and alcohol. However, the examination does not reveal any abnormality in most patients. Nerve conduction studies should exclude large fibre neuropathy, they are normal in SFN. In most patients with burning feet, there is a small fibre neuropathy (SFN) with preferential damage to the small-diameter somatic and autonomic unmyelinated C-fibres and or thinly myelinated A-delta

317

fibres. Skin biopsy shows reduced epidermal neurite density within a 3-mm protein gene product 9.5 (PGP9.5)–immunolabeled lower-leg skin biopsy. [43] Quantitative sensory testing (QST) is recommended, but further study is required to determine the utility of new variations of QST on the diagnosis of SFN. Quantitative sudomotor axon reflex testing (QSART) is a measure of postganglionic sympathetic cholinergic function. It is abnormal in approximately ¾ of patients with SFN. [94]

---

**The aetiology of small fibre neuropathy**.

The reason for placing this in a text box is the suspicion that the aetiology, like many conditions, will change as more is understood about small fibre neuropathy. In as many as 50% of patients, no cause can be established. It is said to occur with:

- diabetes mellitus or impaired glucose tolerance detected either by oral glucose tolerance test [44] or an elevated HBA1c. The HBA1c is less sensitive but more specific in diagnosing diabetes.Some have raised doubt about the association between diabetes and small fibre neuropathy. [93]
- hypothyroidism. [45]
- HIV. [46]
- vitamin B deficiency such as thiamine (B1), riboflavin (B2), nicotinic acid (B3), pantothenic acid (B5) and cyanocobalamin (B12)

*Note:* Vitamin B deficiency may cause burning feet syndrome that may respond to replacement therapy, but the evidence for this is inadequate. [47]

SFN is a rapidly evolving field, and it is imperative to research the literature regularly. The spectrum of clinical conditions attributed to SFN extends well beyond simply burning feet syndrome. The reader can find more information in the excellent reviews by Levine [91} and Oaklander and Nolano. [97]

---

**Symptomatic Treatment of Burning Feet Syndrome**

In essence, there is only symptomatic treatment similar to that of treating neuropathic pain. Neuropathic pain medications include antidepressants (nortriptyline, amitriptyline, duloxetine, milnacipran, venlafaxine), anticonvulsants (gabapentin, pregabalin, lamotrigine, oxcarbazepine, carbamazepine, sodium valproate, lacosamide, zonisamide, topiramate), mexiletine, topical agents (capsaicin, lidocaine, other compound medications), opiates, and neuromodulation. The choice of the drug is based on safety profile, concomitant medication use, and other comorbidities.[95]

In addition, however other treatments include:

**Cold soaks**

Cold soaks are an effective symptomatic treatment for the significant burning, prickling, and tingling in the feet that occurs at night in bed. [47]

- Use cold tap water in a basin and leave the feet in it for 20 minutes.
- Take them out and dry them very thoroughly and use a lotion such as Vaseline Intensive Care massaged into the feet. Often this is needed a couple of times a day to gain good relief.
- In addition, a tricyclic antidepressant, such as amitriptyline or nortriptyline, at night can be used [48], starting with a small dosage and gradually building up to 50–75 mg.

A combination of foot soaking and amitriptyline is effective in the vast majority of patients.

**Aspirin lotion[7]**

Ingredients: 1 x 300-mL pump pack of sorbolene cream; 1 x 100-tablet pack of soluble aspirin (e.g. Disprin)

To make soluble aspirin lotion for skin application:

1. Pump 20 mL (1½ teaspoons) of sorbolene cream into a wide-mouthed glass receptacle or cup.
2. In a spoon dissolve two soluble aspirin in a few drops of water.
3. When the fizzing stops, mix very thoroughly into the sorbolene using a spoon handle in a stirring/beating motion.
4. Apply and rub this cream into the affected skin 3 times a day.

Every morning make a similar quantity for each day's use. Alternatively, aspirin tablets may be crushed to a powder and thoroughly mixed with the cream.

---

7   Aspirin lotion has been shown to be superior to oral aspirin for the burning pain of acute herpes zoster. [49] This recipe was found some years ago by the author who can no longer find the reference. It is an innocuous treatment without side effects and has been used with apparent good effect in patients with burning feet.

# Erythromelalgia

Patients with erythromelalgia complain of *episodic* erythema, intense burning pain, and warmth of the hands and or feet. The aetiology is uncertain, and fortunately, it is rare. When chronic, there is a significant disability. [50] Severe erythromelalgia may spread up the legs and arms, and it can even affect the ears and face. It may be unilateral or bilateral. Symptoms flare-up late in the day and continue overnight.

Erythromelalgia may be a syndrome of dysfunctional vascular dynamics (vasoconstriction and vasodilatation). [51] Exposure to warmth can trigger flaring and increase its severity; symptoms are relieved by cooling in ice water. Occasionally, it may be precipitated by immersing the affected area in hot water for 10–30 minutes. [51] Many patients have either small or large fibre neuropathy (quoted as unpublished data in the article by Kuhnert et al. [52]).

Primary erythromelalgia represents about 5% of patients and is an autosomal dominant disorder in some families. In these families, there are mutations in the gene for sodium channel Na(v)1.7, which is selectively expressed within nociceptive dorsal root ganglion and sympathetic ganglion neurons. Secondary erythromelalgia occurs with myeloproliferative disorders, neuropathies, and autoimmune diseases.

# Unpleasant Sensations in the Feet at Rest Causing Difficulty Walking

## Painful diabetic neuropathy

Diabetes is the commonest cause of peripheral neuropathy. Painful diabetic neuropathy occurs in approximately 16% of patients with diabetes. [106] If the painful diabetic neuropathy is secondary to a large fibre neuropathy objective weakness and sensory loss may cause difficulty walking. If the painful diabetic neuropathy is related to small fibre neuropathy, then this will not cause trouble walking. Patients describe tingling burning sensations, cramps, sharp pains, reduced sensation to pain and temperature. In some patients, there is hyperaesthesia (increased sensitivity to light touch causing discomfort).

| Treatment of painful diabetic neuropathy |
| --- |
| The AAN guidelines recommend four categories of oral medications. [107] These reduce but do not abolish pain. These include the tricyclic (TCAs) antidepressant (amitriptyline[8]), serotonin noradrenaline reuptake( SNRIs) inhibitors (duloxetine and desvenlafaxine), gabapentinoids (gabapentin, pregabalin and mirogabalin) and sodium channel blockers (valproic acid). There is no evidence to assist in the selection of any particular drug. The guidelines stress treating any accompanying depression or sleep disorders, which can influence pain perception. In this setting, TCAs and SNRIs. The guidelines also recommend a combination of SNRI/opioid dual mechanism agents[9] (tapentadol, tramadol). |
| Nonpharmacological approaches include cognitive behaviour therapy, Tai Chi, and mindfulness. Topical therapies include capsaicin, glyceryl trinitrate spray, Citrullus colocynthis and Ginkgo biloba. |

---

8   Although the guidelines state that there is no class evidence affect, my preference is to use nortriptyline as the 25 mg tablet can be cut in half. (I commence with 12.5 mg per day and increasing very gradually by 12.5 mg per day until the minimum effective dose or the maximum tolerated dose, usually 75-100 mg per day.

9   Painful diabetic neuropathy is a lifelong illness and in my opinion opioids should be avoided because of the risk of dependence.

## Tarsal tunnel syndrome

Tarsal tunnel syndrome (TTS) is a controversial entity, and management remains challenging. [96] The posterior tibial nerve is compressed under the flexor retinaculum in the tarsal tunnel, inferior and posterior to the medial malleolus at the ankle. Although it is said to be underdiagnosed, TTS is much rarer than most medical practitioners think[10].

The symptoms consist of:
- Tingling and numbness that MUST be confined to the sole within the distribution of either the medial and or lateral plantar nerves (see Figure 1.21, chapter 1). *Symptoms on the top of the foot excludes the diagnosis.*
- Burning paraesthesia and pain described as sharp, shooting, shock-like or electric radiating either proximally or distally on the sole.
- The symptoms worsen after prolonged standing or walking. [53]
- The symptoms are more intense at the end of the day. Rest and leg elevation can relieve the symptoms.
- Symptoms do not awaken the patient from sleep.
- Rarely, pain confined to the soles of the foot may also occur at rest and in non-weight-bearing positions. [54]
- A positive Tinel's sign with a tapping of the nerve behind the medial malleolus producing tingling into the sole(s) would be diagnostic but is rare. Altered sensation within the distribution of the medial and or lateral plantar nerves is rarely seen.
- Turning the dorsiflexed foot outwards is another provocative test and may precipitate symptoms,

The diagnosis of TTS may be difficult as the symptoms are often vague, as are the physical findings and signs. Bilateral cases are seen occasionally. There is often a long delay in diagnosis of up to 2½ years. [55]

---

**Management of Tarsal Tunnel Syndrome**

The entrapment neuropathy of TTS and its treatment is controversial. Nerve conduction studies are of uncertain value due to the lack of definitive studies and a gold-standard for the diagnosis. There are high false-negative and false-positive rates.[98] Their value is in excluding peripheral neuropathy. The AANEM consensus statement [56] lists the following diagnostic abnormalities in tarsal tunnel syndrome:
An increased distal motor latency over the abductor hallucis and abductor digiti minimi.
Slowed medial and lateral mixed plantar nerve conduction studies across the tarsal tunnel and
Slowed medial and lateral plantar sensory nerve conductions.
Symptoms and signs, operative findings and response to therapy define most cases of TTS reported in the literature. [56] Ultrasound may demonstrate fusiform thickening and loss of the typical vesicular pattern of the tibial nerve. MRI scan can identify the cause of tarsal tunnel. Apart from space-occupying, lesions may show an increased size and signal in the tibial nerve and denervation oedema of the plantar muscles of the foot. However, in most patients, the nerve appears normal on imaging. [98] Many pathologies have been reported with MRI scans [57], although most are idiopathic in origin.
Surgical treatment consists of neurolysis of the tibial nerve in the tarsal tunnel and neurolysis of the medial, lateral plantar, calcaneal nerves in their respective tunnels. Immediate postoperative mobilisation of the posterior tibial nerve through ambulation can achieve a good or excellent outcome in >90% of cases. [58]

---

10 Personal observation based on the number of referrals for nerve conduction studies looking for tarsal tunnel syndrome in patients who have any vague symptom in their feet

# Morton's neuroma and metatarsalgia

Morton's neuroma is perineural fibrosis with thickening and degeneration of an interdigital nerve of the foot. The most commonly affected nerves are between the 3rd and 4th and less commonly the 2nd and 3rd metatarsal heads.

- Patients complain that it feels like a stone or pebble in their shoes.
- There is the gradual onset of pain whilst walking with sudden attacks of throbbing, burning pain and paraesthesia on the *plantar surface of the foot* localised to the webspace that radiates to the corresponding toes.
- It is not associated with altered sensation as opposed to pain of neurological origin.
- Pain is minimal or absent when sitting or lying, in contrast to a calcaneal spur and plantar fasciitis.
- The clue to the diagnosis is that the pain is aggravated by wearing tight shoes and may be relieved by massage to the forefoot and toes. [59]
- There is a localised area of reproducible tenderness between the metatarsal heads.

It occurs most commonly in middle-aged women. Occasional bilateral cases arise. If the pain is severe, it can create difficulties walking because of the pain, referred to as the antalgic gait. A characteristic limp with a very short stance phase may be adopted to avoid pain on weight-bearing structures.

| Management of Morton's Neuroma |
| --- |
| In patients with suspected Morton's neuroma, an ultrasound is more sensitive (85vs 68%) than an MRI scan. It may detect an ovoid, hypoechoic mass located just proximal to the metatarsal heads in the intermetatarsal space in >90% of patients. [60] Current treatment recommendations include modifying the activities that cause pain, anti-inflammatory drugs, avoiding narrow tight and high-heeled shoes, orthotics and icing the inflamed area. In unresponsive cases, local anaesthetic and hydrocortisone injections around the nerve, radiofrequency ablation or surgical excision of neuroma may be necessary. Surgery is said to be more successful with a single neuroma and multiple neuromas. [59], There are no randomised trial results to support this. [61] |

Metatarsalgia is a common overuse injury. It is a common presentation, particularly in middle-aged women and is often confused with Morton's neuroma. The main symptom of metatarsalgia is pain at the end the 2nd, 3rd and 4th metatarsal heads (the ball of the foot). There is the insidious onset of pain over months, either sharp or dull and at times burning in nature. Once again the patient feels like they are walking on a pebble in the pain is exacerbated by walking and running. This pain usually results from disruption of the normal transverse arch created at the region of the metatarsal heads with support from the transmetatarsal ligaments. Conservative management involves modification footwear, use of orthotics and physical therapy. [111-112]

# Calcaneal spur

A calcaneal spur causes:
- sharp, stabbing chronic *heel pain,* particularly in overweight patients [62]
- characteristically worse in the morning
- tenderness to firm palpation at the distal aspect of the heel where the tendon inserts into the calcaneus bone.

Calcaneal spurs can occur in some patients with plantar fasciitis.

## Plantar Fasciitis

Plantar fasciitis is the most common cause of pain on the sole. It is more common in runners, particularly as they increase the distances they run, obesity, and those on their feet most of the day. The condition is self-limiting in most patients and resolves within 12 months. [63]

### Symptoms

- Pain is in the sole.
- Pain is worse when standing after periods of rest or on taking the first steps in the morning.
- The pain improves only to worsen again later in the day after prolonged weight-bearing.
- Nocturnal pain is *not* a feature of plantar fasciitis.
- The pain is searing, throbbing, or piercing, *not* burning or shooting.
- There is tenderness over the origin of the plantar fascia and the anteromedial aspect of the heel.

---

**Treatment for Plantar Fasciitis**

Various treatment regimens have been recommended, but there is no scientific evidence to help guide the choice of a particular therapy.
- First-line treatment consists of the combination of a viscous-elastic heel pad, a stretching program, NSAIDs and a tension night splint. [64]
- Extracorporeal shockwave therapy is also recommended. [65]
- Combined local corticosteroid injections may be given in the form of triamcinolone 2 mL and using a peppering (injecting, withdrawing, redirecting, and reinserting without emerging from the skin) technique. [66]
- Retrospective studies have claimed improvement with surgery in patients who have failed to improve with conservative measures. [67]

---

# Weakness and or Sensory Loss in the Lower Leg
# Foot Drop

A foot drop can result from:
- an L5 radiculopathy
- a lumbosacral plexus problem
- a sciatic nerve problem
- a common peroneal (also called the common fibular) nerve lesion
- a peripheral neuropathy.

A careful examination to establish the pattern of weakness can help differentiate the various causes. The 2*2*4 rule at the end of this chapter can enable anyone to diagnose the cause without detailed knowledge of neuroanatomy.

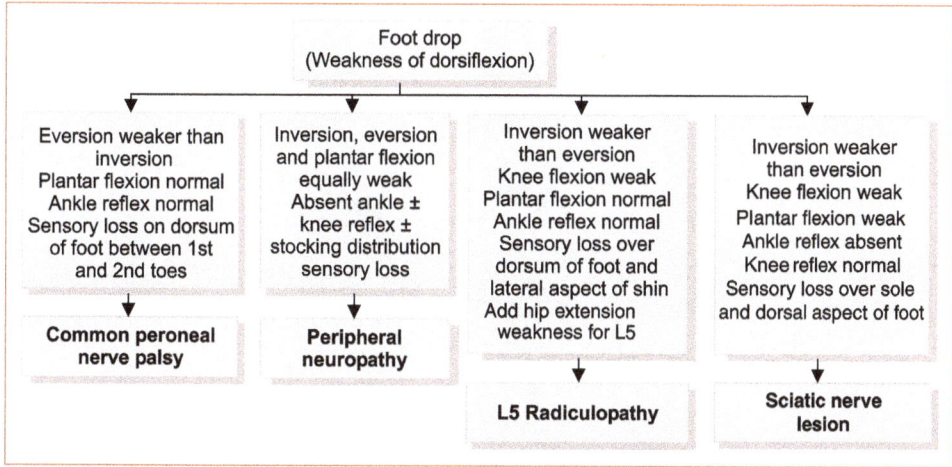

**Figure 12.3** The patterns of weakness that help to differentiate the various causes of foot drop

Figure 12.3 lists the features that help to differentiate the various causes of a foot drop. Figure 12.4 shows how to test these muscles. The crucial thing to note is that the posterior tibialis and anterior tibialis muscles invert the foot at the ankle. The posterior tibialis tendon can be seen and palpated behind, and the anterior tibialis tendon in the front of the medial malleolus (Figure 12.4C).

The neuroanatomy explains the signs:
- Foot drop or weakness of dorsiflexion of the foot relates to the weakness of the anterior tibialis and extensor digitorum muscles. These muscles are supplied by the common peroneal (fibular) nerve, a lateral branch of the sciatic nerve that arises in the popliteal fossa and traverses the neck of the fibula, a common site for compression. The 5th lumbar nerve root (L5) is the primary innervation of these muscles.
- The peroneii muscles evert the foot and are innervated by the common peroneal nerve and the L5 nerve root.
- Inversion of the foot results from the combined action of the anterior and posterior tibialis muscles, both supplied by the L5 nerve root, but the tibialis posterior is supplied by the posterior tibial nerve and the tibialis anterior by the common peroneal nerve.

## Common peroneal (fibular) nerve lesion

A common peroneal nerve lesion at the neck of the fibula is the commonest cause of a foot drop. It is often related to trauma, compression during surgery, in comatose patients, prolonged squatting and in thin patients occasionally occurs in their sleep. In some patients, aetiology cannot be established. [68] In the compressive group, the prognosis for spontaneous recovery is excellent. [68]

Compression can occur during sleep. Here the patient steps out of bed and almost falls due to the weakness of dorsiflexion of the foot. The neurological signs are listed in Figure 12.3. Isolated deep peroneal nerve involvement causes sensory loss limited to the space between the 1st and 2nd toes on the dorsal aspect of the foot. More extensive sensory loss on the dorsum of the foot and lateral aspect of the distal half of the lower leg) is seen when the superficial peroneal nerve is also affected (see Figure 1.19, chapter 1).

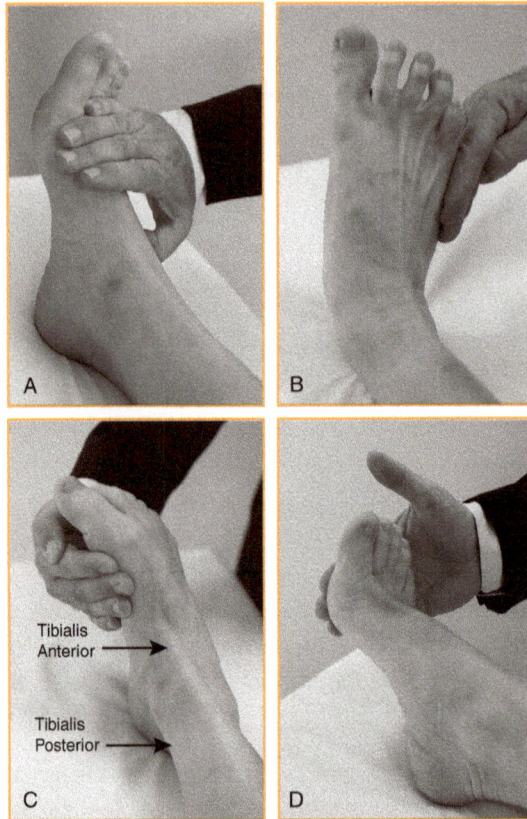

**Figure 12.4** Testing **A** dorsiflexion, note the foot is slightly plantar flexed **B** eversion and **C** inversion of the foot, **D** plantar flexion. When testing inversions and eversion it is best to place the foot in the appropriate position and ask the patient to prevent you from turning the foot in the opposite direction.

# Sciatic nerve lesion

Sciatic nerve lesions are infrequent and usually result from posterior dislocation fracture of the hip or as a complication of total hip joint replacement. They have also been reported as a complication following coronary artery bypass surgery when patients were sat upright while still unconscious. [69]

The neurological signs are listed in Figure 12.3. As opposed to L5 radiculopathy, hip extension is normal. The sensory loss involves the L5 and S1 dermatomes over the lateral aspect of the shin, dorsum, the lateral part of the foot on the plantar surface and the calf.

# L5 radiculopathy

Lumbar nerve root compression is a common cause of leg pain with or without a foot drop. Occasionally patients present with painless radiculopathy. [70] The neurological signs are listed in Figure 12.3. If a sensory loss occurs, it is within the distribution of the 5th lumbar nerve root distribution (see Figure 1.22, chapter 1).

# Peripheral neuropathy

The list of causes of peripheral neuropathy is long and well beyond the scope of this book. Readers can consult more definitive texts. [71] Earlier in this chapter, we referred to significant hip flexion weakness related to the inflammatory demyelinating and IgA and IgG related peripheral neuropathies.

Other causes of peripheral neuropathy typically present with weakness and or sensory loss commencing in the toes ascending from the toes up the foot and leg as the condition worsens. These neuropathies are called length-dependent (because the abnormalities appear first in the longest nerves). The commonest causes are alcohol, where weakness predominates, and diabetes, where distal symmetrical stocking distribution sensory loss is the main clinical feature.

Vitamin $B_{12}$ deficiency is rare, and in most cases, readily diagnosed and treatable. Peripheral neuropathy due to vitamin $B_{12}$ deficiency was recognised in 1958. [99] $B_{12}$ deficiency causes an axonal peripheral neuropathy. The neuropathy is overshadowed by the signs of subacute combined degeneration of the spinal cord that is the cause of the difficulty walking. There is marked vibration and proprioceptive loss in the lower limbs, resulting in significant ataxia and clumsiness exacerbated with eye closure or in the dark. It looks like peripheral neuropathy because the reflexes are absent. The clue is the presence of upgoing plantar responses with absent reflexes. A pattern also seen with Friedreich's ataxia, tabes dorsalis and lesions that affect both the lower end of the spinal cord (conus medullaris) and the descending cauda equina.

The leading cause of B12 deficiency is pernicious anaemia, but it can occur with nitrous oxide poisoning. A normal or only slightly reduced serum $B_{12,}$ the absence of anaemia and normal (not elevated) methylmalonic acid (MMA) or homocysteine levels even with a low $B_{12}$ does not exclude symptomatic $B_{12}$ deficiency. [92] Elevated MMA and homocysteine levels can occur with renal failure. A high homocysteine level is non-specific. It can also occur with folate and $B_6$ deficiency, hypothyroidism, and certain drugs such as metformin, methotrexate, niacin, cholestyramine, and the oral contraceptive pill. [100]

Similar signs occur in paraneoplastic and Sjögren's related neuropathy. The most prevalent symptoms of vitamin $B_{12}$ deficiency are neurologic, such as paraesthesia in hands and feet, muscle cramps, dizziness, cognitive disturbances, ataxia, and erectile dysfunction, as well as fatigue, psychiatric symptoms like depression,

IgM paraprotein related neuropathy is a length-dependent demyelinating neuropathy. Distal sensory loss and paraesthesia and or dysaesthesia predominate with slight weakness.

There are many ways to classify the peripheral neuropathies:

- One way is to differentiate between mononeuropathy (single nerve), multiple single nerves (mononeuritis multiplex), and diffuse peripheral nervous system involvement. In this section, the peripheral neuropathies with diffuse involvement are discussed.
- A second way is how rapidly they evolve—differentiating between acute onset over days to weeks, subacute with onset over months and chronic onset over years.
- A third method is the use of nerve conduction studies. These differentiate between axonal (affecting the axons) and demyelinating (involving the myelin) neuropathies. In the case of demyelinating neuropathies, whether there is uniform slowing or conduction block (see additional information in Table 12.1 below).

Most neuropathies have both an axonal and demyelinating component.

| Management of Patients with Suspected Peripheral Neuropathy |
| --- |
| The initial investigation should be NCS and EMG (Table 12.1). These will confirm the presence of peripheral neuropathy and should help characterise whether it is axonal, demyelinating, or mixed axonal and demyelinating. Conduction block (see definition below) on NCS indicates a demyelinating neuropathy in keeping with the acute and chronic inflammatory demyelinating neuropathies (AIDP, CIDP) or multifocal motor neuropathy with conduction block. If peripheral neuropathy is confirmed, the following screening investigations would be appropriate:<br>• Random blood glucose, HbA1c or GTT<br>• Vitamin B$_{12}$ and folate, thyroid function, and liver function tests<br>• Immunoglobulin quantitation and protein electrophoresis<br>• Bence–Jones proteins.<br>• Anti-MAG and Celiac disease antibodies and HIV when indicated |

In clinical practice, peripheral neuropathy most commonly relates to diabetes or alcohol in western societies; a common cause worldwide is leprosy. Other more common causes include AIDP, CIDP, neuropathy related to monoclonal gammopathies such as IgG, IgM and IgA, drug-related neuropathy, uraemia, familial neuropathy. Although relatively rare, vitamin B$_{12}$ deficiency should not be missed.

- There are many other causes, including hereditary, toxic, metabolic, infectious (including HIV), inflammatory, ischaemic, and paraneoplastic disorders. Occasionally, patients may present with peripheral neuropathy in the setting of malignancy; more often, the neuropathy appears after the diagnosis of the malignancy, and the difficulty is to differentiate neuropathy related to drug therapy of the malignancy and paraneoplastic neuropathy.

- In approximately 20% of patients, a cause may not be established. Careful family history and examination of near relatives (including NCS) will detect familial neuropathy in nearly half of the patients where the initial assessment fails to elucidate the cause.

Currently, peripheral neuropathies are classified as either demyelinating or axonal, mainly based on the results of NCS. [72, 73]

The features on NCS and EMG of demyelinating versus axonal neuropathies are shown in Table 12.1

|  | Demyelinating | Axonal |
| --- | --- | --- |
| **NCS** |  |  |
| **Amplitude of motor response** | Normal or mildly reduced | Markedly reduced |
| **Conduction velocity** | Very slow | Normal or mildly reduced |
| **Conduction block*** | Yes | No |
| **Temporal dispersion**** | Present | Absent |
| **Distal motor latency** | Prolonged | Not prolonged |
| **Absent response** | No | Possible |
| **f-wave latencies** | Prolonged | Not prolonged |
| **EMG** |  |  |
|  | No denervation | Denervation ± reinnervation |

Table 12.1 Electrophysiological findings in axonal vs demyelinating neuropathy. *Conduction block is a >50% reduction in the amplitude of the motor response in a nerve not at a site where it would be predisposed to compression. An absent response with distal stimulation can be a feature of conduction block. The definition varies, but a greater than 50% reduction **Temporal dispersion refers to a reduction in the amplitude and an increase in the duration of the motor response at a more proximal site of stimulation compared to the distal response.

In patients with an acute onset neuropathy, e.g. AIDP, abnormalities on EMG (the study of muscle using a concentric needle electrode) may not be evident for up to 3 weeks although, are usually manifest within 7–10 days of onset of the illness). EMG detects denervation with increased insertional (as the needle enters the muscle) activity, spontaneous activity in the form of fibrillation potentials and positive sharp waves with a reduced recruitment pattern (the diminished number of motor units recruited with voluntary contraction of the muscle) in patients with axonal damage. Fasciculations may be seen but are not synonymous with denervation.

# Diabetes and the Peripheral Nervous System

Diabetes is one of the most common medical problems and it can affect the nervous system in many ways.

### Acute neuropathies
- Diabetic amyotrophy with proximal weakness and pain in the legs
- Third nerve palsy, not involving the pupil
- Truncal neuropathy with pain radiating around the lateral chest and abdominal wall toward the mid-line with sensory loss extending laterally from the mid-line anteriorly

### Chronic neuropathies
- Distal sensory loss to pain and temperature that gradually ascends from the tips of the toes to the feet and legs with increasing duration of diabetes
- Autonomic neuropathy with postural hypotension, anhidrosis, nocturnal diarrhoea, hypothermia, dry eyes and mouth, impotence in males and bladder atony

Chronic proximal motor neuropathy

# Pain in the lower leg
## Radiculopathy

Sciatica (also referred to as radiculopathy) refers to pain from compression of the nerve root, most commonly L5 or S1, less often L2, L3 or L4. Lumbar nerve root compression is a common cause of leg pain, and L5 radiculopathy accounts for 75% and L4 for 15% of these cases.

## Symptoms
- Patients present with severe pain radiating down the back of the thigh to the lateral aspect of the shin to the dorsum of the foot with L5 radiculopathy. The pain is over the medial part of the lower leg with L4 radiculopathy.
- Pain-related to a disc herniation is exacerbated by bending forward, sitting, coughing, or straining and is relieved by lying down or rarely walking. Pain can occur in the absence of any weakness or sensory symptoms.
- Weakness with L5 radiculopathy affects dorsiflexion of the foot, inversion, and eversion of the ankle but not plantarflexion of the foot. Inversion is weaker than eversion. Plantar flexion is normal.
- The area of sensory loss, if present, affects the lateral aspect of the shin and dorsal surface of the foot.

- Many patients with sciatica-like pain radiating from the buttock down to above the knee have no evidence of nerve root compression, and in many patients the aetiology of this pain is unclear. Facet joint disease can produce pain radiating down the leg to no further than the knee. There is a controversial entity called piriformis syndrome, where the sciatic nerve is compressed by the piriformis muscle located in the buttock near the top of the hip joint. [113] The diagnostic criteria include pain with straight leg raising at 45° (Lasègue sign), tenderness at the sciatic notch, increased pain in the sciatic distribution with flexion, adduction, internal rotation of the hip (the FAIR manoeuvre) and electrodiagnostic studies that exclude myopathy or neuropathy.

---

**Management of Sciatica**

Sciatica usually resolves within 12 months in 95% of patients [75] without surgery. If back pain is the primary complaint with little leg pain, back surgery is less likely to relieve back pain symptoms. These patients are best treated conservatively with exercise and cognitive behaviour treatment. [75, 76] Even in patients with predominantly leg pain, the pain may settle with rest, NSAIDs, acetaminophen, skeletal muscle relaxants (for acute low back pain) or tricyclic antidepressants (for chronic low back pain). The anecdotal observation that oral corticosteroids appear to benefit has not been substantiated. [77, 78] Surgical decompression provides better pain relief and improved function in carefully selected patients with spondylolisthesis compared to nonsurgical management. [101]

---

# Exercise-induced leg pain

When a patient says they have pain in the legs, the most critical question often not asked is precisely where the patient is experiencing the pain. Pain confined to the joints exacerbated by weight-bearing or by the movement of the affected joint indicates local pathology within the joint such as arthritis. The diagnosis of acute arthritis is not tricky when associated with swelling, tenderness, redness, and heat emanating from the joint. In long-standing arthritis, there may be associated deformity of the joint; on the other hand, the joints will look normal in most patients presenting for the first time with arthritis. If the pain relates to arthritis, it should be reproduced when the joint is moved during the examination. There may also be a crackling sensation termed crepitus in the affected joint on movement. [79]

---

Localised pain and tenderness in the leg indicates local pathology,
not referred pain from the back.

---

# Lumbar Canal Stenosis vs PVD
## Pain symptoms

The pain resulting from peripheral vascular disease (PVD) and lumbar canal stenosis (also termed cauda equina claudication) are both precipitated by exercise and relieved by rest. What differentiates these two causes of pain is shown in figure 12.5.

- In both, the pain is in the calves, not the joints. It is precipitated by walking and promptly relieved by resting or sitting down.
- The pain from lumbar canal stenosis resolves when the patient lies flat and may be precipitated by simply standing or even sitting.

- Rarely, patients with PVD and severe ischaemia may experience leg pain at rest where the pain of the same intensity lying, sitting, and standing.
- Leg pain exacerbated by an alteration in posture indicates probable lumbar canal stenosis.

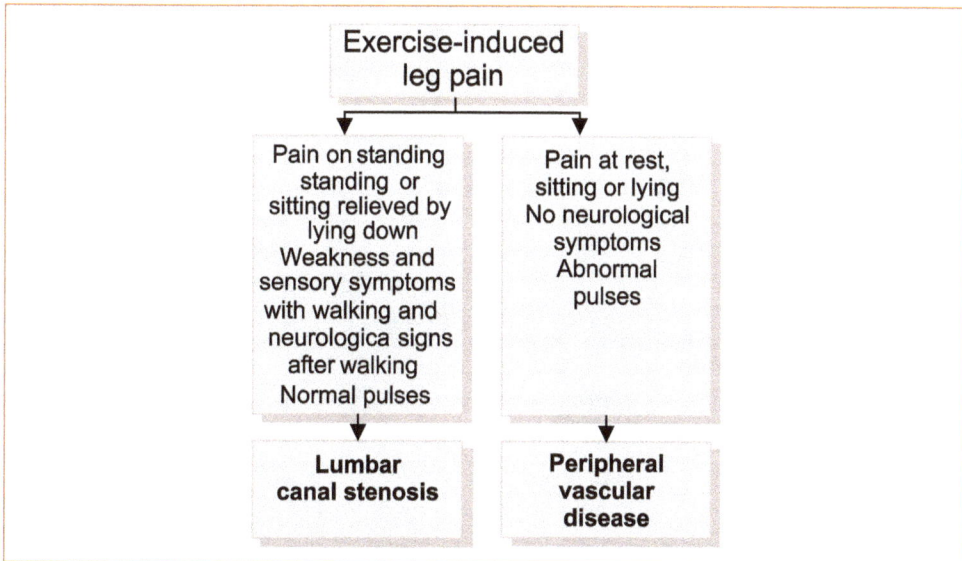

**Figure 12.5** Organisational chart showing the different features of peripheral vascular disease versus lumbar canal stenosis

- The occurrence of exercise-induced neurological symptoms relieved by rest in addition to the exercise-induced leg pain indicates that the pain is secondary to lumbar canal stenosis. The associated neurological symptoms include paraesthesia or numbness in the feet and/or the development of weakness (a foot drop).
- Much less commonly, the pain may be in the genital region, resulting in priapism or vulval pain. The clue to the diagnosis of vulval pain or priapism secondary to lumbar canal stenosis is that the pain is exacerbated by sitting, standing, or walking and relieved by either lying flat or the cessation of walking. Symptoms in the genital region indicate involvement of the sacral nerve roots.
- The pain of lumbar canal stenosis is usually but not always associated with low back pain, whereas the pain of PVD is not. In both conditions, there may the associated buttock pain. In patients with PVD, this relates to disease in the internal iliac vessels.

## Examination

Examination of the lower limbs can differentiate between these two entities:

- In patients with PVD, the peripheral pulses, particularly in the feet, are diminished or absent.
- Often, but not invariably, in patients with lumbar canal stenosis, the ankle reflexes are absent. However, this is not always a helpful sign as many elderly patients have absent ankle reflexes as a normal finding. It is often helpful to send the patient for a walk to induce symptoms and examine them immediately while the symptoms are still present. The development of neurological signs with exercise, in particular sensory loss in the feet, loss of reflexes that were present before activity and the presence of weakness, in particular dorsiflexion of the feet, is strong evidence for a diagnosis of lumbar canal stenosis.

329

# The 2*2*4 Rule for Examining the Lower Limb

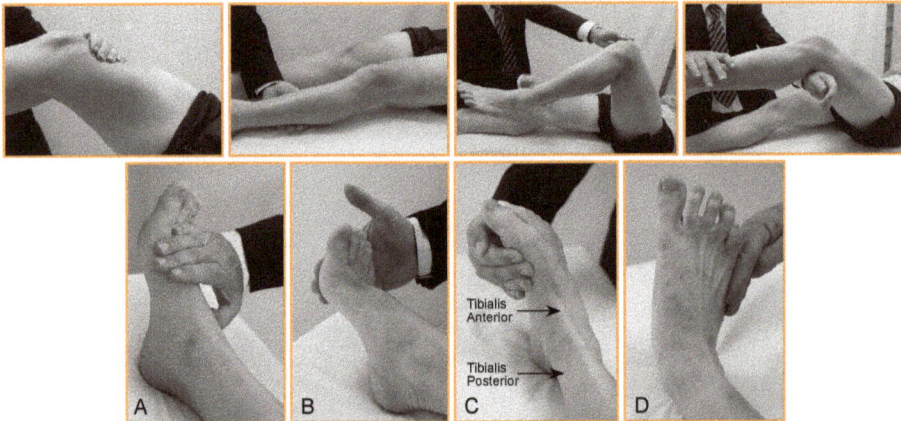

**Figure 12.6** The 2 "muscles" at the hip -flexion & extension) and knee -flexion & extension(top panel) and the 4 muscles at the foot-dorsiflexion, plantarflexion, inversion & eversion (lower panel)

The 2*2*4 rule for examining the lower limbs has been created since the 1st edition. Similar to the 5*3*5 rule of the upper limbs, it should enable the diagnosis of all peripheral nerve and nerve root problems that cause weakness in the lower limbs without the necessity of knowing detailed neuroanatomy.

It does require knowledge of how to correctly examine the muscles (Figure 12.6) to detect weakness when present and not to "detect" weakness when there is none. i.e. a false positive test. Once the weak muscles are defined simply consult table 12.2.

|  | Femoral Nerve | Common Peroneal | Sciatic Nerve | L5 Radiculopathy | UMN * Pattern |
|---|---|---|---|---|---|
| 1 Hip Flexion | Yes | No | No | No | Yes (1st) |
| 2 Hip Extension | No | No | No | Yes | No |
| 1 Knee Flexion | No | No | Yes | Yes | Yes (3rd) |
| 2 Knee Extension | Yes | No | No | No | No |
| 1 Dorsiflexion | No | Yes | Yes | Yes | Yes (2nd) |
| 2 Plantar Flexion | No | No | Yes | No | No |
| 3 Inversion | No | Mild | Yes | Yes | No |
| 4 Eversion | No | Yes | Yes | Mild | No |

**Table 12.2:** The two muscles at the hip, two muscles at the knee and four muscles at the ankle. Yes=weakness, No=no weakness. In patients with an upper motor neurone *(UMN) problem reflecting involvement of the central nervous, a specific pattern of weakness evolves with increasing severity. In the lower limb, the first muscle to become weak is hip flexion, followed by weakness of dorsiflexion of the foot and finally knee flexion. All muscles will be severely weak with a total paralysis (plegia) of the leg.* UMN= upper motor neurone (a central nervous system problem).

Partial weakness that equally affects all muscle groups
usually reflects a non-organic neurological problem.

# References

1   Chou R, et al. Imaging strategies for low-back pain: Systematic review and meta-analysis. *Lancet* 2009;373(9662):463–472.

2   Avrahami E, et al. Early MR demonstration of spinal metastases in patients with normal radiographs and CT and radionuclide bone scans. *J Comput Assist Tomogr* 1989;13(4):598–602.

3   Algra PR, et al. Detection of vertebral metastases: Comparison between MR imaging and bone scintigraphy. *RadioGraphics* 1991;11:219–232.

4   Madigan L, et al. Management of symptomatic lumbar degenerative disk disease. *J Am Acad Orthop Surg* 2009;17(2):102–111.

5   Malmivaara A, et al. The treatment of acute low back pain — bed rest, exercises, or ordinary activity?. *N Engl J Med* 1995;332(6):351–355.

6   Assendelft WJ, et al. Spinal manipulative therapy for low back pain. *Cochrane Database Syst Rev* 2004(1):CD000447.

7   van Tulder MW, Gagnier JJ, Furlan AD. Complementary and alternative therapies for low back pain. *Best Pract Res Clin Rheumatol* 2005;19(4):639–654.

8   Waller B, Lambeck J, Daly D. Therapeutic aquatic exercise in the treatment of low back pain: A systematic review. *Clin Rehabil* 2009;23(1):3–14.

9   Haim A, et al. Meralgia paresthetica: A retrospective analysis of 79 patients evaluated and treated according to a standard algorithm. *Acta Orthop* 2006;77(3):482–486.

10  Khalil N, Nicotra A, Rakowicz W. Treatment for meralgia paraesthetica. *Cochrane Database Syst Rev* 2008(3):CD004159.

11  Ducic I, Dellon AL, Taylor NS. Decompression of the lateral femoral cutaneous nerve in the treatment of meralgia paresthetica. *J Reconstr Microsurg* 2006;22(2):113–118.

12  Krendel DA, Zacharias A, Younger DS. Autoimmune diabetic neuropathy. *Neurol Clin* 1997;15(4): 959–971.

13  Sander HW, Chokroverty S. Diabetic amyotrophy: Current concepts. *Semin Neurol* 1996;16(2): 173–178.

14  Said G, et al. Painful proximal diabetic neuropathy: Inflammatory nerve lesions and spontaneous favorable outcome. *Ann Neurol* 1997;41(6):762–770.

15  Ogawa T, et al. Intravenous immunoglobulin therapy for diabetic amyotrophy. *Intern Med* 2001;40(4):349–352.

16  Courtney AE, McDonnell GV, Patterson VH. Human immunoglobulin for diabetic amyotrophy — a promising prospect?. *Postgrad Med J* 2001;77(907):326–328.

17  Salvarani C, Cantini F, Hunder GG. Polymyalgia rheumatica and giant-cell arteritis. *Lancet* 2008;372(9634):234–245.

18  Salvarani C, et al. Polymyalgia rheumatica and giant cell arteritis: A 5-year epidemiologic and clinical study in Reggio Emilia,. *Italy. Clin Exp Rheumatol* 1987;5(3):205–215.

19  Le Quintrec JS, Le Quintrec JL. Drug-induced myopathies. *Baillieres Clin Rheumatol* 1991;5(1):21–38.

20  Kuncl RW, George EB. Toxic neuropathies and myopathies. *Curr Opin Neurol* 1993;6(5):695–704.

21  Wiendl H. Idiopathic inflammatory myopathies: Current and future therapeutic options. *Neurotherapeutics* 2008;5(4):548–557.

22  Walker UA. Imaging tools for the clinical assessment of idiopathic inflammatory myositis. *Curr Opin Rheumatol* 2008;20(6):656–661.

23  Choy EH, et al. Immunosuppressant and immunomodulatory treatment for dermatomyositis and polymyositis. *Cochrane Database Syst Rev* 2005(3):CD003643.

24  Tran HA. Thyrotoxic periodic paralysis. *Mayo Clin Proc* 2005;80(7):960–961:author reply 961.

25  Lichtstein DM, Arteaga RB. Rhabdomyolysis associated with hyperthyroidism. *Am J Med Sci* 2006;332(2):103–105.

26  Tuncel D, et al. Hoffmann's syndrome: A case report. *Med Princ Pract* 2008;17(4):346–348.

27  Ekbom KA. Restless legs; a report of 70 new cases. *Acta Med Scand Suppl* 1950;246:64–68.

28  Satija P, Ondo WG. Restless legs syndrome: Pathophysiology, diagnosis and treatment. *CNS Drugs* 2008;22(6):497–518.

29  Benes H, et al. Definition of restless legs syndrome, how to diagnose it, and how to differentiate it from RLS mimics. *Mov Disord* 2007;22(Suppl18):S401–S408.

30  Oertel WH, et al. State of the art in restless legs syndrome therapy: Practice recommendations for treating restless legs syndrome. *Mov Disord* 2007;22(Suppl18):S466–S475.

31  *BMJ* 2017; **356**: j104.

32  Silber MH, et al. An algorithm for the management of restless legs syndrome. *Mayo Clin Proc* 2004;79(7):916–922.

33  Conti CF, et al. Levodopa for idiopathic restless legs syndrome: Evidence-based review. *Mov Disord* 2007;22(13):1943–1951.

34  Wagner ML, et al. Randomised, double-blind, placebo-controlled study of clonidine in restless legs syndrome. *Sleep* 1996;19(1):52–58.

35  Ferini-Strambi L, et al. Effect of pramipexole on RLS symptoms and sleep: A randomised, double-blind, placebo-controlled trial. *Sleep Med* 2008;9(8):874–881.

36  Bliwise DL, et al. Randomised, double-blind, placebo-controlled, short-term trial of ropinirole in restless legs syndrome. *Sleep Med* 2005;6(2):141–147.

37  Trenkwalder C, et al. Efficacy of rotigotine for treatment of moderate-to-severe restless legs syndrome: A randomised, double-blind, placebo-controlled trial. *Lancet Neurol* 2008;7(7):595–604.

38  Walters AS, et al. Successful treatment of the idiopathic restless legs syndrome in a randomised double-blind trial of oxycodone versus placebo. *Sleep* 1993;16(4):327–332.

39  Ondo WG. Methadone for refractory restless legs syndrome. *Mov Disord* 2005;20(3):345–348.

40  Dressler D, et al. The syndrome of painful legs and moving toes. *Mov Disord* 1994;9(1):13–21.

41  Walters AS, et al. Painless legs and moving toes: A syndrome related to painful legs and moving toes?. *Mov Disord* 1993;8(3):377–379.

42  Alvarez MV, et al. Case series of painful legs and moving toes: Clinical and electrophysiologic observations. *Mov Disord* 2008;23(14):2062–2066.

43  Tavee J, Zhou L. Small fiber neuropathy: A burning problem. *Cleve Clin J Med* 2009;76(5):297–305.

44  Singleton JR, Smith AG, Bromberg MB. Increased prevalence of impaired glucose tolerance in patients with painful sensory neuropathy. *Diabetes Care* 2001;24(8):1448–1453.

45  Penza P, et al. Painful neuropathy in subclinical hypothyroidism: Clinical and neuropathological recovery after hormone replacement therapy. *Neurol Sci* 2009;30(2):149–151.

46  Gonzalez-Duarte A, Robinson-Papp J, Simpson DM. Diagnosis and management of HIV-associated neuropathy. *Neurol Clin* 2008;26(3):821–832.

47  Makkar RP, et al. Burning feet syndrome: A clinical review. *Aust Fam Physician* 2003;32(12):1006–1009.

48  Vinik AI. Diabetic neuropathy: Pathogenesis and therapy. *Am J Med* 1999;107(2B):17S–26S.

49  Balakrishnan S, et al. A randomised parallel trial of topical aspirin-moisturiser solution vs. oral aspirin for acute herpetic neuralgia. *Int J Dermatol* 2001;40(8):535–538.

50  Buttaci CJ. Erythromelalgia: A case report and literature review. *Pain Med* 2006;7(6):534–538.

51  Cohen JS. Erythromelalgia: New theories and new therapies. *J Am Acad Dermatol* 2000;43(5 Pt 1):841–847.

52　Kuhnert SM, Phillips WJ, Davis MD. Lidocaine and mexiletine therapy for erythromelalgia. *Arch Dermatol* 1999;135(12):1447–1449.

53　Goodgold J, Kopell HP, Spielholz NI. The tarsal-tunnel syndrome: Objective diagnostic criteria. *N Engl J Med* 1965;273(14):742–745.

54　Alshami AM, Souvlis T, Coppieters MW. A review of plantar heel pain of neural origin: Differential diagnosis and management. *Man Ther* 2008;13(2):103–111.

55　Sammarco GJ, Chang L. Outcome of surgical treatment of tarsal tunnel syndrome. *Foot Ankle Int* 2003;24(2):125–131.

56　Patel AT, et al. Usefulness of electrodiagnostic techniques in the evaluation of suspected tarsal tunnel syndrome: An evidence-based review. *Muscle Nerve* 2005;32(2):236–240.

57　Erickson SJ, et al. MR imaging of the tarsal tunnel and related spaces: Normal and abnormal findings with anatomic correlation. *Am J Roentgenol* 1990;155(2):323–328.

58　Mullick T, Dellon AL. Results of decompression of four medial ankle tunnels in the treatment of tarsal tunnel syndrome. *J Reconstr Microsurg* 2008;24(2):119–126.

59　Hassouna H, Singh D. Morton's metatarsalgia: Pathogenesis, aetiology and current management. *Acta Orthop Belg* 2005;71(6):646–655.

60　Redd RA, et al. Morton neuroma: Sonographic evaluation. *Radiology* 1989;171(2):415–417.

61　Thomson CE, Gibson JN, Martin D. Interventions for the treatment of Morton's neuroma. *Cochrane Database Syst Rev* 2004(3):CD003118.

62　Prichasuk S, Subhadrabandhu T. The relationship of pes planus and calcaneal spur to plantar heel pain. *Clin Orthop Relat Res* 1994(306):192–196.

63　Buchbinder R. Plantar fasciitis. *N Engl J Med* 2004;350:2159.

64　Batt ME, Tanji JL, Skattum N. Plantar fasciitis: A prospective randomised clinical trial of the tension night splint. *Clin J Sport Med* 1996;6(3):158–162.

65　Kudo P, et al. Randomised, placebo-controlled, double-blind clinical trial evaluating the treatment of plantar fasciitis with an extracorporeal shockwave therapy (ESWT) device: A North American confirmatory study. *J Orthop Res* 2006;24(2):115–123.

66　Kalaci A, et al. Treatment of plantar fasciitis using four different local injection modalities: A randomised prospective clinical trial. *J Am Podiatr Med Assoc* 2009;99(2):108–113.

67　Cole C, Seto C, Gazewood J. Plantar fasciitis: Evidence-based review of diagnosis and therapy. *Am Fam Physician* 2005;72(11):2237–2242.

68　Berry H, Richardson PM. Common peroneal nerve palsy: A clinical and electrophysiological review. *J Neurol Neurosurg Psychiatry* 1976;39(12):1162–1171.

69　Kempster P, et al. Painful sciatic neuropathy following cardiac surgery. *Aust N Z J Med* 1991;21(5):732–735.

70　Lipetz JS, Misra N, Silber JS. Resolution of pronounced painless weakness arising from radiculopathy and disk extrusion. *Am J Phys Med Rehabil* 2005;84(7):528–537.

71　Dyck PJ, Thomas PK. *Peripheral neuropathy*. 4th edn. Philadelphia: Saunders; 2005.

72　Donofrio PD, Albers JW. AAEM minimonograph No. 34: Polyneuropathy: Classification by nerve conduction studies and electromyography. *Muscle Nerve* 1990;13(10):889–903.

73　Tankisi H, et al. Pathophysiology inferred from electrodiagnostic nerve tests and classification of polyneuropathies: Suggested guidelines. *Clin Neurophysiol* 2005;116(7):1571–1580.

74　Olney RK. Guidelines in electrodiagnostic medicine: Consensus criteria for the diagnosis of partial conduction block. *Muscle Nerve Suppl* 1999;8:S225–S229.

75　Legrand E, et al. Sciatica from disk herniation: Medical treatment or surgery?. *Joint Bone Spine* 2007;74(6):530–535

76　Mirza SK, Deyo RA. Systematic review of randomised trials comparing lumbar fusion surgery to nonoperative care for treatment of chronic back pain. *Spine* 2007;32(7):816–823.

77    Chou R, et al. Correction: Diagnosis and treatment of low back pain. *Ann Intern Med* 2008;148(3): 247–248.

78    Chou R, Huffman LH. Medications for acute and chronic low back pain: A review of the evidence for an American Pain Society/American College of Physicians clinical practice guideline. *Ann Intern Med* 2007;147(7):505–514.

79    Apley AG, Solomon L. Osteoarthritis and related disorders. In: Concise system of orthopaedics and fractures. Oxford: Butterworth—Heinemann; 1994. p. 36–41.

80    Kawagashira Y, Watanabe H, Oki Y, et al. Intravenous immunoglobulin therapy markedly ameliorates muscle weakness and severe pain in proximal diabetic neuropathy. *J Neurol Neurosurg Psychiatry* 2007; 78(8): 899-901.

81    Lundberg IE, Tjärnlund A, Bottai M, et al. 2017 European League Against Rheumatism/American College of Rheumatology classification criteria for adult and juvenile idiopathic inflammatory myopathies and their major subgroups. *Ann Rheum Dis* 2017; 76(12): 1955-64.

82    Lundberg IE, Miller FW, Tjärnlund A, Bottai M. Diagnosis and classification of idiopathic inflammatory myopathies. *J Intern Med* 2016; 280(1): 39-51.

83    Dalakas MC. Inflammatory Muscle Diseases. *New England Journal of Medicine* 2015; 372(18): 1734-47.

84    Lundberg IE, de Visser M, Werth VP. Classification of myositis. *Nature Reviews Rheumatology* 2018; 14(5): 269-78.

85    Buchbinder R, Forbes A, Hall S, Dennett X, Giles G. Incidence of malignant disease in biopsy-proven inflammatory myopathy. A population-based cohort study. *Ann Intern Med* 2001; 134(12): 1087-95.

86    Olazagasti JM, Baez PJ, Wetter DA, Ernste FC. Cancer risk in dermatomyositis: a meta-analysis of cohort studies. *Am J Clin Dermatol* 2015; 16(2): 89-98.

86    Chan YC, Lo YL, Chan ESY. Immunotherapy for diabetic amyotrophy. *Cochrane Database of Systematic Reviews* 2017; (7).

87    Dalakas MC, Illa I, Dambrosia JM, et al. A controlled trial of high-dose intravenous immune globulin infusions as treatment for dermatomyositis. *N Engl J Med* 1993; 329(27): 1993-2000.

88    Dastmalchi M, Grundtman C, Alexanderson H, et al. A high incidence of disease flares in an open pilot study of infliximab In patients with refractory inflammatory myopathies. *Ann Rheum Dis* 2008; 67(12): 1670-7.

89    Winkelman JW. Considering the causes of RLS. *Eur J Neurol* 2006; 13 Suppl 3: 8-14.

90    Pringsheim T, Gardner D, Addington D, et al. The Assessment and Treatment of Antipsychotic-Induced Akathisia. *Can J Psychiatry* 2018; 63(11): 719-29.

91    Levine TD. Small Fiber Neuropathy: Disease Classification Beyond Pain and Burning. *J Cent Nerv Syst Dis* 2018; 10: 1179573518771703.

92    Wolffenbuttel BHR, Wouters H, Heiner-Fokkema MR, van der Klauw MM. The Many Faces of Cobalamin (Vitamin B(12)) Deficiency. *Mayo Clin Proc Innov Qual Outcomes* 2019; 3(2): 200-14.

93    Taloyan M, Momtaz S, Steiner K, Östenson C-G, Salminen H. Burning sensation in the feet and glycosylated haemoglobin levels in Swedish- and non-Swedish-born primary healthcare patients. *Primary Care Diabetes* 2021; 15(3): 522-7.

94    Hovaguimian A, Gibbons CH. Diagnosis and treatment of pain in small-fiber neuropathy. *Curr Pain Headache Rep* 2011; 15(3): 193-200.

95    Farhad K. Current Diagnosis and Treatment of Painful Small Fiber Neuropathy. *Current Neurology and Neuroscience Reports* 2019; 19(12): 103.

96    Doneddu PE, Coraci D, Loreti C, Piccinini G, Padua L. Tarsal tunnel syndrome: still more opinions than evidence. Status of the art. *Neurol Sci* 2017; 38(10): 1735-9.

97    Oaklander AL, Nolano M. Scientific Advances in and Clinical Approaches to Small-Fiber Polyneuropathy: A Review. *JAMA Neurol* 2019; 76(10): 1240-51.

98  Doneddu PE, Coraci D, Loreti C, Piccinini G, Padua L. Tarsal tunnel syndrome: still more opinions than evidence. Status of the art. *Neurol Sci* 2017; 38(10): 1735-9.

99  Singh NN, Thomas FP, Diamond AL, Diamond R. Vitamin B-12 Associated Neurological Diseases. 29/1/2008 2008 (accessed 12/6/2021 2021).

100 Kim J, Kim H, Roh H, Kwon Y. Causes of hyperhomocysteinemia and its pathological significance. *Arch Pharm Res* 2018; 41(4): 372-83.

101 Weinstein JN, Lurie JD, Tosteson TD, et al. Surgical versus Nonsurgical Treatment for Lumbar Degenerative Spondylolisthesis. *New England Journal of Medicine* 2007; 356(22): 2257-70.

102 Garcia-Borreguero D, Garcia-Malo C, Granizo JJ, Ferré S. A Randomized, Placebo-Controlled Crossover Study with Dipyridamole for Restless Legs Syndrome. *Mov Disord* 2021.

103 Romero-Peralta S, Cano-Pumarega I, García-Borreguero D. Emerging Concepts of the Pathophysiology and Adverse Outcomes of Restless Legs Syndrome. *Chest* 2020; 158(3): 1218-29.

104 Earley CJ, Connor J, Garcia-Borreguero D, et al. Altered Brain iron homeostasis and dopaminergic function in Restless Legs Syndrome (Willis–Ekbom Disease). *Sleep Medicine* 2014; 15(11): 1288-301.

105 Natarajan R. Review of periodic limb movement and restless leg syndrome. *J Postgrad Med* 2010; 56(2): 157-62.

106 Daousi C, MacFarlane IA, Woodward A, Nurmikko TJ, Bundred PE, Benbow SJ. Chronic painful peripheral neuropathy in an urban community: a controlled comparison of people with and without diabetes. Diabetic medicine : a journal of the British Diabetic Association 2004; 21(9): 976-82.

107 Price R, Smith D, Franklin G, et al. Oral and Topical Treatment of Painful Diabetic Polyneuropathy: Practice Guideline Update Summary. *Neurology* 2022; 98(1): 31.

108 Leggett, L. E., et al. (2014). "Radiofrequency ablation for chronic low back pain: a systematic review of randomized controlled trials." *Pain Res Manag* 19(5): e146-153.

109 Perolat, R., et al. (2018). "Facet joint syndrome: from diagnosis to interventional management." *Insights into imaging* 9(5): 773-789.

110 Thawrani, D. P., et al. (2019). "Diagnosing Sacroiliac Joint Pain." *J Am Acad Orthop Surg* 27(3): 85-93.

111 Cooke, R., et al. (2021). "Metatarsalgia: anatomy, pathology and management." *Br J Hosp Med (Lond)* 82(9): 1-8.

112 Federer, A. E., et al. (2018). "Conservative Management of Metatarsalgia and Lesser Toe Deformities." *Foot Ankle Clin* 23(1): 9-20.

113 Kirschner, J. S., et al. (2009). "Piriformis syndrome, diagnosis and treatment." *Muscle Nerve* 40(1): 10-18.

114 Mammen, A. L. (2016). "Statin-Associated Autoimmune Myopathy." *N Engl J Med* 374(7): 664-669.

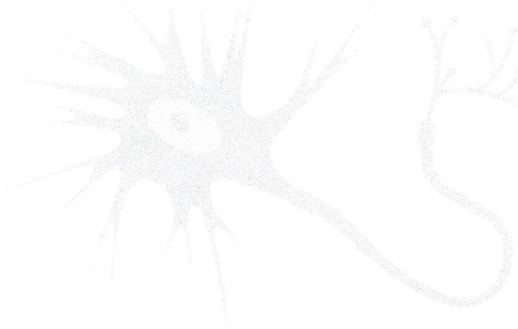

# Abnormal Movements and Difficulty Walking Due to Central Nervous System Problems

Difficulty walking related to peripheral nervous system problems was discussed in the previous chapter. The first half of this chapter deals with the more common central nervous system problems that result in difficulty walking; the second half discusses abnormal movements affecting the face, head, and limbs, with or without difficulty walking.

Difficulty walking related to weakness and sensory disturbances in one or both lower limbs occurs with spinal cord, brainstem or cerebral hemisphere problems affecting the motor and sensory pathways. Unsteadiness in the absence of weakness can occur with vertigo or problems in the cerebellar pathways, including the cerebellar connections in the brainstem. Extrapyramidal problems such as Parkinson's syndrome or a frontal lobe disorder referred to as an apraxic gait can also cause difficulty walking. This chapter does not discuss patients with severe visual impairment due to ocular or occipital lobe problems causing trouble walking.

"My legs are weak, Doc". When a patient states that their legs feel weak, it is crucial to clarify that the legs are weak as many patients often use the term weakness in a non-specific way to say that something is wrong with their legs. In this situation, the difficulty walking is due to another problem.

# Difficulty Walking

When a patient complains that they are having difficulty walking, simply ask if the difficulty relates to a sense of instability in the head, something wrong with their legs or whether they are uncertain why they are having problems. Figure 13.1 shows the diagnostic possibilities in each of these three scenarios.

337

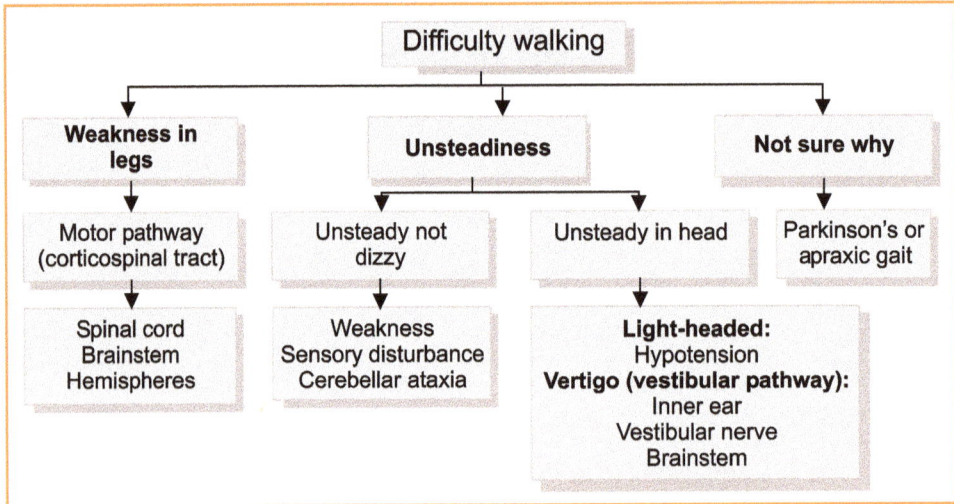

Figure 13.1 A flow chart showing the causes of difficulty walking divided into weakness, unsteadiness and uncertain reason.

> Some elderly patients assume that the gradual onset of difficulty walking results from advancing age and tend not to seek medical attention until the cord compression and limb weakness are severe.

## Difficulty walking related to weakness

The presence of weakness in the legs infers a motor pathway problem somewhere between the motor cortex and muscle.

One needs to determine if the weakness due to a central nervous system problem is related to the spinal cord, brain stem or cerebral hemisphere pathology. This can be very difficult if weakness is the only symptom. Although bilateral leg weakness is more common in patients with spinal cord problems, it can occur in conditions that affect the brainstem and the parafalcine region of the cerebral hemispheres. Unilateral leg weakness is more in keeping with a cerebral hemisphere problem but, once again, can occur with brainstem or spinal cord involvement. Some potential clues that may help determine the site of the pathology are listed below.

**Clues that the *spinal cord is the site of the problem*:**
- Back or neck pain that coincides with the development of neurological symptoms in the lower limbs
- Alteration in sphincter function with constipation and or urinary retention
- Altered sensation with a sensory level on the trunk (a strong indicator)

**Clues that the *brainstem is the site of the problem*:**
- Vertigo
- Diplopia
- Dysphagia (to a lesser extent)
- Ipsilateral facial sensory loss and contralateral loss to pain and temperature affecting the limbs (this pattern of crossed sensory loss only occurs with lateral brainstem involvement)
- A 12th, 6th, or 3rd nerve palsy on the side opposite the weakness points to the medulla, pons, and midbrain, respectively.

338

**Clues that the *cerebral hemisphere is the site of the problem*:**

- When there is upper motor neuron facial weakness in addition to the weakness in the arm and leg, the lesion must be above the mid pons on the contralateral side and, therefore, cannot be in the lower brainstem or the spinal cord. If areas in the hemispheres other than the motor pathway are affected, it is possible to localise the lesion to the hemispheres, particularly the cerebral cortex.
- Dysphasia (dominant hemisphere lesions affecting the cortex)
- Gerstmann's syndrome (dominant parietal lobe)
- Visual field loss (hemianopia or quadrantanopia) if the visual pathways are affected
- Visual inattention if the parietal cortex is affected
- Cortical sensory signs (2-point discrimination, graphaesthesia, impaired stereognosis or sensory inattention) (Other cortical phenomena are described in Chapter 5, 'The cerebral hemispheres and cerebellum'.)

# Spinal Cord Problems

The three common spinal cord problems resulting in leg weakness are cervical spondylitic myelopathy, thoracic cord compression (most often due to malignancy) and transverse myelitis.

Many other rarer conditions can affect the spinal cord and are traditionally divided into:

1. Lesions external to the dura (traumatic spinal cord compression, prolapsed intervertebral discs, epidural abscess)
2. Lesions beneath the dura but external to the spinal cord (neurofibroma, Chiari malformation)
3. Intrinsic spinal cord problems. These include glioma, ependymoma, sarcoidosis, vasculitis, syphilis, arteriovenous malformation, spinal cord infarction and adrenomyeloneuropathy.

The features that point to intrinsic and extrinsic cord pathology are:

- Early development urinary or anal sphincter dysfunction, intrinsic
- Early involvement of the spinothalamic tract, intrinsic
- A suspended sensory loss is a classical feature of an intrinsic spinal cord problem. There is altered pain and temperature sensation in a pattern that resembles a cape with impaired sensation on the upper trunk but sparing the lower trunk and lower limbs.
- Early sacral sensory loss occurs with extrinsic compression, sacral sparing with intrinsic spinal cord lesions.
- The presence of radicular pain indicates lesions extrinsic to the dura.

No neurology textbook would be complete without mentioning the Brown–Sequard hemicord syndrome. There is ipsilateral weakness, impaired vibration, and proprioception with contralateral impairment of pain and temperature sensation. It is indicative of the involvement of one half of the spinal cord. The explanation for this clinical syndrome is that the motor fibres and dorsal columns cross the midline at the level of the foramen magnum. In contrast, the spinothalamic tract crosses in the spinal cord close to the entry into the spinal cord of the dorsal nerve root.

## Cervical Spondylitic Myelopathy (CSM)

Cervical spondylitic myelopathy (CSM) is the commonest cause of spinal cord dysfunction particularly in elderly patients. It is also the most frequent cause of paraparesis or quadriparesis unrelated to trauma.

Repeated occupational trauma, such as carrying axial loads, a genetic predisposition, and Down syndrome, predisposes to an increased cervical spondylosis risk.

Cervical spondylosis is degenerative changes commencing in the cervical discs with subsequent osteophyte (subperiosteal bone) formation. Cervical disc protrusion or extrusion, osteophytes, and hypertrophy of the ligamentum flavum together result in spinal cord compression. Secondary spinal cord ischaemia can occur with severe compression. Rarely spondylolisthesis (one vertebra slipping on the one below) may cause cord compression.

Cervical cord compression (Figure 13.2) is seen in younger patients with congenitally narrow spinal canals (10–13 mm). The spinal cord is stretched during flexion of the cervical spine and buckling of the ligamentum flavum occurs during the cervical spine extension. Thus, repeated flexion and extension in the patient with significant canal narrowing may cause intermittent acute compression of the spinal cord. This mechanism of injury is thought to account for the clinical deterioration seen in many cases of CSM. [1]

The natural course of CSM for any given individual is variable and precise prognostication is not possible. However, once moderate signs and symptoms develop, patients are less likely to improve spontaneously. Worsening occurs more commonly in older patients, whereas patients with mild disability are less likely to worsen. [1]

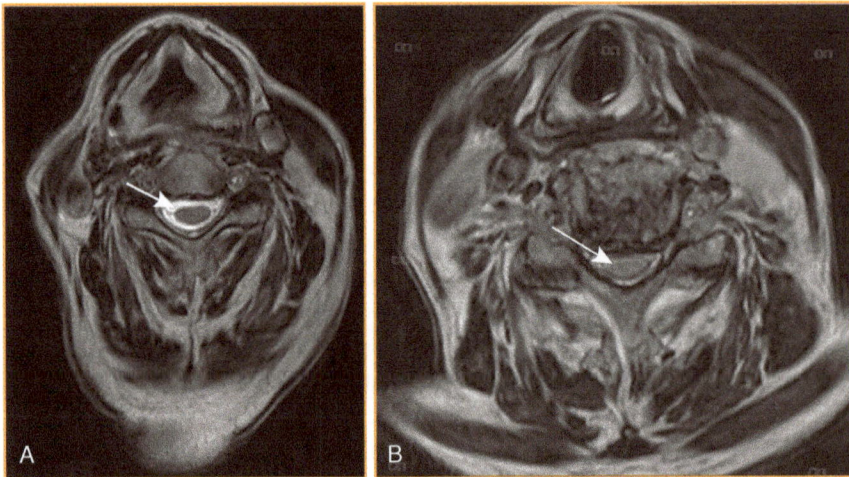

Figure 13.2 MRI scan of A normal cervical spine and B spinal cord compression due to cervical spondylosis. Note the spinal cord flattening and absence of CSF (white) around the spinal cord.

CSM can present in a variety of ways.

1. The most typical presentation is the insidious onset of difficulty walking related to weakness and or stiffness (due to spasticity).
2. Some patients will have neck pain from cervical spondylosis; pain in the arm related to nerve root compression is less common.
3. Older patients, in particular, may present with painless weakness and wasting of the small muscles of the hands related to nerve root compression. The signs of spinal cord compression are detected when they are examined.
4. A presentation that is much less common is central cord syndrome. This results from a hyperextension injury in the setting of cervical canal stenosis. The weakness is greater in the upper than the lower limbs with or without a suspended sensory loss affecting the shoulders and upper torso like a cape. As it is an intrinsic cord lesion, urinary retention may occur.
5. Patients with cervical cord compression may experience an electric shock-like sensation radiating down their back or into their limbs with neck flexion, the so-called Lhermitte phenomenon.

340

The examination will reveal a stiff-legged gait if there is associated spasticity. The tone will be increased with or without sustained ankle clonus; the knee reflexes will be abnormally brisk other than the ankle reflexes that are often absent in the elderly. The plantar should be up-going, but this is not universal. Often there is no sensory deficit at all.

---

**Management of Cervical Spondylitic Myelopathy**

Investigations
- A plain X-ray of the cervical spine may demonstrate degenerative disease. However, this is common in elderly patients without cervical cord compression.
- Similarly, a CT scan of the cervical spine may demonstrate degenerative disease but is not sensitive enough to adequately evaluate the presence of cervical nerve root or cervical spinal cord compression.
- Magnetic resonance imaging (MRI) is the imaging modality of choice in patients suspected of having cervical cord compression.
- If MRI is not available or contraindicated, a CT myelogram is necessary. A CT myelogram is where contrast is injected into the subarachnoid space via a lumbar puncture. The patient is tipped head downwards to allow the contrast to reach the cervical region.

**Treatment**

There are no prospective randomised controlled trials comparing medical management with surgery for CSM. The choice of therapy will be dictated by the patient's attitude to surgery, the severity of the cervical cord compression and the fitness from the medical point of view of the patient to undergo surgery. Patients are advised that the goal of surgery is to prevent worsening and that improvement cannot be guaranteed, although many patients do in fact improve following appropriate surgery. Many neurosurgeons would recommend a period of observation in patients with mild symptoms and signs. Once moderate signs and symptoms develop, however, patients are less likely to spontaneously improve and such patients should consider surgical decompression.

---

# Thoracic Cord Compression

Thoracic spinal cord compression most commonly occurs with metastatic malignancy, less commonly with a thoracic disc, epidural abscess, or extrinsic spinal cord tumours such as a meningioma or neurofibroma. There is an aphorism that 'a thoracic cord lesion in a middle-aged to elderly female is a meningioma (benign tumour arising from the meninges) until proven otherwise'. Back pain is rare with a meningioma, more common but not a universal feature of thoracic discs. *Increasingly severe* back pain occurs for, on average, eight weeks or longer in 80–95% of patients who subsequently develop malignant cord compression. [2] Patients who are not known to suffer from malignancy but who develop increasingly severe midline (especially thoracic) back pain should be investigated promptly in the hope of preventing malignant cord compression.

Although the pain is initially localised to the vertebra, subsequent nerve root compression can result in radicular pain. *A vital clue is that the back pain is often worse after lying down.* Rapidly developing weakness in the legs is the initial and dominant neurological symptom once malignant spinal cord compression occurs. Sensory symptoms are less common, and sphincter disturbance occurs late. A delayed diagnosis of malignant cord compression is common, with many patients only diagnosed after they lose their ability to walk. [2, 3] Unfortunately, once significant cord compression related to malignancy occurs, the prognosis for recovery is poor.

In patients with preexisting malignancy, particularly breast and prostate, the development of thoracic back pain should raise the suspicion of possible secondary malignancy in the spinal column and prompt investigation (Figure 13.3).

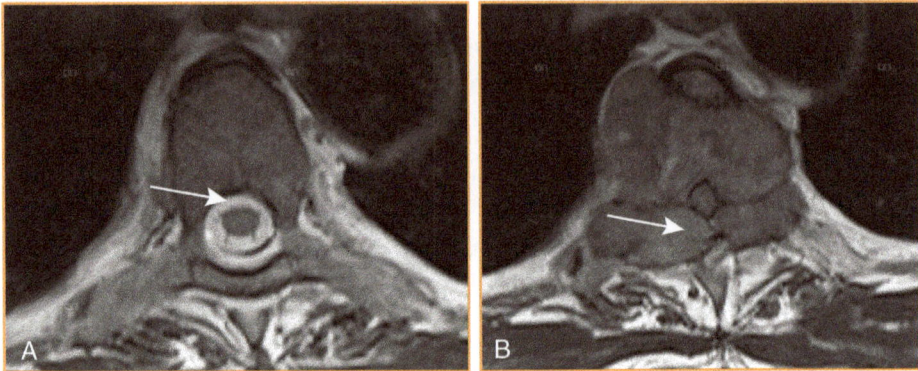

**Figure 13.3** MRI scan of **A** normal thoracic spinal cord (the arrow shows the CSF around the spinal cord) and **B** malignant thoracic spinal cord compression (the arrow points to the malignancy; the CSF space is obliterated)

The following suggest spinal metastases:

- pain in the thoracic spine
- severe unremitting or progressive lumbar spinal pain
- spinal pain aggravated by straining
- nocturnal spinal pain preventing sleep
- localised spinal tenderness. [4]

Some authorities recommend patients with known malignancy should be advised to return urgently within 24 hours for review should they develop thoracic back pain in the midline. [4]

Severe thoracic back pain followed by the rapid development of spinal cord compression can be the initial manifestation of malignancy in as many as one-third of patients with cancer of unknown primary origin, such as non-Hodgkin lymphoma, myeloma, and lung cancer. [2] Metastatic disease less commonly affects the cervical or lumbar spine. Although almost any systemic cancer can metastasise to the spinal column, prostate, breast, and lung are the most common. [2]

| Management of Malignant Cord Compression |
|---|
| Investigations |
| • Plain X-rays and nuclear bone scans may detect metastases in the vertebrae but will not detect cord compression. [5] |
| • MRI is the modality of choice in detecting malignant cord compression. [6, 7] |
| Treatment |
| • High dose corticosteroids result in a significantly better outcome in terms of ambulation in patients undergoing radiotherapy for malignant cord compression. [8] Dexamethasone at a dose in the range of 16–100 mg/day is probably appropriate. [2] |
| • Surgical decompression combined with postoperative radiotherapy results in more patients being able to walk than radiotherapy alone. [9] |

## Intrinsic Spinal Cord Problems

Transverse myelitis is the commonest intrinsic cord lesion resulting in dysfunction in the lower limbs and difficulty walking in younger patients. Spinal cord ischaemia occurs in the elderly. Spinal cord ischaemia can develop abruptly or insidiously. Other intrinsic spinal cord problems such as tumours and the cavitating lesion referred to as syringomyelia are rare and beyond this book's scope.

## Transverse Myelitis

Acute transverse myelitis (ATM) is a focal inflammatory disorder of the spinal cord, resulting in motor, sensory and autonomic dysfunction with many infectious and non-infectious causes. [10] The Transverse Myelitis Consortium Working Group [11] has established diagnostic criteria that require:

- Bilateral signs and or symptoms of spinal cord dysfunction affecting the motor, sensory and autonomic systems
- A clearly defined sensory level
- The exclusion of cord compression
- Inflammatory cells in the cerebrospinal fluid (CSF).

If none of the criteria is met at symptom onset, the MRI and lumbar puncture should be repeated between 2- 7 days following symptom onset.

A febrile illness often precedes the development of neurological symptoms and signs up to 4 weeks before onset. [12] Typically an upper respiratory tract infection. Patients present with an ascending sensory loss, with the development of a sensory level in most patients. There may or may not be paraparesis, paraplegia, quadriplegia, and urinary retention. [12, 13] The *symptoms may develop rapidly over as little as 4 hours or more slowly over several weeks.*

---

An ischaemic aetiology should be presumed when spinal cord symptoms reach their maximal severity in < 4 hours from onset. [1]

---

In one study of acute transverse myelitis, a parainfectious cause was diagnosed in 38% of patients, but the underlying infectious agent was identified in only a minority of patients. In 36% of patients, the aetiology remained uncertain, and in 22%, it was the first manifestation of possible MS. The MRI scan (see Figure 13.4) was abnormal in 96% of cases (i.e. a normal MRI is rare but does not exclude transverse myelitis). [12]

Acute non-compressive myelopathies can also be classified according to their aetiology. [14]

- Multiple sclerosis
- Systemic disease (e.g. Systemic lupus erythematosus [SLE], antiphospholipid syndrome, Sjögren's syndrome
- Parainfectious
- Delayed radiation myelopathy
- Spinal cord infarct
- Idiopathic myelopathy.

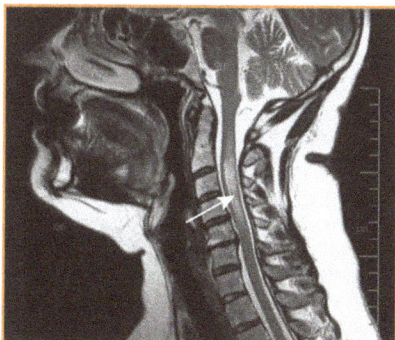

Figure 13.4 MRI scan of transverse myelitis

| Management of Transverse Myelitis |
|---|
| Patients suspected of having transverse myelitis should have an MRI scan and a lumbar puncture. The CSF is abnormal [14] with:<br>• mildly elevated protein (except in postinfectious myelopathy where it may exceed 1 g/L)<br>• lymphocytic pleocytosis (as low as 1 cell/mm³ in delayed radiation myelopathy to as high as 320 cells/mm³ in postinfectious myelopathy)<br>• a normal CSF glucose<br>• negative CSF cytology for malignant cells.<br>MRI scanning usually but not invariably reveals abnormalities that may be restricted to one or many spinal segments. [13] Typically the MRI signal changes extend at least three segments above the sensory level.<br>In western countries transverse myelitis may be the presenting feature of MS or it may manifest during the course of this disease. Patients who are ultimately diagnosed with MS are more likely to have asymmetric clinical findings, predominant sensory symptoms with relative sparing of motor systems, MRI lesions extending over fewer than two spinal segments, abnormal brain MRI and oligoclonal bands in the CSF. [11] It is important to test for oligoclonal bands in the CSF and serum to detect intrathecal synthesis seen with MS. |

## Conus Medullaris and Cauda Equina Syndrome

One very rare syndrome produces both upper and lower motor neuron signs in the lower limbs. This is a lesion at the level of the conus medullaris, the terminal end of the spinal cord at the level of the 2nd lumbar vertebra also involving the cauda equina. The most common cause is a herniated disc. Other causes include epidural abscess, spinal epidural hematoma, diskitis, tumor (either metastatic or a primary CNS tumour), trauma and spinal canal stenosis.

Patients with a pure conus medullaris lesion present with low back pain radiating to the legs and upper motor neuron signs due to compression of the spinal cord from T12-L2. There is increased tone, distal weakness of the legs with increased reflexes, impaired sensation in the perianal area (S3–S5), impotence and either urinary retention or urinary and faecal incontinence.

If the cauda equina is also involved, in addition to low back pain there is asymmetrical weakness, absent reflexes, and radicular sensory loss in the lower limbs (L1-L5–S1). The onset of perineal anesthesia associated with bladder dysfunction is typical of the start of cauda equina syndrome.

Cauda equina syndrome is a neurosurgical emergency, early intervention is associated with a better prognosis. [30]

# Brainstem Problems Causing Leg Weakness

Weakness caused by brainstem problems is either unilateral or bilateral weakness affecting the lower limbs with or without the involvement of the upper limbs and, if above the mid pons, the face. The presence of symptoms and signs pointing to the brainstem (see Chapter 4) is the clue to the site of the pathology.

Brainstem tumours are very rare. The most likely causes of motor weakness related to brainstem pathology are cerebral ischaemia in older patients, where the onset will be sudden, and demyelinating disease in younger patients, where the onset will be over hours to days.

# Cerebral Hemisphere Problems Causing Leg Weakness

Weakness related to cerebral hemisphere problems is almost invariably unilateral. However, bilateral lower limb weakness can occur with involvement of the parafalcine region, typically with cerebral infarction in the anterior cerebral artery distribution. The presence of abulia (a lack of will, drive, or initiative for action, speech and thought) is the clue that the lesion affects the anterior cerebral artery distribution.

Cerebrovascular disease is the most likely cause of motor weakness related to the motor pathways in the cerebral hemispheres, either ischaemia or haemorrhage. Demyelinating diseases and benign and malignant (primary or secondary) tumours are the other more common causes. Imaging with CT scanning or MRI scanning can readily establish the pathology.

# Difficulty Walking due to Unsteadiness

When patients complain that they are unsteady on their feet, it is crucial to clarify whether this sense of instability relates to a feeling of dizziness or instability in the head or whether it relates to something wrong in the legs suggesting a problem in either the spinal cord or peripheral nervous system.

## Unsteadiness Related to Dizziness in the Head

Vertigo is 'an illusion of movement', often rotary, with the sensation as if the room or head is spinning. It renders the patient unable to walk. The presence of vertigo with the head or room spinning indicates the problem must involve the vestibular pathway either in the peripheral vestibular system, where there may be associated tinnitus and or deafness or in the brainstem where the presence of diplopia, weakness, dysarthria, and sensory symptoms may accompany vertigo.

Less severe vertigo includes a sensation of instability, a feeling of disequilibrium like being on a ship, but can also include tipping, tilting, falling etc. The more one strays from the sense of rotation; the less one can be sure that the problem causing instability is within the vestibular system. This sense of dizziness in the head could also relate to hypotension.

## Unsteadiness in the Absence of Weakness or Dizziness

Patients with bilateral vestibular hypofunction (e.g. due to aminoglycoside toxicity) do not present with vertigo but with a sense of disequilibrium.

Patients with marked impairment of proprioception in the lower limbs will be very unsteady on their feet, particularly in the dark and when they close their eyes, e.g. while having a shower or washing their hair. This is often referred to as sensory ataxia. Vitamin $B_{12}$ deficiency with subacute combined degeneration of the cord is probably the commonest cause now that syphilis has largely been eradicated. Very rarely, impairment of proprioception results from a dorsal root ganglionopathy or sensory neuronopathy, seen as a paraneoplastic phenomenon,

[15, 16] Sjögren's syndrome [17] or pyridoxine abuse. [18] The sensory ganglionopathies are rare and may antedate the diagnosis of malignancy. They can also indicate recurrence in a patient with known malignancy and should prompt a search for malignancy. [16]

Nitrous oxide interacts with vitamin $B_{12}$ resulting in selective inhibition of methionine synthase. Nitrous oxide toxicity [77-78] can cause a subacute combined degeneration of the spinal cord. In whipped cream dispensers, the food industry uses nitrous oxide as a foaming agent. Silver canisters containing nitrous oxide known as nangs, bulbs or whippets can readily be purchased over the counter. Nitrous oxide toxicity can also cause an axonal peripheral neuropathy. On magnetic resonance imaging, long segmental hyperintensity changes in the posterior columns can be seen. Homocysteine levels are high.

Another cause of difficulty walking from instability in the absence of dizziness in the head or weakness in the legs is the ataxia related to cerebellar disease. Ataxia in the limbs reflects problems in the cerebellar hemispheres. In contrast, ataxia affecting the trunk (truncal ataxia) is seen in patients with problems related to the midline vermis of the cerebellum.

Truncal ataxia occurs with hypothyroidism [19] and alcoholism. [20] Patients with isolated truncal ataxia walk with a wide-based gait with little in the way of nystagmus or ataxia in the limbs. The commonest cause of ataxia related to cerebellar disease would be cerebellar infarction. Two less common causes of cerebellar ataxia affecting the cerebellar hemispheres are the paraneoplastic cerebellar syndrome [21] and the hereditary spinocerebellar atrophies (SCA). [22] The paraneoplastic cerebellar syndrome may be the initial presenting symptom of malignancy or develop after the diagnosis of malignancy is established. The clinical picture is disabling ataxia affecting the limbs and trunk, with dysarthria and nystagmus evolving rapidly over days to weeks. On the other hand, the hereditary spinocerebellar atrophies present with the insidious onset of ataxia, affecting the limbs with or without nystagmus and dysarthria.

## Difficulty Walking Not Sure Why

There are two conditions, Parkinson's, and apraxia of gait, where patients have increasing difficulty walking in the absence of any apparent weakness or sensory disturbance in the lower limbs or any sensation of instability in the head. These patients are uncertain why they are having difficulty. In both conditions, the patient will appear to walk with short steps: in Parkinson's, the patients shuffle as they walk, whereas, with an apraxic gait, the steps are short, but the patient does not shuffle. It can occasionally be challenging to differentiate mild Parkinson's disease from the apraxic gait.

## Parkinson's Syndrome

Parkinson's syndrome is a term used to describe patients with clinical features that include one or more of:
- A resting tremor
- Stooped posture
- Slowness of movement referred to as bradykinesia
- Cogwheel rigidity (increased tone with the sensation of the muscle giving way in little jerks).

The commonest cause of Parkinson's syndrome is Parkinson's disease. Drugs such as phenothiazines, butyrophenones, metoclopramide, reserpine and tetrabenazine cause reversible Parkinson's syndrome. Toxins such as manganese dust, carbon disulfide and the recreational drug N-methyl-4-phenyl-1,2,3,6-tetrahydropyridine (MPTP) cause an irreversible Parkinson's syndrome [23] by destroying the dopamine neurons in the midbrain.

The term 'Parkinson's disease' is reserved for patients with the above clinical features who have the characteristic neuropathology of loss of pigmentation in the substantia nigra and the presence of Lewy bodies.

Parkinson's is primarily a disease of the elderly, although, in up to 10% of patients, the onset is before 50. The patient with Parkinson's disease affecting both lower limbs walk with small shuffling steps where the shoe's sole can be heard scraping along the ground. As the patient walks, there is a lack of arm swing. More advanced Parkinson's may develop an involuntary sensation where they cannot stop themselves from walking with short accelerating steps, the so-called festinating gait. Occasionally, patients present with unilateral involvement mimicking a hemiparesis and are thought to have had a 'stroke'. The insidious onset and the presence of tremor and cogwheel rigidity on examination should alert the clinician to the correct diagnosis.

As Parkinson's disease becomes more severe, patients will have difficulty getting out of bed and low chairs and will walk with a stooped posture. Patients may have a fixed expression on their face, blink infrequently and lose the ability to smile. Curiously, many patients with Parkinson's can still dance. The other characteristic feature of Parkinson's is the resting tremor, which is discussed in the next section.

# Apraxia of Gait

Apraxia of gait is an inability to walk without weakness, sensory deficit, instability, or incoordination. It is a perseveration of posture and a failure to perform the serial movements necessary for ambulation. There is difficulty initiating walking or changing direction in the initial stage. Patients walk with small steps called the 'marche á petit pas' (walks with little steps); unlike Parkinson's, they do not shuffle but lift their feet off the ground. The features that help differentiate apraxia of gait from Parkinson's disease are listed in Table 13.1.

| Clinical feature | Parkinson's | Frontal lobe apraxia |
|---|---|---|
| Resting tremor | Yes | No |
| Shuffles when walks | Yes | No |
| Lifts feet when walks with small steps | No | Yes |
| Swings arms when walking | No | Yes |
| Smiles spontaneously | No | Yes |
| Bradykinesia | Yes | Yes |
| Difficulty arising from chair | Yes | Yes |
| Grasp and palmo-mental reflexes | No* | Yes |
| Cogwheel rigidity(rigidity constant during testing) | Yes | No |
| Gegenhalten rigidity (rigidity increases with more prolonged testing) | No | Yes |

* May occur late in the course when cognitive decline is present.

**Table 13.1** The clinical features that help differentiate Parkinson's from frontal lobe apraxia, two commonly confused conditions

To the inexperienced clinician, these patients appear to have cogwheel rigidity, but it is, in fact, Gegenhalten or 'an involuntary, voluntary resistance to passive movement'. The way to differentiate between the cogwheel rigidity of Parkinson's and the apparent cogwheel rigidity in frontal lobe disorders is that, in patients with Parkinson's, the cogwheel rigidity is evident from the moment testing begins whereas, in patients with Gegenhalten, the increased tone that has the sensation of cogwheel rigidity is not present initially but, the more the clinician tests for increased tone, the greater the degree of resistance creating the impression of cogwheel rigidity. If testing is momentarily interrupted by simply lowering the hand and wrist and then started again, the increased tone is not present initially but once again appears with further testing.

The method of testing tone in patients with suspected extrapyramidal or frontal lobe apraxia of gait is different from the method when one suspects altered tone due to a problem affecting the motor pathway. One passively extends and then flexes the wrist repeatedly while compacting the wrist as if you are trying to push or compact the hand into the distal aspect of the radius and ulnar. Subtle degrees of increased tone can be detected by using a technique referred to as Jendrassik's manoeuvre. Jendrassik's is a distracting technique in which the patient simultaneously clenches the opposite fist, lifts the arm with the clenched fist in the air and shakes their head from side to side. This is a handy technique when looking for alteration in tone in patients with early suspected Parkinson's.

*Note:* Jendrassik's manoeuvre is also used to elicit reflexes that initially appeared to be absent. While the attention is being diverted, the lower extremity reflexes are tested whilst the patient hooks the flexed fingers of the two hands together, forming a 'monkey grip' and forcibly tries to pull them apart.

Although not confined to frontal lobe pathology, the apraxic gait is characteristic of patients with frontal lobe disorders, most frequently related to degenerative or vascular diseases. There are several treatable causes of an apraxic gait that should always be excluded:
- communicating ('normal pressure') hydrocephalus. [24]
- bilateral subdural haematomas
- sub-frontal meningioma.

## Communicating or 'Normal Pressure' Hydrocephalus

Communicating hydrocephalus also called normal pressure hydrocephalus (NPH) is rare but a potentially treatable condition. The diagnosis is primarily a clinical one based on the triad of:
- gait impairment
- mild cognitive dysfunction
- unwitting urinary incontinence.

The lateral, 3rd and 4th ventricles are enlarged with little or no atrophy of the cerebral hemispheres. NPH presents with a fairly rapid onset over weeks or months of gait apraxia associated with unwitting urinary incontinence and *mild* cognitive impairment. Patients with significant cognitive impairment who subsequently develop apraxia of gait and patients in whom the decline is over several years are less likely to have communicating hydrocephalus.

The term 'normal pressure' is a misnomer as continuous intracranial pressure monitoring has demonstrated intermittent elevation of the intracranial pressure.

**Management of 'Normal Pressure' Hydrocephalus**

The aetiology of normal pressure hydrocephalus is unknown. CT scan of the brain demonstrates enlargement of all the ventricles with little cortical atrophy.

A number of diagnostic tests designed at predicting response to ventricular shunting have been described. These include various MRI abnormalities [25], external continuous lumbar drainage [26], continuous intraventricular pressure monitoring [27] and the CSF tap test [28], where a lumbar puncture is performed and CSF is removed to see if the patient temporarily improves. None have been validated in terms of ruling out a response to surgery. The problem with ventricular-peritoneal CSF drainage is the risk of reducing the intracranial pressure too much, resulting in subdural haematomas or hygromas. This risk has been reduced in recent years with the use of adjustable pressure shunts. [29]

# Abnormal Movements

## Abnormal Movements of the Head, Face, and Neck

Abnormal movements that affect the head, face and neck include:
- essential/familial tremor
- tardive dyskinesia
- Tourette syndrome
- oculogyric crisis
- hemifacial spasm and
- spasmodic torticollis

## Head Tremor

Head tremor also called titubation is usually a manifestation of benign essential/familial tremor or cerebellar disease; it is infrequent in Parkinson's disease. [31] Essential and familial tremor may also affect the mouth and voice. Benign essential and familial tremor is discussed in more detail in the section on abnormal movements of the upper limbs.

## Tardive Dyskinesia

Tardive dyskinesia was first recognised in the 1950s. [32] It consists of repetitive, involuntary, purposeless movements affecting the mouth, lips, and tongue with tongue protrusion; lip smacking, puckering, pursing; facial grimacing and rapid eye blinking. The involuntary movements occur during most of the waking hours. Typically it is a side effect of drugs, although it may occur in the absence of drug therapy, particularly in elderly edentulous patients. Tardive dyskinesia may also affect the limbs and trunk where the abnormal movements are more athetoid (repetitive, involuntary, slow, sinuous, writhing movements) in nature.

**Management of Tardive Dyskinesia**

Tardive dyskinesia is an extrapyramidal syndrome that occurs as a side effect of central dopamine-blocking drugs such as the older antipsychotics such as chlorpromazine, thioridazine and haloperidol. It also occurs as a side effect of drugs used to treat Parkinson's disease and antiemetics such as prochlorperazine. The higher the dose and the longer the duration of treatment, the more likely is this condition to develop. It is less common with the new generation of antipsychotic drugs. [33] Sometimes withdrawing the drug may lead to a resolution of the problem, particularly if the condition is identified very early. However, improvement may take some time, and in some patients, the condition may persist for years after the withdrawal of the offending drug. Tetrabenazine [34] and deep brain stimulation have been reported to be of benefit. [35]

The other extrapyramidal side effects that can occur with the antipsychotic and antidepressant drugs include akathisia (unpleasant sensations of 'inner' restlessness that manifests itself as an inability to sit still or remain motionless), the neuroleptic malignant syndrome [36] and the serotonin syndrome. These entities are discussed below in the section, 'Rare but life-threatening movement disorders'.

# Tourette Syndrome

Tourette syndrome is a condition predominantly seen in school-aged children. [37] The syndrome consists of tics that are sudden, brief, intermittent, involuntary, or semi-voluntary movements (motor tics), such as blinking, nose twitching, head and limb jerking, mouth opening, torticollis, shoulder rotation and sustained eye closure (blepharospasm). More complex motor tics may occur, such as making obscene gestures (copropraxia) and imitating others' gestures (echopraxia). Burping, retching, vomiting, fist-shaking, trunk bending, jumping, or kicking are also seen. Phonic or vocal tics can occur, such as simply sniffing, grunting, coughing, clearing the throat, barking, screaming, shouting obscenities (coprolalia) and repeating one's utterances (echolalia). *One of the diagnostic characteristics is the ability of the patient to suppress their tics.* The motor and phonic tics may persist during sleep. It is much more common in males and often associated with attention-deficit hyperactivity disorder or obsessive-compulsive disorder.

**Management of Tourette Syndrome**

The Tourette Syndrome Classification Study Group has created diagnostic criteria. [38] The aetiology is uncertain, and treatment consists of behaviour therapy, particularly informing people who encounter the patient. Alpha-2 adrenergic agonists (clonidine) or dopamine receptor-blocking drugs (neuroleptics such as haloperidol and pimozide) are used to control the motor tics. [37] Botulinum toxin (Botox) or deep brain stimulation may be useful in severe and disabling motor tics. Vocal cord injections can help phonic tics.

# Oculogyric Crisis

Oculogyric crisis refers to the sudden involuntary contractions of some of the extraocular muscles that result in repetitive, conjugate ocular deviations usually, although not always, in an upward direction. The attack or crisis may last from seconds to minutes. An oculogyric crisis is most commonly seen following exposure to neuroleptic drugs. The incidence of oculogyric crises in patients treated with chronic neuroleptic therapy may be as high as 10%.

| Aetiology and Management of Oculogyric Crisis |
| --- |
| Tetrabenazine, gabapentin, domperidone, carbamazepine and lithium carbonate have all been reported to trigger oculogyric crises. An oculogyric crisis may occur in patients with dopa-responsive dystonia, bilateral paramedian thalamic infarction, herpes encephalitis, cystic glioma of the posterior 3rd ventricle and Wilson's disease. |
|    The acute oculogyric crises can be terminated with intravenous anticholinergics or diphenhydramine injection. Diphenhydramine, 25 or 50 mg IV, is probably the treatment of choice for this condition. Oral clonazepam may be effective for patients with chronic neuroleptic-induced oculogyric crises resistant to anticholinergics. [39] |

# Hemifacial Spasm

Hemifacial spasm consists of unilateral brief clonic movements of the facial muscles. Repetitive blinking occurs if it affects the orbicularis oculi, whilst repetitive upward twitching of the mouth occurs with the involvement of the zygomaticus major. It is believed to be due to a blood vessel irritating the proximal facial nerve near where it emerges from the brainstem.

| Treatment of Hemifacial Spasm |
| --- |
| If mild nothing, most patients do not require treatment. Oral medications can be considered first-line therapy in those unwilling to have botulinum toxin therapy and not good candidates for surgery. Anticonvulsants such as carbamazepine, gabapentin, benzodiazepines (clonazepam), anticholinergics, baclofen and haloperidol all have significant side effects. Botulinum toxin is the treatment of choice, with microvascular decompression of the facial nerve in resistant cases. [79] |

# Abnormal Movements of the Limbs

There are a large number of abnormal movements in the limbs. The more commonly seen in clinical practice are:
- Benign essential or familial tremor
- The tremor of Parkinson's disease
- Cerebellar or intention tremor
- Myoclonus
- Hemiballismus
- Chorea and athetosis
- Orthostatic tremor
- Paroxysmal kinesogenic choreoathetosis.

Some abnormal movements occur only with activity; others occur at rest. (Figure 13.5). Most do not occur during sleep; myoclonus and hemiballismus are the exceptions.

351

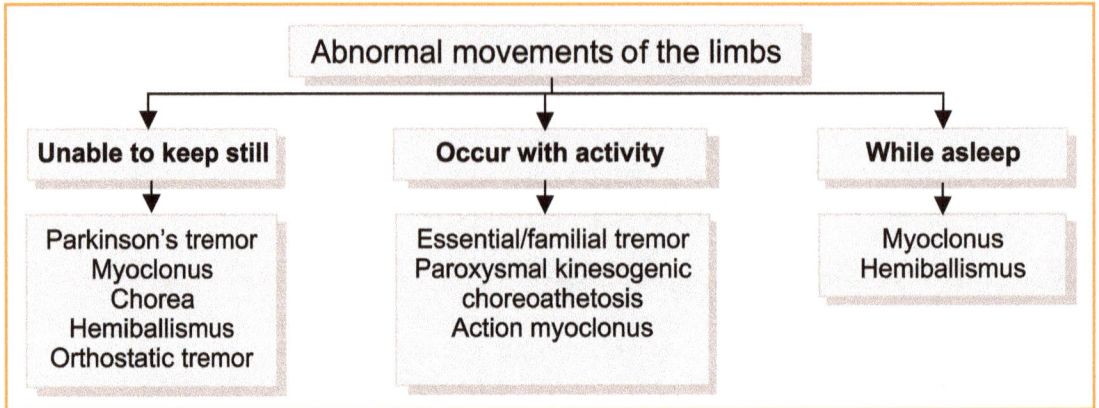

**Figure 13.5** The more common abnormal movements that occur in the limbs

# Abnormal Movements – Cannot Keep Still

## Parkinson's disease

Parkinson's disease was first described by James Parkinson in 1817. [40] Resting tremor abolished by movement is often the initial symptom, although occasional patients with Parkinson's disease may have a non-resting tremor. The associated features of rigidity and bradykinesia characteristic of Parkinson's may be minimal or absent in the very early stages. Patients do not complain that their limbs are rigid or stiff; they tend to say that the muscles in the arms and legs ache and do not work as well. There is an increasing inability to undertake activities of daily living with advanced disease, although patients often assume it is simply the ageing process! Patients with Parkinson's disease walk with a slightly stooped posture and do not swing their arms when they are walking.

| Aetiology and Management of Parkinson's Disease |
| --- |
| The aetiology of Parkinson's disease is unknown, although some patients have a genetic predisposition and mutations in the parkin gene are linked to autosomal recessive juvenile parkinsonism. [41]<br><br>At the time of writing, there is no effective treatment to arrest the progression of the disease. Management is primarily directed towards the alleviation of the symptoms of Parkinson's while trying to minimise the short and long-term side effects of the drugs. In essence, the initial response to levodopa is very gratifying, and the first few years of treatment consist of gradually increasing drug therapy as the condition becomes more severe. In later years, as the disease worsens, increasing dyskinesia and the on-off phenomenon with worsening of the disease leads to the progressive reduction in the doses.<br><br>When reviewing patients with Parkinson's disease, it is important to clarify the exact time of day that they take each of their medications and how long the benefit persists after taking the individual dose. This will help differentiate between the motor fluctuations that represent end-of-dose failure (the beneficial effect of the drug wearing off after a period of time) and the motor fluctuations referred to as the 'on–off phenomenon that can be likened to someone pushing a button and the patient develops increasingly severe symptoms of Parkinson's unrelated to the timing of medication. The former may respond to more frequent doses of levodopa and drugs that prolong the duration of benefit of levodopa; the latter is very difficult to treat but may respond to dopamine agonists.<br><br>Although levodopa is the recognised 'gold standard' drug for the symptomatic relief of Parkinson's disease, the efficacy diminishes after 4–5 years and is supplanted by significant motor fluctuations. [42] Initially, the duration of benefit from a single dose may last several hours; after a period of time, that varies from patient to patient (usually years) the duration of benefit is significantly shorter. The combination of pramipexole and levodopa is superior to levodopa alone. [43] Stereotactic surgery and deep brain stimulation are other treatment modalities in drug-resistant cases. Patients may develop significant depression, dementia, psychosis, and psychosocial issues that need considerable attention in addition to control of the tremor and the other motor manifestations of Parkinson's disease[1]. [44] A detailed discussion of treatment can be found in Appendix J. |

## Myoclonus

Myoclonus refers to sudden, shock-like, involuntary movements that can manifest in various patterns:

- focal, where a few adjacent muscles are involved
- multifocal, where many muscles jerk asynchronously
- generalised, where most of the muscles of the body are affected.

Myoclonic movements may be spontaneous or activated by motion. Myoclonus is most commonly related to epilepsy. Myoclonus might also occur acutely, within 24 hours after hypoxic brain damage, while the patient is still unconscious, or it may manifest as a late complication. The myoclonus related to hypoxia is usually movement-induced, but it can be triggered by noise, touching the patient or tracheal suctioning. The acute form is associated with a poor prognosis. The chronic condition of myoclonus develops days or weeks after the hypoxic insult and predominantly consists of movement induced violent flexion of the body, head, and neck.

*Propriospinal myoclonus (PSM) is a rare movement disorder* characterised by myoclonic jerks arising in muscles corresponding to a single myotome and spreading rostrally and caudally to the other myotomes. PSM can be idiopathic, related to spinal cord lesions, drug use, malignancy, or infection. [45] Patients present with myoclonic jerks involving abdominal wall muscles, which worsen when lying down.

---

1　I give patients a table to complete for each hour of the waking day. I ask them to indicate when they take their medication. They then have to indicate each hour if they have severe symptoms of Parkinson's, severe dyskinesia or if they feel good without severe bradykinesia or dyskinesia. In this way we can differentiate between end of dose faile and the on-off phenomenon.

| Management of Myoclonus |
|---|
| MRI with diffusion tensor imaging with fibre tracking detects abnormalities in patients with PSM. The spinal tracts are disorganised in all patients with a decreased number of total visible fibres in all most patients, mainly seen in the lemniscal posterior or corticospinal posterolateral tracts. [45] Clonazepam, piracetam and valproic acid are the first-line treatments for post-hypoxic action myoclonus or PSM. Propofol and midazolam are used in the acute hypoxic form. [46] Zonisamide has been recommended for PSM. [45] |

## Chorea and Athetosis

Chorea is the ceaseless irregular, rapid, uncontrolled complex body movements that look well-coordinated and purposeful but are involuntary. The term 'chorea' is derived from the Greek word 'choreia' or 'khoreia' for dancing. Chorea can affect the face, arms, or legs. The abnormal movements are almost continuous.

Athetosis consists of repetitive, involuntary, slow, sinuous, writhing movements, especially severe in the hands.

Choreoathetosis is a movement of medium speed, between the quick, flitting movements of chorea and the slower, writhing movements of athetosis.

Chorea is very uncommon; Huntington's disease is the leading cause as Sydenham's chorea has largely disappeared along with rheumatic fever. An infrequent but treatable cause of chorea is Wilson's disease. [47] Several even rarer inherited movement disorders, beyond the scope of this book, can result in dystonia, chorea, or ataxia [48, 49].

## Huntington's Disease

Huntington's disease [50] is a hereditary disorder with a genetic defect on the short arm of chromosome 4. The gene defect leads to the altered function of the ubiquitous protein, huntingtin, that culminates in neuronal loss in the caudate nucleus. The number of tri-nucleotide repeats (cysteine-adenine-guanidine; CAG) influences whether the disease shows incomplete or complete penetrance. The number also affects the onset age, with juvenile-onset Huntington's patients typically having more than 55 tri-nucleotide repeats.

Huntington's disease is characterised by the insidious onset in middle age (35–44 years) of progressive cognitive decline associated with abnormal movements and psychiatric disturbances. The chorea may not be present at the outset; often, the initial symptoms are instability and a lack of coordination with the cognitive decline and psychiatric disturbances appearing later. Chorea is the typical movement disorder, but rigidity, bradykinesia and dystonia may predominate and can be more disabling. Rarely Huntington's develops before 20, so-called juvenile Huntington's disease. In juvenile Huntington's disease, the symptoms are quite different – the patient often presents rigid and akinetic (absence or poverty of movement) – and the progression to disability is more rapid. The inheritance pattern of Huntington's disease is autosomal dominant.

## Sydenham's Chorea

Sydenham's chorea was first described in 1686 by Thomas Sydenham in his work entitled 'Schedula monitoria de novae febris ingress'.[80] It was not until 180 years later (in 1866) that Roger appreciated the association with rheumatic fever.[81] It is a complication of rheumatic fever following infection with group A beta-hemolytic streptococci. It predominantly affects children, although occasionally in adults. It is much rarer these days since the virtual abolition of rheumatic fever.

The antecedent sore throat, polyarthritis, and subcutaneous nodules the size of peas at joints such as the elbows and knees, together with the characteristic pink-red macular rash referred to as erythema marginatum, are the clues to the diagnosis. Sydenham's chorea is a self-limiting illness that initially worsens over 2–4 weeks and then subsequently resolves spontaneously over 3–6 months. Some patients may have waxing and waning symptoms for up to 12 months. [51]

## Wilson's Disease

Wilson's disease results from a mutation in the autosomal recessive ATP7B gene. The mutated gene prevents the transport protein from functioning correctly, allowing copper to accumulate in the liver, brain, kidneys, and skeletal system. [47]

The neurological manifestations are the most common presentation, whilst patients with liver disease present with jaundice. Although chorea occurs in Wilson's disease, it is not the most typical manifestation. The majority present with features of parkinsonism, dystonia, ataxia, pyramidal signs, seizures, myoclonus and athetosis.

---

**Management of Wilson's Disease**

The diagnosis of Wilson's disease is established by the presence of Kayser–Fleischer rings on the cornea, decreased serum ceruloplasmin, elevated 24-hour urine copper or increased hepatic copper content. Unfortunately, none of these findings is entirely sensitive or specific. [48]

Characteristic MRI abnormalities in patients with Wilson's disease consist of axial $T_2$WI bilateral basal ganglionic and thalamic hyperintensity in addition to mild to moderate diffuse atrophy. [47]

Treatment is with zinc acetate, zinc sulfate, or chelating agents such as penicillamine to reduce copper absorption. Liver transplantation is an option in patients who fail to respond or cannot tolerate medical therapy. [52]

Symptomatic treatment for chorea is dopamine-depleting agents such as tetrabenazine or reserpine, benzodiazepines such as clonazepam or diazepam and dopamine antagonists such as haloperidol.

---

# Abnormal Movements – With Activity

## Benign Essential or Familial Tremor

Essential or familial essential tremor [53, 54] is the most common movement disorders in the elderly and the most common cause of action tremor. [55] It can occur in patients in their teens.

Typically, the benign essential/familial tremor occurs when patients are either moving their arms or holding an object such as a book or a cup of liquid. Typically the cup rattles in the saucer and patients have to resort to half-filling their cup in order not to spill the liquid. Eating becomes more difficult as the patient repeatedly spills food off the fork or soup out of the spoon. Although the tremor is bilateral, one side may be more severely affected than the other. The tremor sometimes very slowly leads to physical disability. Many patients are socially disabled as they are too embarrassed to go out. Familial tremor is generally inherited as an autosomal dominant trait but with variable penetrance. Apart from the tremor, the neurological examination is otherwise normal; in particular, there is no rigidity or bradykinesia.

# Differentiating Parkinson's from Essential/Familial Tremor

Table 13.2 shows the differences between Parkinson's and familial or essential tremor.

| Clinical feature | Parkinson's | Essential/familial |
|---|---|---|
| It affects the head and voice | No | Yes |
| Present at rest | Yes | No |
| Present when holding objects | No | Yes |
| Worse with walking | Yes | No |
| Influenced by alcohol | No | Yes |
| Frequency | 3–6 Hz | 5–12 Hz |
| Family history | Occasional | Often (familial) |

Table 13.2 The different features of the tremor of Parkinson's disease and essential/familial tremor

---

**Investigation and Treatment of Essential Tremor**

Hyperthyroidism needs to be excluded in patients with 'essential tremor'. Genetic susceptibility loci have been identified in the FET1 (also known as ETM1) gene located on chromosome 3q1 [56] and ETM mapped to chromosome 2p22–25. [57]

There is no cure and many patients simply require reassurance about the benign nature of the tremor. Small doses of alcohol can be used to reduce the severity of mild tremor. In patients with more severe tremor, low-dose primidone (commencing with ¼ of a tablet or 62.5 mg and increasing to the minimum required or maximally tolerated dose, as much as 250 mg/day) or moderate dose propranolol (commencing with 10 mg and increasing slowly up to 120 mg/day) has been shown to reduce the severity of the tremor. [58] Osteoporosis commonly coexists in the elderly and primidone can exacerbate osteoporosis. Other edications include alprazolam, gabapentin, topiramate, nimodipine, clozapine and clonidine. In patients who are resistant to pharmacological therapy, either thalamotomy or deep brain stimulation may be of benefit. [58]

---

# Cerebellar or Intention Tremor

Cerebellar tremor is also referred to as intention tremor. These patients present with a tremor when using their arms, not at rest. There is little or no tremor with the hands outstretched, but noticeable tremor when the patient is asked to perform finger-to-nose or heel-to-shin testing where instability is noticed as the patient stretches to reach the distant target. The oscillations of intention tremor are perpendicular to the direction of movement and usually of low frequency, less than 5 Hz.

Intention tremor occurs in patients with MS, Friedreich's ataxia, cerebellar infarction, and degeneration.

---

**Treatment for Intention Tremor**

There is no specific treatment for intention tremor. Drugs such as clonazepam, carbamazepine, ondansetron, isoniazid and physostigmine have all been tried with variable success. [59] In refractory cases, deep-brain stimulation may be of benefit. [60, 61]

---

# Orthostatic Tremor

Orthostatic tremor is a condition where the patient finds it impossible to stand still for any length of time. They develop an increasingly severe sensation of instability (not dizziness) with their body developing a shaky feeling. Patients rarely fall and usually hang on to something, sit down or commence walking. Many patients avoid stopping while walking to avoid this sensation. The neurological examination is otherwise normal. Most cases are idiopathic [62], but it has been described in progressive supranuclear palsy [63] and following head injury. [64]

| Treatment of Orthostatic Tremor |
|---|
| Clonazepam and primidone, particularly a combination of both drugs [65], and pramipexole [66] have been reported to reduce the severity of orthostatic tremor although none has been subjected to randomised controlled trials. A benefit from deep brain stimulation has also been described. [67] |

# Action Myoclonus

Myoclonus is the one abnormal movement that occurs at rest and persists in sleep. Action myoclonus refers to sudden arrhythmic muscular jerking induced by voluntary movement. The condition is usually associated with diffuse neuronal disease, such as post-hypoxic encephalopathy [68], uraemia and various forms of progressive myoclonic epilepsy such as the Ramsay–Hunt syndrome. [69]

# Paroxysmal Kinesogenic Choreoathetosis

Paroxysmal kinesogenic choreoathetosis (PKC) has its onset in childhood or early adulthood. The characteristic feature is discrete episodes of *abnormal movements precipitated by sudden movement* such as standing up from sitting or being startled. Chorea occurs, as does hyperkinesia, dystonia, athetosis and ballism. The neurological exam is normal between the events. The attacks are brief (< 5 minutes) and may occur several times a day.

| Management of Paroxysmal Kinesogenic Choreoathetosis |
|---|
| Linkage has been established in eight Japanese families to chromosome 16p11.2-q12.1. [70] The condition responds very well to low-dose anticonvulsant therapy such as carbamazepine or phenytoin. [71] |

# Abnormal Movements During Sleep

Myoclonus has already been discussed; the other abnormal movement during sleep is hemiballismus.

# Hemiballismus

Hemiballismus (derived from the Greek word 'ballismos' which means jumping about or dancing) is considered a rare form of chorea. It is almost a continuous, violent, coordinated involuntary motor restlessness of half (very rarely bilateral, referred to as paraballism) of the body. The movements are usually continuous contorting movements and often rotatory. It is most marked in the upper extremities and is usually caused by a lesion involving the subthalamic nucleus of the opposite side of the brain. However, it can arise from contralateral lesions in the cortex, basal ganglia, and thalamus. [72] The commonest cause is an infarct, but it has been reported with demyelinating disease.

Although spontaneous remission is common, hemiballismus is a potentially life-threatening disorder, and therapy is essential.

| Management of Hemiballismus |
|---|
| An MRI scan, in particular a diffusion-weighted MRI scan, may define the site of the pathology in patients with hemiballismus. Pharmacological agents include haloperidol, risperidone, clonazepam, and baclofen. Pallidotomy or thalamotomy may be necessary in intractable cases. |

# Rare Life-Threatening Movement Disorders

These have also been referred to as movement disorder emergencies and are defined as any movement disorder that evolves over hours to days and includes acute parkinsonism, dystonia, chorea, tics, and myoclonus. The commonest is drug-induced (neuroleptics and antiemetics) parkinsonism. Cyanide, methanol, carbon monoxide, carbon disulfide, organophosphate pesticides, and the designer drug MPTP are some toxins that may produce severe encephalopathy with clinical features of parkinsonism. Only neuroleptic malignant syndrome and serotonin syndrome will be discussed here. For an excellent review of movement disorder emergencies, see the review by Poston. [39]

## Neuroleptic Malignant Syndrome

Neuroleptic malignant syndrome is a very rare, potentially life-threatening but treatable idiosyncratic response to $D_2$-dopamine receptor agonists such as antiemetics, droperidol, anaesthetic agents and antipsychotic drugs. A rapid increase in the dose may increase the risk of the neuroleptic malignant syndrome. It can also occur if treatment for Parkinson's is suddenly withdrawn.

The clinical features consist of rigidity, fever, sweating, severe hypertension, and altered consciousness. Creatinine kinase is elevated, and liver function abnormalities occur. Dehydration leads to renal impairment. Features of parkinsonism and the presence of fever should alert the clinician to the possibility of this condition. It can occur at any age and in either sex.

| Treatment of Neuroleptic Malignant Syndrome2 |
|---|
| Neuroleptic Malignant Syndrome is a neurological emergency. The initial step is to withdraw the offending neuroleptic medication. If the syndrome has occurred in the setting of an abrupt withdrawal of dopaminergic medication, then this medication should be reinstituted as quickly as possible. |
| Treatment consists of lowering the body temperature, IV fluids to correct hypotension and nutrients. Short-term dantrolene (an initial bolus dose of 1 to 2.5 mg/kg followed by 1 mg/kg every 6 hours up to a maximum amount of 10 mg/kg/day until symptoms resolve) or the dopamine agonists such as bromocriptine ( 2.5 mg 2 or 3 times daily and increasing doses by 2.5 mg every 24 hours until a response or until reaching a maximum dose of 45 mg/day) are the drugs of 1st choice. Once patients have recovered from neuroleptic malignant syndrome, about 87% will be able to tolerate an antipsychotic at some point in the future. Usually a different antipsychotic class and an atypical antipsychotic. [76] |

---

2   NORD https://rarediseases.org/rare-diseases/neuroleptic-malignant-syndrome/
   And BMJ Best Practice https://bestpractice.bmj.com/topics/en-gb/3000227

# Serotonin Syndrome

Serotonin syndrome [73] is caused by the serotonin-specific reuptake inhibitors (sertraline, fluoxetine, paroxetine, and fluvoxamine), clomipramine, ecstasy and the combination of monoamine oxidase inhibitors and meperidine that increase the biological activity of serotonin.

Serotonin syndrome consists of fever with confusion, hypomania, agitation, tachycardia, sweating, shivering, tremor, diarrhoea, hypertension, incoordination, myoclonus, and rigidity hyperreflexia. The clinical features of serotonin syndrome and neuroleptic malignant syndrome overlap. The presence of myoclonus in serotonin syndrome distinguishes it from the neuroleptic malignant syndrome.

| Treatment of Serotonin Syndrome |
| --- |
| If symptoms are minor, ceasing the offending medication is appropriate. In more severe cases, IV fluids and oxygen may be required. IV benzodiazepines (e.g. lorazepam 2 to 4 mg or diazepam 5 to 10 mg) for the agitation. These doses can be repeated every 8 to 10 minutes based upon patient response. Esmolol, a cardioselective beta-1 adrenergic antagonist or nitroprusside, are used for autonomic instability (severe hypertension and tachycardia). Hyperthermia should be treated; if extreme (temperature > 41ºC), intubation sedation and paralysis may be required. Severe hypotension is treated with phenylephrine, epinephrine, or norepinephrine. Cyproheptadine (4-16mg/day) is a histamine-1 receptor antagonist and is an antidote[3]. [74, 75] |

# References

1   Baron EM, Young WF. Cervical spondylotic myelopathy: A brief review of its pathophysiology, clinical course, and diagnosis. *Neurosurgery* 2007;60(Supp1 1):S35–S41.

2   Prasad D, Schiff D. Malignant spinal-cord compression. *Lancet Oncol* 2005;6(1):15–24.

3   Husband DJ. Malignant spinal cord compression: Prospective study of delays in referral and treatment. *BMJ* 1998;317(7150):18–21.

4   White BD, et al. Diagnosis and management of patients at risk of or with metastatic spinal cord compression: Summary of NICE guidance. *BMJ* 2008;337:a2538.

5   Portenoy RK, et al. Identification of epidural neoplasm. Radiography and bone scintigraphy in the symptomatic and asymptomatic spine. *Cancer* 1989;64(11):2207–2213.

6   Hyman RA, et al. 0.6 T MR imaging of the cervical spine: Multislice and multiecho techniques. *Am J Neuroradiol* 1985;6(2):229–236.

7   Loblaw DA, et al. Systematic review of the diagnosis and management of malignant extradural spinal cord compression: The Cancer Care Ontario Practice Guidelines Initiative's Neuro-Oncology Disease Site Group. *J Clin Oncol* 2005;23(9):2028–2037.

8   Sorensen S, et al. Effect of high-dose dexamethasone in carcinomatous metastatic spinal cord compression treated with radiotherapy: A randomised trial. *Eur J Cancer* 1994;30A(1):22–27.

9   Patchell RA, et al. Direct decompressive surgical resection in the treatment of spinal cord compression caused by metastatic cancer: A randomised trial. *Lancet* 2005;366(9486):643–648.

10  al Deeb SM, et al. Acute transverse myelitis: A localised form of postinfectious encephalomyelitis. *Brain* 1997;120(Pt 7):1115–1122.

11  Transverse Myelitis Consortium Working Group. Proposed diagnostic criteria and nosology of acute transverse myelitis. *Neurology* 2002;59(4):499–505.

12  Harzheim M, et al. Discriminatory features of acute transverse myelitis: A retrospective analysis of 45 patients. *J Neurol Sci* 2004;217(2):217–223.

3   Up-to-date https://www.uptodate.com/contents/serotonin-syndrome-serotonin-toxicity

13    Misra UK, Kalita J, Kumar S. A clinical, MRI and neurophysiological study of acute transverse myelitis. *J Neurol Sci* 1996;138(1–2):150–156.

14    de Seze J, et al. Acute myelopathies: Clinical, laboratory and outcome profiles in 79 cases. *Brain* 2001;124(Pt 8):1509–1521.

15    Croft P. Neuromuscular syndromes associated with malignant disease. *Br J Hosp Med* 1977;17(4): 360–362:356.

16    Rudnicki SA, Dalmau J. Paraneoplastic syndromes of the peripheral nerves. *Curr Opin Neurol* 2005;18(5):598–603.

17    Malinow K, et al. Subacute sensory neuronopathy secondary to dorsal root ganglionitis in primary Sjögren's syndrome. *Ann Neurol* 1986;20(4):535–537.

18    Schaumburg H, et al. Sensory neuropathy from pyridoxine abuse: A new megavitamin syndrome. *N Engl J Med* 1983;309(8):445–448.

19    Jellinek EH, Kelly RE. Cerebellar syndrome in myxoedema. *Lancet* 1960;2(7144):225–227.

20    Skillicorn SA. Presenile cerebellar ataxia in chronic alcoholics. *Neurology* 1955;5(8):527–534.

21    Bariety M, et al. ["Paraneoplastic" psychic and cerebellar syndrome reversible by radiotherapeutic treatment of its cause: "Anaplastic bronchial epithelioma".]. *Bull Mem Soc Med Hop Paris* 1960;76: 650–661.

22    Richter R. The hereditary nature of late cortical cerebellar atrophy. *Trans Am Neurol Assoc* 1948;73(73 Annual Meet):85–78.

23    Davis GC, et al. Chronic parkinsonism secondary to intravenous injection of meperidine analogues. *Psychiatry Res* 1979;1(3):249–254.

24    Messert B, Baker NH. Syndrome of progressive spastic ataxia and apraxia associated with occult hydrocephalus. *Neurology* 1966;16(5):440–452.

25    Dixon GR, et al. Use of cerebrospinal fluid flow rates measured by phase-contrast MR to predict outcome of ventriculoperitoneal shunting for idiopathic normal-pressure hydrocephalus. *Mayo Clin Proc* 2002;77(6):509–514.

26    Panagiotopoulos V, et al. The predictive value of external continuous lumbar drainage, with cerebrospinal fluid outflow controlled by medium pressure valve, in normal pressure hydrocephalus. *Acta Neurochir (Wien)* 2005;147(9):953–958:discussion 958.

27    Pfisterer WK, et al. Continuous intraventricular pressure monitoring for diagnosis of normal-pressure hydrocephalus. *Acta Neurochir (Wien)* 2007;149(10):983–990:discussion 990.

28    Wikkelso C, et al. Normal pressure hydrocephalus. Predictive value of the cerebrospinal fluid tap-test. *Acta Neurol Scand* 1986;73(6):566–573.

29    Bret P, et al. [Clinical experience with the Sp[hy adjustable valve in the treatment of adult hydrocephalus: A series of 147 cases.]. *Neurochirurgie* 1999;45(2):98–108:discussion 108–109.

30    Rider, L. S. and E. M. Marra (2021). Cauda Equina And Conus Medullaris Syndromes. *StatPearls* StatPearls Publishing.

31    Gan J, et al. Possible Parkinson's disease revealed by a pure head resting tremor. *J Neurol Sci* 2009;279(1–2):121–123.

32    Schonecker VM. Ein eigentumliches syndrom in oralen Bereich bei Negaphenapplikation. *Nervenarzt* 1957;28:35.

33    Tarsy D, Baldessarini RJ. Epidemiology of tardive dyskinesia: Is risk declining with modern antipsychotics?. *Mov Disord* 2006;21(5):589–598.

34    Kenney C, Jankovic J. Tetrabenazine in the treatment of hyperkinetic movement disorders. *Expert Rev Neurother* 2006;6(1):7–17.

35    Sun B, et al. Subthalamic nucleus stimulation for primary dystonia and tardive dystonia. *Acta Neurochir Suppl* 2007;97(Pt 2):207–214.

36  Nisijima K, Shioda K, Iwamura T. Neuroleptic malignant syndrome and serotonin syndrome. *Prog Brain Res* 2007;162:81–104.

37  Jankovic J. Tourette's syndrome. *N Engl J Med* 2001;345(16):1184–1192.

38  The Tourette Syndrome Classification Study Group. Definitions and classification of tic disorders. *Arch Neurol* 1993;50(10):1013–1016.

39  Poston KL, Frucht SJ. Movement disorder emergencies. *J Neurol* 2008;255(Suppl 4):2–13.

40  Parkinson J. *An essay on the shaking palsy*. London: Whittingham and Roland; 1817.

41  Polymeropoulos MH, et al. Mutation in the alpha-synuclein gene identified in families with Parkinson's disease. *Science* 1997;276(5321):2045–2047.

42  Miyasaki JM, et al. Practice parameter: Initiation of treatment for Parkinson's disease: An evidence-based review: Report of the Quality Standards Subcommittee of the American Academy of Neurology. *Neurology* 2002;58(1):11–17.

43  Parkinson Study Group. Pramipexole vs levodopa as initial treatment for Parkinson disease: A randomised controlled trial. *JAMA* 2000;284(15):1931–1938.

44  Miyasaki JM, et al. Practice parameter: Evaluation and treatment of depression, psychosis, and dementia in Parkinson disease (an evidence-based review): Report of the Quality Standards Subcommittee of the American Academy of Neurology. *Neurology* 2006;66(7):996–1002.

45  Roze E, et al. Propriospinal myoclonus revisited: Clinical, neurophysiologic, and neuroradiologic findings. *Neurology* 2009;72(15):1301–1309.

46  Venkatesan A, Frucht S. Movement disorders after resuscitation from cardiac arrest. *Neurol Clin* 2006;24(1):123–132.

47  Taly AB, et al. Wilson disease: Description of 282 patients evaluated over 3 decades. *Medicine (Baltimore)* 2007;86(2):112–121.

48  Sharma N, Standaert DG. Inherited movement disorders. *Neurol Clin* 2002;20(3):759–778:vii.

49  Jen JC, et al. Primary episodic ataxias: Diagnosis, pathogenesis and treatment. *Brain* 2007;130(Pt 10):2484–2493.

50  Huntington G. On chorea. The Medical and Surgical Reporter:. *A Weekly Journal* 1872;26(15): 317–321.

51  Gordon N. Sydenham's chorea, and its complications affecting the nervous system. *Brain Dev* 2009;31(1):11–14.

52  Cox DW, Roberts E. Wilson's disease. 2006. Gene Tests website. Available: http://www.ncbi.nlm.nih. gov/bookshelf/br.fcgi?book=gene&part=wilson#wilson (14 Dec 2009).

53  Critchley M. Observations on essential (heredofamial) tremor. *Brain* 1949;72(Pt 2):113–139.

54  Davis CH, Kunkle EC. Benign essential (heredofamilial) tremor. *Trans Am Neurol Assoc* 1951;56: 87–89.

55  Thanvi B, Lo N, Robinson T. Essential tremor — the most common movement disorder in older people. *Age Ageing* 2006;35(4):344–349.

56  Gulcher JR, et al. Mapping of a familial essential tremor gene, FET1, to chromosome 3q13. *Nat Genet* 1997;17(1):84–87.

57  Higgins JJ, Pho LT, Nee LE. A gene (ETM) for essential tremor maps to chromosome 2p22-p25. *Mov Disord* 1997;12(6):859–864.

58  Zesiewicz TA, et al. Practice parameter: Therapies for essential tremor: Report of the Quality Standards Subcommittee of the American Academy of Neurology. *Neurology* 2005;64(12):2008–2020.

59  Bhidayasiri R. Differential diagnosis of common tremor syndromes. *Postgrad Med J* 2005;81(962): 756–762.

60  Nandi D, Aziz TZ. Deep brain stimulation in the management of neuropathic pain and multiple sclerosis tremor. *J Clin Neurophysiol* 2004;21(1):31–39.

61  Wishart HA, et al. Chronic deep brain stimulation for the treatment of tremor in multiple sclerosis: Review and case reports. *J Neurol Neurosurg Psychiatry* 2003;74(10):1392–1397.

62  Gates PC. Orthostatic tremor (shaky legs syndrome). *Clin Exp Neurol* 1993;30:66–71.

63  de Bie RM, Chen R, Lang AE. Orthostatic tremor in progressive supranuclear palsy. *Mov Disord* 2007;22(8):1192–1194.

64  Sanitate SS, Meerschaert JR. Orthostatic tremor: Delayed onset following head trauma. *Arch Phys Med Rehabil* 1993;74(8):886–889.

65  Poersch M. Orthostatic tremor: Combined treatment with primidone and clonazepam. *Mov Disord* 1994;9(4):467.

66  Finkel MF. Pramipexole is a possible effective treatment for primary orthostatic tremor (shaky leg syndrome). *Arch Neurol* 2000;57(10):1519–1520.

67  Guridi J, et al. Successful thalamic deep brain stimulation for orthostatic tremor. *Mov Disord* 2008;23(13):1808–1811.

68  Fahn S. Posthypoxic action myoclonus: Literature review update. *Adv Neurol* 1986;43:157–169.

69  Lance JW. Action myoclonus, Ramsay Hunt syndrome, and other cerebellar myoclonic syndromes. *Adv Neurol* 1986;43:33–55.

70  Tomita H, et al. Paroxysmal kinesigenic choreoathetosis locus maps to chromosome 16p11.2-q12.1. *Am J Hum Genet* 1999;65(6):1688–1697.

71  Wein T, et al. Exquisite sensitivity of paroxysmal kinesigenic choreoathetosis to carbamazepine. *Neurology* 1996;47(4):1104–1106.

72  Dewey Jr RB, Jankovic J. Hemiballism-hemichorea: Clinical and pharmacologic findings in 21 patients. *Arch Neurol* 1989;46(8):862–867.

73  Sternbach H. The serotonin syndrome. *Am J Psychiatry* 1991;148(6):705–713.

74  Lappin RI, Auchincloss EL. Treatment of the serotonin syndrome with cyproheptadine. *N Engl J Med* 1994;331(15):1021–1022.

75  Graudins A, Stearman A, Chan B. Treatment of the serotonin syndrome with cyproheptadine. *J Emerg Med* 1998;16(4):615–619.

76  Berman BD. Neuroleptic malignant syndrome: a review for neurohospitalists. N*eurohospitalist* 2011; 1(1): 41-7.

77  Lan SY, Kuo CY, Chou CC, et al. Recreational nitrous oxide abuse related subacute combined degeneration of the spinal cord in adolescents - A case series and literature review. *Brain Dev* 2019; 41(5): 428-35.

78  Xiang Y, Li L, Ma X, et al. Recreational Nitrous Oxide Abuse: Prevalence, Neurotoxicity, and Treatment. *Neurotox Res* 2021; 39(3): 975-85.

79  Jannetta, P. J. (1975). "The cause of hemifacial spasm: definitive microsurgical treatment at the brainstem in 31 patients." *Trans Sect Otolaryngol Am Acad Ophthalmol Otolaryngol* 80(3 Pt 1): 319-322.

80  Sydenham, T. (1848). *On St Vitus's dance. The works of Thomas Sydenham.* London, Sydenham Society.

81  Roger, H. (1866). " [Recherches cliniques sur la choree, sur le rheumatisme et surles maladies du coeur chez les enfants]." *Arch Gen Med* 2: 641-665.

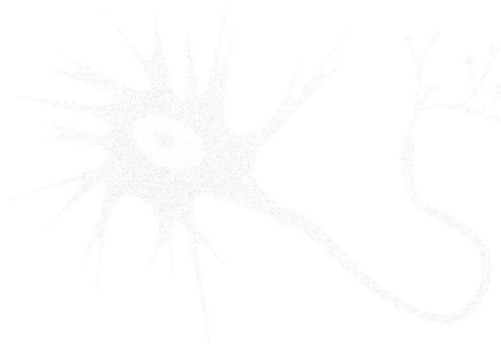

# Miscellaneous Neurological Disorders

The principal aim of this textbook has been to introduce simple concepts, basic principles and rules that I have developed over many years to assist the 'student of neurology'. The second aim was to discuss the more common neurological problems encountered in everyday clinical practice using a symptom-oriented rather than a disease-oriented approach .

No neurology textbook however, would be complete without discussing specific less common neurological problems.

- assessment of patients with a depressed conscious state
- assessment of the confused or demented patient
- disorders of muscle and the neuromuscular junction
- multiple sclerosis
- tumours and the nervous system
- infections of the nervous system.

# Depressed Consciousness

Fred Plum and Jereme Posner have written the definitive text on this subject in a superb monograph, entitled *The Diagnosis of Stupor and Coma.* [1] It should be required reading for every neurologist in training.

Essentially there are three patterns of a depressed conscious state:

1. **Diffuse Symptoms** – consciousness is depressed in the absence of neurological signs. The leading causes include:
   - drugs (alcohol, opiates and sedatives)
   - hypothermia (may cause coma if the temperature is less than 31°C),
   - meningitis, encephalitis
   - subarachnoid haemorrhage, acute hydrocephalus
   - severe hypotension from any cause
   - metabolic disturbances such as hypoxaemia, hepatic coma, hyponatraemia, hypernatraemia, hypercapnia, hypoglycaemia.

2. **Cerebral hemisphere symptoms** – the depressed conscious state is associated with hemiparesis or hemiplegia. Conditions that produce a mass effect cause downward herniation of the brain through the tentorium with secondary brainstem compression. Such conditions include:
   - extradural, subdural and intracerebral haemorrhage
   - tumours
   - brain abscess
   - herpes simplex encephalitis.

3. **Diseases in the brainstem** – the conscious state is depressed with abnormalities in the brainstem reflexes. These include:
   - brainstem infarction secondary to basilar artery occlusion
   - pontine haemorrhage

In an unconscious patient, even before a neurological examination, it is vital to ensure
   - The *airway* is not obstructed.
   - The patient is *breathing* adequately; if not, intubate them.
   - Check the *circulation* – pulse and blood pressure. If the patient is hypotensive, treat with appropriate fluids and, if necessary pharmacological agents.
   - Check the blood glucose to exclude hypoglycaemia or hyperglycaemia.

Hypotension suggests possible drug overdose, severe internal bleeding into a body cavity such as the chest or abdomen, sepsis, severe hypothyroidism or an Addisonian crisis.
   1. *Look at the pupils.* If the pupils are pinpoint, administer naloxone. (pontine haemorrhage and narcotic or barbiturate overdose result in pinpoint pupils.)
   2. *Smell the breath* for alcohol or ketones.
   3. *Check the blood alcohol.*
   4. Look for IV needle puncture marks.

Once the patient is stabilised, it is imperative to obtain as much information as possible to provide clues to the cause of the coma. Often patients are found unconscious, and a detailed history is not possible. In this setting, question the person who found the patient.
   - Attempt to establish when the patient was last seen well and narrow down the time they may have been unconscious.
   - Were there empty bottles or syringes to indicate possible overdose from prescription medications (e.g. insulin or hypoglycaemics) or illicit drugs.
   - Was there a suicide note?
   - Question ambulance officers rather than rely on the ambulance report.
   - Telephone relatives, neighbours or anybody who might provide clues to the diagnosis.
   - Ask about evidence to suggest trauma, e.g. overturned furniture, blood on the floor.
   - See if there is anything in the past medical history that may provide a clue.

# Examination of Patients with Depressed Consciousness

The neurological examination in patients with a depressed conscious state is entirely different to the standard neurological examination. It ascertains
   1. the level of arousal
   2. the response to pain
   3. abnormalities within the cranial nerves that indicate brainstem involvement.

*Look for spontaneous movements of the limbs* or lack thereof, the latter suggesting possible paralysis. Observe whether they are opening their eyes and looking around, indicating a lesser degree of depression of the conscious state. *Look for focal seizure activity* in the face or limbs.

## Level of Arousal

The next step is to *attempt to arouse the patient with verbal stimuli* and, if that fails, *painful stimuli* (Figure 14.1). One of the most valuable techniques is to pinch the skin between your fingernails on the medial aspect of the elbows and knees. A normal response is abduction of the limbs away from the painful stimulus; an abnormal response is extension of the limbs or adduction of the limbs towards the painful stimulus. Before testing the reaction to painful stimuli in front of the family, explain that it is the best way to test when someone is unconscious. The family should also be warned that this technique may leave bruises.

*Examine the brainstem reflexes*. The region tested is shown in brackets.
* The *pupillary reflex* – the afferent pathway is the 2nd nerve; the efferent pathway is the parasympathetic pathway on the surface of the 3rd nerve (midbrain and 3rd nerve)
* *The corneal and nasal tickle reflexes* – the afferent pathway is the 5th cranial nerve; the efferent pathway is the 7th nerve in the pons.
* *Doll's eye reflexes* – spontaneous and head movement-evoked eye movements. Moving the head up and down tests vertical eye movements and the midbrain. Moving the head side to side tests horizontal eye movements and the pons.
* *The gag reflex* – use a tongue depressor and apply it to the back of the throat on each side. The afferent pathway is the 9th cranial nerve; the efferent pathway is the 10th cranial nerve in the medulla.

Normal pupil responses, doll's eye testing and corneal or nasal tickle reflexes indicate that the brainstem is intact and that the cause of the coma is either in the cerebral hemispheres or a diffuse problem. A 3rd or 6th nerve palsy does not necessarily indicate brainstem involvement. A 3rd can occur with a hemisphere lesion with downward herniation, and a 6th can occur with raised intracranial pressure as a false localising sign.

## Response to Pain

If the patient abducts or withdraws the limb away from the painful stimulus applied to the medial aspect of the elbow or knee, this implies that the motor pathway is intact. On the other hand, if the patient does not withdraw the limb, but the arm or leg moves towards the painful stimulus or straightens, the motor pathway is affected.

Decorticate and decerebrate rigidity are two terms used to describe specific postures that may occur in the unconscious patient. Decorticate rigidity is flexion of the elbows and wrists and supination of the arms. Decorticate rigidity occurs with bilateral damage above (rostral) to the midbrain. Decerebrate rigidity consists of the extension of the elbows and wrists with pronation of the forearms. It indicates damage to the motor pathways in the midbrain or lower part (caudal) of the diencephalon (thalamus and hypothalamus). These abnormal postures were thought to have localising value, although this is now in question. Similarly, the pattern of respiration is not of great localising value. Cyclic breathing with periods of apnoea referred to as Cheyne–Stokes respiration can occur with bilateral hemisphere damage or metabolic suppression of the conscious state.

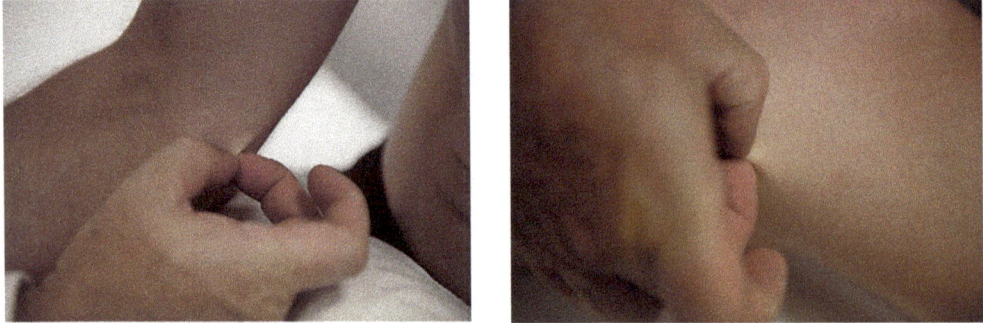

**Figure 14.1** Method of applying painful stimuli to the limbs

# The Corneal and Nasal Tickle Reflexes

The cornea of the eye or the nostril are stimulated using cotton wool (not tissue paper as this may damage the cornea), and reflex closure of the eyelids indicates that the pons is intact. Absent reflexes may occur with hemisphere lesions, drug overdose or structural brainstem lesions and, thus, absent corneal reflexes are not particularly useful for localising the problem (figure 14.2).

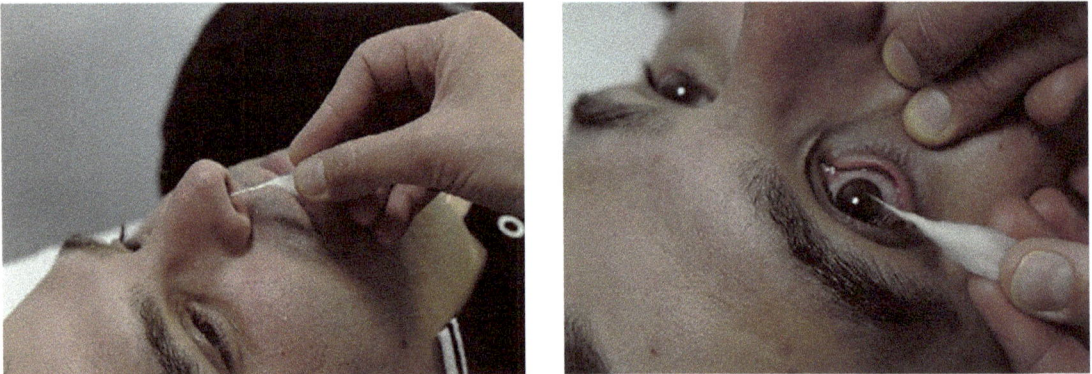

**Figure 14.2** Method of testing the nasal and corneal reflexes

# The Eye Movements

Divergent eyes during sleep is normal.

- Spontaneous movements of the eyes, referred to as 'roving eyes', excludes damage to the midbrain and pons.
- Eyes deviated to one side indicate ipsilateral hemisphere or contralateral pontine pathology. In hemisphere lesions, the eyes deviate away from the side of the paralysis and towards the side of the lesion. In brainstem lesions, the opposite is the case. The eyes deviate away from the side of the lesion and towards the side of the hemiparesis. One exception to this rule is that with irritating hemisphere lesions, the eyes may be deviated away from the side of the lesion and towards the side of the paralysis.
- Ocular bobbing indicates bilateral pontine damage, most often with basilar artery thrombosis. It consists of the absence of horizontal eye movements, a characteristic brisk downward movement of both eyes, and a slow upward movement to return to the normal position.

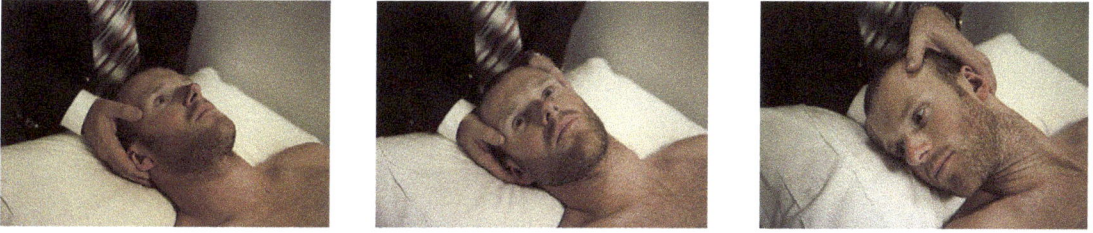

**Figure 14.3** Method of testing eye movements using the doll's eye procedure.

> Eyes that spontaneously deviate away from the side of the paralysis indicate a hemisphere lesion on the side opposite to the paralysis; eyes that deviate to the side of the paralysis indicate a brainstem lesion on the side opposite the paralysis.

The oculocephalic reflex or doll's eye test (Figure 14.3) also assesses the brainstem.
- The head is moved rapidly, initially horizontally and then vertically, while the movement of the eyes in the opposite direction is observed.
- If the brainstem is not affected, when the head is turned to the right, the eyes deviate fully to the left and vice versa.
- If the eye movements are complete, i.e. the eyes move in the orbits to their full extent so that no sclera can be seen, the brainstem is intact and therefore not the site of the pathology causing the impaired consciousness.
- If the eyes fail to move in one direction, this suggests damage to the ipsilateral brainstem nuclei.
- In patients with severe depression of the conscious state due to drug overdose, the oculocephalic reflexes may be abnormal and not indicate any structural damage to the brainstem. In this setting, the pupils would usually be of normal size and react to light, which would not occur in destructive brainstem lesions.

More intense stimulation of the oculocephalic reflex can be produced with caloric stimulation. Before performing this test, it is essential to ensure that the external ear canal is not occluded by wax. Tonic deviation of the eyes with nystagmus to the opposite side with cold water and the same side with warm water indicates that the brainstem is intact. If the eyes fail to deviate, this points to brainstem damage.

## The Pupil Reflex

The pupil reflex is tested with a bright light. It is one of the most critical aspects of the examination (Figure 14.4). It may be necessary to use a magnifying glass to see slight reactions. Pupil size and the response to light helps exclude or localise pathology affecting the midbrain and pons of the brainstem.
- Bilateral normal size (2.5–5mm) and reactive pupils:
  Essentially excludes midbrain damage
- Unilateral dilated (> 6 mm) and non-reactive pupil + contralateral weakness: Compression of the ipsilateral 3rd cranial nerve with herniation due to a mass lesion (tumour, haemorrhage, oedema related to a cerebral infarct) in the cerebral hemisphere
- Bilateral dilated and non-reactive pupils: Bilateral midbrain pathology

- Bilateral small (1–2.5 mm) and reactive pupils:     Metabolic encephalopathy or bilateral deep hemisphere lesions
- Bilateral pinpoint pupils that react to light: Pontine haemorrhage, narcotic or barbiturate overdose

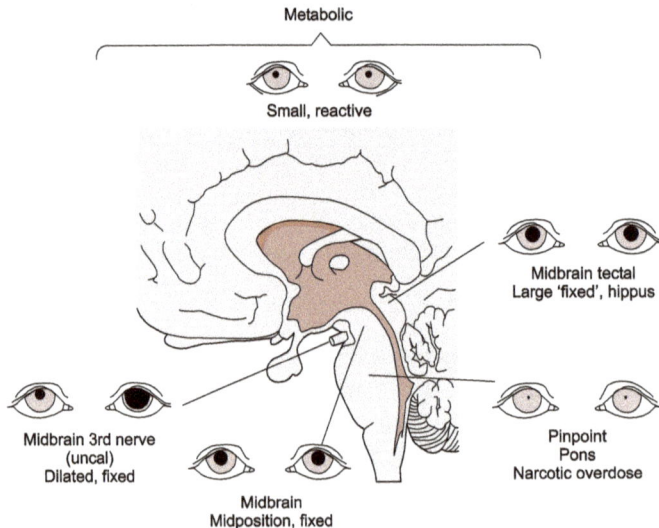

**Figure 14.4** Abnormal pupil responses in the unconscious patient
Reproduced from Diagnosis of Stupor and Coma. 2nd edn, by F Plum, JB Posner, 1972, FA Davis.

# Assessment of the Confused Patient

Many students have difficulty understanding the difference between delirium and dementia because of their similar symptoms. Patients with delirium become agitated rapidly and lapse in and out of consciousness. Delirium is usually reversible, and memory symptoms are typically short-term. Dementia develops gradually, and the effects on memory are more permanent.

## Confusion and Delirium

Delirium is characterised by a disturbance of attention, orientation, and awareness that develops within a short period, with transient symptoms that may fluctuate depending on the underlying cause. Delirium often includes disturbance of behaviour and emotion and may consist of impairment in multiple cognitive domains. A sleep-wake cycle disruption may also be present, including reduced arousal of acute onset or total sleep loss with reversal of the sleep-wake cycle. Delirium may be caused by the direct physiological effects of a medical condition, a substance or medication, including withdrawal, or by multiple or unknown etiological factors.

The International Classification of Diseases, 11th edition [2] defines delirium as:
- Impairment of consciousness and attention.
- Global disturbances of cognition, including illusions, hallucinations, delusions and disorientation.
- Psychomotor disturbances.
- Disturbances of the sleep-wake cycle.
- Emotional disturbances.

There are many causes of delirium, and it is often multifactorial. Even after extensive investigation, it is not always possible to establish the particular aetiology in all patients. Delirium usually resolves spontaneously. Delirium in the absence of any definable alternative explanation is not uncommon in hospital in the postoperative period following prolonged anaesthesia. Delirium can occur with a chest or urinary tract infection, electrolyte disturbance, cardiac, liver or renal failure, drug toxicity and drug withdrawal in patients with mild cognitive impairment. It can occur when individuals are admitted to a hospital simply because they are in an unfamiliar environment.

It is essential to review all medications, particularly those recently commenced or ceased. Clinical signs of chronic liver disease and the characteristic odour on the breath referred to as 'fetor hepaticus' (the breath of the dead with a sweet or faecal smell related to mercaptans, ammonia and ketones) identifies patients with portal hypertension and hepatic encephalopathy. Patients with metabolic encephalopathy due to any cause may have a short, flapping tremor called asterixis elicited by having patients hold their arms out in front of them with their wrists extended. Asterixis may occur in patients with hypercapnia (elevated carbon dioxide) and anticonvulsant overdose. A tremor and myoclonic jerks are seen in patients with renal failure or patients exposed to antipsychotic drugs. Delirium may also be a manifestation of hypoxia in the setting of cardiac or respiratory failure or a chest infection.

Patients with delirium should have a complete workup for sepsis. This involves looking for fever and tachycardia, examining the chest for evidence of infection, palpating the abdomen to look for tenderness that might suggest intraabdominal pathology and checking for neck rigidity by flexing the neck. Check the urine with a dipstick to look for evidence of a urinary tract infection (protein, blood and nitrites) and request a full blood examination, ESR, CRP and urine, blood and, if appropriate, sputum cultures. In the absence of apparent infection, hepatic and renal function, blood gases and electrolytes (sodium, calcium and magnesium) should be tested. Very rarely, delirium may be the presenting feature of meningitis or encephalitis, and a lumbar puncture may be necessary.

It is not uncommon for patients with hemisphere lesions affecting the parietal lobes to be diagnosed with confusion or delirium. One clue is that patients with confusion and delirium are usually restless and agitated, whereas patients with symptoms related to parietal lobe pathology are not, as a rule, agitated. Patients with symptoms in the dominant parieto-temporal lobe appeared to be very confused because they have fluent dysphasia, word salad, literal and verbal paraphasic errors and neologisms (see Chapter 5, 'The cerebral hemispheres and cerebellum'). Patients with symptoms in the non-dominant parietal lobe appeared to be confused because they are "lost in space". A quick screening examination (if the patient can cooperate) with double simultaneous stimuli in the visual fields and asking the patient to hold their arms out could detect the visual inattention and parietal drift that would alert one to focal rather than diffuse brain pathology.

| Management of Delirium |
|---|
| The main goal in managing delirium is keeping each patient comfortable and safe. Place patients in a quiet, well-lit room with familiar people and objects, a visible clock and a wall calendar.<br><br>Alcohol withdrawal or delirium tremens, 'the DT's', is a common cause of delirium. Benzodiazepines are the treatment of choice. A meta-analysis of nine prospective controlled trials [3] concluded that sedative-hypnotic agents (diazepam, chlordiazepoxide, pentobarbital paraldehyde and barbital) are more effective at reducing the duration of delirium and mortality than neuroleptic agents (chlorpromazine, promazine and thioridazine). The doses used should aim to maintain light sleepiness for the duration of delirium. Combined with comprehensive supportive medical care, this approach is highly effective in reducing morbidity and mortality. In general, it is best to use one drug at a time, use the minimal effective dose, increase the dose as required, and review the treatment regularly. [4] The atypical antipsychotics such as risperidone and olanzapine have the advantage of producing less sedation and are less likely to be associated with extrapyramidal side effects.<br><br>There are no randomised trials for patients with delirium unrelated to alcohol withdrawal, but most clinicians would follow the same management principles. [5] Imaging in the form of a CT or MRI scan is often performed but rarely rewarding. |

# Dementia

The term dementia is derived from the Latin' de-', meaning apart or away, + 'mens' (genitive mentis), meaning mind. It consists of a progressive global deterioration of intellectual and cognitive function with defects in orientation, memory, intellect, judgement and affect. Dementia is often associated with depression and apathy. As cognitive function declines, the patient develops problems with activities of daily living.

There are many causes of dementia; the more common include Alzheimer's disease (AD), vascular dementia, dementia with Lewy bodies (DLB), frontotemporal dementia (FTD) alcoholism and Parkinson's disease.

Potentially treatable rarer causes of dementia include: [108, 159]
- Hypothyroidism, hyperthyroidism
- vitamin $B_1$ or vitamin $B_{12}$ deficiency
- normal pressure hydrocephalus
- subdural haematoma
- drug intoxication
- depression (pseudodementia)
- cerebral vasculitis
- neurosyphilis
- heavy metal intoxication
- brain tumours
- intracranial empyema or abscess
- meningitis related to tuberculosis, cryptococcus, sarcoidosis and
- the extremely rare entities of Whipple's and Wilson's disease.
- Immune-mediated encephalitis, e.g. Limbic & Hashimoto's

# Alzheimer's disease

Alzheimer's disease (AD ) is the commonest cause of dementia. Although there are several biomarkers such as CSF (amyloid β and tau), serum (Plasma Phospho-tau217), and Positron emission tomography (PET) scan (amyloid β and tau) [109,110], none are included in the current diagnostic guidelines [110-112] because they lack specificity. They can be detected in individuals with normal cognitive function and minimal cognitive impairment. The definitive diagnosis requires histopathological demonstration of sufficient numbers of amyloid plaques and neurofibrillary tangles in a patient with the clinical syndrome of AD. The same pathology can be present in cognitively normal individuals and those with minimal cognitive impairment (MCI). Current evidence about the natural history of asymptomatic people at risk with positive biological markers is insufficient to predict subsequent cognitive decline and dementia. [111] If the serum biomarker [110] proves to be reliable, it may add confirmation in an individual with a clinically definite AD diagnosis

The risk of Alzheimer's increases with advancing age, 20–40% of patients over 85 will have Alzheimer's disease. Positive family history is not uncommon. Patients with Down syndrome (trisomy 21) have an increased risk of Alzheimer's disease after 40 years of age.

Most patients with AD have an insidious onset of memory impairment over many years, particularly short-term memory. As cognitive function declines, the patient develops increasing difficulties with daily activities, and it is this difficulty that differentiates mild cognitive impairment from true dementia. A reversal of the sleep cycle with patients sleeping during the day and wandering at night is not uncommon. Some patients with AD are often unaware of their cognitive impairment, and it is concerned relatives that urge them to seek medical attention. Patients may cope well in their home environment, but often the dementia is unmasked when patients are placed in unfamiliar environments, e.g. admission to the hospital. As the disease relentlessly progresses, patients get lost when they go for walks or when driving, and they have difficulty with finances, housekeeping, shopping and following instructions. Leaving the stove on is a common complaint. Some patients may develop a characteristic disorder called apraxic gait (Chapter 13) where walking becomes increasingly difficult. Language function deteriorates with problems naming objects, comprehension, and subsequently the development of aphasia. In advanced Alzheimer's, patients can no longer care for themselves in dressing, bathing, and feeding and eventually lose control of their bladder and bowels.

Depression can present with many of the clinical features of dementia. This is an entity called pseudodementia. These patients often complain of memory disturbance yet can often recant the history of their 'cognitive decline' without much difficulty. The correct diagnosis may only reveal itself when the patient improves with treatment for depression. In a small study, Reynolds et al. [6] found significantly greater pretreatment for depression, early morning awakening, higher ratings of psychological anxiety, and more severe libido impairment were features of pseudodementia. In contrast, patients with dementia showed significantly more disorientation to time, increased difficulty finding their way about familiar streets or indoors and more impairment with dressing.

There are several rare syndromes where dementia may begin with focal neurological deficits. [7–10] These include posterior cortical atrophy (P.C.A.), corticobasal syndrome (C.B.S.), behavioural variant frontotemporal dementia (bvFTD), progressive non-fluent aphasia (PNFA) (or mixed aphasia) and semantic dementia (S.D.). In some instances, these patients will have the pathological features of Alzheimer's disease. These focal syndromes may remain pure for many years before the subsequent appearance of other signs of dementia. The underlying neuropathology does not uniquely associate the clinical syndromes with distinctive patterns of pathological markers. A detailed discussion of these entities is beyond the scope of this textbook. [7, 9, 10]

# Rapidly Progressive Dementia (RPD)

Rapidly progressive dementia develops subacutely over months, weeks or even days. Prion disease (Creutzfeldt–Jakob disease) is the commonest cause. Rarely frontotemporal dementia (FTD), corticobasal degeneration (CBD), Alzheimer's disease, dementia with Lewy bodies (D.L.B.) and progressive supranuclear palsy may present in a fulminant form with death occurring in less than three years. [11]

Immune-mediated encephalitis (IME) can present with dementia. [108] IME can be associated with cancer (paraneoplastic) or occur without cancer (non-paraneoplastic). Immune-mediated encephalopathy and Hashimoto's encephalopathy (HE) with associated antineuronal antibodies are potentially treatable causes of rapidly progressive dementia. Multiple sclerosis and neurosarcoidosis may also cause rapidly progressive dementia.

Limbic encephalitis is another immune-mediated encephalitis. It presents with rapid memory loss, depression, anxiety, personality changes, impaired cognitive function and seizures. Table 14.3 lists the currently identified anti-neuronal antibodies in the serum or cerebrospinal fluid.

Creutzfeldt–Jakob disease (CJD) presents with rapid dementia, cerebellar ataxia and behavioural disturbances. There is a variant of CJD, called 'mad-cow disease, bovine spongiform encephalopathy (B.S.E.) or variant CJD. The initial manifestations are significant psychiatric symptoms with ataxia and dementia associated with chorea and myoclonus occurring later in the course. An outbreak of mad-cow disease in the U.K. originated from supplementing protein in cattle that were fed a meat-and-bone meal manufactured from the remains of other animals.*

# Forgetfulness vs Early Dementia

Forgetfulness or absent-mindedness is a feature of the ageing process. Most patients over the age of 70 complain of memory problems. Many patients with minimal cognitive impairment seek medical attention concerned about the possibility of dementia. It can, at times be challenging to differentiate between these two processes. [12] Episodic memory loss precedes the widespread cognitive decline in early AD. [13] Screening tests include the Mini-Mental state, Montreal Cognitive Assessment( MoCA) and the Saint Louis University Mental Status (SLUMS ). [113-116] These screening tests are all very similar, and in general, the one used is a personal preference. Detailed neuropsychological testing is more definitive.

---

**Management of Alzheimer's Disease**

The management of patients with Alzheimer's disease involves providing support for the family and the patient, treatment of depression and treatment of seizures if they occur. In the early stages, patients can write lists or create notes as reminders to see what they need to do that day. It is also helpful if patients with Alzheimer's develop a daily routine, including physical exercise. Caring for patients with Alzheimer's disease day in and day out is very demanding. Organising a period of family relief where the patient is admitted to an interim care facility, allowing the supportive family member a break will often enable the patient to remain at home for a more extended period1. Several cholinesterase inhibitors provide symptomatic benefit, but whether they decrease the rate of cognitive decline in the first few years is unclear. In June 2021, the Federal Drug Administration (FDA) approved the use of aducanumab, a monoclonal antibody that reduces amyloid deposits in the brain. A huge controversy erupted. The FDA advisory committee, along with an independent think tank and several prominent experts — including some Alzheimer›s doctors who worked on the aducanumab clinical trials — said the evidence raised significant doubts about whether the drug is effective. More drugs are expected to be developed in the not too distant future.

---

1   Personal observation

# Disorders of Muscle and Neuromuscular Junction

Many patients use the word weakness to describe their symptoms, yet they may not have actual muscle weakness. It is essential to establish that the complaint of weakness refers to weakness of muscles, not a sense of general fatigue. Diseases of muscle and conditions affecting the neuromuscular junction are infrequent. For example, the prevalence of inflammatory muscle disease is 1 in 100,000, and myasthenia gravis is 8 in 100,000. A complete discussion of all muscle disorders is well beyond the scope of this text, and interested readers will find many excellent reviews, textbooks and websites. [15–18]

Muscle disease should be suspected when patients complain of weakness with or without wasting muscles in the absence of other neurological symptoms. The weakness develops very slowly over the years in most muscle disorders other than inflammatory myopathies. However, even in the inflammatory myopathies where the weakness usually evolves over weeks to months, occasionally, the onset may be more gradual. As many muscle diseases are hereditary, one should always enquire about the family history.

Although symptoms such as myalgia (muscle pain), muscle cramps, muscle stiffness, fatigue and exercise intolerance may occur in patients with muscle disease, many of these are non-specific

- *Frailty and sarcopenia* are clinical syndromes occurring in older people that can present with generalised weakness
- *Muscle pain* or *myalgia* is rare in muscle diseases apart from iatrogenic drug-induced muscle pain. Pain more often relates to rheumatological, psychiatric or orthopaedic disorders. However, it may occur in patients with congenital or endocrine myopathies and myositis. It is essential to question patients presenting with muscle pain on whether they are taking prescription and non-prescription medications.
- *Fatigue* is also a very non-specific symptom. Patients with depression, for example, often complain of fatigue; however, increased or decreased weakness with exercise may point to the involvement of the neuromuscular junction with conditions such as myasthenia gravis and the Lambert–Eaton syndrome. Fatigue is also a prominent symptom in patients with motor neuron disease.
- *Muscle cramps* occur with hyponatraemia, renal failure, hypothyroidism, and other conditions affecting peripheral nerves. Often a cause cannot be identified.
- *Myotonia* is the inability to relax a muscle after forced voluntary contraction, for example gripping an object with the hands. It occurs in hereditary muscle disorders such as myotonic dystrophy, Thompson's disease and acquired conditions such as neuromyotonia (Isaac's syndrome).

There are many approaches to patients with suspected muscle disease. One method is shown in Figure 14.5.

1. The initial step is to ask about the **family history**, as many muscle diseases, such as muscular dystrophies, congenital, metabolic and mitochondrial myopathies, are inherited. A negative family history does not exclude hereditary diseases of muscle. Some patients are so mildly affected that they are unaware of the problem or have not sought medical attention, a common scenario in patients with muscular dystrophy. Specific genetic testing for conditions such as myotonic dystrophy, facioscapulohumeral muscular dystrophy, Duchenne muscular dystrophy, oculopharyngeal muscular dystrophy, oculopharyngodistal myopathy facioscapulohumeral dystrophy and mitochondrial myopathy can eliminate the need for muscle biopsy. [120, 168] In other phenotypes, whole exome or RNA sequencing is available. [168]

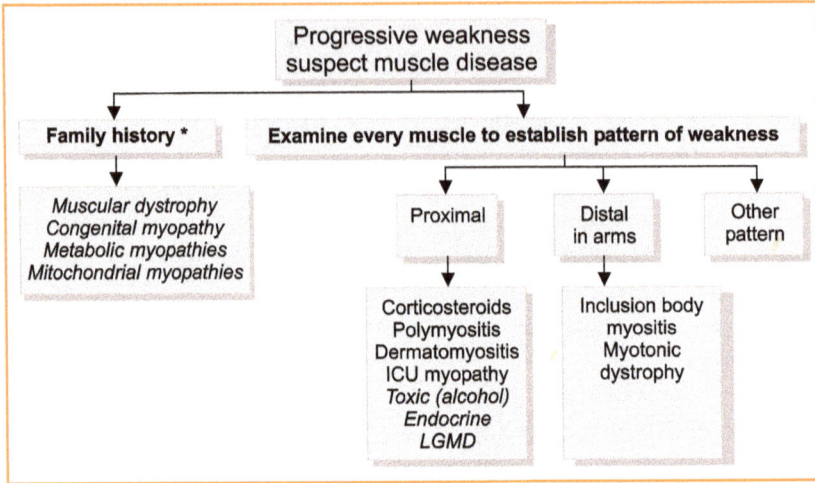

**Figure 14.5** An approach to patients with suspected muscle disease. Note: The uncommon diseases are in italics. *A 'negative' family history does not exclude inherited disorders of muscle. 'Other' pattern refers to patterns of weakness other than proximal or distal, for example, facioscapulohumeral. ICU = intensive care unit; LGMD = limb-girdle muscular dystrophy

2. The **age of onset** can provide another clue, e.g. congenital myopathies may be present at birth. The muscular dystrophies often develop in the first few years of life, and inclusion body myositis occurs mainly in elderly patients.

3. Consider the **rapidity of onset of the weakness**. Many muscle disorders, particularly inherited muscle disorders, develop gradually over many years; most of the acquired muscle diseases, such as inflammatory myopathies, usually progress rapidly over months. Patients with congenital myopathies may not progress at all. *Fluctuating weakness* suggests neuromuscular junction disorders, such as myasthenia gravis and Lambert–Eaton syndrome. Recurrent attacks of weakness are a feature of the periodic paralyses and certain glycolytic pathway disorders.

4. **Define the pattern of weakness**. Many muscle conditions have been labelled according to the pattern of weakness—muscle diseases such as limb-girdle muscular dystrophy (LGMD) and facioscapulohumeral dystrophy (FSH). As the underlying genetic basis for the muscle diseases is defined, it is increasingly apparent that there is significant variability in the phenotypic expression (the pattern of weakness), reflecting the severity of the underlying genetic defect. For example, with mutations in the dysferlin gene, patients can present with a limb-girdle muscular dystrophy pattern, a distal anterior compartment myopathy, or the classic Miyoshi myopathy with multifocal weakness and wasting. [20] The 2018 gene table of monogenic neuromuscular disorders contains 16 categories, 884 diseases involving 492 genes and many proteins. It includes 71 loci that await identification of the corresponding gene[2]. Every year new gene loci and different phenotypes are added. The classification of limb-girdle dystrophies continues to be revised based on the underlying protein and genetic abnormalities. [121] The online version[3] is up to date. In everyday clinical practice, other than 'proximal myopathy', which is probably the most common pattern and distal weakness in the forearms, most of the other muscle disorders are extremely rare.

---

2 https://www.emjreviews.com/neurology/article/diagnosing-neuromuscular-diseases/

3 On Line versio http://www.musclegenetable.fr/

Disease caused by mitochondrial genome mutations see https://www.mitomap.org/MITOMAP

5. **Associated phenomena** may help differentiate one condition from another.
   - Muscle hypertrophy: is seen with Duchenne and Becker muscular dystrophy, hypothyroidism
   - Respiratory failure: occurs with myotonic dystrophy, centronuclear myopathy, nemaline myopathy and acid maltase deficiency
   - Cardiac disease: occurs with Myotonic dystrophy, Duchenne or Becker muscular dystrophies. Limb-girdle muscular dystrophies 1B, 2I, 2C–F, 2G, Emery–Dreifuss muscular dystrophy.
   - Scoliosis, a rigid spine and contractures in the elbows and ankles point to specific congenital muscular dystrophies (e.g., laminin alpha deficiency, collagen VI syndromes)
   - Hepatomegaly: suggests metabolic or alcoholic myopathies
   - Characteristic facial features with frontal baldness, ptosis, bilateral facial weakness and neck weakness in myotonic dystrophy
   - Skin rash: a red or purple rash on sun-exposed skin and eyelids in dermatomyositis.
   - Central nervous system involvement may occur in patients with mitochondrial myopathies [15]
6. Check for drug use such as alcohol, cocaine, heroin and prescription drugs such as statins and corticosteroids that can cause muscle toxicity.
7. Blood tests
   - **Creatinine kinase** (C.K.). CK is elevated in most but not all muscle disorders and in itself is not a particularly useful test to differentiate one disease of muscle from another; however, a markedly elevated CK occurs with Duchenne muscular dystrophy and the dysferlinopathies. A normal CK does not exclude muscle disease.
   - **Thyroid function tests and electrolytes** should be routine investigations: parathyroid hormone and human immunodeficiency virus (HIV ) in selected cases.
   - **25 hydroxyvitamin D** to exclude osteomalacia.
   - Antinuclear factor (ANF), double-stranded DNA, rheumatoid factor, anti-cyclic citrullinated peptide antibody (anti-CCP), Scl-70 antibody (scleroderma antibody, anti-topoisomerase I antibody) and centromere antibody (ACA)/centromere for connective tissue diseases such as systemic lupus erythematosus, scleroderma and rheumatoid arthritis that can be associated with inflammatory myopathies.
8. The **urine** should be tested for **myoglobinuria** in patients with exercise-induced muscle pain.
9. A **forearm ischaemic lactate test** is performed in patients suspected of having a metabolic myopathy; a less than threefold increase in the lactate is abnormal.
10. **Nerve conduction studies and electromyography**.Nerve conduction studies (NCS) are normal in patients with muscle disease (exceptions include mitochondrial disorders, myotonic dystrophy and inclusion body myositis). Electromyography (EMG) can confirm the presence of myopathy with the demonstration of brief small-amplitude polyphasic potentials (BSAPPs) and a full recruitment pattern with minimal effort. NCS and EMG can exclude other conditions such as motor neuron disease, peripheral neuropathy, and neuromuscular junction disorders. Occasionally, nerve conduction studies and EMG can be completely normal in patients with muscle disease. Fibrillation potentials and positive sharp waves with the myopathic changes on EMG described above indicate an inflammatory myositis. The sound of a motorbike or dive-bomber on EMG indicates myotonia in myotonic and congenital muscular dystrophies.

11. ***Myositis-specific and myositis-associated autoantibodies*** (MS A, MAA) are present in 25-50% of patients with polymyositis and dermatomyositis. These autoantibodies can also identify the antisynthetase syndrome. Whether the antibodies play a role in tissue injury remains unknown.[123,124] Myositis-specific autoantibodies and myositis-associated autoantibodies have a high specificity of 94.2 and 99.9% respectively but a low sensitivity of 0-12.9%. [124] They are found primarily in patients with idiopathic inflammatory myopathies. Myositis-associated autoantibodies are not specific for the disease but are important diagnostic markers, e.g. anti-PMS cl autoantibodies are found in polymyositis and scleroderma overlap. Anti-HMGCR antibodies occur in statin immune-mediated necrotising myopathy with 92.3 and 100% sensitivity and specificity. [125]

12. ***Muscle biopsy*** of an affected muscle using an open or a needle biopsy. A needle biopsy is less invasive, and multiple samples can be taken, but the individual piece size is small. It is important to remember that pathological changes may be focal, and thus, a normal (particularly needle) biopsy does not necessarily exclude muscle disease. Suresh argues that an open biopsy is the preferred method. [117] Formalin-fixed paraffin-embedded muscle samples alone almost always lead to inconclusive or unspecific results. Liquid nitrogen frozen muscle sections are imperative for neuromuscular diagnosis. Three-dimensional axial T1, fat-suppressed and short tau inversion recovery MRI are valuable tools to determine the optimal site for biopsy. [122] It is more rewarding to biopsy an affected muscle, but not one so severely affected that the likely pathology will be non-diagnostic end-stage muscle. It is also essential not to biopsy a muscle at the site of EMG as the EMG needle will cause abnormal pathology. Increasingly sophisticated pathological methods, such as immunohistochemical staining with a panel of antibodies, quantitative analysis of proteins by western blotting and DNA analysis, are now a routine part of the pathological examination of muscle and help determine the cause of muscle weakness in most patients.

In clinical practice, there are two common clinical presentations of patients with muscle disease: proximal (proximal myopathy) and distal weakness. (Figure 14.5)

# Proximal Weakness-'Proximal Myopathy'

Patients with proximal muscle weakness complain of difficulty getting out of chairs, getting up off the floor, climbing up and downstairs, lifting objects above their head or brushing their hair. The term 'proximal myopathy' is very non-specific, and both hereditary and acquired conditions can result in weakness of the proximal muscles (shoulder abduction and hip flexion). The list of causes is extensive [117] and includes drugs, alcohol, thyroid disease, osteomalacia, idiopathic inflammatory myopathies (IIM ), hereditary myopathies, malignancy, infections and sarcoidosis. The commonest causes would be iatrogenic corticosteroid use, critical illness or ICU myopathy, inflammatory myopathies and thyroid disease, although weakness is increasingly uncommon with earlier detection of thyroid disease.

Desmin-related myopathy can cause both distal and proximal weakness. It is also associated with cardiomyopathy and or complete heart block requiring a pacemaker. The cardiac abnormalities may be the presenting feature. [162]

# Muscle Diseases with Distal Weakness

Patients with distal weakness will have difficulty opening jars, turning the key in the lock, or doing buttons. Distal weakness in the legs related to muscle disease is extremely rare and is more common in patients with peripheral neuropathies. If present, distal weakness in the legs causes patients to complain of difficulty walking on uneven surfaces, often associated with tripping due to a foot drop. Several very rare hereditary distal myopathies, including Laing's, GNE, Myoshi's, Udd's and Markesbery-Griggs myopathy, cause distal weakness in the arms and legs. [169] Although there are many causes of distal weakness in the arms [16], myotonic dystrophy and inclusion body myositis are the two commonest. Some of the limb-girdle muscular dystrophies may cause distal and proximal muscles. [21]

---

**Treatment of Muscular Dystrophies**

Genetic testing for some of the more common types of dystrophies, including Duchenne muscular dystrophy (DMD), Becker muscular dystrophy (BMD), facioscapulohumeral muscular dystrophy (FSHD) and myotonic dystrophy (MD), if available, can establish the diagnosis and prevent the need for a muscle biopsy in some patients. The current state-of-the-art treatment is oligonucleotide-based gene therapy that restores disease-related protein.

This approach has limited efficacy and is unlikely to be curative. Myogenic stem cell transplantation and artificial skeletal muscle generated by myogenic cells and muscle resident cells are alternative approaches currently being explored. [126]

Corticosteroids have a defined role in patients with Duchenne muscular dystrophy but not in other muscular dystrophies. They reduce the risk of developing scoliosis and subsequent surgical correction, improve cardiac health and increase long-term survival. [23,142 ]

---

# The Idiopathic Inflammatory Myopathies

The list of idiopathic inflammatory myopathies (IIM) has been expanded from polymyositis (PM), dermatomyositis (DM) and inclusion body myositis(IBM) to include HMG-CoA reductase autoantibody immune-mediated necrotising myopathy (NM),anti-synthetase syndrome (ASS) and overlap syndromes with myositis. Patients with necrotising myopathy progress rapidly to disability within months. HMG-CoA reductase autoantibodies are seen in NM patients who may or may not be taking a statin. [128] ASS is a severe condition with myositis, non-erosive arthritis, interstitial lung disease and multiple organ involvement. PM and D.M. cause the insidious onset over months of symmetrical proximal muscle weakness. The weakness affects shoulder abduction, hip flexion and neck flexion (the latter is a clue to the diagnosis). Rarely, the bulbar respiratory muscles may be affected. Patients with DM may have characteristic skin changes. These include the heliotrope rash resulting in violaceous discolouration of the eyelids; scaly erythema over the joints on the dorsal aspect of the hands; macular erythema on the posterior neck and shoulders or the anterior neck and chest or violaceous erythema associated with increased pigment and telangiectasia on the anterior neck, chest, behind the shoulders, back and buttocks. Twenty to twenty-five per cent of PM and DM patients have an underlying malignancy. [127] Myositis may precede the detection of the malignancy for up to three years. Myositis-specific (MS A) and myositis-associated antibodies (MAA) are present in some patients.

| Treatment of Polymyositis and Dermatomyositis |
|---|
| Treatment of polymyositis and dermatomyositis is mainly empirical. A 2012 Cochrane review stated a lack of high-quality randomised trials to assess the efficacy of immunosuppression. [143] Corticosteroids remain the first choice agent, despite the lack of randomised controlled data. [24] Other immunosuppressive agents are recommended for patients who fail to respond to corticosteroids or combined with corticosteroids to reduce side effects from the steroids.<br>• The initial prednisolone dose is 1–2 mg/kg body weight for 2–4 weeks, slowly reducing the dose over six months and changing to an alternate day regimen as maintenance therapy.<br>• If at three months the response to corticosteroids is suboptimal, other immunosuppression with azathioprine (it may take 3–6 months before seeing any benefit), cyclophosphamide, cyclosporine, methotrexate and mycophenolate is recommended. [25-27] Long-term use of azathioprine, in particular, increases the risk of certain malignancies such as lymphoma and nonmelanoma skin cancer<br>• Plasma exchange was better than sham apheresis in a randomised controlled trial [28] and is recommended in acute myositis if other therapy fails.<br>• Two trials of IVIG found conflicting results. [29, 145] It may have a role if steroids and immunosuppressives are contraindicated. The recommended dose is 1–2 g/kg every 3–6 weeks. [146]<br>• Another randomised controlled trial has confirmed the efficacy of intravenous immunoglobulin in corticosteroid-resistant polymyositis [29] and is currently recommended by the European Federation of Neurological Societies. [30] Treatment may need to continue for 1–3 years to prevent relapse. |

# Inclusion Body Myositis

Inclusion body myositis (IBM) is mainly a sporadic condition, with rare hereditary cases referred to as IBM type 2 seen in patients over 50. IBM has a pathognomonic pattern of weakness affecting the quadriceps muscle with severe weakness of knee extension resulting in frequent falls as the knees give way. There is distal weakness in the forearms and hands with weakness of flexion of the fingers. Hip flexion weakness is much less severe than knee extension weakness. Dysphagia is common, but the involvement of the respiratory muscles is rare. [31] The muscle biopsy demonstrates inflammatory cells and vacuoles in muscle fibres.

| Treatment of Inclusion Body Myositis |
|---|
| Many immunosuppressive drugs have been tried in IBM, including corticosteroids, azathioprine, cyclosporine, methotrexate and intravenous immunoglobulin and interferon-beta-1a, all to no avail. Current recommendations encourage exercise for patients with IBM. [32] Several experimental drugs are currently being trialled, including arimoclomol, bimagrumab, follistatin, and rapamycin.[4] |

# Drug-Induced Myopathies

Side effects from prescription drugs are rare and occur in less than 0.5% of patients. They include muscle pain that can be mild and not require cessation of the drug or severe and associated with fatigue and elevation of the CK to more than ten times the upper limit of normal. Other complications include proximal muscle weakness and rhabdomyolysis, which at times is fatal. Myopathy is more common in patients on multiple therapeutic agents and may relate to drug-drug interactions. Although the CK is usually elevated, a normal value does not

---

4 Myositis Association. https://www.myositis.org/about-myositis/treatment-disease-management/potential-treatments-sporadic-inclusion-body-myositis/

exclude a drug-induced myopathy. [33] Myopathy may take months or even years to develop, and symptoms may persist for some time after cessation of the drug. [34]

Drug-induced myopathy, including rhabdomyolysis, can be caused by statins, fibrates, antidepressants, antipsychotic drugs, benzodiazepines, calcium channel blockers, corticosteroids, alcohol, cocaine, amphetamines, colchicine and heroin. Amiodarone induces a vacuolar myopathy associated with neuropathy. [129] Anti-HMGCR antibody-induced myopathy resembling limb-girdle muscular dystrophy is seen in patients, on and not on statins.

Statins, one of the most widely prescribed lipid-lowering agents, can affect muscle in several ways:

- Myalgia with an elevated CK,
- Rhabdomyolysis with a very high CK, myoglobinuria and renal failure
- A self-limiting toxic myopathy with myalgia, a high CK and proximal weakness
- A very severe immune-mediated anti-HMGCR antibody-induced necrotising myopathy that, unlike the other muscle symptoms, does NOT improve when statins are ceased. [141]

| Treatment of Necrotising Myositis |
|---|
| Cessation of the statin. Early and prompt treatment with either steroids or induction with IVIG and steroid-sparing immunosuppressives in patients with a +ve HMGCR antibody, a high CK with or without proximal weakness.[144] |

# HyperCKaemia

An isolated elevation of the CK is not uncommon, and investigations are usually unrewarding, particularly if the nerve conduction studies and EMG are normal. An aetiological diagnosis is more likely the higher the level of CK and the younger the patient, particularly if there is associated weakness. [148]

# Fluctuating Weakness with Exercise

## Myasthenia Gravis and Lambert–Eaton Syndrome

The term 'myasthenia' literally means muscle weakness and is derived from the Latin' myos', meaning muscle, and the Greek' asthenes', meaning a- (without) + sthenos (strength).

| |
|---|
| Disorders of the neuromuscular junction should be suspected in patients with weakness that is either temporarily worsened or improved with exercise. |

The two currently recognised disorders that affect the neuromuscular junction (NMJ) are myasthenia gravis [35] and the Lambert–Eaton syndrome, also referred to as the Lambert–Eaton myasthenic syndrome. [36] Patients with myasthenia gravis observe that their weakness is exacerbated by exercise, whereas patients with Lambert–Eaton syndrome complain of weakness and fatigue that may temporarily lesson after exercise or exertion. Patients with amyotrophic lateral sclerosis (motor neuron disease) often experience a significant worsening of weakness with exercise. However, they have severe fixed weakness, wasting and fasciculations not seen in disorders of the NMJ. [37]

Both are immune-mediated disorders.[1] Lambert–Eaton syndrome is often associated with malignancy, particularly small cell carcinoma of the lung [40], but may also occur as an autoimmune disease in the absence of malignancy. [41] Myasthenia gravis may be associated with a tumour of the thymus [42], either benign or malignant; this is more common in elderly patients, whilst younger patients tend to have thymic hyperplasia or aplasia of the thymus.

Myasthenia gravis is classified as either purely ocular if it only affects the ocular muscles (including the eyelids) or generalised if it affects the facial, bulbar and limb muscles. The characteristic feature is exacerbation of weakness with exercise or prolonged use of the muscles. Variable ptosis (drooping of the eyelid) and variable diplopia with a mixture of horizontal and vertical diplopia at different times occur with ocular myasthenia gravis. However, the occasional patient does not observe variable diplopia and an incorrect diagnosis of a 3rd, 4th or 6th nerve palsy or an internuclear ophthalmoplegia (a lesion of the median longitudinal fasciculus in the brainstem) is suspected. The ocular muscles may also be affected in patients with generalised myasthenia gravis. Patients with generalised myasthenia may complain of difficulty holding their head up while watching television due to weakness of the extensor muscles of the neck; increasing dysarthria the more they speak; difficulty chewing or swallowing food, again worse with prolonged chewing; increasing weakness leading to difficulty holding the arms above their head when washing their hair or putting clothes on the clothes line. Patients have to rest momentarily before they can continue this activity. Increasing degrees of ptosis and diplopia can be elicited during the examination by asking the patient to look up for a prolonged period; fatiguable weakness in the limbs can be produced with repetitive exercise. A quick test in patients with suspected ocular myasthenia is to place ice on the eyelid and see the temporary resolution of the ptosis. [43] Changes in the degree of diplopia with the ice test should be interpreted with caution. [44]

The reflexes are normal and are not influenced by exercise. Several diagnostic tests for myasthenia gravis have variable sensitivity but high specificity (Table 14.1).

| Test | Sensitivity (%) (95% CI) | Specificity (%) (95% CI) |
|---|---|---|
| Tensilon test [45] | 92 (83–100%) | 97 (91–100) |
| Ice test [43] | 95 (87–100) | 97 (90–100) |
| ACHR antibody* [46] | 54 (44–63) | 98 (96–100) |
| Repetitive nerve stimulation [47] | 26 (15–44) | 95 (94–100) |
| SFEMG [48] | 89 (83–95) | 88 (78–96) |

*The figures for the ACHR antibody assay are at variance with the accepted figure of approximately 85% sensitivity. [50] The explanation for this is unclear.

**Table 14.1** Sensitivity and specificity of diagnostic tests in myasthenia gravis. ACHR-Acetylcholine receptor antibodies. SFEMG-single fibre electromyography

# Diagnostic Tests

## The Tensilon Test

The tensilon (edrophonium hydrochloride) test demonstrates transient improvement lasting 30–60 seconds.

1. The patient should be pre-treated with atropine 600 µg to reduce the gastrointestinal side effects of the edrophonium hydrochloride.
2. 10 mg (1mL) of edrophonium is mixed with 9 mL of normal saline (1 mg of edrophonium per mL).
3. Initially, 2 mg is injected; if the patient fails to respond to 2 mg, the other 8 mg is injected.
4. Observe the patient for at least 3 minutes after the injection (longer in older patients due to a slower circulation time).

In some patients, 2mg is too much, and 8mg may be insufficient in other patients. [51] In normal patients, the tensilon test does not produce any change in strength.

## Acetylcholine Receptor, MUSK and other Antibodies

Acetylcholine receptor (ACHR) antibodies are positive in 85% of patients with myasthenia gravis. [50] ACHR antibodies may be detected with repeat testing in some patients with myasthenia gravis, in whom they are initially negative. [52] In the future other antibodies will likely be discovered in the seronegative (the ACHR antibody negative) patients with myasthenia gravis.

MuSK, low-density lipoprotein receptor–related protein 4 (LRP4) and agrin antibodies have been found in patients who are -ve for AChR antibodies. MuSk antibodies are IgG antibodies against muscle-specific kinase (MuSK). The presence of MuSK antibodies appears to define a subgroup of patients with seronegative myasthenia gravis. In many cases, these individuals have predominantly localised bulbar, muscle weakness (face, tongue, pharynx, etc.) and reduced response to conventional immunosuppressive treatments. [53] Anti-titin antibodies may identify patients with a thymoma. [39] On the other hand LRP4 and agrin antibodies are associated with generalised myasthenia gravis

## Nerve Conduction Studies

Nerve conduction studies can differentiate between myasthenia gravis and Lambert–Eaton syndrome.

A repetitive stimulation study is where the nerve is stimulated at 3 per second for eight impulses immediately before and immediately after 20 seconds sustained exercise, and then at intervals of 1 minute for several minutes. The test may demonstrate a decremental response (the 5th response is of lower amplitude than the 1st response) in patients with myasthenia gravis and an incremental response in patients with the Lambert–Eaton syndrome.

Single fibre electromyography (SFEMG) demonstrates instability at the neuromuscular junction (referred to as increased jitter). It cannot differentiate between Lambert–Eaton syndrome, myasthenia gravis and increased jitter that occurs in motor neuron disease.

---

**Treatment of Myasthenia Gravis**

Treatment of myasthenia gravis is primarily determined by the presence or absence of a thymic tumour. Most authorities would recommend thymectomy [54] in patients with thymic tumours as it is difficult to differentiate between benign and malignant tumours before surgery. Thymic tumours are locally malignant, invading the lung and or pericardium; they do not metastasise.

In patients with isolated ocular myasthenia gravis, the treatment options include nothing, symptomatic relief with pyridostigmine[3], other anticholinesterase drugs and immunosuppressive treatment. In patients with generalised myasthenia gravis, thymectomy in the presence of thymic hyperplasia may be curative. If not, immunosuppression, IVIG or plasma exchange are recommended. Although a randomized trial found little difference between IVIG and plasma exchange [149], some patients who have not responded to IVIG have responded to plasma exchange[5].

In generalised myasthenia gravis, corticosteroids are often the drug of first choice, and limited evidence from randomised controlled trials has demonstrated short-term benefit. [56] Small randomised controlled trials suggest that cyclosporine, as monotherapy or with corticosteroids, or cyclophosphamide with corticosteroids significantly improve myasthenia gravis. Azathioprine, either as monotherapy or with steroids, has not been beneficial in randomised controlled trials. Mycophenolate mofetil (as monotherapy or with either corticosteroids or cyclosporine) or tacrolimus (with corticosteroids or plasma exchange) has also been advocated in resistant cases. [57] Intravenous immunoglobulin (IVIG) is superior to placebo but no different to plasma exchange. The ease of use means that intravenous immunoglobulin is regarded by most as the treatment of choice. IVIG and plasma exchange are used for a myasthenic crisis. They are also employed preoperatively in patients undergoing thymectomy or other surgery if the myasthenia is unstable. Pyridostigmine may provide some symptomatic benefit but often causes gastrointestinal upset. It is difficult to use because an excess dose can cause similar symptoms to worsening myasthenia gravis. Excess salivation and abdominal discomfort with diarrhoea are the clues that there may be an excess of pyridostigmine. A tensilon test will exacerbate symptoms due to excess pyridostigmine.

Currently, corticosteroids, azathioprine, plasma exchange, intravenous immunoglobulins and 3,4-diaminopyridine are used in the treatment of Lambert–Eaton myasthenic syndrome with limited success. Some evidence from randomised controlled trials shows that either 3,4-diaminopyridine or intravenous immunoglobulin improves muscle strength scores and compound muscle action potential amplitudes in patients with Lambert–Eaton myasthenic syndrome. [58] 3,4 diaminopyridine works by blocking $K^+$ channel efflux in nerve terminals so that action potential duration is increased. $Ca^{2+}$ channels thus remain open for a longer period of time, which allows greater acetylcholine release to stimulate the muscle at the end plate.

Efgartigimod (ARGX-113), a human IgG1 antibody Fc fragment engineered to reduce pathogenic IgG autoantibody levels [130] Zilucoplan, a subcutaneously (SC) self-administered macrocyclic peptide inhibitor of complement component 5 [147] and Rozanolixizumab, a high-affinity anti-FcRn monoclonal antibody [130] have all been shown to be effective. Rituximab initiated early in new-onset myasthenia gravis, can lead to faster and more sustained remission, particularly MuSK-positive myasthenia gravis. [130]

# Post-Viral fatigue

Post-viral fatigue syndrome is common. It was initially described at the Royal Free Hospital [59] and labelled benign myalgic encephalomyelitis. [60] The aetiology remains obscure. A similar fatigue syndrome is common following infectious mononucleosis [61] and recently with covid 19 caused by the coronavirus, SARS-CoV-2 [170] suggesting a possible viral aetiology.

Although post-viral fatigue can occur in epidemics, it is usually sporadic. It appears at any age but is more common in young and middle-aged females. The overwhelming complaint is severe fatigue with muscle aches and pains developing after a flu-like illness. Other symptoms include depression, excessive sleep, poor memory and difficulty concentrating. [62]

---

5   Personal observation

| Management of Post-Viral Fatigue |
| --- |
| There is no specific test. The diagnosis is clinical and requires a definite viral infection followed by severe fatigue. There is no specific treatment. Fortunately, it is a self-limiting illness in most patients, although some may be troubled for months or even years. In 2021 The National Institute for Health and Care Excellence (NICE) said that it had been unable to produce a document on diagnosis and treatment of the condition "that is supported by all".[6] In a small, eight-week randomised trial, Co-enzyme Q10 and nicotinamide adenine dinucleotide combination improved the fatigue but did not benefit pain and excessive sleep. [135] |

# Multiple Sclerosis

In the first edition, I stated: "that everything written in this section is likely to be outdated rapidly". There have been enormous advances in multiple sclerosis that prove this statement to be correct.

Multiple sclerosis was first described in 1868 by the French neurologist Charcot. After more than a century of study, the aetiology of multiple sclerosis (MS) remains unknown. There is no gold-standard test to confirm the diagnosis, and there is no curative treatment. MS is an immune-mediated, chronic inflammatory demyelinating disease of the central nervous system. There is secondary axonal loss with progressive neurodegeneration even in the early stages.

Currently, the diagnosis is based on the clinical features, the results of MRI, analysis of the cerebral spinal fluid and visual evoked potentials [63] (see Appendix I). These criteria have been modified on several occasions and are likely to change in the future. The diagnosis of MS can be challenging as several conditions can result in multifocal involvement of the central nervous system and thus mimic MS. These include central nervous system or systemic vasculitis, acute disseminated encephalomyelitis, immune-mediated encephalitis, antiphospholipid antibody syndrome, sarcoidosis, Wilson's disease, paraneoplastic syndromes and central nervous system lymphoma.

MS is more common in women and younger patients between the ages of 15 and 50, with a mean age of onset of 29–33 years. It can rarely occur in children or adults over the age of 50. There is probably a genetic predisposition. [64] The natural history is highly variable from the very benign, incidentally discovered at autopsy, to the very malignant with death within the first few years of onset. This variability makes it challenging to assess therapeutic interventions. In general, at ten years, 50% of patients with MS will have a neurological deficit requiring the use of a cane to walk, while 15% will be in a wheelchair. [65]

MS may present as a clinically isolated syndrome (one episode confined to one part of the central nervous system), a relapsing/remitting course with or without secondary progressive MS or primary progressive MS where progression to disability occurs without remission.

# Variability of Multiple Sclerosis
## Clinically Isolated Syndrome

The clinically isolated syndrome tends to occur in younger patients. It is a single episode of demyelination affecting a specific part of the central nervous system. The commonest isolated syndromes are optic or retrobulbar neuritis affecting the optic nerve, transverse myelitis of the spinal cord and an internuclear ophthalmoplegia in the brainstem. These episodes are

---

6    Personal observation. As many are depressed it seems logical to recommend an antidepressant.

usually self-limiting with resolution over several weeks. The presence of gadolinium-enhancing abnormalities or juxtacortical lesions on an MRI scan and or the presence of oligoclonal bands in the CSF increases the risk of progression to clinically definite MS in patients with clinically isolated syndromes.[63]

## Relapsing-Remitting Multiple Sclerosis

The course in most patients is a relapsing and remitting (RRMS) one with initially complete resolution of symptoms and signs. In other patients, residual deficits may occur and accumulate with subsequent relapses.

## Secondary Progressive Multiple Sclerosis

Many patients with the relapsing-remitting form of MS will subsequently develop a secondary progressive course with increasing disability in the absence of any apparent relapses. They also accumulate a cumulative neurological deficit when the relapses do not entirely resolve.

## Primary Progressive Multiple Sclerosis

There is a primary progressive form of MS where the increasing disability occurs without apparent relapses or attacks. The primary progressive form of MS typically occurs in patients of middle age who develop progressive cervical spinal cord involvement.

# When to Suspect Multiple Sclerosis

MS should be suspected in patients with gradual onset over hours to days of focal neurological symptoms associated with impaired function.

## Optic or Retrobulbar Neuritis

The unilateral blurring of vision associated with pain on movement of the eye evolving over hours to days is a very typical initial presentation. It represents optic or retrobulbar neuritis. As described in Chapter 4, 'The cranial nerves and understanding the brainstem', patients with optic neuritis will have markedly impaired visual acuity with a swollen optic disc and an afferent pupillary defect with or without impaired colour vision. In contrast, patients with retrobulbar neuritis will have the same features without optic disc swelling. Impaired colour vision detected by the Ischiari colour charts suggests asymptomatic optic nerve involvement.

Not all patients with optic neuritis develop MS.

## Transverse Myelitis

Weakness commencing in the lower limbs that may spread to affect the upper limbs or an ascending sensory disturbance once again starting in the lower limbs and spreading up onto the trunk and sometimes into the arms represents the involvement of the spinal cord and is referred to as transverse myelitis. The word transverse is a misnomer as the lesions tend to involve the spinal cord vertically over several segments. Sphincter disturbance is common in patients with spinal cord involvement with either acute urinary retention or incontinence of either urine and or faeces.

It is important to remember that transverse myelitis is a syndrome and not a diagnosis. Although MS is a common cause of transverse myelitis, transverse myelitis also occurs with infectious and post-infectious diseases, as a paraneoplastic phenomenon and in collagen vascular diseases. Patients with transverse myelitis and a normal brain MRI scan have a low risk of developing clinically definite MS. [66]

## Neuromyelitis Optica Spectrum Disorder (NMOSD)

The term neuromyelitis optica spectrum disorder is an immune-mediated disorder that affects the optic nerves, spinal cord and brainstem. An entity where severe optic neuritis and transverse myelitis attacks occur simultaneously or in succession. Although a monophasic form exists, the tendency is for recurrent episodes of optic neuritis and transverse myelitis. The original description was transverse myelitis with bilateral optic or bilateral retrobulbar neuritis. MS, systemic lupus erythematosus, acute disseminated encephalomyelitis, and Behçet's have clinical features resembling NMOSD. NMOSD is a distinct disorder separate from MS. [67] On MRI, T2 lesions span several longitudinal segments in the central spinal cord. CSF oligoclonal bands are usually negative. Patients clinically diagnosed as NMOSD may include aquaporin 4 (AQP4)-antibody-seropositive autoimmune astrocytopathic disease, myelin oligodendrocyte glycoprotein (MOG)-antibody-seropositive inflammatory demyelinating disease, and double-seronegative disease. [165] Patients with NMOSD may succumb to respiratory failure.

In contrast, in patients with MS, the spinal cord abnormality on MRI usually involves fewer than two segments, is asymmetrical and in the peripheral aspect of the spinal cord.

## Bilateral Internuclear Ophthalmoplegia

Another classical presentation is horizontal diplopia with or without vertigo due to involvement of the medial longitudinal fasciculus in the brainstem. The ipsilateral failure of adduction (looking towards the nose) and leading eye nystagmus in the opposite eye is called an internuclear ophthalmoplegia. Bilateral internuclear ophthalmoplegia is almost pathognomonic of MS. Pseudo-internuclear ophthalmoplegia can occur with the Miller-Fisher variant of acute inflammatory demyelinating peripheral neuropathy, myasthenia gravis and thyroid eye disease. In these conditions, other signs are the clue to the diagnosis.

## Sphincter Disturbance

Neurologists are often asked to see young patients with disturbances of micturition and, although this can be a presenting symptom in a small number of patients with MS, most of these patients do not have MS.

## Uhthoff's Phenomenon

Transient worsening of symptoms in patients with MS is not uncommon in excessive heat or an infection that causes fever. This is referred to as Uhthoff's phenomenon. Patients with established MS will often confuse this with a relapse of their MS. The clue is that it is a transient worsening of <u>pre-existing symptoms</u> and signs rather than the appearance of new symptoms or signs indicating the involvement of a different part of the nervous system.

## LHermitte's Phenomenon

Electric shock-like sensations radiate from the neck down the body and into the limbs with neck flexion are referred to as LHermitte's phenomenon. Although characteristic of MS, it is not pathognomonic and can occur with severe cervical cord compression.

## Trigeminal Neuralgia

Although trigeminal neuralgia (see Chapter 4, 'The cranial nerves and understanding the brainstem') can occur in patients, MS is rarely the cause but should be suspected in young patients with trigeminal neuralgia. Having said this, dental pain is often confused with trigeminal neuralgia as both have severe pain in the distribution of the trigeminal nerve.

# Investigation in suspected multiple sclerosis

MRI has revolutionised the management of patients with MS. It is a powerful tool for diagnosis and a surrogate endpoint in therapeutic trials. The current McDonald criteria [63] used for the diagnosis of MS rely heavily on the MRI scan findings. The current criteria can be found in Appendix I.

> The MRI scan must not be used in isolation to diagnose M.S.
> MRI findings must be carefully correlated with the clinical presentation.

## Treatment of Multiple Sclerosis

The ultimate goal of treatment of RRMS is to choose the right drug for the right patient at the right time. In 2021 the Multiple Sclerosis Therapy Consensus Group, based on several large observational and registry studies stated that modern MS therapy could and should prevent the accumulation of disability and, thus, possible neurodegeneration.[172] It is generally agreed that disease-modifying treatments (DMT's) have a better effect early in the course of MS, acknowledging that the individual patient's course is extremely difficult to predict. [172]

There is little evidence to help determine which patient should receive what therapy. [164] The 2018 AAN Practice Guidelines [164] advise respecting patients preferences and informing them to be realistic as DMTs reduce but do not eliminate MS relapses and MRI activity.

The traditional approach was referred to as escalation therapy, starting with lower risk, lower efficacy DMT's and switching to high risk higher efficacy DMT when relapses occurred. Many centres now institute the hit-hard-and-early concept and recommend higher risk higher efficacy DMT therapy much earlier on in the disease, before any significant disability develops. Early treatment may prevent progression from relapsing-remitting MS to secondary progressive MS. [151-152] The newer DMT's significantly reduce the relapse rate and the accumulation of T2 lesions on MRI scan. They also reduce progression to disability in the short term, at this stage their ability to prevent progression to disability over the long-term is uncertain.

In individual cases, a wait-and-see approach with regular neurological and imaging checks may also be considered in patients with very low lesion burden and complete remission of mild clinical symptoms. [172]

In isolated optic neuritis with a normal MRI, it is reasonable to withhold treatment and monitor.

Interferon-b-1a i.m., Interferonb-1a s.c., Interferon-b-1b s.c. and in the USA, siponimod are recommended in patients with clinically isolated syndromes (CIS) with ongoing careful monitoring.

In patients with CIS and a high lesion burden and or infratentorial lesions on diagnostic MRI, high efficacy immunotherapy should be actively recommended given the presumed unfavourable prognosis.

The first-line therapies in MS include interferon-ß1a, interferon-ß1b, and glatiramer acetate that have fewer serious adverse side effects. Mitoxantrone and cyclophosphamide carry a significant risk of adverse side effects.

The newer generation high efficacy DMT's include the cell-replication inhibitor teriflunomide and the oral sphingosine-1-phosphate antagonists fingolimod, siponimod, ponesimod and ozanimod, inhibitors of cell trafficking, and cell-deleting therapies such as oral (cladribine) and intravenous (alemtuzumab, ocrelizumab ocrelizumab, ofatumumab,) are all associated with potentially serious adverse side-effects.

Ocrelizumab (Ocrevus®), the humanized anti-CD20 monoclonal antibody, has been shown to reduce clinical relapses and the total number of gadolinium-enhanced T1 lesions observed on MRI scans in relapsing-remitting MS. The reduction of MRI lesions was 89-96% in the 600mg and 2,000mg groups respectively. Clinical relapses were reduced by 80% and 73% in the 600mg and 2,000mg groups, respectively. [166] Relapses and new gadolinium-enhancing T1 lesions on MRI scans were not totally abolished.

Ocrelizumab is the first drug to be approved for primary progressive MS after it was shown to reduce disability progression. [167, 171]

The main concern with some of the DMT's is the development of progressive multifocal leucoencephalopathy (PML) due to the JC virus, particularly with natalizumab and to a lesser extent fingolimod and dimethyl fumarate. [150] All patients with MS should have a JC virus-detecting test prior to commencing therapy with these agents[7]. Although a positive test does not indicate the patient will develop PML, it has only been seen in JC positive patients. Serum, urine and CSF can all be tested for the JC virus.

Patients receiving these drugs require careful monitoring and patients should be managed in centres of excellence.[8]

Bone marrow transplantation and autologous haematopoietic stem cell transplantation are recommended for patients with progressive disease not responding to DMT.[153-154]

As knowledge accumulates, recommendations will change, and it is crucial to check the latest guidelines regularly.

---

7   The Australian product information recommends JC virus DNA on the CSF
8   Personal opinion, but I suspect shared by many

# Tumours and the Nervous System

Neurological symptoms in patients with malignancy may relate to:

1.  direct effects of the malignancy on the central nervous system – patients present with focal neurological deficits, seizures or headache.
2.  remote effects of the malignancy, the paraneoplastic syndrome – patients present with diffuse neurological symptoms.
3.  complications of therapy (chemotherapy or radiotherapy) of the malignancy.

Just because a patient has malignancy does not mean they cannot develop an unrelated neurological problem.

## Direct Effects of Malignancy

### Primary Tumours of the Nervous System

Primary tumours of the nervous system can affect the brain, spinal cord or rarely the peripheral nervous system. They are named according to their cell of origin (Table 14.2).

Classifications of tumours of the nervous system, such as that of the World Health Organization [68, 69], will continue to evolve with new discoveries. [70] Primary central nervous system tumours declare themselves with seizures, headaches or a progressive focal neurological deficit.

Gliomas can affect any part of the nervous system but are less common in the brainstem and spinal cord. They can infiltrate the corpus callosum, spread to both hemispheres and form a butterfly glioma, or infiltrate throughout the entire brain (gliomatosis cerebri) rather than a discrete mass.

Tumours of the pituitary gland represent about 10% of primary central nervous system tumours. Symptoms arise from pituitary tumours in three ways:

1.  a direct result of the tumour (visual loss due to compression of the optic chiasm or optic nerves and headache).
2.  destruction of the pituitary gland and loss of hormone function, in particular, hypothyroidism and amenorrhoea.
3.  excess hormone secretion, e.g. growth hormone causing either gigantism or acromegaly or prolactin causing galactorrhoea.

Most pituitary tumours are macroadenomas, whereas hormone-secreting tumours such as prolactinomas are microadenomas.

| Central nervous system | Cell of origin | Name of tumour |
|---|---|---|
| | Astrocytes | Astrocytoma* |
| | Ependyma | Ependymoma* |
| | Oligodendrocytes | Oligodendrogliomas* |
| | Neuroectoderm | Medulloblastoma, pinealoblastoma |
| | Meninges | Meningioma |
| | Schwann cell | Neurofibroma |
| Peripheral nervous system | | |
| | Schwann cell | Neurofibroma |
| | Neuroectoderm | Ewing's sarcoma |

* Astrocytomas, ependymomas and oligodendrogliomas are collectively called gliomas.

**Table 14.2 Primary tumours of the nervous system named according to their cell of origin**

## Secondary Tumours of the Nervous System

In non-central nervous system malignancy, the neurological manifestations may be the presenting symptom or may develop after the diagnosis of malignancy. Any tumour can potentially metastasise to the brain, but the common ones are lung and breast, while the paired organs (thyroid, lung, breast, kidney and prostate) metastasise to the spinal column, predominantly the thoracic region. Secondaries tend to occur in patients between the ages of 40 and 60. Spinal cord compression due to malignancy is discussed in Chapter 13.

# Paraneoplastic syndromes

Paraneoplastic syndromes refer to neurological symptoms and signs in a patient with malignancy that are not the direct result of the tumour but rather an immune-mediated remote effect. They are rare. Paraneoplastic syndromes can affect the neuromuscular junction, the central and peripheral nervous systems. (tables 14.3 and 14.4) *Similar antibody-mediated clinical syndromes occur in the absence of malignancy.*[9] Limbic encephalitis and subacute sensory neuropathy are more often non-paraneoplastic. Approximately 50% of subacute cerebellar ataxia cases and 40% of Lambert-Eaton myasthenic syndrome cases are not paraneoplastic. [137]

Psychiatric symptoms are the initial manifestation in up to 60% of patients. Seizures, catatonia, autonomic instability, or hyperkinesia occur in psychiatric patients with immune-mediated encephalitis. [140]

Myasthenia gravis usually occurs with thymic hyperplasia but may occur with a benign or malignant thymoma. Two of the more common paraneoplastic syndromes include Lambert–Eaton syndrome (small cell carcinoma of the lung) and demyelinating peripheral neuropathy (osteosclerotic plasmacytoma).

Increasing numbers of antibodies are being identified, and the type of malignancy underlying a paraneoplastic syndromes can vary considerably (Tables 14.3 and 14.4). It is now recognised that pure presentations of these syndromes are the exception rather than the rule. Similarly, the same antibody can cause different paraneoplastic syndromes. Hu (ANNA-1), for example, can

---

9   Bhagavati has written an excellent review of the autoimmune disorders of the nervous system. [139]

cause sensory neuronopathy, encephalomyelitis and limbic encephalitis. It is not uncommon for patients with malignancy and paraneoplastic phenomena to have multifocal symptoms and signs. In 2021 an expert panel developed a modified set of diagnostic criteria. [132] They stratified the risk of cancer with some antibodies high-risk (>70%), some intermediate-risk (30-70%) and others low-risk (<30%). The paper by Pelosof and Gerber contains an excellent summary and detailed description of the clinical features of paraneoplastic syndromes. [135]

| Clinical syndrome | Antibodies | Underlying malignancy |
|---|---|---|
| Carcinoma-associated retinopathy* | Retinal | SCLC, melanoma, gynaecologic |
| Limbic encephalitis | Hu, Ma2, Ma, AMPAR, GABABR, LGI1, GlyR | SCLC, testicular, malignant thymoma |
| Anti-NMDAR Encephalitis | NMDAR | Ovarian or extraovarian teratoma |
| Encephalitis | mGluR5, GABAAR, DPPX | Hodgkin lymphoma |
| Brainstem encephalitis | Ma, Ma2, Ri(ANNA-2), KLHL11 | Lung, testicular |
| Encephalomyelitis | Amphiphysin,PCA-2, CRMP5, ANNA-3, NMDA-receptor | SCLC, breast, thymoma, ovarian |
| Meningoencephalitis | GFAP | Ovarian teratomas and adenocarcinomas |
| Cerebellar ataxia | mGluR1 | Haematological |
| Rapidly progressive cerebellar degeneration | Yo, Hu, Tr (DNER), Ma1, mGluR1, PCA-2, CRMP5, SOX1, P/Q VGCC | SCLC, ovarian, breast, bladder, Hodgkin's lymphoma |
| Opsoclonus–myoclonus | Ri | Ovarian, breast, bladder, lung |
| Neuromyelitis Optica spectrum disorder | AQP4 | Adenocarcinoma |
| MOG antibody-associated diseases | IgG antibodies to myelin oligodendrocyte glycoprotein (MOG) | Ovarian teratomas |
| Chorea | CRMP5 (CV2) | SCLC, breast, thymoma |
| Progressive encephalomyelitis with rigidity and myoclonus; | GlyR, DPPX | |
| Necrotising myelopathy | None identified | Not specific |
| Stiff-person syndrome | Amphiphysin | SCLC, breast |

Table 14.3 Central nervous system paraneoplastic syndromes * There are several other ocular paraneoplastic syndromes. [138] Compiled from Darnell and Posner [71], Dalmau [72], Anderson and Barber [73] and Graus et al. [132]

| Clinical syndrome | Antibodies | Underlying malignancy |
|---|---|---|
| Dorsal root ganglionopathy | Anti-Hu, anti-CRMP5 (anti-CV2), ANNA-3 | Lung, SCLC, thymoma |
| Peripheral neuropathy | MAG | Waldenstrom's |
| Autonomic neuropathy | Hu, nicotinic AchR | SCLC, bladder, thyroid |
| Myasthenia gravis | AchR, titin | Thymoma |
| Lambert–Eaton syndrome | VGCC, anti-PCA-2. P/Q VGCC | SCLC |
| Dermatomyositis | None identified | Ovarian, breast, lung |
| Necrotising myopathy | None identified | No specific neoplasm |
| Morvans syndrome * | SASPR2, CASPR2 | Malignant thymoma |
| Neuromyotonia | VGKC, CASPR2 | SCLC, malignant thymoma |
| Stiff-person syndrome | Amphiphysin, GAD65 | SCLC, breast |

**Table 14.4 Peripheral nervous system paraneoplastic syndromes** * Morvans has both central and peripheral nervous system involvement. Compiled from Darnell and Posner [71], Dalmau [72], Rudnicki [74], Anderson and Barber [73] and Graus et al. [132]

These neurological syndromes are severe, often disabling, and sometimes fatal. They can develop rapidly over days but more commonly weeks to months. The neurological symptom and signs often, but not invariably, precede the diagnosis of malignancy for months and sometimes years. The malignancy may, despite extensive investigations, elude detection. The probable reason is that effective antitumour immunity prevents tumour growth but causes autoimmune brain disease. [71, 75–81]

Patients with paraneoplastic syndromes should be screened every 4-6 months for two years after the initial diagnosis. [132] A relapse of the paraneoplastic syndrome may herald a recurrence of the tumour years after the initial presentation and should prompt further tests to detect the underlying malignancy.

| Investigation and Management of Paraneoplastic Syndromes |
|---|
| The paraneoplastic syndromes arise from immune cross-reactivity between malignant and normal tissues. [135] In patients with malignancy, onconeural antibodies and onconeural antigen-specific T lymphocytes inadvertently attack components of the nervous system.<br><br>PET scanning can detect malignancy even in patients where a CT scan is negative. In patients with paraneoplastic syndromes, PET scanning has an 80% and 67% sensitivity and specificity, respectively. [82] Self-examination, mammography, ultrasound, MRI and elasticity imaging (a non-invasive medical imaging technique that helps determine the stiffness of organs and other structures) are all used to detect breast cancer. [83]<br><br>As new anti-neuronal antibodies are identified, it has become clear that a particular antibody is often a guide to the site of the underlying malignancy (see Tables 14.3 and 14.4).<br><br>The most effective treatment is removing the antigen by treatment of the underlying malignancy. This may not necessarily remove the onconeural antibodies, and the mainstay of therapy is immunosuppression with corticosteroids, corticosteroid-sparing agents (e.g., azathioprine, cyclophosphamide), the anti-CD20 monoclonal antibody rituximab, IV immunoglobulin (IVIG), and plasma exchange. Unfortunately, many patients are severely disabled at the time of presentation. |

# Complications of Therapy

When neurological symptoms develop in a patient undergoing therapy for malignancy, it is essential to consider side effects due to the treatment. There are many recognised complications of radiotherapy and chemotherapy. The list of neurological complications is expanding due to newer chemotherapeutic agents, including monoclonal antibodies and proteasome inhibitors.

## Complications of Chemotherapy

The most common neurological side effect of chemotherapeutic agents is peripheral neuropathy. [84, 85] The neuropathy is dose-dependent, develops gradually and increases in severity with subsequent doses. It is almost invariably a length-dependent peripheral neuropathy in which patients develop a distal sensory loss in the lower limbs with or without distal weakness. Very rarely, the autonomic nervous system may be affected, for example, with vincristine. Oxaliplatin can cause an acute reversible peripheral neuropathy developing within hours of commencing intravenous therapy. [86] Improvement often but not invariably occurs if treatment is ceased. Peripheral neuropathy occurs with many of the currently employed chemotherapeutic agents. These include thalidomide, lenalidomide (an analogue of thalidomide), vinca alkaloids (vincristine and vinblastine), platinum compounds (cisplatin, carboplatin and oxaliplatin), taxanes (paclitaxel and docetaxel) and cytarabine. *Cognitive decline* may occur with chemotherapy and is called 'chemobrain'. [85] Other neurological complications of chemotherapy include encephalopathy, seizures, headache, vision changes, cerebellar dysfunction, and spinal cord damage with myelopathy.

## Complications of Intrathecal Therapy

Intrathecal methotrexate and cytarabine can induce *chemical meningitis, myelopathy* (spinal cord involvement) or *seizures. Multifocal leucoencephalopathy* has been reported with capecitabine. [87] The inadvertent intrathecal administration of vincristine causes severe and often fatal myelopathy. [88]

## Complications of Radiotherapy

The neurological complications of radiotherapy can be early (within days) or delayed. [89] The early complications are usually mild and transient, whereas the delayed complications are typically progressive and disabling. Complications occur when central nervous system tumours are irradiated or from incidental damage with radiation of soft tissue tumours adjacent to the nervous system. The site of the neurological complications will relate directly to the location of radiotherapy.

Immediate radiation damage to the spinal cord is usually transient, developing within weeks of radiation with numbness and paraesthesia without weakness or objective neurological signs. These sensory symptoms spread from the radiation site to the limbs and are often associated with the LHermitte phenomena. Symptoms usually resolve within months.

The onset of delayed symptoms usually commences 1–3 years after therapy but may begin as early as three months or as late as 12 years. Necrosis resulting in swelling and a mass effect may occur with radiation to the brain. The symptoms and signs relate to the mass. It can sometimes be challenging to differentiate between recurrent tumour and radiation necrosis. Radiation necrosis-induced masses may, like tumours, enhance with contrast on a CT scan of the brain.

Careful correlation with the sight of maximum irradiation may sometimes help to differentiate recurrent tumours from radiation necrosis. Magnetic resonance spectroscopy or computer-assisted stereotactic biopsy can differentiate tumour recurrence from radiation necrosis. [90, 91]

Non-reversible radiation myelopathy with paraplegia or quadriplegia evolving over days secondary to arterial occlusion can occur acutely. [92] This acute form of myelopathy is rare. Chronic progressive myelopathy, developing about one year after treatment, is more common. However, it may occur as early as four months or as late as 13 years after radiation. The patient develops ascending sensory loss and weakness, often associated with sphincter disturbance. The symptoms and signs are usually bilateral but may be unilateral. The myelopathy progresses over months, often to severe disability. An MRI scan demonstrates swelling of the spinal cord, focal contrast enhancement, low signal over several segments on T1-weighted images and high signal on T2-weighted images. [93, 94]

Radiation injury may also occur to single or multiple cranial nerves. The brachial plexus is another site where radiation damage can occur. It can be challenging to differentiate between radiation injury to the brachial plexus and malignant infiltration. Pain is more common with the tumour that usually affects the lower brachial plexus, while radiation damage affects the upper brachial plexus.

**Treatment of Radiation Necrosis**

There is little effective treatment for radiation damage to the nervous system. The use of more focused radiation, e.g. Stereotactic radiosurgery, can reduce the risk. Treatment with corticosteroids, surgery or antioxidants is often ineffective, and the role of anticoagulation remains unclear. [95, 96] Uncontrolled studies claim a benefit with hyperbaric oxygen. [156] As did a small controlled trial of the vascular endothelial growth factor-A-specific angiogenesis inhibitor bevacizumab. [157]

# Infections of the Nervous System

Meningitis, one of the more common nervous system infections, was discussed in Chapter 9. Patients with HIV or on immunosuppressive therapy are at increased risk of opportunistic infections. A complete discussion of central nervous system infections is beyond the scope of this book[10].

# Encephalitis

Encephalitis is inflammation of the brain; meningoencephalitis is encephalitis associated with meningitis. The essential clinical features of encephalitis are fever, headache, confusion, focal or generalised seizures and focal neurological signs. It can occur in HIV, related to malignancy, as a paraneoplastic phenomenon or secondary to viral infection. Viral encephalitis can be epidemic (Murray–Valley, Japanese encephalitis, West Nile virus, enterovirus, coxsackievirus, varicella-zoster virus and tick-borne encephalitis virus) or sporadic.

Various viruses affect different parts of the brain. Herpes simplex virus (HSV), varicella-zoster and human herpesvirus 6 (in post-transplant limbic encephalitis) typically affect the temporal lobes. West Nile virus, Japanese encephalitis virus, respiratory viruses, rabies,

10 See (2000). Infectious Diseases of the Nervous System. London, Butterworth-Heinemann.
  Scheld, W. M., et al. (2014). Infections of the central nervous system. Philadelphia, Wolters Kluwer.

and Rocky Mountain spotted fever affect the basal ganglia and thalamus as can the bacterium mycobacterium tuberculosis. Varicella-zoster virus, West Nile virus, Powasson virus and the bacterium mycoplasma pneumonia affect the cerebellum. Brainstem encephalitis occurs with enteroviruses, West Nile virus, Japanese encephalitis virus, rabies, listeria monocytogenes and mycoplasma pneumonia. Arun Venkatesan from Baltimore has written an excellent review of encephalitis and brain abscess. [158]

## Herpes Simplex Encephalitis

The mortality of untreated herpes simplex encephalitis (HSE) approaches 70%. Morbidity is severe, with only 10% of patients resuming everyday life. [97] Effective therapy (see below) has reduced mortality to approximately 20%. [97] Rates as low as 7% have been reported. [98] A poor outcome still occurs in 30–40% of patients. [98]

Herpes simplex encephalitis presents with fever, focal deficit and seizures. Dysphasia, hemiparesis and either focal or generalised seizures occur. An altered mental state is common, coma may ensue, but headache, nausea and vomiting are uncommon. Treatment should be initiated immediately the diagnosis is suspected and before investigations confirm or exclude the diagnosis.

---

As no test has a sensitivity of 100%, if the clinical picture is strongly suggestive of HSE, a full course of treatment is recommended.

Imaging should be performed immediately prior to a lumbar puncture as swelling of the temporal lobe can occur in patients with HSE without obvious clinical deterioration, and an LP could result in transtentorial herniation11.

---

### Management of Herpes Simplex Encephalitis

Periodic lateralised epileptiform discharges and focal temporal slowing can be seen on the electroencephalogram in the first 24–48 hours. While low-density abnormalities may be present on the CT scan, the findings are not always present in the early stages. [99] MRI scanning enables the early diagnosis of HSE [100] and is abnormal in more than 80% of patients in the first 24–48 hours. [101] A repeat MRI scan is indicated in suspected cases if the initial scan is normal. MRI demonstrates increased signal on T2-weighted images in one or both temporal lobes. The diagnosis is confirmed by polymerase chain reaction (PCR) for the herpes simplex type 1 or 2 viral genome in the CSF. [102]

Treatment consists of supportive measures. The antiviral agent acyclovir 10–15 mg/kg 8-hourly for ten days is the treatment of choice for HSE. [97, 103] Although corticosteroids have been recommended based on a retrospective study [104], uncertainty remains regarding their use in HSE. [105] Acyclovir has reduced mortality from 60–70% down to 30%.

---

11 Personal experience

# The Immunocompromised Patient

Human or acquired immune deficiency (HIV, AIDS) virus results in severe immune deficiency. Immune deficiency also occurs in patients with malignancy on chemotherapy and vasculitis treated with immunosuppressants.

The HIV virus also directly results in various peripheral nervous system complications, such as painful peripheral neuropathy, vacuolar myelopathy, and inflammatory myopathy. [106] Direct invasion of the virus into the central nervous system results in the AIDS dementia complex[12]. [107]

Immunosuppressed patients develop opportunistic infections of the central nervous system, such as toxoplasmosis, cytomegalovirus, tuberculous and cryptococcal meningitis. Primary central nervous system lymphoma and progressive multifocal encephalopathy (PML) also occur. Toxoplasmosis, primary central nervous system lymphoma and progressive multifocal encephalopathy (PML) are the commonest causes of focal disease in immunosuppressed patients, particularly those with AIDS.

Patients present with meningitis or intracerebral and brainstem symptoms secondary to mass lesions. In patients with malignancy, it can sometimes be challenging to differentiate between recurrent malignancy, primary lymphoma, toxoplasmosis and PML.

MRI and stereotactic biopsy is recommended in patients with mass lesions who are alert. Open biopsy and decompression are necessary if there is imminent herniation. Analysis of CSF, MRI and empirical treatment for toxoplasmosis is the approach if there are multiple lesions and the patient is alert and stable.

# Covid-19 and the Nervous System

In 2020 the Covid-19 virus caused a worldwide pandemic. In many reports, it is difficult to know if the CNS problem was directly related to Covid-19 or whether these conditions occurred in patients with Covid-19 coincidentally. Thus, our understanding of the effects on the nervous system is still evolving, and therefore the information is in a text box.

---

**Covid19 and Covid 19 Vaccines**

The nervous system is involved in 22.5-36.4% of patients with Covid-19.

Encephalopathy due to direct brain invasion by the virus has been described. Seizures, ischaemic and haemorrhagic stroke, meningoencephalitis and acute disseminated encephalomyelitis are other possible central nervous system manifestations.

Although acute inflammatory demyelinating peripheral neuropathy and other peripheral neuropathies have been reported, the causal link is unclear.

Anosmia and dysgeusia are common complications. Optic neuritis and third nerve palsies can occur, as can a Miller-Fisher syndrome-like illness with multiple cranial nerve palsies. [160,162] Transverse myelitis has been reported. [173]

Cerebral vein thrombosis secondary to thrombotic, immune-mediated thrombocytopenia is a rare complication from vaccination with the recombinant adenoviral vector encoding the spike protein antigen.[163]

Long Covid is prolonged symptoms after the acute infection that resembles chronic fatigue syndrome. Brain fog, fatigue, cognitive dysfunction and headaches can last months. It occurs in a third of patients during the first six months after infection.

---

12 These are beyond the scope of this book; please refer to the book entitled AIDS and the Nervous System by Rosenblum, Levy and Bredesen (New York: Raven Press; 1998). In particular, Chapter 19 of that book contains excellent algorithms to aid in the management of patients with AIDS and neurological symptoms.

# References

1   Plum F, Posner JB. *Diagnosis of stupor and coma*. 2nd edn Philadelphia: FA Davis; 1972, 286.

2   World Health Organization. International Classification of Diseases and Related Health Symptoms 2003, 11th Revision. adopted by the Seventy-second World Health Assembly in May 2019 and comes into effect on 1 January 2022. Available: https://icd.who.int/en

3   Mayo-Smith MF, et al. Management of alcohol withdrawal delirium: An evidence-based practice guideline. *Arch Intern Med* 2004;164(13):1405–1412.

4   Attard A, Ranjith G, Taylor D. Delirium and its treatment. *C.N.S. Drugs* 2008;22(8):631–644.

5   Lonergan E, et al. Benzodiazepines for delirium. *Cochrane Database Syst Rev* 2009(1):CD006379.

6   Reynolds 3rd C.F., et al. Bedside differentiation of depressive pseudodementia from dementia. *Am J Psychiatry* 1988;145(9):1099–1103.

7   Kertesz A. Clinical features and diagnosis of frontotemporal dementia. *Front Neurol Neurosci* 2009;24:140–148.

8   Alladi S, et al. Focal cortical presentations of Alzheimer's disease. *Brain* 2007;130(Pt 10):2636–2645.

9   Mesulam MM. Primary progressive aphasia. *Ann Neurol* 2001;49(4):425–432.

10  Petersen RC. Focal dementia syndromes: In search of the gold standard. *Ann Neurol* 2001;49(4): 421–423.

11  Geschwind MD, et al. Rapidly progressive dementia. *Ann Neurol* 2008;64(1):97–108.

12  Pokorski RJ. Differentiating age-related memory loss from early dementia. *J Insur Med* 2002;34(2): 100–113.

13  Linn RT, et al. The 'preclinical phase' of probable Alzheimer's disease: A 13-year prospective study of the Framingham cohort. *Arch Neurol* 1995;52(5):485–490.

14  Meyer JS, Huang J, Chowdhury MH. MRI confirms mild cognitive impairments prodromal for Alzheimer's, vascular and Parkinson–Lewy body dementias. *J Neurol Sci* 2007;257(1–2):97–104.

15  Jackson CE. A clinical approach to muscle diseases. Semin Neurol 2008 Apr. Available: http://www.medscape.com/viewarticle/572269 (28 Feb 2009).

16  Washington University. Myopathy and neuromuscular junction disorders: Differential diagnosis. Available: http://neuromuscular.wustl.edu/maltbrain.html (3 Jul 2009).

17  Karpati G, Hilton-Jones D, Griggs RD. *Disorders of voluntary muscle*. 7th edn New York: Cambridge University Press; 2001.

18  Mendell JR. Approach to the patient with muscle disease. In: Hauser SL, editor. *Harrison's neurology in clinical medicine*. San Francisco: McGraw–Hill; 2006.

19  Klopstock T. Drug-induced myopathies. *Curr Opin Neurol* 2008;21(5):590–595.

20  Klinge L, et al. New aspects on patients affected by dysferlin deficient muscular dystrophy. *J Neurol Neurosurg Psychiatry* 14 Jun 2009:[Epub ahead of print].

21  Norwood F, et al. EFNS guideline on diagnosis and management of limb girdle muscular dystrophies. *Eur J Neurol* 2007;14(12):1305–1312.

22  Hilton-Jones D, Kissel JT. The examination and investigation of the patient with muscle disease. In: Karpati G, Hilton-Jones D, Griggs R, editors. *Disorders of voluntary muscle*. New York: Cambridge University Press; 2001. p. 349–373.

23  Moxley 3rd R.T., et al. Practice parameter: Corticosteroid treatment of Duchenne dystrophy: Report of the Quality Standards Subcommittee of the American Academy of Neurology and the Practice Committee of the Child Neurology Society. *Neurology* 2005;64(1):13–20.

24  Choy EH, et al. Immunosuppressant and immunomodulatory treatment for dermatomyositis and polymyositis. *Cochrane Database Syst Rev* 2012 Aug 15;2012(8):CD003643.

25  Wiendl H. Idiopathic inflammatory myopathies: Current and future therapeutic options. *Neurotherapeutics* 2008;5(4):548–557.

26  Fries JF, et al. Cyclophosphamide therapy in systemic lupus erythematosus and polymyositis. *Arthritis Rheum* 1973;16(2):154–162.

27  Vencovsky J, et al. Cyclosporine A versus methotrexate in the treatment of polymyositis and dermatomyositis. *Scand J Rheumatol* 2000;29(2):95–102.

28  Miller FW, et al. Controlled trial of plasma exchange and leukapheresis in polymyositis and dermatomyositis. *N Engl J Med* 1992;326(21):1380–1384.

29  Dalakas MC, et al. A controlled trial of high-dose intravenous immune globulin infusions as treatment for dermatomyositis. *N Engl J Med* 1993;329(27):1993–2000.

30  Elovaara I, et al. EFNS guidelines for the use of intravenous immunoglobulin in treatment of neurological diseases: EFNS task force on the use of intravenous immunoglobulin in treatment of neurological diseases. *Eur J Neurol* 2008;15(9):893–908.

31  Oldfors A, Lindberg C. Diagnosis, pathogenesis and treatment of inclusion body myositis. *Curr Opin Neurol* 2005;18(5):497–503.

32  Greenberg SA. Inclusion body myositis: Review of recent literature. *Curr Neurol Neurosci Rep* 2009;9(1):83–89.

33  Phillips PS, et al. Statin-associated myopathy with normal creatine kinase levels. *Ann Intern Med* 2002;137(7):581–585.

34  Sailler L, et al. Increased exposure to statins in patients developing chronic muscle diseases: A 2-year retrospective study. *Ann Rheum Dis* 2008;67(5):614–619.

35  Willis T. *De anima brutorum*. Oxford: Oxonii Theatro Sheldoniano; 1672, 404–407.

36  Eaton LM, Lambert EH. Electromyography and electric stimulation of nerves in diseases of motor unit: Observations on myasthenic syndrome associated with malignant tumors. *J Am Med Assoc* 1957;163(13):1117–1124.

37  Mulder DW, Lambert EH, Eaton LM. Myasthenic syndrome in patients with amyotrophic lateral sclerosis. *Neurology* 1959;9:627–631.

38  Hoch W, et al. Auto-antibodies to the receptor tyrosine kinase MuSK in patients with myasthenia gravis without acetylcholine receptor antibodies. *Nat Med* 2001;7(3):365–368.

39  Aarli JA, et al. Patients with myasthenia gravis and thymoma have in their sera IgG autoantibodies against titin. *Clin Exp Immunol* 1990;82(2):284–288.

40  Kennedy WR, Jimenez-Pabon E. The myasthenic syndrome associated with small cell carcinoma of the lung (Eaton–Lambert syndrome). *Neurology* 1968;18(8):757–766.

41  Gutmann L, et al. The Eaton–Lambert syndrome and autoimmune disorders. *Am J Med* 1972;53(3): 354–356.

42  Ackerman LV, et al. Thymoma in a case of myasthenia gravis. *Mo Med* 1949;46(4):270–272.

43  Sethi KD, Rivner MH, Swift TR. Ice pack test for myasthenia gravis. *Neurology* 1987;37(8):1383–1385.

44  Larner AJ, Thomas DJ. Can myasthenia gravis be diagnosed with the 'ice pack test'? A cautionary note. *Postgrad Med J* 2000;76(893):162–163.

45  Osserman KE, Kaplan LI. Rapid diagnostic test for myasthenia gravis: Increased muscle strength, without fasciculations, after intravenous administration of edrophonium (tensilon) chloride. *JAMA* 1952;150(4):265–268.

46  Aharonov A, et al. Humoral antibodies to acetylcholine receptor in patients with myasthenia gravis. *Lancet* 1975;2(7930):340–342.

47  Schwartz MS , Stalberg E. Single fibre electromyographic studies in myasthenia gravis with repetitive nerve stimulation. *J Neurol Neurosurg Psychiatry* 1975;38(7):678–682.

48  Stalberg E, Ekstedt J, Broman A. Neuromuscular transmission in myasthenia gravis studied with single fibre electromyography. *J Neurol Neurosurg Psychiatry* 1974;37(5):540–547.

49  Benatar M. A systematic review of diagnostic studies in myasthenia gravis. *Neuromuscul Disord* 2006;16(7):459–467.

50    Vincent A, et al. Antibodies in myasthenia gravis and related disorders. *Ann N Y Acad Sci* 2003;998:324–335.

51    Osserman KE, Genkins G. Critical reappraisal of the use of edrophonium (tensilon) chloride tests in myasthenia gravis and significance of clinical classification. *Ann N Y Acad Sci* 1966;135(1):312–334.

52    Vincent A, Newsom-Davis J. Acetylcholine receptor antibody as a diagnostic test for myasthenia gravis: Results in 153 validated cases and 2967 diagnostic assays. *J Neurol Neurosurg Psychiatry* 1985;48(12):1246–1252.

53    Vincent A, et al. Seronegative generalised myasthenia gravis: Clinical features, antibodies, and their targets. *Lancet Neurol* 2003;2(2):99–106.

54    Sonett JR, Jaretzki 3rd A. Thymectomy for nonthymomatous myasthenia gravis: A critical analysis. *Ann N Y Acad Sci* 2008;1132:315–328.

55    Walker MB. Treatment of myasthenia gravis with physostigmine. *Lancet* 1934;1:1200–1201.

56    Schneider-Gold C, et al. Corticosteroids for myasthenia gravis. *Cochrane Database Syst Rev* 2005(2):CD002828.

57    Hart IK, Sathasivam S, Sharshar T. Immunosuppressive agents for myasthenia gravis. *Cochrane Database Syst Rev* 2007(4):CD005224.

58    Maddison P, Newsom-Davis J. *Treatment for Lambert–Eaton myasthenic syndrome. Cochrane Database Syst Rev* 2003(2):CD003279.

59    Ramsay AM, O'Sullivan E. Encephalomyelitis simulating poliomyelitis. *Lancet* 1956;270(6926):761–764.

60    Galpine JF, Brady C. Benign myalgic encephalomyelitis. *Lancet* 1957;272(6972):757–758.

61    Petersen I, et al. Risk and predictors of fatigue after infectious mononucleosis in a large primary-care cohort. *Q J Med* 2006;99(1):49–55.

62    Behan PO, Bakheit AM. Clinical spectrum of postviral fatigue syndrome. *Br Med Bull* 1991;47(4):793–808.

63    Thompson, A.J. Banwell, B.L. Barkhof, F. et al. Diagnosis of multiple sclerosis: 2017 revisions of the McDonald criteria. Lancet neurology 2018;17(2):162-173

64    Ebers GC, et al. A population-based study of multiple sclerosis in twins. *N Engl J Med* 1986;315(26):1638–1642.

65    Courtney AM, et al. Multiple sclerosis. *Med Clin North Am* 2009;93(2):451–476:ix–x.

66    Scott TF, Kassab SL, Singh S. Acute partial transverse myelitis with normal cerebral magnetic resonance imaging: Transition rate to clinically definite multiple sclerosis. *Mult Scler* 2005;11(4):373–377.

67    Weinshenker BG. Neuromyelitis optica is distinct from multiple sclerosis. *Arch Neurol* 2007;64(6):899–901.

68    Brat DJ, et al. Surgical neuropathology update: A review of changes introduced by the WHO classification of tumours of the central nervous system, 4th edn. *Arch Pathol Lab Med* 2008;132(6):993–1007.

69 Villa C, Miquel C, Mosses D, Bernier M, Di Stefano AL. The 2016 World Health Organization classification of tumours of the central nervous system. *La Presse Médicale* 2018; **47**(11, Part 2): e187-e200.

70    Rousseau A, Mokhtari K, Duyckaerts C. The 2007 WHO classification of tumors of the central nervous system – what has changed?. *Curr Opin Neurol* 2008;21(6):720–727.

71    Darnell RB, Posner JB. Paraneoplastic syndromes involving the nervous system. *N Engl J Med* 2003;349(16):1543–1554.

72    Dalmau J, et al. Anti-NMDA-receptor encephalitis: Case series and analysis of the effects of antibodies. *Lancet Neurol* 2008;7(12):1091–1098.

73    Anderson NE, Barber PA. Limbic encephalitis – a review. *J Clin Neurosci* 2008;15(9):961–971.

74    Rudnicki SA, Dalmau J. Paraneoplastic syndromes of the spinal cord, nerve, and muscle. *Muscle Nerve* 2000;23(12):1800–1818.

75 Posner JB, Dalmau J. Paraneoplastic syndromes. *Curr Opin Immunol* 1997;9(5):723–729.

76 Bennett JL, et al. Neuro-ophthalmologic manifestations of a paraneoplastic syndrome and testicular carcinoma. *Neurology* 1999;52(4):864–867.

77 Saiz A, et al. Anti-Hu-associated brainstem encephalitis. *J Neurol Neurosurg Psychiatry* 2009;80(4): 404–407.

78 Chiang YZ, Tjon Tan K, Hart IK. Lambert–Eaton myasthenic syndrome. *Br J Hosp Med (Lond)* 2009;70(3):168–169.

79 Duddy ME, Baker MR. Stiff person syndrome. *Front Neurol Neurosci* 2009;26:147–165.

80 Ferreyra HA, et al. Management of autoimmune retinopathies with immunosuppression. *Arch Ophthalmol* 2009;127(4):390–397.

81 Mehta SH, Morgan JC, Sethi KD. Paraneoplastic movement disorders. *Curr Neurol Neurosci Rep* 2009;9(4):285–291.

82 Hadjivassiliou M, et al. P.E.T. scan in clinically suspected paraneoplastic neurological syndromes: A 6-year prospective study in a regional neuroscience unit. *Acta Neurol Scand* 2009;119(3):186–193.

83 Sarvazyan A, et al. Cost-effective screening for breast cancer worldwide: Current state and future directions. *Breast Cancer* 2008;1:91–99.

84 Young DF. Neurological complications of cancer chemotherapy. In: Silverstein A, editor. *Neurological complications of therapy*. New York: Futura Publishing; 1982. p. 57–113.

85 Kannarkat G, Lasher EE, Schiff D. Neurologic complications of chemotherapy agents. *Curr Opin Neurol* 2007;20(6):719–725.

86 Grolleau F, et al. A possible explanation for a neurotoxic effect of the anticancer agent oxaliplatin on neuronal voltage-gated sodium channels. *J Neurophysiol* 2001;85(5):2293–2297.

87 Jabbour E, et al. Neurologic complications associated with intrathecal liposomal cytarabine given prophylactically in combination with high-dose methotrexate and cytarabine to patients with acute lymphocytic leukemia. *Blood* 2007;109(8):3214–3218.

88 Schochet Jr. SS, Lampert PW, Earle KM. Neuronal changes induced by intrathecal vincristine sulfate. *J Neuropathol Exp Neurol* 1968;27(4):645–658.

89 Berger PS. Neurological complications of radiotherapy. In: Silverstein A, editor. *Neurological complications of therapy*. New York: Futura Publishing; 1982. p. 137–185.

90 Schlemmer HP, et al. Differentiation of radiation necrosis from tumor progression using proton magnetic resonance spectroscopy. *Neuroradiology* 2002;44(3):216–222.

91 Forsyth PA, et al. Radiation necrosis or glioma recurrence: Is computer-assisted stereotactic biopsy useful?. *J Neurosurg* 1995;82(3):436–444.

92 Di Chiro G, Herdt JR. Angiographic demonstration of spinal cord arterial occlusion in postradiation myelomalacia. *Radiology* 1973;106(2):317–319.

93 de Toffol B, et al. Chronic cervical radiation myelopathy diagnosed by MRI *J Neuroradiol* 1989;16(3): 251–253.

94 Wang PY, Shen WC, Jan JS. Serial MRI changes in radiation myelopathy. *Neuroradiology* 1995;37(5):374–377.

95 Glantz MJ, et al. Treatment of radiation-induced nervous system injury with heparin and warfarin. *Neurology* 1994;44(11):2020–2027.

96 Happold C, et al. Anticoagulation for radiation-induced neurotoxicity revisited. *J Neurooncol* 2008;90(3):357–362.

97 Herpes simplex encephalitis. Lancet. 1986:1(8480):535–536.

98 Shoji H. Can we predict a prolonged course and intractable cases of herpes simplex encephalitis?. *Intern Med* 2009;48(4):177–178.

99 Dutt MK, Johnston ID. Computed tomography and E.E.G. in herpes simplex encephalitis: Their value in diagnosis and prognosis. *Arch Neurol* 1982;39(2):99–102.

100  Schroth G, et al. Early diagnosis of herpes simplex encephalitis by MRI *Neurology* 1987;37(2):179–183.

101  Al-Shekhlee A, Kocharian N, Suarez JJ. Re-evaluating the diagnostic methods in herpes simplex encephalitis. *Herpes* 2006;13(1):17–19.

102  Domingues RB, et al. Diagnosis of herpes simplex encephalitis by magnetic resonance imaging and polymerase chain reaction assay of cerebrospinal fluid. *J Neurol Sci* 1998;157(2):148–153.

103  Whitley RJ, Roizman B. Herpes simplex virus infections. *Lancet* 2001;357(9267):1513–1518.

104  Kamei S, et al. Evaluation of combination therapy using aciclovir and corticosteroid in adult patients with herpes simplex virus encephalitis. *J Neurol Neurosurg Psychiatry* 2005;76(11):1544–1549.

105  Openshaw H, Cantin EM. Corticosteroids in herpes simplex virus encephalitis. *J Neurol Neurosurg Psychiatry* 2005;76(11):1469.

106  Price R.W. Neurological complications of HIV infection. *Lancet* 1996;348(9025):445–452.

107  Clifford DB. AIDS dementia. *Med Clin North Am* 2002;86(3):537–550:vi.

108  Bastiaansen A.E.M., van Steenhoven R.W., de Bruijn MAAM, et al. Autoimmune Encephalitis Resembling Dementia Syndromes. *Neurology – Neuroimmunology Neuroinflammation* 2021; 8(5): e1039.

109  Jack CR, Jr., Bennett DA, Blennow K, et al. NIA-AA Research Framework: Toward a biological definition of Alzheimer's disease. *Alzheimers Dement* 2018; 14(4): 535-62.

110  Palmqvist S, Janelidze S, Quiroz YT, et al. Discriminative Accuracy of Plasma Phospho-tau217 for Alzheimer Disease vs Other Neurodegenerative Disorders. *Jama* 2020; 324(8): 772-81.

111  Dubois B, Villain N, Frisoni GB, et al. Clinical diagnosis of Alzheimer's disease: recommendations of the International Working Group. *The Lancet Neurology* 2021; 20(6): 484-96.

112  Jagust WJ. The changing definition of Alzheimer's disease. *The Lancet Neurology* 2021; 20(6): 414-5.

113  Folstein MF, Folstein SE, McHugh PR. "Mini-mental state". A practical method for grading the cognitive state of patients for the clinician. *J Psychiatr Res* 1975; 12(3): 189-98.

114  Nasreddine ZS, Phillips NA, Bédirian V, et al. The Montreal Cognitive Assessment, MoCA: a brief screening tool for mild cognitive impairment. *J Am Geriatr Soc* 2005; 53(4): 695-9.

115  Tariq SH, Tumosa N, Chibnall JT, Perry MH, 3rd, Morley JE. Comparison of the Saint Louis University mental status examination and the mini-mental state examination for detecting dementia and mild neurocognitive disorder--a pilot study. *Am J Geriatr Psychiatry* 2006; 14(11): 900-10.

116  Cummings-Vaughn LA, Chavakula NN, Malmstrom TK, Tumosa N, Morley JE, Cruz-Oliver DM. Veterans Affairs Saint Louis University Mental Status examination compared with the Montreal Cognitive Assessment and the Short Test of Mental Status. *J Am Geriatr Soc* 2014; 62(7): 1341-6.

117  Suresh E, Wimalaratna S. Proximal myopathy: diagnostic approach and initial management. *Postgrad Med J* 2013; 89(1054): 470-7.

118  Bönnemann CG, Wang CH, Quijano-Roy S, et al. Diagnostic approach to the congenital muscular dystrophies. *Neuromuscul Disord* 2014; 24(4): 289-311.

119  Cotta A, Carvalho E, da-Cunha-Júnior AL, et al. Muscle biopsy essential diagnostic advice for pathologists. *Surgical and Experimental Pathology* 2021; 4(1): 3.

120  Walters J, Baborie A. Muscle biopsy: what and why and when? *Practical Neurology* 2020; 20(5): 385.

121  Bonne G, Rivier F, Hamroun D. The 2018 version of the gene table of monogenic neuromuscular disorders (nuclear genome). *Neuromuscul Disord* 2017; 27(12): 1152-83.

122  Lassche S, Janssen BH, T IJ, et al. MRI-Guided Biopsy as a Tool for Diagnosis and Research of Muscle Disorders. *J Neuromuscul Dis* 2018; 5(3): 315-9.

123  Targoff IN. Update on myositis-specific and myositis-associated autoantibodies. *Curr Opin Rheumatol* 2000; 12(6): 475-81.

124  Lackner A, Tiefenthaler V, Mirzayeva J, et al. The use and diagnostic value of testing myositis-specific and myositis-associated autoantibodies by line immuno-assay: a retrospective study. *Therapeutic Advances in Musculoskeletal Disease* 2020; 12: 1759720X20975907.

125 Lundberg IE, Tjärnlund A, Bottai M, et al. 2017 European League Against Rheumatism/American College of Rheumatology classification criteria for adult and juvenile idiopathic inflammatory myopathies and their major subgroups. *Ann Rheum Dis* 2017; 76(12): 1955-64.

126 Motohashi N, Shimizu-Motohashi Y, Roberts TC, Aoki Y. Potential Therapies Using Myogenic Stem Cells Combined with Bio-Engineering Approaches for Treatment of Muscular Dystrophies. *Cells* 2019; 8(9): 1066.

127 Mende M, Borchardt-Lohölter V, Meyer W, Scheper T, Schlumberger W. Autoantibodies in Myositis. How to Achieve a Comprehensive Strategy for Serological Testing. *Mediterr J Rheumatol* 2019; 30(3): 155-61.

128 Werner JL, Christopher-Stine L, Ghazarian SR, et al. Antibody levels correlate with creatine kinase levels and strength in anti-3-hydroxy-3-methylglutaryl-coenzyme A reductase-associated autoimmune myopathy. *Arthritis Rheum* 2012; 64(12): 4087-93.

129 Pulipaka U, Lacomis D, Omalu B. Amiodarone-induced neuromyopathy: three cases and a review of the literature. *J Clin Neuromuscul Dis* 2002; 3(3): 97-105.

130 Howard JF, Jr., Bril V, Vu T, et al. Safety, efficacy, and tolerability of efgartigimod in patients with generalised myasthenia gravis (ADAPT): a multicentre, randomised, placebo-controlled, phase 3 trial. *Lancet Neurol* 2021; 20(7): 526-36.

131 Dalakas MC. Progress in the therapy of myasthenia gravis: getting closer to effective targeted immunotherapies. *Curr Opin Neurol* 2020; 33(5): 545-52.

132 Graus F, Vogrig A, Muñiz-Castrillo S, et al. Updated Diagnostic Criteria for Paraneoplastic Neurologic Syndromes. *Neurology - Neuroimmunology Neuroinflammation* 2021; 8(4): e1014.

133 Abbatemarco JR, Clardy SL. The Pursuit of Precision in Paraneoplastic Neurologic Disease. *Neurology – Neuroimmunology Neuroinflammation* 2021; 8(4): e1015.

134 Reindl M, Rostasy K. MOG antibody-associated diseases. *Neurol Neuroimmunol Neuroinflamm* 2015; 2(1): e60.

135 Pelosof LC, Gerber DE. Paraneoplastic syndromes: an approach to diagnosis and treatment. *Mayo Clin Proc* 2010; 85(9): 838-54.

136 Castro-Marrero J, Sáez-Francàs N, Segundo MJ, et al. Effect of coenzyme Q10 plus nicotinamide adenine dinucleotide supplementation on maximum heart rate after exercise testing in chronic fatigue syndrome - A randomized, controlled, double-blind trial. *Clin Nutr* 2016; 35(4): 826-34.

137 Honnorat J, Antoine JC. Paraneoplastic neurological syndromes. *Orphanet J Rare Dis* 2007; 2: 22.

138 Przeździecka-Dołyk J, Brzecka A, Ejma M, et al. Ocular Paraneoplastic Syndromes. *Biomedicines* 2020; 8(11).

139 Bhagavati S. Autoimmune Disorders of the Nervous System: Pathophysiology, Clinical Features, and Therapy. *Frontiers in Neurology* 2021; 12(539).

140 Herken J, Prüss H. Red Flags: Clinical Signs for Identifying Autoimmune Encephalitis in Psychiatric Patients. *Front Psychiatry* 2017; 8: 25.

141 Selva-O'Callaghan A, Alvarado-Cardenas M, Pinal-Fernández I, et al. Statin-induced myalgia and myositis: an update on pathogenesis and clinical recommendations. *Expert Rev Clin Immunol* 2018; 14(3): 215-24.

142 Thangarajh M. The Dystrophinopathies. *Continuum (Minneap Minn)* 2019; 25(6): 1619-39.

143 Gordon PA, Winer JB, Hoogendijk JE, Choy EH. Immunosuppressant and immunomodulatory treatment for dermatomyositis and polymyositis. *Cochrane Database Syst Rev* 2012; 2012(8): Cd003643.

144 Meyer A, Troyanov Y, Drouin J, et al. Statin-induced anti-HMGCR myopathy: successful therapeutic strategies for corticosteroid-free remission in 55 patients. *Arthritis Research & Therapy* 2020; 22(1): 5.

145 Miyasaka N, Hara M, Koike T, Saito E, Yamada M, Tanaka Y. Effects of intravenous immunoglobulin therapy in Japanese patients with polymyositis and dermatomyositis resistant to corticosteroids: a randomized double-blind placebo-controlled trial. *Mod Rheumatol* 2012; 22(3): 382-93.

146 Glaubitz S, Zeng R, Schmidt J. New insights into the treatment of myositis. *Therapeutic Advances in Musculoskeletal Disease* 2020; 12: 1759720X19886494.

147 Howard JF, Jr., Nowak RJ, Wolfe GI, et al. Clinical Effects of the Self-administered Subcutaneous Complement Inhibitor Zilucoplan in Patients With Moderate to Severe Generalized Myasthenia Gravis: Results of a Phase 2 Randomized, Double-Blind, Placebo-Controlled, Multicenter Clinical Trial. *JAMA Neurol* 2020; 77(5): 582-92.

148 Venance SL. Approach to the Patient With HyperCKemia. *Continuum (Minneap Minn)* 2016; 22(6, Muscle and Neuromuscular Junction Disorders): 1803-14.

149 Bril V, Barnett-Tapia C, Barth D, Katzberg HD. IVIG and PLEX in the treatment of myasthenia gravis. *Ann N Y Acad Sci* 2012; 1275: 1-6.

150 Berger JR. Classifying PML risk with disease modifying therapies. *Mult Scler Relat Disord* 2017; 12: 59-63.

151 Brown JWL, Coles A, Horakova D, et al. Association of Initial Disease-Modifying Therapy With Later Conversion to Secondary Progressive Multiple Sclerosis. *Jama* 2019; 321(2): 175-87.

152 Jalkh G, Abi Nahed R, Macaron G, Rensel M. Safety of Newer Disease Modifying Therapies in Multiple Sclerosis. *Vaccines* 2021; 9(12): 1-30.

153 Burt RK, Burns W, Hess A. Bone marrow transplantation for multiple sclerosis. *Bone Marrow Transplant* 1995; 16(1): 1-6.

154 Muraro PA, Pasquini M, Atkins HL, et al. Long-term Outcomes After Autologous Hematopoietic Stem Cell Transplantation for Multiple Sclerosis. *JAMA Neurol* 2017; 74(4): 459-69.

155 Kannarkat G, Lasher EE, Schiff D. Neurologic complications of chemotherapy agents. *Curr Opin Neurol* 2007; 20(6): 719-25.

156 Co J, De Moraes MV, Katznelson R, et al. Hyperbaric Oxygen for Radiation Necrosis of the Brain. *Can J Neurol Sci* 2020; 47(1): 92-9.

157 Levin VA, Bidaut L, Hou P, et al. Randomized double-blind placebo-controlled trial of bevacizumab therapy for radiation necrosis of the central nervous system. *Int J Radiat Oncol Biol Phys* 2011; 79(5): 1487-95.

158 Venkatesan A. Encephalitis and Brain Abscess. *CONTINUUM: Lifelong Learning in Neurology* 2021; 27(4): 855-86.

159 Tripathi M, Vibha D. Reversible dementias. *Indian J Psychiatry* 2009; 51 Suppl 1(Suppl1): S52-5.

160 Guerrero JI, Barragán LA, Martínez JD, et al. Central and peripheral nervous system involvement by COVID-19: a systematic review of the pathophysiology, clinical manifestations, neuropathology, neuroimaging, electrophysiology, and cerebrospinal fluid findings. *BMC Infectious Diseases* 2021; 21(1): 515.

161 Bodro M, Compta Y, Sánchez-Valle R. Presentations and mechanisms of CNS disorders related to COVID-19. *Neurology - Neuroimmunology Neuroinflammation* 2021; 8(1): e923.

162 Shelly S, Talha N, Pereira NL, Engel AG, Johnson JN, Selcen D. Expanding Spectrum of Desmin-Related Myopathy, Long-term Follow-up, and Cardiac Transplantation. *Neurology* 2021; 97(11): e1150.

163 Greinacher A, Thiele T, Warkentin TE, Weisser K, Kyrle PA, Eichinger S. Thrombotic Thrombocytopenia after ChAdOx1 nCov-19 Vaccination. *New England Journal of Medicine* 2021; 384(22): 2092-101.

164 Rae-Grant A, Day GS, Marrie RA, et al. Practice guideline recommendations summary: Disease-modifying therapies for adults with multiple sclerosis. *Neurology* 2018; 90(17): 777.

165 Hor JY, Asgari N, Nakashima I, et al. Epidemiology of Neuromyelitis Optica Spectrum Disorder and Its Prevalence and Incidence Worldwide. *Frontiers in Neurology* 2020; 11(501).

166 Hauser SL, Bar-Or A, Comi G, et al. Ocrelizumab versus Interferon Beta-1a in Relapsing Multiple Sclerosis. *N Engl J Med* 2017; 376(3): 221-34.

167 Montalban X, Hauser SL, Kappos L, et al. Ocrelizumab versus Placebo in Primary Progressive Multiple Sclerosis. *N Engl J Med* 2017; 376(3): 209-20.

168 Nicolau S, Milone M, Liewluck T. Guidelines for genetic testing of muscle and neuromuscular junction disorders. *Muscle & Nerve* 2021; 64(3): 255-69.

169 Felice KJ. Differential Diagnosis of Distal Myopathies. The era of clinical molecular genetics has refined diagnosis and will hopefully lead to disease-modifying treatments. *Practical Neurology* 2019; 19(July-August): 82-91.

170 Fowler-Davis S, Platts K, Thelwell M, Woodward A, Harrop D. A mixed-methods systematic review of post-viral fatigue interventions: Are there lessons for long Covid? *PLOS ONE* 2021; 16(11): e0259533.

171 Turner B, Cree BAC, Kappos L, et al. Ocrelizumab efficacy in subgroups of patients with relapsing multiple sclerosis. *J Neurol* 2019; 266(5): 1182-93.

172 Wiendl H, Gold R, Zipp F, et al. Multiple sclerosis therapy consensus group (MSTCG): answers to the discussion questions. *Neurological Research and Practice* 2021; 3(1): 44.

173 Chow, C. C. N., et al. (2020). "Acute transverse myelitis in COVID-19 infection." *BMJ case reports* 13(8): e236720.

# Chapter 15 Keeping up-to-date and Retrieving Information

This textbook is not a comprehensive discussion of neurology. It contains the simple concepts that have been developed over more than 40 years of clinical practice and teaching. The aim of this book is to make the learning (and the practice) of clinical neurology more interesting and less intimidating for the non-neurologist (medical students, hospital medical officers, physician trainees, general physicians[1] and general practitioners) and as an introductory text for neurology trainees. I am aware that a number of neurologists use the principles in this book in their teaching[2]. Most of the chapters have been written from a symptom rather than a disease-oriented approach, discussing the more commonly encountered neurological disorders.

The basics of practising medicine will not change dramatically because of innovative technologies or the World Wide Web, but these will change the way healthcare is delivered. This is not because of the technology itself or the attention it receives, but because patients will need and demand this kind of knowledge and expertise. Doctors of the 21st century must be ready and qualified to meet these expectations.

This chapter suggests techniques that can be employed to 'keep up-to-date' that, with the rapidly expanding knowledge base and the vast array of journals and websites, at times seems an almost impossible task. It contains links to many websites[3] and recommendations for further reading, including other books that this author has constantly referred to for additional information.

## Keeping up to date

The amount of information available to the clinician is mindboggling. Typing the word 'stroke' into Google[4] retrieves 687,000,000 hits! This is reduced to 3,070,000 for Google Scholar and 392,737 in PubMed. The numbers have more than doubled in a little over a decade. In 2010 the numbers

---

1 One general physician commented that the rule of four of the brainstem had demystified the brainstem for the general physician.

2 Personal communication

3 Many of the URLs in the first edition have changed. It may be necessary to search the name if the link does not work.

4 My own personal experience is that google is useful to find obscure topics and rarities, whilst google scholar and pubmed are better at retrieving more reliable and scientific papers.

were 49,000,000, 1,580,000 and 145,200, respectively. This has been referred to as 'information overload' [1].

---

Although it is impossible to read every article this should not be used as an excuse to read none.

---

As Paul Glasziou, Director of the Institute for Evidence based Healthcare at Bond University pointed out, only 1 in 18 articles fulfil evidence-based medicine criteria, indicating that for the uninitiated there are vast numbers of potentially misleading papers in the literature. There are several books [2, 3][5] and articles in journals [4–23] that discuss how to read the medical literature. Unfortunately, most medical practitioners never acquire the skills or have the time to read journal articles thoroughly. The McMaster[6] group devised a simple and effective strategy for filtering papers [24]. They suggested the approach illustrated in Figure 15.1.

---

Learning does not end the day a medical student graduates. All clinicians must, for the benefit of their patients commit to a lifelong learning process to keep up to date.

---

5   A review of "How to Read a Paper" stated this is one of the bestselling texts on evidence-based medicine, used by health care professionals and medical students worldwide. Trisha Greenhalgh's ability to explain the basics of evidence-based medicine in an accessible and readable way means the book is an ideal introduction for all, from first year students to experienced practitioners.

   This is a text that explains the meaning of critical appraisal and terms such as 'numbers needed to treat', 'how to search the literature', 'evaluate the different types of papers' and 'put the conclusions to clinical use'.

6   I was fortunate to be able to undertake the introduction to clinical epidemiology course on how to read a paper at McMaster University in 1983.

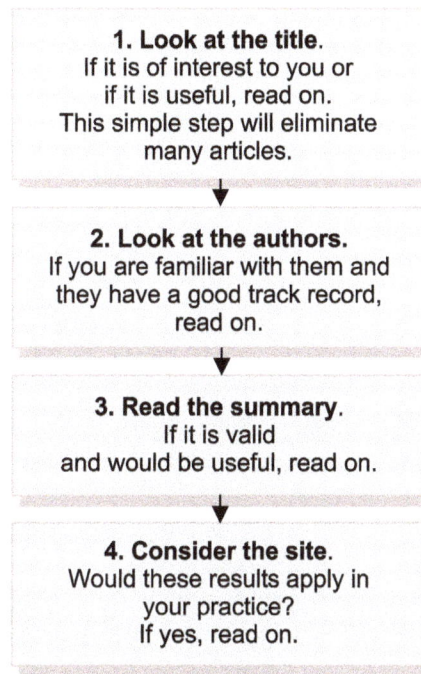

> **1. Look at the title.**
> If it is of interest to you or
> if it is useful, read on.
> This simple step will eliminate
> many articles.
>
> ↓
>
> **2. Look at the authors.**
> If you are familiar with them and
> they have a good track record,
> read on.
>
> ↓
>
> **3. Read the summary.**
> If it is valid
> and would be useful, read on.
>
> ↓
>
> **4. Consider the site.**
> Would these results apply in
> your practice?
> If yes, read on.

**FIGURE 15.1** The McMaster group devised a simple and effective strategy for filtering papers, Adapted from *Clinical Epidemiology. A Basic Science for Clinical Medicine,* by DL Sackett, RB Haynes, P Tugwell, 1985, Littlfe, Brown, p 370

The next step depends on the nature of the paper:

- **A** **Diagnostic test**. Was there an independent 'blind' comparison with a 'gold standard' of diagnosis?
- **B** **Clinical course and prognosis.** Was there an 'inception cohort'?[7]
- **C** **Determining aetiology.** Were the basic methods used to study causation strong?
- **D** **Distinguishing useful from useless or harmful therapy**. Was the assignment of patients to treatments really randomised?[8]

If the answer to the relevant question was 'yes,' the next step is to read the patients and methods section to see if the study has been well conducted. In the end, after reading the paper you must decide whether you will allow the results of this paper to influence the management of your patients.

---

7 An inception cohort is where patients are identified at an early and uniform point in the course of the disease.

8 If the natural history of a disease is unpredictable, and if spontaneous remission can occur the only way to assess whether a therapy is of benefit in these patients is to randomly allocate half of the patients to the active treatment and the other half to an alternative treatment or to a placebo.

# Ways of Keeping up to Date

**Collaborating with colleagues** who meet on a regular basis to discuss cases and papers in the literature is one of the most effective ways of keeping up to date. If each person has a different subspecialty area of interest, they keep abreast of the literature in that area and can share their knowledge with the others. This often occurs in the setting of hospital-based meetings and when discussing cases in corridor conversations.

**Attendance at national and international meetings** is a second way of keeping abreast of the latest developments.

**Pharmaceutical company sponsored guest speakers** is common. It is important to remember that this guest speaker usually has a point of view that is positive towards the products that the company markets; otherwise, they would not be invited to speak[9].

Another useful technique is to **peruse the contents page of a journal** for articles of interest, particularly those that have an associated editorial. Every week I retrieve neurology-related and other articles of interest from the three major journals. The British Medical Journal, the Lancet, and the New England Journal of Medicine.

The **clinicopathological conferences** held in one's own institution and in the New England Journal of Medicine are a wonderful learning resource.[10]

**Patient-oriented research** is perhaps the most effective method of gaining new knowledge is retrieving information about a particular problem that you are dealing with at that time. Research can be undertaken during[11] or after the consultation. Ready access to the internet makes it possible to find relevant papers even during a consultation with the patient. The internet can help sort out a difficult diagnostic problem such as that discussed in Chapter 6, 'After the history and examination, what next?' Most frequently, the question that arises relates to the latest diagnostic test, the criteria for a particular diagnosis or the optimal treatment for a particular condition. It is not possible to retrieve and evaluate all this information at the time of consultation. Another approach is to undertake a review of the literature on a particular disease on a regular basis.

A major issue is the growing number of institutions and companies vying to provide online information. In essence all these entities are retrieving the same literature and trying to put it into a digestible form. It is suggested that you sample a few and find one that meets your needs before committing to a subscription.

---

9 I was once told by a pharmaceutical company that they would withdraw the invitation to talk if they could not vet my talk. I very much enjoyed teaching in this format but after this incident I declined further requests.

10 I read every neurological CPC in the NEJM. It is an excellent method of keeping abreast of recent developments and observe the logical approach of the discussants.

11 I have no qualms saying to patients that it I want to search the internet to see if there is anything new that might alter what our diagnostic or treatment approach. This approach helped me recommend a curative thymectomy in a man over the age of 60. Prior to me seeing the latest research the accepted dogma was not undertake a thymectomy in elderly patients with myasthenia gravis.

# Internet Resources

## Pubmed

Pubmed is the database used by most clinicians. A more detailed description on free-access and biomedical databases other than PubMed can be found in the article by Giglia [25].

**(https://pubmed.ncbi.nlm.nih.gov/?db=PubMed)**

## Biomed–Central

Biomed–Central is an open-access publisher. **(https://www.biomedcentral.com/)** It maintains a catalogue of more than 1000 databases. Some databases contain experimental data, others provide synopses of public information, and most are freely accessible. Journals can be accessed **(https://www.biomedcentral.com/journals)**

In the subject area there are options to search neurology or neuroscience and under the content section the options include disease, experimental data, images, journal articles and links to other sources, to mention only a few.

## Evidence-Based Medicine Databases

There are numerous evidence-based medicine databases, most require payment for access.

- Abstracts are available on the **Cochrane Review**, access to the full article requires a payment. **(http://www.cochrane.org/index.htm)**
- **Netting the Evidence** is a British-based website facilitates evidence-based healthcare by providing support and access to helpful organisations and useful learning resources, such as an evidence-based virtual library, software, and journals. The resources can be browsed by type, and a search facility is available. **(http://www.shef.ac.uk/scharr/ir/netting)**
- The aim of the **Turning research into practice (TRIP)** database **(http://www.tripdatabase. com/index.html)** is to allow health professionals to easily find the highest quality material available on the web – to help support evidence-based practice. This is an interesting and user-friendly tool.
- The **QuickClinical (QC)** information retrieval system **(http://www.chi.unsw.edu.au/CHIweb.nsf/ page/QuickClinical)** is a new type of evidence-access technology that utilises intelligent search filter technology to model typical clinical tasks such as 'diagnosis' or 'prescribing' to ensure that only the most relevant evidence is retrieved. This means clinicians are more likely to search and, when they do search, are more likely to find information that changes their practice.
- The aim of the **Centre for Evidence Based Medicine** **(www.cebm.net)** is to develop, teach and promote evidence-based health care and provide support and resources to doctors and healthcare professionals to help maintain the highest standards of medicine.
- The **National Guideline Clearinghouse™ (NGC)** **(http://www.ahrq.gov/)** is a public resource for evidence-based clinical practice guidelines. NGC is an initiative of the Agency for Healthcare Research and Quality (AHRQ), US Department of Health and Human Services. NGC was originally created by AHRQ in partnership with the American Medical Association and the American Association of Health Plans (now America's Health Insurance Plans [AHIP]). It also offers synthesis of selected guidelines **(http://www.guideline.gov/compare/ synthesis.aspx)** and expert commentary on issues **(http://www.guideline.gov/resources/ expert_commentary.aspx)**

- **Up-to-Date** is an excellent resource that was expensive. Now an annual subscription costs as little as A$1.48 per day[12]. **(https://www.uptodate.com)**
- **Clinicians Health Channel (http://www.use.hcn.com.au/profiles/shared/component/use/ query.%7B%7D/search.html)** is sponsored by the Victorian Department of Health and is for the benefit of clinicians working in the Victorian public health sector. It provides access to journals, books, evidence-based practice resources, drug information resources and citation databases.

## Searching PubMed and Other Search Engines

The traditional approach to searching the literature has been with PubMed **(http://www. ncbi.nlm.nih.gov/pubmed/),** which is a service of the US National Library of Medicine and the National Institutes of Health. It is the integrated, text-based search-and-retrieval system used at The National Centre for Biotechnology Information (NCBI) for the major databases, including PubMed, Nucleotide and Protein Sequences, Protein Structures, Complete Genomes, Taxonomy, and others. MeSH (Medical Subject Headings) is the National Library of Medicine controlled vocabulary thesaurus used for indexing articles for PubMed.

There are tutorials available for using PubMed (PubMed® Online Training). **(http://www.nlm. nih.gov/bsd/disted/pubmed.html)** There is also a PDF designed to print and trifold. PubMed is the main database that most to retrieve the **(http://nnlm.gov/training/resources/pmtri.pdf)** clinicians would use more scientifically valid information.

## Finding a Neurology Journal

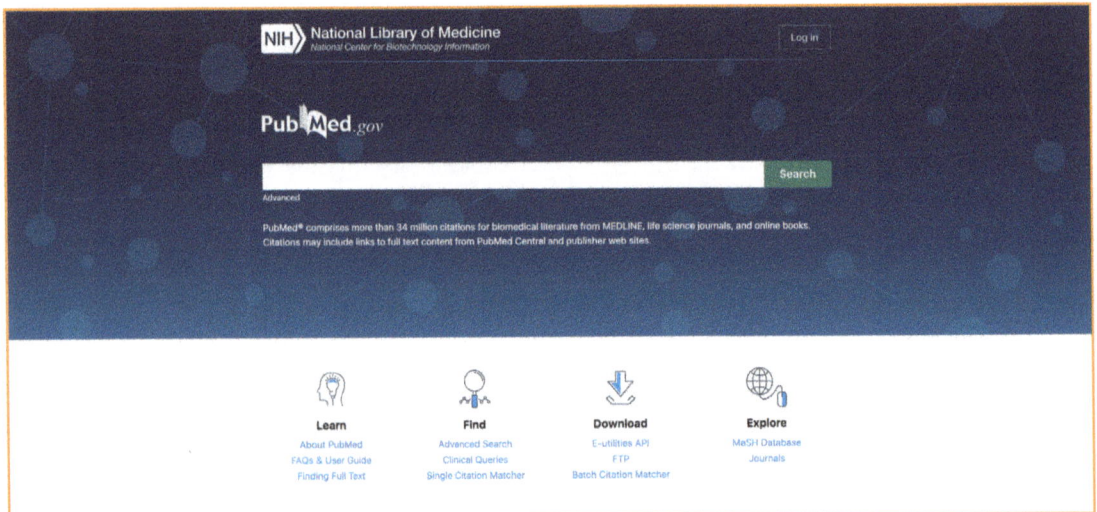

**Figure 15.2** Pubmed Main Website.

Pubmed is the free access to Medline, upgraded since the first edition. Figure 15.2 shows the basic Pubmed website. **A** is the basic search section. **(https://pubmed.ncbi.nlm.nih.gov/)** **B** is the advanced search option that enables restricting the search with more specific parameters, e.g., an author, certain years etc. **(https://pubmed.ncbi.nlm.nih.gov/advanced/)** When searching for an author use their surname and follow with their initials without any punctuation, e.g., gates pc. **C**

---

12 To subscribe visit (https://www.uptodate.com/login?&redirect=true)

is the icon to click on when undertaking clinical queries (https://pubmed.ncbi.nlm.nih.gov/clinical/) and **D** is where one can search for journals. Typing the word neurology in the journals section (https://www.ncbi.nlm.nih.gov/nlmcatalog/journals/) will retrieve an astonishing 657 neurology related journals compared to 461 in 2010 at the time of the first edition.

When a subject is entered into the search section often many thousands of references are retrieved. On the left-hand side of the page will there are options to limit the search criteria either by article type (clinical trial, review, meta-analysis et cetera) or publication date with options to choose one year five years 10 years or a custom range. At the very bottom of this list is a section called additional filters, clicking on this brings up a pop-up window with many more options to refine the research question.

## Finding Practice Guidelines

Using the advanced search option of PubMed, enter the word guidelines and add the search the topic you wish to retrieve, e.g., epilepsy treatment creates the following search criteria: (epilepsy treatment) AND (guidelines)

## Finding the Latest Information on a Particular Disease

Use the advanced option and type in the item of interest. To limit the results to possibly more useful or more recent articles add controlled trials, clinical trials, meta-analyses, reviews, and systematic reviews. Unfortunately, the word 'review' is included in so many papers it often retrieves numerous and at times irrelevant references that are not true reviews of the subject of interest. One can limit the search to one, five or ten years or alternatively create a custom range[13].

## Related references in Pubmed

Another particularly useful function of PubMed is the related references link. If, as you peruse the initial list of references, you see a particular article that seems to be close to what you want, view the related references below listed under the heading related articles.

## Exporting References to a Reference Manager

It is possible to export the references retrieved from PubMed into a reference management program such as *Endnotes, Reference Manager etc*. In the past references often misquoted in papers or contained significant errors. Reference management programs eliminate these problems. Reference management programs also allow different format depending on the requirements of specific journals.

In recent years, a "cite" option or export citation icon has been added to Pubmed. When one clicks on this icon often a download nbib option appears, clicking on this will either result in the paper being imported directly into the reference program or download to the C drive of your computer. Other websites create a list of citation manager formats which one can choose. These include Bib TeX, Bookends, EasyBib, Endnote (tagged). Endnote 8 (xml), Medlars, Mendeley, Papers, Refworks Tagged, Ref Manager, RIS and Zotero. Clicking on one of these will create the option to import into the reference management program.

PubMed and MedlinePlus allow searching by topics, authors, or journals.

---

13 I use the custom range to retrieve articles published since the last time I reviewed the topic. I look at the articles I have stored from prior searches, take note of the date that I last searched and restrict the search to after that date.

# Alternative Search Engines Using the Semantic Web

The vision of the originator of the world wide web Tim Berners-Lee was that the semantic web would become a playground for intelligent "agents." These agents would automate much of the work that the world had only just learned to do on the web. [27] Most of the semantic-based alternative search engines (GoPubmed, Hakia, Pubmed hakia, Searchmedia and Webicina) described in the first edition are no longer available. These include. Semantic Scholar **(https://www.semanticscholar.org/)** is a web-based search engine that contains 205,469,176[14] papers from all fields of science. Entering the term migraine treatment retrieves twenty-one citations, however most are old, this makes one suspect it has not been kept up to date.

## General Neurology Websites

- **Cochrane Collaboration (http://www.cochrane.org/index.htm)** The aim of the Cochrane Collaboration is improving healthcare decision making globally, through systematic reviews of the effects of healthcare interventions. Unfortunately, many reviews conclude that there is insufficient evidence and that further studies are required.
- **European Academy of Neurology** The European Academy of Neurology Federation of Neurological Societies has replaced the European Federation of Neurological Societies and represents the national neurological societies of 40 European countries. **(https://www.ean.org/home)**
- **Internet Drug Index (http://www.rxlist.com/)** This provides an alphabetical list of drugs, a pill identifier and an explanation of diseases, conditions, and tests.
- **World Federation of Neurology (WFN) (http://www.wfneurology.org/).** The WFN is the international body representing the specialty of neurology in more than one hundred countries/regions of the globe. The WFN has these neurological societies as its members, and their individual members are in turn WFN members through the association. The purpose of the WFN is to improve human health worldwide by promoting prevention and the care of persons with disorders of the entire nervous system by:
  - fostering the best standards of neurological practice.
  - educating, in collaboration with neuroscience and other international public and private organisations.
  - facilitating research through its research groups.

## Country-Based Neurology Websites

The World Federation of Neurology has a marvellous website with links to the neurological societies in Asia-Oceania, Europe, Latin America, North America, Pan-Africa and Pan-Arab. **(https://wfneurology.org/member-societies)** Hopefully this will be kept up to date. Whilst revising this section many societies either changed their name or the URL.

## North American Websites

- American Academy of Neurology. **(http://www.aan.com/)**
- American Neurological Association. **(https://myana.org/)**
- Canadian Neurological Sciences Federation. **(https://www.cnsf.org/)**
- National Institutes of Health – Brain and Nervous System. **(https://www.ninds.nih.gov/)**

---

14 Accessed 26th February 2022

## Central American Websites

- El Salvador: Asociación de Ciencias Neurológicas de El Salvador. **(https://neurologiaelsalvador.com/)**
- Nicaragua: Asociación de Ciencias Neurologicas de Nicaragua. **(no website, contact siriasmd@hotmail.com)**
- Costa Rica: Asociación Costarricense de Ciencias Neurológicas **(no website, contact asoneurocienciascr@gmail.com)**
- Cuba: Instituto de Neurología y Neurocirugía de Cuba. **(no website, contact rmusteli@ infomed.sld.cu)**
- Dominican Neurological and Neurosurgical Society **(http://www.neuro.do)**
- Guatemala: Asociación Guatemalteca de Neurología. **(no website, contact drmecordon@yahoo.com)**
- Honduras: Asociación Hondureña de Neurología. **(no website, contact marcotmedina@yahoo.com)**
- Mexico: Academia Mexicana de Neurologia, A.C. **(http://www.neurologia.org.mx)**
- Panamanian Society of Neurology & Neurosurgery. **(no website, contact luisc@castillo.net)**
- Puerto Rico: Puerto Rican Academy of Neurology. **(no website, contact Academianeurologia@gmail.com)**

## South American Websites

- Argentina Neurological Society. **(http://www.sna.org.ar)**
- Bolivian Society of Neurology. **(no website, contact soboneuro-lpz@outlook.com)**
- Brazilian Academy of Neurology. **(http://abneuro.org.br/ )**
- Society of Neurology, Psychiatry and Neurosurgery, Chile. **(http://www.sonepsyn.cl)**
- Colombian Association of Neurology. **(http://www.acdn.org)**
- Ecuadorian Society of Neurology. **(no website, contact arturocarpio@etapanet.net)**
- Paraguayan Society of Neurology. **(http://www.sociedadparaguayadeneurologia.org)**
- Peruvian Society of Neurology. **(no website, contact sociedadperuananeurologiaspn@hotmail.com)**
- Uruguay. **(http://www.neurologiauruguay.org)**
- Venezuela, Bolivarian Republic of. **(no website, contact neurologia.v@gmail.com)**

## Asia and Pacific Websites

- Neurology ASIA. **(https://www.neurology-asia.org/index.php)**
- Australian and New Zealand Association of Neurologists. **(http://www.anzan.org.au/index.asp)**
- Hong Kong Neurological Society. **(https://www.hkns.org/)**
- Japanese Society of Psychiatry and Neurology. **(https://www.jspn.or.jp/modules/english/index.php?content_id=1)**
- Korean Neurological Association. **(https://www.neuro.or.kr/english/)**
- Malaysian Society of Neurosciences. **(https://www.neuro.org.my/)**
- Neurological Society of India. **(https://neurosocietyindia.org/site/index.html)**
- Thai Neuroscience Society. **(https://www.facebook.com/)**
- Pakistan Society of Neurology-PSN. **(https://www.facebook.com/PakistanSocietyOfNeurologyPsn/)**

- Philippine Neurological Association.
(**https://www.philippineneurologicalassociation.com/**)
- Clinical Neuroscience Society, Singapore. (**http://www.cns.org.sg/**)
- Asian and Oceanic Association of Neurology. Has links to twenty-one countries and includes many not listed above. (**http://www.aoaneurology.org/aoan-delegate.html**)

## European Websites

- European Federation of Neurological Societies (**https://www.ean.org/**) has links to the neurological societies of forty-seven countries.

  (**https://www.ean.org/home/members/national-neurological-societies**)

## Middle East Websites

- Egypt: Egyptian Society of Neurology, Psychiatry and Neurosurgery
(**https://www.omicsonline.org/societies/egyptian-society-of-neurology-psychiatry-and-neurosurgery/**).
- Israel: Israel Society for Neuroscience עמותה שילארשי למדעי המוח (**https://www.isfn.org.il/**)
- Saudi Arabia: Saudi Neurological Society. (**http://www.saudineurology.org/**)
- Tunisian Society of Neurology. (**http://www.stneuro.tn/en/**)

# Websites Related to Common Neurological Problems

## Clinical Trials

The following are especially useful and readily accessible resources.

- **The National Institutes of Health** has a website (**http://www.clinicaltrials.gov/**) dedicated to clinical trials that has more than 70,000 registered trials. These can be searched by topic and country, e.g., headache, stroke etc. The website comments on whether the trial is recruiting or not and whether completed. Links are provided to the most up-to-date information, including when the results have been published linked to abstracts on PubMed.
- The NIH also has a website dedicated to *neurological disorders* listed alphabetically (**http://www.ninds.nih.gov/index.htm**).
- There is a section dedicated to *patient resources,* also listed alphabetically (**http://www.ninds.nih.gov/find_people/voluntary_orgs/organizations_index.htm**).

## Cerebral Vascular Disease

- American Stroke Association. (**https://www.stroke.org/**)
- Stroke Trials Registry. (**https://clinicaltrials.gov/**)
- Washington University Internet Stroke Centre, St Louis. (**https://stroke.wustl.edu/**)
- Cochrane Library Stroke Reviews,
(**http://www.cochrane.org/reviews/en/topics/93_reviews.html**)

## Epilepsy

- International League against Epilepsy. (**http://www.ilae-epilepsy.org/**)
- Scottish Intercollegiate Guidelines Network.
(**http://www.sign.ac.uk/guidelines/fulltext/70/index.html**).
- American Epilepsy Society. (**http://www.aesnet.org/**)
- Epilepsy Society of Australia. (**https://www.epilepsy-society.org.au/**)

## Epilepsy Treatment Guidelines

- American Epilepsy Society Clinical Guidance.
  **(http://www.aesnet.org/clinical-care/clinical-guidance)**
- American Academy of Neurology Epilepsy Guidelines.
  **(https://www.aan.com/Guidelines/home/ByTopic?topicId=23)**
- The College of Psychiatric and Neurologic Pharmacists (CPNP).
  **(https://cpnp.org/guideline/external/seisure)**
- The United Kingdom National Clinical Guideline Centre.
  **(https://www.nice.org.uk/guidance/cg137/evidence/full-guideline-pdf-4840753069)**

## Headache

- American Headache Society. **(https://americanheadachesociety.org/)**
- The Migraine Trust. **(http://www.migrainetrust.org)**
- The National Headache Foundation. **(http://www.headaches.org)**
- National Institute of Neurological Disorders and Stroke
  **(https://www.ninds.nih.gov/Disorders/All-Disorders/Migraine-Information-Page)**

## Parkinson's and Movement Disorders

- National Institute of Neurological Disorders and Stroke. **(https://www.ninds.nih.gov/Disorders/All-Disorders/Parkinsons-disease-Information-Page)**
- Parkinson's Disease Foundation (USA). **(http://www.pdf.org/)**
- Parkinson's Disease Society (UK). **(http://www.parkinsons.org.uk/)**
- Tourette syndrome. **(http://www.tsa-usa.org/)**

## Multiple Sclerosis

- Multiple Sclerosis Society (UK). **(https://www.mssociety.org.uk/)**
- National Multiple Sclerosis Society (USA). **(http://www.nationalmssociety.org/index.aspx)**
- MS Australia. **(http://www.msaustralia.org.au/)**

## Neurophysiology

- American Association of Neuromuscular and Electrodiagnostic Medicine.
  **(http://www.aanem.org/)**
- British Society for Clinical Neurophysiology. **(http://www.bscn.org.uk/)**

# Major Neurology Journal Websites

The major general medical journals listed below frequently have neurology-related editorials, original research, review articles and neurology cases or clinical pathological conferences.

The most significant website is of course PubMed **(http://www.ncbi.nlm.nih.gov/sites/entrez?db=pubmed)** supported by the US National Library of Medicine and the National Institutes of Health in the USA.

# General Journal with Neurology Content

- The Lancet (UK). **(http://www.thelancet.com/)**
- Lancet Neurology (UK). **(https://www.thelancet.com/journals/laneur/home)**
- British Medical Journal (UK). **(http://www.bmj.com/)**
- New England Journal of Medicine. **(https://www.nejm.org/)**

## Specific Neurology Journal Websites

The journals marked with an asterisk (*) were rated as the top 5 in a questionnaire of members of the World Federation of Neurology [26].

- **com/journal/16000404)**
- Annals of Indian Academy of Neurology. (India), **(http://www.annalsofian.org/)**
- Annals of Neurology.* (USA), **(https://onlinelibrary.wiley.com/journal/15318249)**
- Archives of Neurology (now JAMA Neurology) (USA). **(https://jamanetwork.com/journals/jamaneurology)**
- Brain* (UK). **(http://brain.oxfordjournals.org/)**
- Cerebrovascular Diseases. **(https://www.karger.com/Journal/Home/224153**)
- Chinese Journal of Cerebrovascular Diseases. **(https://ores.su/en/journals/chinese-journal-of-cerebrovascular-diseases/)**
- Chinese Journal of Neurology. **(https://ores.su/en/journals/chinese-journal-of-neurology/)**
- Epilepsia (USA). **(https://onlinelibrary.wiley.com/journal/1528116)**
- European Journal of Neurology **(https://onlinelibrary.wiley.com/journal/14681331)**
- Headache (USA). **(https://headachejournal.onlinelibrary.wiley.com/)**
- Journal of Clinical Neuroscience (Australia). **(http://www.elsevier.com/wps/find/journaldescription.cws_home/623056/description#description)**
- Journal of Neurology, Neurosurgery, and Psychiatry (UK), **(http://jnnp.bmj.com/)**
- Journal of the Neurological Sciences (USA). **(http://www.elsevier.com/wps/find/journaldescription.cws_home/506078/description#description)**
- Journal für Neurologie, Neurochirurgie und Psychiatrie (Austria). **(http://www.kup.at/journals/neurologie/index.html)**
- Journal of Neurotrauma* (USA). **(https://www.scijournal.org/impact-factor-of-j-neurotraum.shtml)**
- Movement Disorders (USA). **(https://www.movementdisorders.org/MDS/Journals/Online-MD-Journal.htm)**
- Multiple Sclerosis. (USA). **(http://msj.sagepub.com/)**
- Neurology* (USA). **(http://www.neurology.org/)**
- Neurology Asia. **(http://neurologyasia.org/journal.php)**
- Pakistan Journal of Neurology. **(http://www.pakmedinet.com/PJNeuro)**
- Stroke* (USA). **(http://stroke.ahajournals.org/)**

## Resources for Patients

There are literally thousands of disease-oriented consumer organisations around the world striving to raise money for research into their ailment of interest and to keep their members abreast of the latest developments. The American Academy of Neurology produces regular practice guidelines for both the treating clinician and the patient.

Probably one of the most authoritative is the site sponsored by the United States National Library of Medicine and the National Institutes of Health titled **MedlinePlus** (http://medlineplus.gov/). MedlinePlus website states that it 'brings together authoritative information from National Library of Medicine (NLM), the National Institutes of Health (NIH), and other government agencies and health-related organisations. Preformulated MEDLINE searches are included in MedlinePlus and give easy access to medical journal articles. MedlinePlus has extensive information about drugs, an illustrated medical encyclopaedia, health topics, drugs and supplements, genetics, medical test, and healthy recipes. The help topics section links to the National Institute of Neurological Disorders and Stroke website. It also provides health information in sixty-seven languages. **(http://www.nlm.nih.gov/medlineplus/languages/languages.html).**

# Recommended Books[15]

Medical practitioners often possess large numbers of medical books, most of which they never read and to some of which they occasionally refer. The problem with textbooks is that most of the information is rapidly out of date; this is particularly the case with investigations and treatment.

Although this book has primarily been written for students and the non–neurologist, it is also potentially suitable for the neurology trainee in the initial stages of training. What follows is a list of books (not in any order) that this author has collected and enjoyed reading. Many have been useful resources to which he has constantly referred.

*Gray's Anatomy,* 42nd edn, Susan Standring, Churchill Livingstone. This is a book that one refers to when detailed neuroanatomy is required.

*Mechanism and Management of Headache.* 7th edn, J Lance, PJ Goadsby, Elsevier Butterworth–Heinemann, 2004. One of those books to which you will constantly refer.

*Aids to the Examination of the Peripheral Nervous System,* 4th edn[16], Brain, WB Saunders Company, 2000. This is a thin paperback book that should be on every desktop. It shows how to examine each muscle, the nerve and nerve root supply and contains excellent illustrations of the individual nerves supplying muscles, the sensory supply to the skin of the nerves and the nerve roots (dermatomes).

*Seizures and Epilepsy,* J Engel, Jr, FA Davis Company, 1989. An excellent clinical textbook about epilepsy[17].

*The Diagnosis of Stupor and Coma,* Fred Plum, Jerome Posner, Oxford University Press, 2007. One of the neurological classics with a superb description of how to examine the comatose patient and how to use those findings to establish the cause of the coma.

*Neurological Aspects of Substance Abuse,* 2nd edn, JCM Brust, Elsevier Butterworth–Heinemann, 2004. An excellent reference source for dealing with patients admitted with complications from using recreational drugs.

*Cerebrospinal Fluid in Diseases of the Nervous System,* 2nd edn, RA Fishman, WB Saunders Company, 1992. An invaluable resource to check the cerebrospinal fluid abnormalities in particular diseases.

*McAlpine's Multiple Sclerosis,* 1st edn, WB Matthews, ED Acheson, JR Batchelor, RO Weller, Churchill Livingstone, 1985.

*McAlpine's Multiple Sclerosis,* 4th edn, A Compstan, I McDonald, J Noseworthy, H Lassmnaa, D Miller, K Smith, H Wekerle, C Confravreux, Churchill Livingstone, 2005. Both these books are excellent resources on multiple sclerosis.

*Neurological Complications of Therapy,* A Silverstein (ed), Futura Publishing Company, 1982. Although old nothing has been written that has replaced it. This book has excellent chapters on the neurological complications of chemotherapy and radiotherapy.

*Principles and Practice of Movement Disorders,* S Fahn S, J Jankovic, Churchill Livingstone, Elsevier, 2007. Written by two world experts who have clearly seen many patients

---

15 This is the books that I have enjoyed reading, many of which I still consult. Bookauthority lists one hundred "best neurology books of all time." https://bookauthority.org/books/best-neurology-books

16 A fifth edition was published in 2010

17 A second edition was published in 2013

with movement disorders. Described by a colleague with subspecialty interest in this area as the best book he has ever read on the subject.

*Neurological Complications of Renal Disease,* CF Bolton, GB Young, Butterworth Publishers, 1990. An excellent description of the neurological complications of renal disease.

*Handbook of Neurologic Rating Scales*, RM Herndon (ed), Demos Vermande, 1997. Describes and discusses the neurological rating scales applicable to many disorders of the nervous system.

*Primer on the Autonomic Nervous System*, D Robertson, I Biaggioni, G Burnstock, PA Low, Elsevier Academic Press, 2004. This has been written by one of the world's authorities on the autonomic nervous system.

*AIDS and the Nervous System*, 1st edn, ML Rosenblum, RM Levy, DE Bresdesen, Raven Press, 1988; 2nd edn, JR Berger, RM Levy, 1997. Excellent description of the approach to the patient with AIDS and neurological symptoms.

*The Clinical Practice of Critical Care Neurology*, E Wijdicks, Oxford University Press, 2003. An excellent book to aid the neurologist who is called upon to see patients in the intensive care unit.

*Neurologic Catastrophes in the Emergency Department,* E Wijdicks, Butterworth–Heinemann, 1999. A useful book for every neurologist attached to a hospital who must attend the accident and emergency department.

*Infectious Diseases of the Central Nervous System*, KL Tyler, JB Martin, (Contemporary Neurology Series), FA Davis Co., 1993.

*Posterior Circulation Disease: Clinical Findings, Diagnosis, and Management*, LR Kaplan, Blackwell Science, 1996.

*Peripheral Neuropathy*, 4th edn, P Dyck, PK Thomas (eds), Elsevier Saunders, 2005.

*The Treatment of Epilepsy – Principles and Practice*, 3rd edn, E Wyllie (ed), Lippincott Williams & Wilkins, 2001.

*Cranial Neuroimaging and Clinical Neuroanatomy*, H-J Kretschmann, W Weinrich, Georg Thieme Verlag, 2004.

*Handbook of Epilepsy Treatment*, 2nd edn, SD Shorvon, Blackwell Science, 2005.

*Handbook of Clinical Neurology*, PJ Vinken, GW Bruyn, HL Klawans (eds), Elsevier, 1986. This is the encyclopaedia of clinical neurology, currently into the revised edition. Each chapter is detailed and a good place to look for those neurological oddities[18].

## General Neurology Books

There are many excellent textbooks of general neurology; the author does not own all of these but reviews in the literature have been positive.

*Neurology in Clinical Practice,* W Bradley et al, Butterworth–Heinemann
*Practical Neurology,* J Biller, Lippincott, Williams & Wilkins
*Textbook of Clinical Neurology,* C Goetz, WB Saunders Company
*Merritt's Neurology,* RL Lewis, HH Merritt, Lippincott, Williams & Wilkins
*Harrison's Neurology in Clinical Practice*, S Hauser, McGraw Hill
*Neurological Differential Diagnosis,* J Patten, Springer–Verlag
*Adams and Victor's Manual of Neurology,* 7th edn, M Victor, AH Ropper, McGraw–Hill
*Introductory Neurology*, JG McLeod, JW Lance, L Davies, Blackwell Science

---

18 An example is the patient with severe muscle hypertrophy such that he was bursting out of his clothes. This author consulted the handbook and was able to find the cause of the patient's problem: it was hypothyroidism.

# References

1   Glasziou PP. Information overload: What's behind it, what's beyond it? *Med J Aust* 2008;189(2):84–85.

2   Greenhalgh T. *How to read a paper: The basics of evidence-based medicine*. 2nd edn London: BMJ Books; 2001.

3   Sackett DL, et al. *Evidence-based medicine: How to practise and teach EBM*. Toronto: Churchill Livingstone; 2000.

4   Richardson WS, et al. Users' guides to the medical literature: XXIV. How to use an article on the clinical manifestations of disease. Evidence-Based Medicine Working Group. *JAMA* 2000;284(7):869–875.

5   Giacomini MK, Cook DJ. Users' guides to the medical literature: XXIII. Qualitative research in health care B. What are the results and how do they help me care for my patients? Evidence-Based Medicine Working Group. *JAMA* 2000;284(4):478–482.

6   Giacomini MK, Cook DJ. Users' guides to the medical literature: XXIII. Qualitative research in health care A. Are the results of the study valid? Evidence-Based Medicine Working Group. *JAMA* 2000;284(3):357–362.

7   McGinn TG, et al. Users' guides to the medical literature: XXII. How to use articles about clinical decision rules. Evidence-Based Medicine Working Group. *JAMA* 2000;284(1):79–84.

8   Hunt DL, Jaeschke R. McKibbon KA. Users' guides to the medical literature: XXI. Using electronic health information resources in evidence-based practice. Evidence-Based Medicine Working Group. *JAMA* 2000;283(14):1875–1879.

9   Bucher HC, et al. Users' guides to the medical literature: XIX. Applying clinical trial results. A. How to use an article measuring the effect of an intervention on surrogate end points. Evidence-Based Medicine Working Group. *JAMA* 1999;282(8):771–778.

10  Randolph AG, et al. Users' guides to the medical literature: XVIII. How to use an article evaluating the clinical impact of a computer-based clinical decision support system. *JAMA* 1999;282(1):67–74.

11  Barratt A, et al. Users' guides to the medical literature: XVII. How to use guidelines and recommendations about screening. Evidence-Based Medicine Working Group. *JAMA* 1999;281(21):2029–2034.

12  Guyatt GH, et al. Users' guides to the medical literature: XVI. How to use a treatment recommendation. Evidence-Based Medicine Working Group and the Cochrane Applicability Methods Working Group. *JAMA* 1999;281(19):1836–1843.

13  Richardson WS, et al. Users' guides to the medical literature: XV. How to use an article about disease probability for differential diagnosis. Evidence-Based Medicine Working Group. *JAMA* 1999;281(13):1214–1219.

14  Dans AL, et al. Users' guides to the medical literature: XIV. How to decide on the applicability of clinical trial results to your patient. Evidence-Based Medicine Working Group. *JAMA* 1998;279(7):545–549.

15  O'Brien BJ, et al. Users' guides to the medical literature: XIII. How to use an article on economic analysis of clinical practice. B. What are the results, and will they help me in caring for my patients? Evidence-Based Medicine Working Group. *JAMA* 1997;277(22):1802–1806.

16  Drummond MF, et al. Users' guides to the medical literature: XIII. How to use an article on economic analysis of clinical practice. A. Are the results of the study valid? Evidence-Based Medicine Working Group. *JAMA* 1997;277(19):1552–1557.

17  Guyatt GH, et al. Users' guides to the medical literature: XII. How to use articles about health-related quality of life. Evidence-Based Medicine Working Group. *JAMA* 1997;277(15):1232–1237.

18  Naylor CD, Guyatt GH. Users' guides to the medical literature: XI. How to use an article about a clinical utilization review. Evidence-Based Medicine Working Group. *JAMA* 1996;275(18):1435–1439.

19  Naylor CD, Guyatt GH. Users' guides to the medical literature: X. How to use an article reporting variations in the outcomes of health services. The Evidence-Based Medicine Working Group. *JAMA* 1996;275(7):554–558.

20   Guyatt GH, et al. Users' guides to the medical literature: IX. A method for grading health care recommendations. Evidence-Based Medicine Working Group. *JAMA* 1995;274(22):1800–1804.

21   Wilson MC, et al. Users' guides to the medical literature: VIII. How to use clinical practice guidelines. B. what are the recommendations, and will they help you in caring for your patients? The Evidence-Based Medicine Working Group. *JAMA* 1995;274(20):1630–1632.

22   Hayward RS, et al. Users' guides to the medical literature: VIII. How to use clinical practice guidelines. A. Are the recommendations valid? The Evidence-Based Medicine Working Group. *JAMA* 1995;274(7):570–574.

23   Richardson WS, Detsky AS. Users' guides to the medical literature: VII. How to use a clinical decision analysis. B. What are the results and will they help me in caring for my patients? Evidence Based Medicine Working Group. *JAMA* 1995;273(20):1610–1613.

24   Sackett DL, Haynes RB, Tugwell P. *Clinical epidemiology: A basic science for clinical medicine.*: Little, Brown; 1985, 370.

25   Giglia E. Beyond PubMed. Other free-access biomedical databases. *Eur Medicophys* 2007;43(4): 563–569.

26   Yue W, Wilson CS, Boller F. Peer assessment of journal quality in clinical neurology. *J Med Libr Assoc* 2007;95(1):70–76.

27   Berners-Lee, T. and J. Hendler (2001). "Publishing on the semantic web." *Nature* 410(6832): 1023-1024.

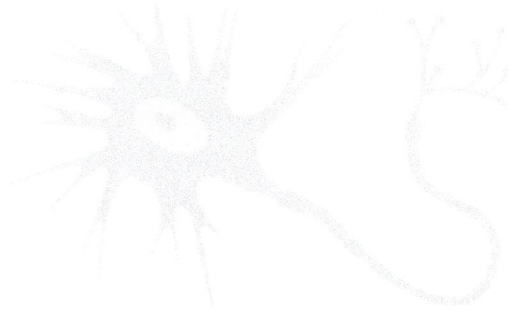

# Appendices

# MONTREAL COGNITIVE ASSESSMENT (MOCA)

NAME :
Education :
Sex :

Date of birth :
DATE :

| VISUOSPATIAL / EXECUTIVE | Copy cube | Draw CLOCK (Ten past eleven) ( 3 points ) | POINTS |
|---|---|---|---|

(E) End   (A)
(5)
(1)   (B)   (2)
Begin
(D)   (4)   (3)
(C)

[ ]

[ ]

[ ] [ ] [ ]
Contour  Numbers  Hands

__/5

## NAMING

[ ]  [ ]  [ ]   __/3

| MEMORY | Read list of words, subject must repeat them. Do 2 trials. Do a recall after 5 minutes. | | FACE | VELVET | CHURCH | DAISY | RED | No points |
|---|---|---|---|---|---|---|---|---|
| | | 1st trial | | | | | | |
| | | 2nd trial | | | | | | |

| ATTENTION | Read list of digits (1 digit/ sec.). | Subject has to repeat them in the forward order | [ ] 2 1 8 5 4 | |
|---|---|---|---|---|
| | | Subject has to repeat them in the backward order | [ ] 7 4 2 | __/2 |

Read list of letters. The subject must tap with his hand at each letter A. No points if ≥ 2 errors

[ ] F B A C M N A A J K L B A F A K D E A A A J A M O F A A B   __/1

| Serial 7 subtraction starting at 100 | [ ] 93 | [ ] 86 | [ ] 79 | [ ] 72 | [ ] 65 | |
|---|---|---|---|---|---|---|
| | 4 or 5 correct subtractions: **3 pts**, 2 or 3 correct: **2 pts**, 1 correct: **1 pt**, 0 correct: **0 pt** | | | | | __/3 |

| LANGUAGE | Repeat : I only know that John is the one to help today. [ ] | |
|---|---|---|
| | The cat always hid under the couch when dogs were in the room. [ ] | __/2 |

| Fluency / Name maximum number of words in one minute that begin with the letter F | [ ] ____ (N ≥ 11 words) | __/1 |
|---|---|---|

| ABSTRACTION | Similarity between e.g. banana – orange = fruit [ ] train – bicycle [ ] watch – ruler | __/2 |
|---|---|---|

| DELAYED RECALL | Has to recall words | FACE | VELVET | CHURCH | DAISY | RED | Points for UNCUED recall only | __/5 |
|---|---|---|---|---|---|---|---|---|
| | WITH NO CUE | [ ] | [ ] | [ ] | [ ] | [ ] | | |
| Optional | Category cue | | | | | | | |
| | Multiple choice cue | | | | | | | |

| ORIENTATION | [ ] Date | [ ] Month | [ ] Year | [ ] Day | [ ] Place | [ ] City | __/6 |
|---|---|---|---|---|---|---|---|

© Z.Nasreddine MD  Version November 7, 2004

www.mocatest.org

Normal ≥ 26 / 30

TOTAL __/30

Add 1 point if ≤ 12 yr edu

# Montreal Cognitive Assessment (MoCA)
# Administration and Scoring Instructions

The Montreal Cognitive Assessment (MoCA) was designed as a rapid screening instrument for mild cognitive dysfunction. It assesses different cognitive domains: attention and concentration, executive functions, memory, language,visuoconstructional skills, conceptual thinking, calculations, and orientation. Time to administer the MoCA is approximately 10 minutes. The total possible score is 30 points; a score of 26 or above is considered normal.

## 1. Alternating Trail Making:

Administration: The examiner instructs the subject: *"Please draw a line, going from a number to a letter in ascending order. Begin here* [point to (1)] *and draw a line from 1 then to A then to 2 and so on. End here* [point to (E)]."

Scoring: Allocate one point if the subject successfully draws the following pattern:

1 –A- 2- B- 3- C- 4- D- 5- E, without drawing any lines that cross. Any error that is not immediately self-corrected earns a score of 0.

## 2. Visuoconstructional Skills (Cube):

Administration: The examiner gives the following instructions, pointing to the cube: *"Copy this drawing as accurately as you can,in the space below"*.

Scoring: One point is allocated for a correctly executed drawing.
* Drawing must be three-dimensional
* All lines are drawn
* No line is added
* Lines are relatively parallel and their length is similar (rectangular prisms are accepted) A point is not assigned if any of the above-criteria are not met.

## 3. Visuoconstructional Skills (Clock):

Administration: Indicate the right third of the space and give the following instructions: *"Draw a clock. Put in all the numbers and set the time to 10 past 11"*.

Scoring: One point is allocated for each of the following three criteria:
* Contour (1 pt.): the clock face must be a circle with only minor distortion acceptable (e.g.,slight imperfection on closing the circle);
* Numbers(1pt.): all clock numbers must be present with no additional numbers; numbers must be in the correct order and placed in the approximate quadrants on the clock face; Roman numerals are acceptable; numbers can be placed outside the circle contour;
* Hands (1 pt.): there must be two hands jointly indicating the correct time; the hour hand must be clearly shorter than the minute hand; hands must be centred within the clock face with their junction close to the clock centre.

A point is not assigned for a given element if any of the above-criteria are not met.

## 4. Naming:

Administration: Beginning on the left, point to each figure and say: "Tell me the name of this animal".

Scoring: One point each is given for the following responses: (1) lion (2) rhinoceros or rhino (3) camel or dromedary.

## 5. Memory:

Administration: The examiner reads a list of 5 words at a rate of one per second, giving the following instructions: *"This is a memory test. I am going to read a list of words that you will have to remember now and later on. Listen carefully. When I am through, tell me as many words as you can remember. It doesn't matter in what order you say them"*. Mark a check in the allocated space for each word the subject produces on this first trial. When the subject indicates that(s) he has finished (has recalled all words), or can recall no more words, read the list a second time with the following instructions: *"I am going to read the same list for a second time. Try to remember and tell me as many words as you can, including words you said the first time."* Put a check in the allocated space for each word the subject recalls after the second trial.

At the end of the second trial, inform the subject that (s)he will be asked to recall these words again by saying, *"I will ask you to recall those words again at the end of the test."*

Scoring: No points are given for Trials One and Two.

## 6. Attention:

Forward Digit Span: Administration: Give the following instruction: "I am going to say some numbers and when I am through, repeat them to me exactly as I said them". Read the five number sequence at a rate of one digit per second.

Backward Digit Span: Administration: Give the following instruction: "Now I am going to say some more numbers, but when I am through you must repeat them to me in the backwards order."Read the three number sequence at a rate of one digit per second.

Scoring: Allocate one point for each sequence correctly repeated, (N.B.: the correct response for the backwards trial is 2-4-7).

Vigilance: Administration: The examiner reads the list of letters at a rate of one per second, after giving the following instruction: *"I am going to read a sequence of letters. Every time I say the letter A, tap your hand once. If I say a different letter, do not tap your hand"*.

Scoring: Give one point if there is zero to one errors (an error is a tap on a wrong letter or a failure to tap on letter A).

Serial 7s: Administration: The examiner gives the following instruction: *"Now, I will ask you to count by subtracting seven from 100, and then, keep subtracting seven from your answer until I tell you to stop."* Give this instruction twice if necessary.

Scoring: This item is scored out of 3 points. Give no (0) points for no correct subtractions, 1point for one correction subtraction, 2 points for two-to-three correct subtractions, and 3 points if the participant successfully makes four or five correct subtractions. Count each correct subtraction of 7 beginning at 100. Each subtraction is evaluated independently; that is, if the participant responds with an incorrect number but continues to correctly subtract 7 from it, give a point for each correct subtraction. For example, a participant may respond "92–85–78–71– 64" where the "92" is incorrect, but all subsequent numbers are subtracted correctly. This is one error and the item would be given a score of 3.

## 7  Sentence repetition:

Administration: The examiner gives the following instructions: *"I am going to read you a sentence. Repeat it after me,exactly as I say it* [pause]: ***I only know that John is the one to help today."*** Following the response, say: *"Now I am going to read you another sentence. Repeat it after me, exactly as I say it* [pause]: ***The cat always hid under the couch when dogs were in the room."***

Scoring: Allocate 1 point for each sentence correctly repeated. Repetition must be exact. Be alert for errors that are omissions (e.g., omitting "only", "always") and substitutions/additions(e.g.,"John is the one who helped today;" substituting" hides" for "hid", altering plurals, etc.).

## 8  Verbal fluency:

Administration: The examiner gives the following instruction: *"Tell me as many words as you can think of that begin with a certain letter of the alphabet that I will tell you in a moment. You can say any kind of word you want, except for proper nouns (like Bob or Boston), numbers, or words that begin with the same sound but have a different suffix, for example, love, lover,loving. I will tell you to stop after one minute. Are you ready? [Pause] Now, tell me as many words as you can think of that begin with the letter F.* [time for 60 sec]. *Stop."*

Scoring: Allocate one point if the subject generates 11 words or more in 60 sec. Record the subject's response in the bottom or side margins.

## 9.  Abstraction:

Administration: The examiner asks the subject to explain what each pair of words has in common, starting with the example: *"Tell me how an orange and a banana are alike".* If the subject answers in a concrete manner, then say only one additional time: *"Tell me another way in which those items area like".* If the subject does not give the appropriate response *(fruit),* say, *"Yes, and they are also both fruit."* Do not give any additional instructions or clarification. After the practice trial, say: *"Now, tell me how a train and a bicycle are alike".* Following the response, administer the second trial, saying: *"Now tell me how a ruler and a watch are alike".*Do not give any additional instructions or prompts.

Scoring: Only the last two item pairs are scored. Give 1 point to each item pair correctly answered. The following responses are acceptable:
Train-bicycle = means of transportation, means of travelling, you take trips in both;
Ruler-watch = measuring instruments, used to measure.
The following responses are **not** acceptable: Train-bicycle = they have wheels;
Ruler-watch = they have numbers.

## 10. Delayed recall:

Administration: The examiner gives the following instruction: *"I read some words to you earlier, which I asked you to remember. Tell me as many of those words as you can remember."* Make a check mark ( √ ) for each of the words correctly recalled spontaneously without any cues, in the allocated space.

Scoring: **Allocate 1 point for each word recalled freely without any cues.**

---

## Optional:

Following the delayed free recall trial, prompt the subject with the semantic category cue provided below for any word not recalled. Make a check mark ( √ ) in the allocated space if the subject remembered the word with the help of a category or multiple-choice cue. Prompt all non-recalled words in this manner. If the subject does not recall the word after the category cue, give him/her a multiple choice trial, using the following example instruction, *"Which of the following words do you think it was, NOSE, FACE, or HAND?"*

Use the following category and/or multiple-choice cues for each word, when appropriate:

| | | |
|---|---|---|
| FACE: | category cue: part of the body | multiple choice: nose, face, hand |
| VELVET: | category cue: type of fabric | multiple choice: denim, cotton, velvet |
| CHURCH: | category cue: type of building | multiple choice: church, school, hospital |
| DAISY: | category cue: type of flower | multiple choice: rose, daisy, tulip |
| RED: | category cue: a colour | multiple choice: red, blue, green |

Scoring: No points are allocated for words recalled with a cue. A cue is used for clinical information purposes only and can give the test interpreter additional information about the type of memory disorder. For memory deficits due to retrieval failures, performance can be improved with a cue. For memory deficits due to encoding failures, performance does not improve with a cue.

---

## 11. Orientation:

Administration: The examiner gives the following instructions: "Tell me the date today". If the subject does not give a complete answer, then prompt accordingly by saying: *"Tell me the [year, month, exact date, and day of the week]."* Then say: *"Now, tell me the name of this place, and which city it is in."*

Scoring: Give one point for each item correctly answered. The subject must tell the exact date and the exact place (name of hospital, clinic, office). No points are allocated if subject makes an error of one day for the day and date.

**TOTAL SCORE:** Sum all subscores listed on the right-hand side. Add one point for an individual who has 12 years or fewer of formal education, for a possible maximum of 30 points. A final total score of 26 and above is considered normal.

# VAMC
# SLUMS ExaMination

Questions about this assessment tool? E-mail aging@slu.edu

Name_____ Age_____

Is the patient alert?_____ Level of education_____

__/1   **①** **1. What day of the week is it?**

__/1   **①** **2. What is the year?**

__/1   **①** **3. What state are we in?**

**4. Please remember these five objects. I will ask you what they are later.**
     Apple      Pen      Tie      House      Car

**5. You have $100 and you go to the store and buy a dozen apples for $3 and a tricycle for $20.**
   **①**   How much did you spend?
__/3   **②**   How much do you have left?

**6. Please name as many animals as you can in one minute.**
   **⓪** 0-4 animals    **①** 5-9 animals    **②** 10-14 animals    **③** 15+ animals
__/3

__/5   **7. What were the five objects I asked you to remember? 1 point for each one correct.**

**8. I am going to give you a series of numbers and I would like you to give them to me backwards. For example, if I say 42, you would say 24.**
   **⓪** 87    **①** 648    **①** 8537
__/2

**9. This is a clock face. Please put in the hour markers and the time at ten minutes to eleven o'clock.**
   **②**   Hour markers okay
__/4   **②**   Time correct

**①** **10. Please place an X in the triangle.**

**①**   Which of the above figures is largest?
__/2

**11. I am going to tell you a story. Please listen carefully because afterwards, I'm going to ask you some questions about it.**
Jill was a very successful stockbroker. She made a lot of money on the stock market. She then met Jack, a devastatingly handsome man. She married him and had three children. They lived in Chicago. She then stopped work and stayed at home to bring up her children. When they were teenagers, she went back to work. She and Jack lived happily ever after.

   **②** What was the female's name?      **②** What work did she do?
__/8   **②** When did she go back to work?    **②** What state did she live in?

_____   **TOTAL SCORE**

| SCORING | | |
|---|---|---|
| **HigH ScHooL EdUcation** | | **Less tHan HigH ScHooL EdUcation** |
| 27-30 | Normal | 25-30 |
| 21-26 | mild NeurocogNitive disorder | 20-24 |
| 1-20 | demeNtia | 1-19 |

CLINICIAN'S SIGNATURE        DATE        TIME

SH Tariq, N Tumosa, JT Chibnall, HM Perry III, and JE Morley. The Saint Louis University Mental Status (SLUMS) Examination for detecting mild cognitive impairment and dementia is more sensitive than the Mini-Mental Status Examination (MMSE) - A pilot study. *Am J Geriatr Psych* 14:900-10, 2006.

| Name of patient: | | DOB: | / / | Name of examiner: | | Date of test: | / / |
|---|---|---|---|---|---|---|---|

# Standardised Mini-Mental State Examination (SMMSE)

**Please see accompanying guidelines for administration and scoring instructions**

**Say:** *I am going to ask you some questions and give you some problems to solve. Please try to answer as best you can.*

1. Allow ten seconds for each reply. **Say:**
   a) *What year is this?* (accept exact answer only) /1
   b) *What season is this?* (during the last week of the old season or first week of a new season, accept either) /1
   c) *What month is this?* (on the first day of a new month or the last day of the previous month, accept either) /1
   d) *What is today's date?* (accept previous or next date) /1
   e) *What day of the week is this?* (accept exact answer only) /1

2. Allow ten seconds for each reply. **Say:**
   a) *What country are we in?* (accept exact answer only) /1
   b) *What state are we in?* (accept exact answer only) /1
   c) *What city/town are we in?* (accept exact answer only) /1
   d) <At home> *What is the street address of this house?* (accept street name and house number or equivalent in rural areas) /1
      <In facility>*What is the name of this building?* (accept exact name of institution only) /1
   e) <At home>*What room are we in?* (accept exact answer only) /1
      <In facility>*What floor of the building are we on?* (accept exact answer only) /1

3. **Say:** I am going to name three objects. When I am finished, I want you to repeat them. Remember what they are because I am going to ask you to name them again in a few minutes (say slowly at approximately one-second intervals).

   **Ball      Car      Man**

   For repeated use: Bell, jar, fan; bill, tar, can; bull, bar, pan

   **Say:** *Please repeat the three items for me* (score one point for each correct reply on the first attempt) /3

   Allow 20 seconds for reply; if the person did not repeat all three, repeat until they are learned or up to a maximum of five times (but only score first attempt)

4. **Say:** *Spell the word WORLD* (you may help the person to spell the word correctly). **Say:** Now spell it backwards please (allow 30 seconds; if the person cannot spell world even with assistance, score zero). Refer to accompanying guide for scoring instructions (score on reverse of this sheet) /5

5. **Say:** *Now what were the three objects I asked you to remember?* /3
   (score one point for each correct answer regardless of order; allow ten seconds)

6. Show wrist watch. **Ask:** *What is this called?* /1
   (score one point for correct response; accept 'wristwatch' or 'watch'; do not accept 'clock' or 'time', etc.; allow ten seconds)

429

7. **Show pencil**. Ask: *What is this called?*                              /1
   (score one point for correct response; accept 'pencil' only; score zero for pen; allow ten seconds for reply)

8. **Say:** *I would like you to repeat a phrase after me: No ifs, ands, or buts*                              /1
   (allow ten seconds for response. Score one point for a correct repetition. Must be exact, e.g. no ifs or buts, score zero)

9. **Say:** *Read the words on this page and then do what it says*                              /1

   Then, **hand** the person the sheet with CLOSE YOUR EYES (score on reverse of this sheet) on it. If the subject just reads and does not close eyes, you may repeat: *Read the words on this page and then do what it says*, a maximum of three times. See point number three in Directions for Administration section of accompanying guidelines. Allow ten seconds; score one point only if the person closes their eyes. The person does not have to read aloud.

10. **Hand** the person a pencil and paper. **Say:** *Write any complete sentence on that piece of paper* (allow 30 seconds. Score one point. The sentence must make sense. Ignore spelling errors). /1

11. **Place** design (see page 3), pencil, eraser and paper in front of the person. **Say:** *Copy this design please.* Allow multiple tries.                              /1
    Wait until the person is finished and hands it back. Score one point for a correctly copied diagram. The person must have drawn a four-sided figure between two five-sided figures. Maximum time: one minute.

12. **Ask** the person if he is right or left handed. **Take** a piece of paper, hold it up in front of the person and **say** the following: *Take this paper in your right/left hand* (whichever is non-dominant), *fold the paper in half once with both hands and put the paper down on the floor.*

| | | |
|---|---|---|
| Takes paper in correct hand_____ | | /1 |
| Folds it in half_____ | | /1 |
| Puts it on the floor_____ | | /1 |
| **TOTAL TEST SCORE:**<br>ADJUSTED SCORE: | / | **/30** |

Molloy DW, Alemayehu E, Roberts R. Reliability of a standardized Mini-Mental State Examination compared with the traditional Mini-Mental state Examination. *American Journal of Psychiatry*, Vol.148, 1991a, pp.102-105. A guide to the Standardized Mini-Mental State Examination: https://www.cambridge.org/core/journals/international-psychogeriatrics/article/abs/guide-to-the-standardizedminimentalstate-examination/E28A67ABD498D7CE938C6DF604058B38

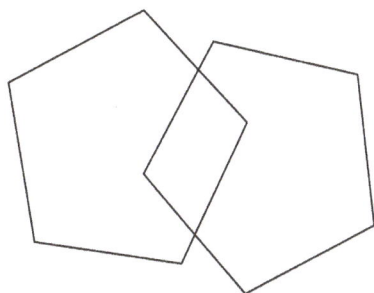

Time:

- - - - - - - - - - - - - - - - - - - - - - - - - - - - - - - - - - - - - - - - - - - - - - - - - - - - - - - - - - -

| D | L | R | O | W | = | |
|---|---|---|---|---|---|---|
| | | | | | | |

- - - - - - - - - - - - - - - - - - - - - - - - - - - - - - - - - - - - - - - - - - - - - - - - - - - - - - - - - - -

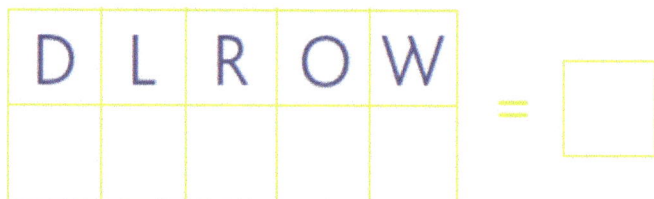

# CLOSE YOUR EYES

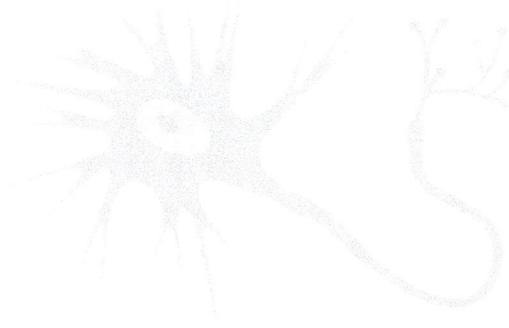

# Rare Seizures of Infancy and Childhood

## Epileptic Spasms

Epileptic spasms consist of brief (1-3 second) events of an arm, leg and head flexion (arms and legs pull into the body) or extension. Epileptic spasms are seen most commonly in children less than two years of age. The term infantile spasms describes this seizure type in infants. Spasms typically occur in clusters with events every 5-10 seconds over a 5-10-minute period. Most children with spasms will have several clusters per day. The spasms are most commonly seen in infants with serious epilepsies such as West syndrome or Ohtahara syndrome but may also occur in Lennox-Gastaut syndrome.

## Rolandic Epilepsy

These are focal seizures consisting of unilateral facial sensory-motor symptoms. Motor manifestations are clonic contractions sometimes concurrent with an ipsilateral tonic deviation of the mouth and the lower lip. They may spread to the ipsilateral hand (the same side as the face is affected). The sensory symptoms are numbness or paraesthesia (tingling, prickling or freezing) inside the mouth, associated with strange sounds, such as death rattle, gargling, grunting and guttural sounds. The speech is affected by anarthria, with the child being unable to utter a single intelligible word and attempting to communicate with gestures. There may or may not be impaired consciousness, but many of these seizures occur during sleep, and the child awakes hemiparetic and anarthric [1].

Although rolandic seizures are usually brief, lasting 1–3 minutes, opercular status epilepticus may persist for hours to months. Opercular status epilepticus causes unilateral or bilateral contractions of the mouth, tongue or eyelids, positive or negative subtle perioral or other myoclonus, dysarthria, speech arrest, difficulties in swallowing, buccofacial apraxia and hypersalivation [1].

# Panayiotopoulos Syndrome

The first apparent ictal symptom is usually nausea ± vomiting, although this may occur long after the onset of other manifestations. Pallor, urinary ± faecal incontinence, hypersalivation, difficulty breathing and even cyanosis are other autonomic manifestations. The seizures are usually lengthy, lasting more than 6 minutes, and almost half of them last for 30 minutes to many hours, thus constituting autonomic status epilepticus [1].

# Idiopathic Childhood Occipital Epilepsy

In idiopathic childhood occipital epilepsy of Gastaut seizures are usually frequent and brief and manifest with elementary visual hallucinations, blindness or both [1]. Elementary visual hallucinations are frequently the first and often the only seizure symptom and consist mainly of small multicoloured circular patterns that often appear in the periphery of a visual field, becoming more prominent and multiplying during the seizure, frequently moving towards the other side. Unlike in migraine, the visual disturbance develops rapidly within seconds. Ictal blindness is probably the second most common symptom after visual hallucinations. It is sudden and usually total. Complex formed visual hallucinations, such as faces and figures, and visual illusions, such as micropsia (objects appear undersize), palinopsia (the hallucinatory persistence of an object after the viewer has turned away) and metamorphopsia (images appear distorted in various ways), occur in < 10% of patients and mainly after the appearance of elementary visual hallucinations [1].

Post-ictal headache, mainly diffuse but severe, or unilateral, pulsating and indistinguishable from migraine headache, occurs in half the patients, in 10% of whom may be associated with nausea and vomiting. These headaches arise immediately or 5–10 minutes after the end of the visual hallucinations. The duration and severity of the headache appears to be proportional to the duration and severity of the preceding seizure, although it may also occur after brief, simple visual episodes.

# References

1.  Panayiotopoulos CP, et al. Benign childhood focal epilepsies: Assessment of established and newly recognized syndromes. *Brain 2008*;131(Pt 9):2264–2286.

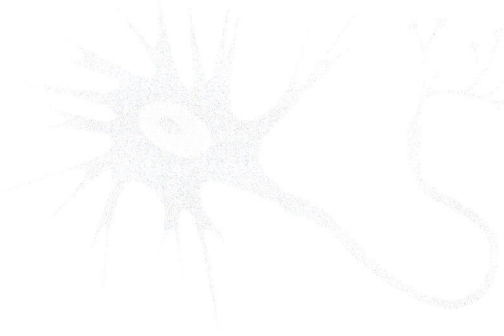

| Warning |
| :---: |
| The information in this appendix will be rapidly out of date. Always check the latest guidelines. |

# Epilepsy Nomenclature

# Currently Recommended Drugs and their Common Side Effects

## Focal Onset

### Generalised Onset

### Unknown

**Aware**

**Impaired awareness**

**Motor**
Tonic-clonic
Clonic
Tonic
Myoclonic
Myoclonic-tonic-clonic
(JME) Myoclonic-
atonic (DS)
Atonic
Epileptic spasms

**Motor**
Tonic-clonic
Epileptic spasms

**Non-motor**
Behaviour arrest

**Motor Onset**
Automatisms
Atonic
Clonic
Epileptic spasms
Hyperkinetic
Myoclonic
Tonic

**Non-motor onset**
Autonomic
Behaviour arrest
Cognitive
Emotional
Sensory

**Non-Motor (absence)**
Typical
Atypical
Myoclonic
Eyelid myoclonia
(JS)

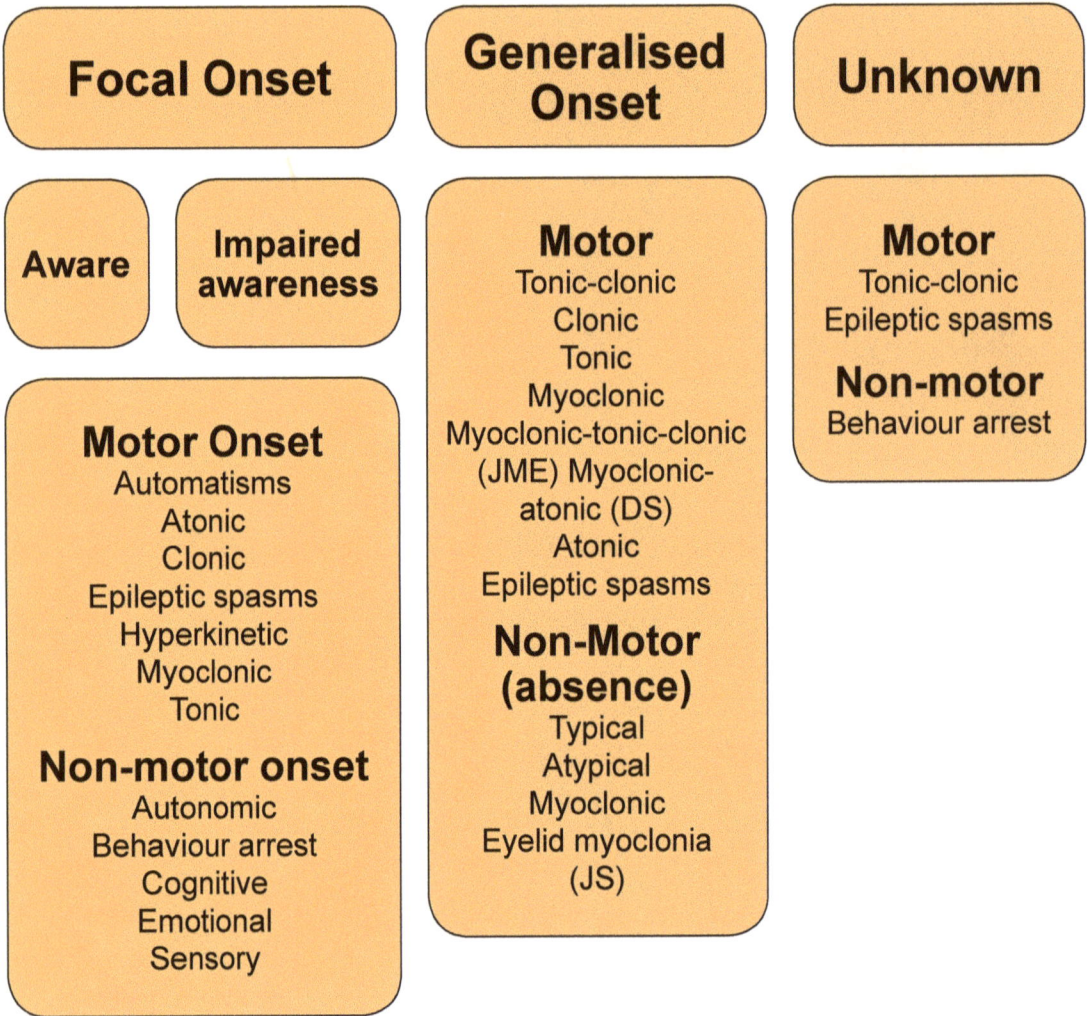

**Figure D1** The ILAE 2017 Classification of Seizures . Abbreviations: JME = Juvenile Myoclonic Epilepsy, DS = Doose syndrome [20], JS = Jeavons syndrome [21].

Figure D1 shows the 2017 revised International League Against Epilepsy (ILAE) classification of seizures. [15] To those of us brought up in the era of the old terminology, the changes are difficult to understand. Seizures have been divided into focal, generalised and unknown onset. The focal onset seizures are further sub-divided into aware and impaired awareness, both with motor and non-motor onset. Generalised onset has been divided into a motor and non-motor onset. In chapter 8 I have used the old nomenclature in the graphs but have added the new terminology to the headings.

---

1 Cognitive seizures imply impaired language or other cognitive domains or positive features such as déjà vu, hallucinations, illusions or perceptual distortions. Emotional seizures involve anxiety, fear, joy, other emotions or appearance of affect without subjective emotions. An absence is atypical because of slow onset or termination or significant changes in tone supported by atypical, slow, generalized spike and wave on the EEG. Automatisms are nonpurposeful, stereotyped, and repetitive behaviors that commonly accompany focal impaired awareness seizures

# Currently Available Drugs

An analysis of 525 patients in 2000 found that only 60% were free of seizures after one year. Cryptogenic or symptomatic epilepsy as opposed to generalised and the number of seizures before commencing treatment predicted a poorer outcome. [22] Many more antiepileptic drugs (AED's) drugs have come onto the market since the 1st edition of this book, sadly only 50% of patients remain seizure-free for one year or longer with the initial AED, and only about 2/3 are seizure-free with the addition of a 2nd and 3rd AED. [16]

The following recommendations are based on the guidelines of the American Epilepsy Society [1, 2], the International League Against Epilepsy [3], the European Federation of Neurological Societies [4], the Cochrane database [5], the SANAD trial [6, 7], the UK Epilepsy Society,[14] and the Epilepsy Foundation of the USA. [15] Many more drugs are in development, and clinicians treating patients with epilepsy must continue to monitor new developments. [16,17]

## General Principles

- Formulations of antiepileptic drugs (AEDs) are not interchangeable, and generic substitution should not be employed.
- Lamotrigine and oxcarbazepine seem to be better tolerated and may produce fewer long-term side effects and adverse interactions.
- Lamotrigine may have advantages in young women, adolescents and the elderly. It is well-tolerated, does not cause weight gain, has a favourable cognitive and behavioural profile and does not induce the metabolism of lipid-soluble drugs (such as the hormonal components of the oral contraceptive agents).
- Side effects may also occur due to drug interactions, and the MIMS interact (or any similar program) should be used to check potential drug interactions before prescribing an anticonvulsant.
- The SANAD study [6, 7], a pragmatic randomised clinical trial, found that:
- Carbamazepine is the drug of choice for partial or focal seizures.
- Valproic acid is the drug of choice for generalised seizures.

# New-onset epilepsy
## Generalised Onset Tonic-Clonic Seizures

Carbamazepine, phenytoin and valproic acid have the most evidence to support their use. The newer AEDs such as lamotrigine, oxcarbazepine, phenobarbital, topiramate are efficacious in adults. Carbamazepine, phenobarbital, phenytoin, topiramate and valproic acid are efficacious in children.

## Absence Seizures

The drugs of choice are ethosuximide, lamotrigine and valproic acid. Drugs such as carbamazepine, oxcarbazepine, phenytoin, gabapentin and tiagabine should be avoided as they may precipitate or aggravate absence seizures.

# Juvenile Myoclonic Epilepsy

Some authorities regard valproic acid as the drug of choice. [1] Clonazepam can suppress the myoclonic but not the tonic-clonic seizures, which is a disadvantage as it removes the warnings jerks of a tonic-clonic seizure. [8]

Carbamazepine, oxcarbazepine, phenytoin, gabapentin and tiagabine may precipitate or aggravate absence and myoclonic seizures and should be avoided.

# Partial (Focal) with or without Secondary Generalised Seizures

Carbamazepine, phenytoin, valproic acid, gabapentin, lamotrigine, topiramate and oxcarbazepine have efficacy as monotherapy in newly diagnosed adolescents and adults with either partial or mixed seizure disorders.

# Refractory or Drug-Resistant Epilepsy

Control of seizures is inadequate in more than 30% of patients with epilepsy. Only a small percentage of patients who have many seizures before commencing therapy and patients who fail to respond to the first drug will become seizure-free. The seizure-free rate for monotherapy is the same with established and newer drugs [9].

Limited evidence suggests that lamotrigine and topiramate are also effective for adjunctive treatment of idiopathic generalised epilepsy in adults and children and treatment of the Lennox–Gastaut syndrome. In adults with refractory partial seizures, gabapentin, lamotrigine, topiramate, tiagabine, oxcarbazepine, levetiracetam, and zonisamide are all appropriate for adjunctive treatment. Gabapentin, lamotrigine, oxcarbazepine and topiramate are for the treatment of refractory partial seizures in children. A 2018 AAN guideline [23] states that there is level A evidence for pregabalin, perampanel and vigabatrin as add-on therapy for treatment-resistant focal epilepsy, whilst rufinamide is effective add-on therapy for the Lennox-Gastaut syndrome.

# Status Epilepsy

Intravenous (IV) lorazepam is the drug of choice in both adults [10] and children. [5] Others include IV diazepam or IV phenytoin. If IV access is unavailable, 30 mg of rectal diazepam gel is an alternative. [10]

In recent years IV, valproic acid, and IV levetiracetam have become available. Small studies suggest that IV levetiracetam [11] and IV valproic acid [12] may be effective in benzodiazepine refractory status epilepsy. However, as yet, there are no randomised controlled trials.

# Side Effects of the Antiepileptic Drugs

Patients are often horrified; some are terrified when they are informed of the potential side effects of drugs. It is important to stress to patients that drugs remain on the market because more patients benefit than those who experience side effects. In general, side effects commence soon after initiation of therapy. Table C1 list the common side effects of the currently available anticonvulsants.

| Generic Drug Name | Type of Seizure | More Common Side Effects |
|---|---|---|
| Acetazolamide [19] | As adjunctive therapy for RE | Dizziness, lightheadedness, or increased urination may occur, especially during the first few days as your body adjusts to the medication. Blurred vision, dry mouth, drowsiness, loss of appetite, nausea, vomiting, diarrhoea, or changes in taste |
| Brivaracetam | FC, FG, FS | Drowsiness, sedation, dizziness, fatigue, nausea, vomiting, loss of balance or coordination, irritability |
| Cannabidiol [23] | D, LG | Dry mouth, diarrhoea, reduced appetite, drowsiness and fatigue. |
| Carbamazepine | FC, FG | Skin rash (rarely, Stevens-Johnson syndrome), drowsiness and fatigue, hepatic toxicity, blood dyscrasias |
| Cenobamate | FS | Tiredness, dizziness, double vision, headache |
| Clobazam | Add on for LG | Tiredness, problems with coordination, difficulty speaking or swallowing, drooling, change in appetite, vomiting, Constipation, cough |
| Clonazepam | FA, LG, M | Drowsiness, Depression, Dependence Behavioural disturbances (agitation, aggression) |
| Diazepam* | A, FA, FS, FC, G, LG, M | Drowsiness, dizziness, tiredness, muscle weakness, headache, dry mouth, nausea, constipation |
| Eslicarbazepine acetate | FC | Clumsy, problems with coordination, dizziness, double or blurred vision, headache, nausea, problems with thinking, memory or attention (cognitive problems), sleepiness, tremors. |
| Ethosuximide | FA, JME | Drowsiness, skin rash, blood dyscrasias, personality changes, dependence |
| Everolimus | TSS | Diarrhoea, constipation, change in the ability to taste food, weight loss, dry mouth, weakness, headache, difficulty falling asleep or staying asleep |
| Ezogabine | FC, FG, FS | Urinary retention, hallucinations, irritability, anxiety, depression, dizziness, sleepiness, mild changes in heart rhythm, suicide thoughts, withdrawal seizures |
| Felbamate | FC, LG | Decreased appetite, weight loss, nausea insomnia, headache, tremor, vision problems, dizziness, vomiting, mood changes or anxiety, sleepiness |
| Fenfluramine | D | Decreased appetite, diarrhoea, weight loss, tiredness |
| Gabapentin | FA, FC | Drowsiness and fatigue, weight gain, leucopenia, dry mouth, gastrointestinal upset |
| Lacosamide | FA, FC, FG | Coordination problems, dizziness, double vision, headache, nausea, vomiting, sleepiness, unsteady walking |
| Lamotrigine | FA, FG, G, JME, LG | Skin rash (including Stevens-Johnson syndrome and toxic epidermal necrolysis), fever, blood dyscrasias, hepatic dysfunction |
| Levetiracetam | FA, FC, FG, JME, M | Drowsiness and fatigue, headache, memory impairment, aggression, confusion, irritability and suicidal thoughts. blood dyscrasias (thrombocytopenia) |

| Generic Drug Name | Type of Seizure | More Common Side Effects |
|---|---|---|
| Lorazepam* | A, BR, D, FA, FC, FG, FS, G, JME, LG, LK, M, RA, RC, W | Allergic reactions (rashes, hives, difficulty breathing, swallowing), aggressive behaviour, suicidal thoughts, chest congestion, tremors, hallucinations, memory loss, shortness of breath |
| Oxcarbazepine | FC, FG, FS, G | Dizziness, drowsiness, tiredness, nausea/vomiting, stomach/abdominal pain, headache, trouble sleeping, or constipation |
| Perampanel | FA, FC, FG, G | Anxiety, dizziness, falls, headache, irritability, problems with coordination, sleepiness, nausea, vomiting |
| Phenobarbital | C, FA, FC, FG, FS, G, LG, RA, T | Drowsiness, bradycardia, hypotension, dependence, osteoporosis, blood dyscrasias |
| Phenytoin | FC, FG, FS, G | Gum hyperplasia, hirsutism, coarse features, osteomalacia |
| Piracetam | M | Diarrhoea, weight gain, drowsiness, insomnia, nervousness, depression, muscle spasms, hyperactivity |
| Pregabalin | FC, FS | Drowsiness, confusion and hallucinations, weight gain, tremor, gastrointestinal upset, pancreatitis, rhabdomyolysis, renal failure |
| Primidone | G, JME, G | Tiredness, dizziness, difficulty coordinating movements, nausea, loss of appetite, double vision, uncontrollable eye movements |
| Rufinamide | LG | Sleepiness, headache, loss of coordination, difficulty walking, excessive movement, uncontrollable shaking, uncontrollable movements of the eyes, difficulty paying attention |
| Sodium Valproate or Valproic acid | FA, FC, FS, FG, G, JME, LG, M | Stomach pain, nausea or vomiting, diarrhoea, dry or sore mouth, swollen gums, tremor, unusual eye movements, tiredness, headache, weight gain, thinning hair, or changes to the colour or texture of hair |
| Stiripentol | D | Confusion, drowsiness, difficulty concentrating, dizziness, muscle tremors, loss of muscle coordination, decreased appetite, weight loss |
| Tiagabine | FC, FS | Drowsiness, restlessness, exacerbation of seizures, tremor |
| Topiramate | FC, FS, G, LG | Drowsiness and fatigue, depression and suicidal thoughts, personality changes, anorexia and weight loss, blood dyscrasias (leucopenia) |
| Vigabatrin | FC, FG, FS, W | Drowsiness and fatigue, depression, visual field defects, weight gain, gastrointestinal upset |

**Table C.1** Antiepileptic drugs, the type of seizure they treat and their more common potential side effects.[2] Detailed information can be accessed for drugs that are underlined by pasting the following url into a browser: **https://www.medicines.org.uk/emc/search?q=** then adding the drug of interest to the end of the url directly after the = character. *Diazepam and Lorazepam are used for treating seizures, not for prophylaxis. Not all drugs are available in every country. Abbreviations: **A** = Atonic seizures, **BR** = Benign Rolandic, **C** = Clonic, **D** = Dravet syndrome, **FA** = Focal (absence) seizures, **FC** = Focal (complex-partial ) seizures, **FS** = Focal (simple-partial) seizures, **FG** = Focal with secondary generalised seizures, **G** = Primary generalised (tonic-clonic) seizures, **JME** = Juvenile myoclonic epilepsy, **LG** = Lennox-Gastaut, **LK** = Landau-Kleffner Syndrome, **M**= Myoclonic seizures, **RA** = Rasmussen's Syndrome, **RE** = Refractory epilepsy, **RC** = Ring Chromosome 20 Syndrome, **T** = Tonic, **TSS** = Seizures associated with Tuberous sclerosis, **W** = West's syndrome

2  Sources: MIMS database, [13] the Epilepsy Foundation of the USA https://www.epilepsy.com/medications/ and the Epilepsy Society UK https://epilepsysociety.org.uk/list-anti-epileptic-drugs

The commonest side effects of all the drugs would include dizziness and ataxia with excess doses. One significant drug interaction is the interaction between valproic acid and lamotrigine. Lamotrigine increases the serum levels of valproic acid. Therefore, the lamotrigine dose needs to be increased slowly, commencing with 25 mg every 2nd day for 2 weeks, then 25 mg daily for two weeks, increasing more rapidly as required.

# References

1   French JA, et al. Efficacy and tolerability of the new antiepileptic drugs. II: Treatment of refractory epilepsy: Report of the Therapeutics and Technology Assessment Subcommittee and Quality Standards Subcommittee of the American Academy of Neurology and the American Epilepsy Society. *Neurology* 2004;62(8):1261–1273.

2   French JA, et al. Efficacy and tolerability of the new antiepileptic drugs. I: Treatment of new-onset epilepsy: Report of the Therapeutics and Technology Assessment Subcommittee and Quality Standards Subcommittee of the American Academy of Neurology and the American Epilepsy Society. *Neurology* 2004;62(8):1252–1260.

3   Glauser T, et al. ILAE treatment guidelines: Evidence-based analysis of antiepileptic drug efficacy and effectiveness as initial monotherapy for epileptic seizures and syndromes. *Epilepsia* 2006;47(7):1094–1120.

4   Meierkord H, et al. EFNS guideline on the management of status epilepticus. *Eur J Neurol* 2006;13(5):445–450.

5   Appleton R, Macleod S, Martland T. Drug management for acute tonic-clonic convulsions including convulsive status epilepticus in children. *Cochrane Database Syst Rev* 2008(3): CD001905.

6   Marson AG, et al. The SANAD study of effectiveness of valproate, Lamotrigine, or Topiramate for generalised and unclassifiable epilepsy: An unblinded randomised controlled trial. *Lancet* 2007;369(9566):1016–1026.

7   Marson AG, et al. The SANAD study of effectiveness of carbamazepine, Gabapentin, Lamotrigine, oxcarbazepine, or Topiramate for treatment of partial epilepsy: An unblinded randomised controlled trial. *Lancet* 2007;369(9566):1000–1015.

8   Obeid T, Panayiotopoulos CP. Clonazepam in juvenile myoclonic epilepsy. *Epilepsia* 1989;30(5):603–606.

9   Kwan P, Brodie MJ. Early identification of refractory epilepsy. *N Engl J Med* 2000;342(5):314–319.

10  Prasad K, et al. Anticonvulsant therapy for status epilepticus. *Cochrane Database Syst Rev* 2005(4): CD003723.

11  Knake S, et al. Intravenous levetiracetam in the treatment of benzodiazepine refractory status epilepticus. *J Neurol Neurosurg Psychiatry* 2008;**79**(5):588–589.

12  Agarwal P, Kumar N, Chandra R, Gupta G, Antony AR, Garg N. Randomized study of intravenous valproate and phenytoin in status epilepticus. *Seizure* 2007; 16(6): 527-32.

13  MIMS. Available: http://www.mims.com.au/index.php?option=com_content&task=view&id=98&Itemid=133 (14 Dec 2009).

14  The United Kingdom Epilepsy Society https://epilepsysociety.org.uk/list-anti-epileptic-drugs

15  Scheffer IE, Berkovic S, Capovilla G, et al. ILAE classification of the epilepsies: Position paper of the ILAE Commission for Classification and Terminology. *Epilepsia* 2017; 58(4): 512-21

16  Chen Z, Brodie MJ, Liew D, Kwan P. Treatment Outcomes in Patients With Newly Diagnosed Epilepsy Treated With Established and New Antiepileptic Drugs: A 30-Year Longitudinal Cohort Study. *JAMA Neurology* 2018; 75(3): 279-86.

17  Bialer M, Johannessen SI, Koepp MJ, et al. Progress report on new antiepileptic drugs: A summary of the Fifteenth Eilat Conference on New Antiepileptic Drugs and Devices (EILAT XV). I. Drugs in preclinical and early clinical development. *Epilepsia* 2020; 61(11): 2340-64.

18    Bialer M, Johannessen SI, Koepp MJ, et al. Progress report on new antiepileptic drugs: A summary of the Fifteenth Eilat Conference on New Antiepileptic Drugs and Devices (EILAT XV). II. Drugs in more advanced clinical development. *Epilepsia* 2020; 61(11): 2365-85.

19    Reiss WG, Oles KS. Acetazolamide in the treatment of seizures. Ann Pharmacother 1996; 30(5): 514-9.

20    Kelley SA, Kossoff EH. Doose syndrome (myoclonic-astatic epilepsy): 40 years of progress. *Dev Med Child Neurol* 2010; 52(11): 988-93.

21    Striano S, Capovilla G, Sofia V, et al. Eyelid myoclonia with absences (Jeavons syndrome): a well-defined idiopathic generalised epilepsy syndrome or a spectrum of photosensitive conditions? *Epilepsia* 2009; 50 Suppl 5: 15-9.

22    Kwan P, Brodie MJ. Early identification of refractory epilepsy. *N Engl J Med* 2000; 342(5): 314-9.

23    Arzimanoglou A, Brandl U, Cross JH, et al. Epilepsy and cannabidiol: a guide to treatment. *Epileptic Disord* 2020; 22(1): 1-14.

# Classification and Treatment of Migraine

| Warning |
|---|
| The information in this appendix will be rapidly out of date. Always check the latest guidelines. |

## The International Classification of Headache Disorders, 3rd edition. *Cephalalgia* 2018

**1.1  Migraine without aura**

**1.2  Migraine with aura**

    1.2.1  Migraine with typical aura

        1.2.1.1  Typical aura with headache

        1.2.1.2  Typical aura without headache

    1.2.2  Migraine with brainstem aura

    1.2.3  Hemiplegic migraine

        1.2.3.1  Familial hemiplegic migraine (FHM)

            1.2.3.1.1  Familial hemiplegic migraine type 1

            1.2.3.1.2  Familial hemiplegic migraine type 2

            1.2.3.1.3  Familial hemiplegic migraine type 3

            1.2.3.1.4  Familial hemiplegic migraine, other loci

        1.2.3.2  Sporadic hemiplegic migraine

    1.2.4  Retinal migraine

**1.3  Chronic migraine**

**1.4  Complications of migraine**

    1.4.1  Status migrainosus

    1.4.2  Persistent aura without infarction

    1.4.3  Migrainous infarction

    1.4.4  Migraine aura-triggered seizure

**1.5  Probable migraine**

    1.5.1  Probable migraine without aura

    1.5.2  Probable migraine with aura

## 1.6  Episodic syndromes that may be associated with migraine

    1.6.1  Recurrent gastrointestinal disturbance

        1.6.1.1  Cyclical vomiting syndrome

        1.6.1.2  Abdominal migraine

    1.6.2  Benign paroxysmal vertigo

    1.6.3  Benign paroxysmal torticollis

**Source:** American Headache Society [1] In an appendix on the IHS website, there is a proposed alternative classification scheme designated intended for research. In this appendix is the entity vestibular migraine is listed under the code A1.6.6 To view the new classification click on the footnote below1.

# Acute Treatment of Migraine

Many new drugs have been added since the 1st edition of this book. The list of drugs in the next two tables is current as of May 2021. Many more are likely to be added in the future. A suggested source to keep up to date is The Migraine Trust at: https://www.migrainetrust.org/living-with-migraine/treatments/

| Acute Treatments for Migraine | | |
|---|---|---|
| **Agent** | **Route** | **Dose** |
| **Analgesics** | | |
| Acetylsalicylic Acid | Oral | 650-1300mg QQH** |
| Ibuprofen | Oral | 400-800mg QID** |
| Naproxen | Oral | 275-550mg QID |
| **Triptans** | | |
| Rizatriptan, | Oral | 10mg |
| Eletriptan, | Oral | 80mg |
| Almotriptan | Oral | 12·5mg |
| Sumatriptan | Oral | 50-100mg (repeat twice in 24 hours) |
| Sumatriptan | S/C | 6mg (repeat once in 24 hours) |
| Sumatriptan | IN | 10mg and 20 mg/0.1 ml (into 1 nostril) |
| Naratriptan | Oral | 2.5mg |
| Zolmatriptan | Oral | 2.5mg |
| **Ergotamines** | | |
| Cafergot | Oral | 1-2mg |
| Cafergot | Rectal | 2mg (max 3 doses/24 hours) |
| Ergotamine | Oral | 1-2mg (repeat 1 hour max 3 doses/24 hours) |
| Dihydroergotamine | S/C, IM, IV | 0.5-1.0mg (repeat at 1hour, max 4mg/24 hours |
| Dihydroergotamine (INP104) | Intranasal | |

---

1    Accessed 16 May 2021https://journals.sagepub.com/doi/pdf/10.1177/0333102417738202

| Acute Treatments for Migraine | | |
|---|---|---|
| **Antiemetics** | | |
| Metoclopramide | IV | 10mg |
| Prochlorperazine | Rectal | 25mg (max 3 doses/24 hours) |
| **Major Tranquillisers** | | |
| Chlorpromazine | IM, IV | 50mg IM or 0.1mg/kg over 20 minutes, repeat after 15 minutes (pre-treat with IV normal saline |
| **Opiates** | | |
| Butorphanol | IN | 1 mg in 1 nostril (repeat 3-5 hours later) |
| **NSAID** | | |
| Celecoxib oral solution | Oral | 120mg once only |
| **Corticosteroids** | | |
| Dexamethasone | IV | 10-20mg |
| **CGRP receptor. Antagonists (Gepants)** | | |
| Rimegepant | 75mg | 75mg |
| Ubrogepant | 50mg | 100mg |
| Zavegepant | 10mg 20mg | 20mg |
| **Ditans (selective serotonin 5-HT1F agonist** | | |
| Lasmiditan | 50,100 or 200mg | 50,100 or 200mg once (ne benefit of 2nd dose) |
| **External Trigeminal Nerve Stimulation** | 2 hours | Continuous stimulation of supratrochlear and supraorbital nerves bilaterally |

**Table D.1** Acute treatment of migraine.

# Preventative Treatment of Migraine

| Prophylactic Therapy for Migraine | | |
|---|---|---|
| Agent | Dose | Maximum Daily Dose |
| **Serotonin receptor Antagonists** | | |
| Methysergide | 1-2mg TDS | 8mg (max 5 months, 1 month off) |
| Pizotifen | 0.5mg | 1.5mg |
| **Tricyclic Antidepressants** | | |
| Amitriptyline | 10-150mg | 150mg |
| Nortriptyline | 10-150mg | 150mg |
| **Beta blockers** | | |
| Propranolol | 40-240mg/day | 240mg |
| Atenolol | 50-150mg/day | 150mg |
| Metoprolol | 100-200mg/day | 200mg |
| Nadolol | 40mg | 240mg |
| Timolol eye drops (0.5%) | 1 drop both eyes | 2nd dose 30 minutes later |
| **Anticonvulsants** | | |
| Valproic acid | 500-1500mg | 1500mg |
| Topiramate | 25 mg initially | 200mg |
| **Calcium channel blockers** | | |
| Verapamil | 240-320mg | 320mg |
| Flunarizine | 5-10mg | 10mg |
| **Angiotensin II blockers** | | |
| Candesartan | 16mg | 32mg |
| **CGRP Monoclonal Antibodies** | | |
| Erenumab | 70mg SC/month | 140mg SC/month |
| Fremanezumab | 225mg SC/month | 675mg SC every 3 months |
| Galcanezumab | 240mg SC loading dose | 120mg SC/month |
| Eptinezumab | 100mg IV/3 months | 300mg IV/3 months |
| OnabotulinumtoxinA | 155 U | 155 U at 12-week intervals |
| Abbreviations mg = milligram, max = maximum[2] | | |

**Table D. 2** Prophylactic treatment of migraine.

---

2   The Migraine Trust:

# References

1   Headache Classification Committee of the International Headache Society (IHS) The International Classification of Headache Disorders, 3rd edition. *Cephalalgia* 2018; 38(1): 1-211.

2   Pryse-Phillips, W.E., et al., Guidelines for the diagnosis and management of migraine in clinical practice. Canadian Headache Society. *Cmaj*, 1997. 156(9): p. 1273-87.

3   Evers, S., et al., EFNS guideline on the drug treatment of migraine – report of an EFNS task force. *Eur J Neurol*, 2006. 13(6): p. 560-72.

4   Geraud, G., A. Compagnon, and A. Rossi, Zolmitriptan versus a combination of acetylsalicylic acid and metoclopramide in the acute oral treatment of migraine: a double-blind, randomised, three-attack study. *Eur Neurol*, 2002. 47(2): p. 88-98.

5   Sorge, F. and E. Marano, Flunarizine v. placebo in childhood migraine. A double-blind study. *Cephalalgia*, 1985. 5 Suppl 2: p. 145-8.

6   Diener, H.C., et al., Efficacy, tolerability and safety of oral eletriptan and ergotamine plus caffeine (Cafergot) in the acute treatment of migraine: a multicentre, randomised, double-blind, placebo-controlled comparison. *Eur Neurol*, 2002. 47(2): p. 99-107.

7   Ferrari, M.D., et al., Oral triptans (serotonin 5-HT(1B/1D) agonists) in acute migraine treatment: a meta-analysis of 53 trials. *Lancet*, 2001. 358(9294): p. 1668-75.

8   Charles A, Pozo-Rosich P. Targeting calcitonin gene-related peptide: a new era in migraine therapy. *Lancet* 2019; 394(10210): 1765-74.

9   Ashina M, Vasudeva R, Jin L, et al. Onset of Efficacy Following Oral Treatment with Lasmiditan for the Acute Treatment of Migraine: Integrated Results From 2 Randomized Double-Blind Placebo-Controlled Phase 3 Clinical Studies. *Headache* 2019; 59(10): 1788-801.

10  Schoenen J, Jacquy J, Lenaerts M. Effectiveness of high-dose riboflavin in migraine prophylaxis. A randomized controlled trial. *Neurology* 1998;50(2):466–470.

11  MacLennan SC, et al. High-dose riboflavin for migraine prophylaxis in children: A double-blind, randomized, placebo-controlled trial. *J Child Neurol* 2008;23(11):1300–1304.

12  Dodick DW, et al. Topiramate versus amitriptyline in migraine prevention: A 26-week, multicenter, randomized, double-blind, double-dummy, parallel-group noninferiority trial in adult migraineurs. *Clin Ther* 2009;31(3):542–559.

13  Louis P, Spierings EL. Comparison of flunarizine (Sibelium) and pizotifen (Sandomigran) in migraine treatment: A double-blind study. *Cephalalgia* 1982;2(4):197–203.

14  Pryse-Phillips WE, et al. Guidelines for the diagnosis and management of migraine in clinical practice. Canadian Headache Society. *CMAJ* 1997;156(9):1273–1287.

15  Evers S, et al. EFNS guideline on the drug treatment of migraine – report of an EFNS task force. *Eur J Neurol* 2006;13(6):560–572.

16  Geraud G, Compagnon A, Rossi A. Zolmitriptan versus a combination of acetylsalicylic acid and metoclopramide in the acute oral treatment of migraine: A double-blind, randomised, three-attack study. *Eur Neurol* 2002;47(2):88–98.

17  Sorge F, Marano E. Flunarizine v. placebo in childhood migraine. A double-blind study. *Cephalalgia* 1985;5(Suppl 2):145–148.

18  Diener HC, et al. Efficacy, tolerability and safety of oral eletriptan and ergotamine plus caffeine (Cafergot) in the acute treatment of migraine: A multicentre, randomised, double-blind, placebo-controlled comparison. *Eur Neurol* 2002;47(2):99–107.

19  Ferrari MD, et al. Oral triptans (serotonin 5-HT(1B/1D) agonists) in acute migraine treatment: A meta-analysis of 53 trials. *Lancet* 2001;358(9294):1668–1675.

20  Ashina M, Vasudeva R, Jin L, et al. Onset of Efficacy Following Oral Treatment with Lasmiditan for the Acute Treatment of Migraine: Integrated Results From 2 Randomized Double-Blind Placebo-Controlled Phase 3 Clinical Studies. *Headache* 2019; 59(10): 1788-801.

21  Charles, A., Pozo-Rosich P. Targeting calcitonin gene-related peptide: a new era in migraine therapy. *Lancet* 2019; 394(10210): 1765-74.

22  American Headache Society. The American Headache Society Position Statement on Integrating New Migraine Treatments into Clinical Practice. *Headache: The Journal of Head and Face Pain* 2019; 59(1): 1-18.

23  Ailani, J., et al. (2021). "The American Headache Society Consensus Statement: Update on integrating new migraine treatments into clinical practice." *Headache* 61(7): 1021-1039

24  Dodick DW, Turkel CC, DeGryse RE, et al. OnabotulinumtoxinA for treatment of chronic migraine: pooled results from the double-blind, randomized, placebo-controlled phases of the PREEMPT clinical program. *Headache* 2010; 50(6): 921-36.

25  Lipton RB, Nye BL, Hirman J, Aurora SK, Shrewsbury SB. Treatment consistency across multiple migraine attacks: Results from the phase 3 open label STOP 301 study. *Headache* 2021; 61(Abstract P-183): 148.

26  Croop R, Madonia J, Conway CM, al. e. Intranasal zavegepant is effective and well tolerated for the acute treatment of migraine: A phase 2/3 dose-ranging clinical trial. *Headache 2021;61(S1):104-105*; 61: 1-4-105.

27  Kuruvilla DE, Starling AJ, Tepper SJ, Mann JI, Johnson M. A phase 3 randomized, double-blind, sham-controlled trial of e-TNS for the acute treatment of migraine (TEAM) *Headache* 2021; 61(Abstract IOR-02).

28  Geraud G, Compagnon A, Rossi A. Zolmitriptan versus a combination of acetylsalicylic acid and metoclopramide in the acute oral treatment of migraine: a double-blind, randomised, three-attack study. *Eur Neurol* 2002; 47(2): 88-98.

29  Sorge F, Marano E. Flunarizine v. placebo in childhood migraine. A double-blind study. Cephalalgia: an international journal of headache 1985; 5 Suppl 2: 145-8. 30 Diener HC, Jansen JP, Reches A, Pascual J, Pitei D, Steiner TJ. Efficacy, tolerability and safety of oral eletriptan and ergotamine plus caffeine (Cafergot) in the acute treatment of migraine: a multicentre, randomised, double-blind, placebo-controlled comparison. *Eur Neurol* 2002; 47(2): 99-107.

31  Ferrari MD, Roon KI, Lipton RB, Goadsby PJ. Oral triptans (serotonin 5-HT(1B/1D) agonists) in acute migraine treatment: a meta-analysis of 53 trials. Lancet (London, England) 2001; 358(9294): 1668-75.

32  Pryse-Phillips WE, Dodick DW, Edmeads JG, et al. Guidelines for the diagnosis and management of migraine in clinical practice. Canadian Headache Society. *CMAJ: Canadian Medical Association Journal* 1997; 156(9): 1273-87.

33  Evers S, Afra J, Frese A, et al. EFNS guideline on the drug treatment of migraine – report of an EFNS task force. *Eur J Neurol* 2006; 13(6): 560-72.

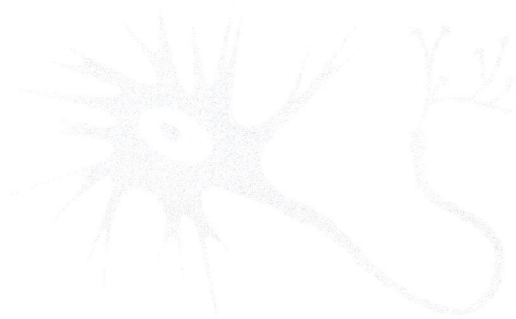

| Warning |
|---|
| The information in this appendix will be rapidly out of date. Always check the latest guidelines. |

# Epidemiology and Primary Prevention of Stroke

Increasing age, hypertension, atrial fibrillation, hyperlipidaemia, diabetes, obesity, and smoking are the major risk factors for cerebral vascular disease. **Increasing age is by far the most significant risk factor for stroke.** Beyond the age of 55 years, the prevalence of stroke almost doubles every ten years. [1, 2]

A family history of stroke or transient ischaemic attack (TIA) increases the risk by 1.4–2.4 times (95% CI 0.60–6.03). [3] The relative risk of stroke with a paternal history is 2.4 (95% CI 0.96–6.03), while with a maternal history, it is 1.4 (95% CI 0.60–3.25). [3]

The relative risk of stroke with the other currently recognised risk factors is shown in Table E.1. The high prevalence of hypertension, diabete and smoking makes these risk factors the most significant. Fortunately, in the western world, the prevalence of smoking is declining. Sadly, this is not the case in Asia.

| Risk factor | Prevalence (%) | Relative risk of stroke |
|---|---|---|
| Hypertension | 20–60 | 1–4* |
| Cigarette smoking | 12–18 | 1.8 |
| Diabetes | 5–27 | 1.8–6 |
| Non-valvular atrial fibrillation | 1.5–23.5** | 2.6–4.5 |
| Dyslipidaemia | 15 | 1.5–2.5 |
| Coronary artery disease | 5.6–8.4 | 1.55–1.73 |
| Asymptomatic carotid stenosis | 2–7 | 2.0 |

**Table E.1** Influence of risk factors on the relative risk of stroke. *The influence of hypertension diminishes with increasing age. The relative risk of stroke in patients with hypertension is 4 at 50, 3 at 60, 2 at 70, 1.8 at

80 and 1.0 at 90 years of age. **The prevalence of AF increases dramatically after 80; the prevalence is 1.5 at 50–59, 2.8 at 60–69, 9.9 at 70–79 and 23.5 at 80–89 years of age. Hypertension, smoking, and alcohol abuse are risk factors for subarachnoid haemorrhage. [4] Increasing age, hypertension, high alcohol intake and male sex are risk factors for intracerebral haemorrhage. [5]

The risk of atrial fibrillation (AF) -related stroke can be estimated using either the $CHADS_2$, the $CHA_2DS_2$-VASc score [6] or the score derived from the Framingham study. [7] The $CHADS_2$ score, and the risk of stroke are shown in tables E.2 and E.3. The $CHA_2DS_2$-VASc score, and risk of stroke are shown in tables E.4 and E.5.

Primary prevention refers to the institution of therapy for those risk factors that can be modified. There a many risk factors that increase the risk of cerebral vascular disease, some, such as a genetic predisposition and ageing, cannot be altered. Hypertension and AF are the two most significant risk factors for which primary prevention is most effective.

# Lifestyle Advice

The following lifestyle modifications[1] are encouraged for all:
1. Weight reduction if overweight.
2. Limitation of alcohol intake (men 1–2, women one standard drink per day)
3. Increased aerobic physical activity (30–45 minutes daily, or at least <u>150 minutes of moderate physical activity</u> or 75 minutes of vigorous physical exercise (or an equivalent combination of both) each week. )
4. Reduction of sodium intake (< 2.30g) [47]
5. Maintenance of adequate dietary potassium (260 mmol/L.4,700mg/dL)
6. Smoking cessation
7. Dietary Approaches to Stop Hypertension (DASH) diet. DASH is a diet rich in fruit, vegetables, whole grains, low-fat dairy products, skinless poultry and fish, nuts, and legumes, reduced in saturated and total fat and the use of non-tropical vegetable oils). [8, 9]

# Hypertension

In the early 1960s, insurance companies identified the link between hypertension and stroke. [10] The relative risk of death due to vascular lesions of the nervous system was 1.6 for blood pressure (BP) of 130–147/83–92 mmHg, rising to as high as 6.2 for a BP of 148–177/93–102 mmHg.

The 1967 Veterans Administration study [11] of only 143 patients with a diastolic BP above 115 mmHg resulted in a relative risk reduction (RRR) of 83%, an absolute risk reduction (ARR) of 36% with numbers needed to treat (NNT) of only 3.3! Contrast this with the SPRINT study of 9361 comparing intensive (systolic BP < 120 mm Hg) versus standard care (systolic BP<140mm Hg) at increased risk of cardiovascular disease.[2] [43] The RRR for myocardial infarction, other acute coronary syndromes, stroke, heart failure, or death from cardiovascular causes was 25%.

---

1 AHA Recommendations: <u>https://www.heart.org/en/healthy-living/healthy-eating/eat-smart/nutrition-basics/aha-diet-and-lifestyle-recommendations</u>
2 Increased cardiovascular risk was defined by one or more of the following: clinical or subclinical cardiovascular disease other than stroke; chronic kidney disease, excluding polycystic kidney disease, with an estimated glomerular filtration rate (eGFR) of 20 to less than 60 ml per minute per 1.73 m2 of bodysurface area, calculated with the use of the fourvariable Modification of Diet in Renal Disease equation; a 10-year risk of cardiovascular disease of 15% or greater on the basis of the Framingham risk score; or an age of 75 years or older.

However, the ARR was only 1.6 % over 3.26 years or 0.49% per year. The NNT was 185! Side effects were more common in the intensive group. The relative risk increase (RRI) was 88%, the absolute risk increase (ARI) was 2.2% A study of intensive treatment (BP <130 vs < 150) in 8511 elderly (60-80yo) Chinese patients, the RRR was 33% for stroke over 3.34 years. The ARR was only 0.6% (0.2% per year) with NNT 193. [48]

The definition of what constitutes hypertension has evolved as further studies on the effect of treatment with various levels of BP have been undertaken. At one stage, a normal systolic BP was 100 plus the age of the patient! The Progress Study [12] demonstrated a benefit from lowering the BP in patients defined as not having hypertension. Although systolic and diastolic blood pressure increases the risk, systolic BP has a more significant prognostic effect. [39] Current guidelines recommend lowering systolic blood pressure to 120-130 mm Hg systolic patients < 65 years and to ≤ 140/90 mmHg. Many elderly patients will not be able to tolerate the medications required to achieve this level, nor will they achieve this level of BP. [9] To complicate matters further, the Berlin Initiative Study in patients over 70, particularly over 80, demonstrated increased mortality if the systolic blood pressure was reduced to less than 140/90 mm Hg. [40]

---

### Treatment of Hypertension

Initial treatment is lifestyle advice, as detailed above.

In most patients, pharmacological intervention is necessary. At least five classes of drugs, thiazide and thiazide-type diuretics, angiotensin-converting enzyme inhibitors (ACEIs), angiotensin receptor blockers (ARBs), beta-blockers and calcium antagonists (CCB), have been proven to reduce mortality. The American Guidelines state that comorbidities influence the choice of antihypertensive. They recommend ACEIs and ARBs in patients with chronic renal disease, diabetes, heart failure, and post-myocardial infarction; and BBs in those with angina pectoris, arrhythmias, post-myocardial infarction, and heart failure. [45] The European guidelines state that beta-blockers are first-line agents. Both guidelines advocate for the preferential use of thiazide and thiazide-like diuretics. Only the ACC/AHA guidelines recommend preferential use of chlorthalidone versus hydrochlorothiazide. Combination therapy is needed in many if not most patients to achieve optimal BP control; sometimes, as many as two or three drugs are required. [8] Both the American and European guidelines now recommend initiating treatment with combination therapy instead of the traditional approach using monotherapy and adding additional drugs if BP is not controlled. Both recommend combining either an ACEI or ARB with either a diuretic or calcium channel blocker. Triple therapy is recommended in non-responders with either an ACEI or ARB combined with a diuretic and a calcium channel blocker. Compliance is better when the dual or triple-drug therapy are formulated into a single pill.

In the long-term prevention of hypertension-related cardiovascular events, there is no difference between ARBs and ACE inhibitors used as monotherapy. Adverse effects are lower with ARBs. [42]

The level of blood pressure that one should initiate treatment varies depending on whether patients have a high cardiovascular risk, diabetes, kidney disease, in the general population or greater the age of 75. The Australian [44], American [45] and European guidelines [46] also differ slightly in their recommendations. These are shown in table E3 below

Many elderly patients may not tolerate the drugs or a BP < 140/90 mmHg, and it may be necessary to compromise and accept the lowest possible BP.

The TRIUMPH trial demonstrated significant benefit with modification of lifestyle (dietary counselling, behavioural weight management, and exercise) most likely because of weight loss. [49]

A pragmatic approach is to attempt to lower the blood pressure to as close as possible to 120/80 mm Hg in all patients at high risk and under the age of 75. This will ensure maximum risk reduction. One often must accept a higher systolic blood pressure because not all patients can tolerate such a significant reduction.

| | Australia 2016[44] | | USA 2017[45] | | Europe 2018[46] | |
|---|---|---|---|---|---|---|
| Hypertension definition (mmHg) | ≥140/90 | | ≥130/80 | | ≥140/90 | |
| | Start | Target | Start | Target | Start | Target |
| When to treat | ≥160/100* | <140/90 | ≥140/90 | <130/80 | ≥160/90* | <130/80 |
| | | | | | | |
| High CVD risk | ≥140/90 | <120/– | ≥130/80 | <130/80 | ≥140/90† | <130/80 |
| Older age ‡ | – | <120/– | ≥130/– | <130/– | ≥140/90 Age 80+ ≥160/90 | <130/80 |
| Diabetes | ≥140/90 | <120/90 | ≥130/80 | <130/80 | ≥140/90 | <130/80 |
| Kidney disease | ≥140/90 | <120/90 | ≥130/80 | <130/80 | ≥140/90 | <140/80 |

**Table E3** A comparison of the Australian, American and European Guidelines[3].
* For those with a systolic blood pressure of 140–159 mmHg, treatment may begin after a period of lifestyle advice.
† Treatment may be considered in those with coronary disease or stroke with a systolic blood pressure of 130–140 mmHg.
‡ Older people are ≥75 years in Australian guidelines, ≥65 years in US guidelines, while the European guidelines include separate recommendations for 65–79 years and ≥80 years.

# Atrial Fibrillation

In patients with atrial fibrillation the annual risk of stroke can be estimated from the $CHADS_2$ (see tables E.2 and E.3) or the $CHA_2DS_2$-VASc score (see tables E.4 and E.5). Anticoagulation is recommended for patients with AF who have valvular heart disease (particularly those with mechanical heart valves). Patients with non-valvular AF with a $CHA_2DS_{2\text{-VASc}}$ score of ≥1 in men and ≥ 2 in women provided no contraindications [13]. Others would argue that, although patients with a $CHADS_2$ score of 2 or more derive more significant benefit, even patients with a $CHADS_2$ score of 1 benefit from oral anticoagulant therapy with a low risk of bleeding. [14] Anticoagulation reduces the risk of stroke by as much as 60–70%. [15]

Some would argue that many of the factors perceived to be barriers to anticoagulant therapy in older persons with AF should not influence the choice of stroke prevention in these patients. [16] Impaired cognitive function is only a contraindication if the patient's medication is not supervised. The risk of falls is also a relative, not an absolute, contraindication. In patients with a high annual risk of stroke, for example, a $CHADS_2$ $CHA_2DS_2$-VASc or score of 3 or more, the slightly increased risk associated with anticoagulation is outweighed by the significant reduction in the subsequent risk of stroke. [17] There is conflicting evidence that increasing age, a propensity to falls, activities that could cause trauma and prior gastrointestinal bleeding influence the risk of anticoagulant-related bleeding. The degree of anticoagulation is the main factor influencing the risk of intracranial bleeding. [18]

The only absolute contraindications to anticoagulants are active peptic ulcer disease and the risk of bleeding. These include severe alcoholic liver disease with an elevated PT INR, epistaxis, or gastrointestinal bleeding of any cause. If the bleeding source can be identified and treated, anticoagulation could then be commenced. The HAS-BLED (see below) score can estimate a patient's risk of bleeding.

3   Atkins, E.R and Perkovic, V. Australian Prescriber 2019;42:127-130 Reproduced with permission Australian Prescriber

# How to Detect and is it Useful to Screen for AF?

Stroke and AF are more common with increasing age. Thus, many patients with CVD will have AF. The question is whether it is a mere association or whether the AF is the cause of symptoms. This is discussed below. AF may be present when the patient is first seen with their symptoms of CVD, or it may be detected if they are monitored whilst they are an inpatient. The longer the monitoring, the more likely one is to detect AF. The advent of loop recorders has increased the rate of AF detection in patients with CVD (31.8% versus 12.2%. [55] In the LOOP study, the detection of AF and commencement of anticoagulation did not significantly reduce the risk of stroke, systemic arterial embolism, death, or cardiovascular death. In the StrokeStop study [56], daily ECGs for 14 days detected AF in 12.1%, not much different from the 12.8% in the control group who did not have regular ECGs. Although the study claims there was a risk reduction in those who had AF detected with the daily ECGs, the confidence intervals reached 1.0; thus, level of benefit is negligible. Smartphones can detect an irregular pulse, but the sensitivity and specificity have yet to be determined, and caution is recommended before adopting this technology.[57]

| | Condition | Points |
|---|---|---|
| C | Congestive heart failure (in last 3 months) | 1 |
| H | Hypertension (untreated or treated) | 1 |
| A | Age > 75 years | 1 |
| D | Diabetes | 1 |
| $S_2$ | Prior stroke or TIA | 2 |

**Table E.2** $CHADS_2$ score – points allocated for each of the five entities that make up the score

| | Condition | Points |
|---|---|---|
| C | Congestive heart failure (in last 3 months) | 1 |
| H | Hypertension (untreated or treated) | 1 |
| A2 | Age 65-75 years | 1 |
| A2 | Age > 75 | 2 |
| D | Diabetes | 1 |
| $S_2$ | Prior stroke or TIA | 2 |
| VASc | Vascular disease history (prior MI, PVD, or aortic plaque) | |

**Table E.3** The $CHA_2DS_2$-VASc Score for AF Stroke Risk

| CHADS$_2$ score | Stroke risk % | 95% CI |
|---|---|---|
| 0 | 1.9 | 1.2–3.0 |
| 1 | 2.8 | 2.0–3.8 |
| 2 | 4.0 | 3.1–5.1 |
| 3 | 5.9 | 4.6–7.3 |
| 4 | 8.5 | 6.3–11.1 |
| 5 | 12.5 | 8.2–17.5 |
| 6 | 18.2 | 10.5–27.4 |

**Table E.4** The annual risk of stroke in patients with AF using the CHADS$_2$ criteria [6]*
*This score is particularly useful in explaining the balance between risk versus benefit of treatment with anticoagulants.

| CHA$_2$DS$_2$-VASc score | Ischaemic Stroke risk % | Stroke/TIA/systemic embolism |
|---|---|---|
| 0 | 0.2 | 0.3 |
| 1 | 0.6 | 0.9 |
| 2 | 2.2 | 2.9 |
| 3 | 3.2 | 4.6 |
| 4 | 4.8 | 6.7 |
| 5 | 7.2 | 10.0 |
| 6 | 9.7 | 13.6 |
| 7 | 11.2 | 15.7 |
| 8 | 10.8 | 15.2 |
| 9 | 12.2 | 17.4 |

**Table E.5** The annual risk of stroke in patients with AF using the CHA$_2$DS$_2$-Vasc criteria. [120-121] The explanation for a lower risk with a score of 8 is unclear.

## Treatment of Atrial Fibrillation

Anticoagulation is recommended for all patients with non-valvular atrial fibrillation or atrial flutter, whether paroxysmal, persistent, or permanent, who have a $CHA_2DS_2$-VASc score of 2 or greater in men or three or greater in women. That is, provided there are no absolute contraindications. [50] The absolute and relative contraindications have been discussed in the text.

If using warfarin[4] the PT INR should be maintained somewhere between 2.0 and 3.0.

A higher level of anticoagulation (PT INR 3.0–3.5) is recommended in patients with a mechanical heart valve. [20] Subsequent studies using moderate and low-dose warfarin have suggested that lower intensity anticoagulation may effectively reduce the risk of haemorrhagic complications in this group of patients. [21–23]

Warfarin is a challenging drug to use because, in most patients, the PT INR fluctuates wildly, requiring careful monitoring and frequent blood tests. The PT INR should be checked weekly during initiation and NO patient should go longer than four weeks between tests of PT INR. [50]

Since the first edition of this book, several factor Xa inhibitors apixaban, betrixaban, edoxaban, fondaparinux, idraparinux, or rivaroxaban, collectively referred to as **N**ovel (or **D**ual) **O**ral **A**nti**C**oagulants (NOAC's) and the direct thrombin inhibitors dabigratrin and ximelagatran have largely supplanted warfarin, except in patients with mechanical heart valves.

NOAC's have several advantages, not the least being that they do not require regular blood tests. They are equally effective as warfarin in reducing ischaemic stroke and are associated with a lower risk of major bleeding events. The major disadvantage in the early years was that there was no way of reversing the drugs should bleeding occur. Subsequently specific antidotes have been developed, idarucizumab for dabigatran and andexanet alfa for the FXa inhibitors. [24] If these antidotes are not available oral activated charcoal should be given if there has been recent ingestion of these drugs, and four-factor prothrombin complex concentrate (4F-PCC) should be administered.

NOAC's are now recommended over warfarin for patients with AF except for those with moderate-severe mitral stenosis or mechanical heart valves. [50]

Vitamin K and 4F-PCC are recommended to reverse warfarin.

In patients in whom anticoagulation is contra-indicated percutaneous left atrial appendage (LAA) occlusion may be considered. [50] The current American College of Cardiology/American Heart Association Task Force on Clinical Practice Guidelines and the Heart Rhythm Society guidelines suggest that AF catheter ablation may be reasonable in selected patients with symptomatic AF and heart failure reduced left ventricular (LV) ejection fraction. [50] A meta-analysis of randomised clinical trials including first-line therapy of patients with paroxysmal AF found that catheter ablation compared with antiarrhythmic drugs was associated with reductions in recurrence of atrial arrhythmias and hospitalization's, with no difference in major adverse events. [51]

The European Society of Cardiology, European Heart Rhythm Association and European Association for Cardio-Thoracic Surgery (EACTS) 2020 guidelines [52] suggest that catheter ablation can be considered as first line therapy rather than in those who fail anti-arrhythmic drug control of rhythm. Anticoagulation is recommended even after catheter ablation in high-risk patients. Catheter ablation is more effective when performed in the first year and in patients with paroxysmal AF.

At this point in time there is no unambiguous evidence to help choose between the various NOAC's in terms of efficacy nor to advocate ablation therapy as first line treatment. A 2021 study found that rivaroxaban has a slightly higher risk (HR, 1.40[CI 1.01 to 1.94]) of gastrointestinal bleeding than other NOAC's. [80]

---

4    *The name warfarin stems from the acronym WARF, for Wisconsin Alumni Research Foundation + the ending -arin, indicating its link with coumarin, the first naturally occurring anticoagulant discovered in mouldy sweet clover [19]*

| Contrarian thought |
|---|
| If we look at the CHA$_2$DS$_2$-VASc scoring systems, the annual risk of stroke with isolated AF (no other risk factors) is 0.2-0.3%, i.e., negligible. The factors that increase the risk are the very same factors that increase the risk of stroke in patients without AF. Could this be the reason anticoagulation needs to be continued in high-risk patients after catheter ablation? Interrogation of loop recorders, defibrillators and pacemakers has shown that only 2% of patients have subclinical AF > 6 minutes duration at the time of their stroke. [53] |
|     Is AF the significant risk factor for stroke that we have all been taught to believe? Is it time we did a trial of anticoagulation in patients with high CHA$_2$DS$_2$-VASC scores in the absence of AF? I am not the only one who has had this same contrarian thought. [54] |

# HAS-BLED Score for Major Bleeding

The HAS-BLED score can be used to estimate and advise patients of the risk of major bleeding.

| HAS-BLED Score | % Risk of Major Bleeding |
|---|---|
| 0 | 0.9 |
| 1 | 3.4 |
| 2 | 4.1 |
| 3 | 5.8 |
| 4 | 8.9 |
| 5 | 9.1 |

**Table E6.** The risk of major bleeding.

Score 1 point for:
- Uncontrolled hypertension (greater than 160 mm Hg systolic)
- Renal disease (dialysis, transplant creatinine greater than 2.26 mg/dL or greater than 200 μmol per litre)
- Liver disease (cirrhosis, bilirubin twice normal, AST/ALT/AP greater than three times normal)
- Stroke history and
- Major bleeding or predisposition to bleeding. [125,126]

# Asymptomatic Carotid Stenosis

The 5-year-risk of stroke is 11.8% for all strokes and 6.1% for fatal or disabling strokes in patients with asymptomatic carotid stenosis. [25] Thus, the risk of severe or disabling stroke is incredibly low (1.2% per annum). The absolute risk reduction of carotid endarterectomy (CEA) over five years is similar in asymptomatic carotid stenosis to that of symptomatic patients with a moderate degree of stenosis (50–69%). In patients with asymptomatic stenosis of 50–69%, ARR was 5.8% in the Asymptomatic Carotid Atherosclerosis Study (ACAS) [26] and 6% in the Asymptomatic Carotid Surgery Trial (ACST) [25], i.e., approximately 1% per year.

In 2009 the European Society of Vascular Surgeons (ESVS) published guidelines recommended: [28]

- CEA in asymptomatic men < 75 years old with 70–99% stenosis if the perioperative stroke/death risk is < 3%.
- The benefit in women with asymptomatic stenosis is significantly less than in men; CEA should therefore be considered only in younger, fit women.
- Aspirin at a dose of 75–325 mg daily and statins should be given before, during and following CEA.
- Carotid artery stenting (CAS) is recommended for patients at high risk with CEA.

The American Society for vascular surgery guidelines recommends carotid endarterectomy and maximal medical therapy for asymptomatic carotid stenosis greater than 75% in low-risk surgical patients! [59]

The Cochrane review suggests that there is insufficient evidence to conclude if endarterectomy should be performed in asymptomatic patients. [29]

Since the first edition, many [74-78] have questioned whether patients with asymptomatic carotid stenosis should be subjected to carotid endarterectomy or carotid stenting. The US Preventive Services Task Force has concluded with moderate certainty that the harms of screening for asymptomatic carotid stenosis outweigh the benefits. [58,75] The American Heart Association (AHA) advises against long-term follow-up imaging of the extracranial carotid circulation with carotid duplex Ultrasound. [79]

*This is yet another example where physicians and surgeons can read precisely the same literature and come to different conclusions.*

---

**Management of Asymptomatic Carotid Stenosis**

Patients with asymptomatic carotid stenosis should be offered maximum medical therapy for their risk factors. An acceptable stroke complication rate of endarterectomy for patients with asymptomatic stenosis is < 3%. There is no evidence that complication rates of CEA have been lower in recent years; on the contrary, they may be a little higher than those reported in the randomised controlled trials. This higher complication rate may reflect the older age of patients undergoing endarterectomy. [27] The published complication rates are irrelevant to the individual patient Every institution should continuously monitor its complication rate. If too high, they need to reduce it or abandon carotid endarterectomy in their institution.

The practical reality is that many patients with high-grade asymptomatic carotid stenosis feel like they are walking around with a timebomb in their neck. They often seek surgery even when advised against surgery.[5] CEA may be unavoidable in patients with high-grade (>80% stenosis)

---

# Hyperlipidaemia

High total cholesterol and low high-density lipoprotein (LDL) cholesterol are associated with an increased risk of stroke. Treatment can result in a significant relative risk reduction. [30] To put this into perspective, let us use the American College of Cardiology/American Heart Association ASCVD risk calculator[6] in a patient with no other risk factors other than elevated cholesterol. If we take a hypothetical 60-year-old man with a BP of 130/90 with normal cholesterol of 130 mg/dL

---

5   Personal observation, I describe the symptoms they might experience, i.e., transient blindness in the eye on the same side, weakness, and numbness on the opposite and if a left carotid stenosis a transient inability to speak. I inform the patient that if they experience these symptoms, they should seek urgent medical attention as the risk of stroke is much higher in patients who develop symptoms.

6   http://www.cvriskcalculator.com/

(7.2 mmol/L) and a normal high-density lipoprotein (HDL) of 60 mg/dL. (3.3 mmol/L) His 10-year-risk of heart attack and stroke is 5.2%. If his total cholesterol is exceedingly high at 240 mg/dL (13.3 mmol/L), his HDL is low 30 mg/dL (1.7 mmol) and his BP 130/80, his 10-year-risk increases to 14.9%. This almost threefold relative increased risk equates to an absolute risk increase of only 0.97% per year greater than someone without elevated cholesterol. This is relevant when dealing with patients who cannot tolerate statins.

Several statins have been studied in patients with atherosclerotic vascular disease, and there is no evidence supporting one more than another. High-dose atorvastatin (80 mg) resulted in a modest 5-year ARR of 2.2% or 0.44% per year (adjusted hazard ratio, 0.84; 95% confidence interval, 0.71–0.99; P=0.03; unadjusted P=0.05) and a RRR of 14.5% in patients with high cholesterol and cerebral ischaemia but without known coronary artery disease. [31]

Recent data demonstrate that apolipoprotein B (apo B) is a better measure of circulating LDL particle numbers (LDL-P) and is a more reliable risk indicator than LDL-C. It has been recommended that the measurement of apo B be added to the routine assessment of patients at risk [32].

It has been assumed that the reduction in risk demonstrated in the statin trials reflects the reduction in cholesterol, but this may not be the case. Rosuvastatin 20 mg/day has been shown to reduce myocardial infarction, stroke, arterial revascularisation, hospitalisation for unstable angina or death from cardiovascular causes in patients with high-sensitivity C-reactive protein (CRP) levels of 2.0 mg/L or higher in the absence of elevated cholesterol (a low-density glycoprotein cholesterol level < 3.4 mmol/L). The hazard ratio for stroke was 0.18 in the treatment group and 0.34 in the control group (hazard ratio, 0.52; 95% CI, 0.34–0.79; P = 0.002). [33]

A systematic review and meta-analysis of randomised controlled trials of statins for the primary prevention of CVD (94,283 participants) concluded that there was a statistically significant relative risk reduction in non-fatal myocardial infarction (RRR 38%), CVD mortality (RRR 20%) and non-fatal stroke (RRR 17%). The ARR is approximately 1% for primary prevention. This reduction was associated with a slightly increased risk of intracerebral haemorrhage. The NNT is approximately 200 for primary prevention. Each mmol/L reduction of LDL equates to a RRR of 25%. [34] The absolute risk reduction of fatal and non-fatal stroke in the SPARCL trial was 2.2 % over five years (0.44% per year). [66] Ezetimibe at a dose of 10 mg per day reduces LDL cholesterol by 20%. Combined with simvastatin, it resulted in a 17% RRR and a negligible 0.7% ARR over six years, representing a little over 0.1% annual absolute risk reduction. [68] This minimal ARR can be used to reassure patients that they are not walking with a Sword of Damocles over their head if they cannot tolerate their statins due to side effects. Muscle pain is the main side-effect of statins. Two other rarer complications include HMG-CoA antibody-induced myositis and rhabdomyolysis. [69]

| Treatment of Hyperlipidaemia-Current Guidelines |
|---|
| Modification of lifestyle is the first step. Lifestyle changes are recommended if (a) the 10-year ASCVD risk is ≤ 7.5%, (b) ≥ 7.5 and ≤ 20% with the possible addition of a statin. If the 10-year-risk is ≥ 20% in addition to lifestyle changes a statin is recommended to reduce the LDL-C ≥ 50%. The cholesterol decreases by 0.23 mmol/L (8.69 mg/dL) for every 10 kg weight loss. [64] |
| A review of dietary treatment found that diet reduced the LDL levels by approximately 15% (although the range varies from 0% to 37%). [65] |
| Lipid-modifying medications can reduce the relative risk of stroke in high-risk patients with coronary heart disease. [9] **Statins** (3-hydroxy-3-methylglutaryl-coenzyme A reductase inhibitors), **ezetimibe** (blocks cholesterol absorption from the gastrointestinal tract) and the **PCSK9** inhibitors (reduce the degradation of LDL receptors and increases the clearance of LDL cholesterol). |
| The current American Heart Association/American College of Cardiology (AHA/ACC) guidelines [67] recommend high-intensity statin therapy for primary prevention in patients with severe primary hypercholesterolaemia (LDL-C level ≥ 10.6 mmol/L (190 mg/dL). A more aggressive approach is recommended in patients with diabetes aged 40-75. Moderate-intensity statin is recommended if the LDL-C is ≥ 3.9 mmol/L (70 mg/dL). The current American Heart Association/American Stroke Association guidelines do not specify a target LDL level. The AHA/ACC guidelines recommend lowering the LDL cholesterol to <3.9 mmol/L (70 mg/dL) Ezetimibe and the PCSK9 inhibitors are not discussed in the current guidelines. The European Society of Cardiology (ESC) and European Atherosclerosis Society (EAS) guidelines [69] recommend the addition of ezetimibe if maximum tolerated statins do not lower the LDL-C ≥ 50% and the addition of the PCSK9 inhibitors if this combination does not achieve a lower LDL-C. |

# Diabetes

The relative risk of stroke with diabetes is 1.8–6. [35] In the Diabetes Control and Complications Trial (DCCT) and the Epidemiology of Diabetes Interventions and Complications (EDIC) study, lower levels of HbA1c were associated with thinner carotid IMT, less coronary calcification, and a lower incidence of clinical cardiovascular events, including myocardial infarction, stroke, and cardiac death. [81] In reality, endocrinologists attempt to optimise diabetes control in all patients.

# Obesity

The relative risk of stroke with obesity is 1.75–2.37 [36]. The benefit of treatment is unknown and relates to the difficulty patients experience with weight reduction. The lowering of BP with weight loss will reduce the incidence of stroke. [37]

All patients should be encouraged to lose weight, and a dietician should see the patient and their spouse. In clinical practice, a pragmatic approach is required. Suppose attempts to lose weight make both the patient and their family utterly miserable. In that case, it is wise to encourage a more modest amount of weight reduction or accept that it is not possible. Several drugs are approved in some countries that induce a modest weight loss. These include phentermine-topiramate (Qsymia), orlistat (Xenical), naltrexone-bupropion (Contrave), glucagon-like peptide-1receptor agonist (GLP-1RA), liraglutide (Saxenda) and semaglutide (Wegovy). [82] Bariatric surgery reduces the risk of TIA, myocardial infarction but not ischaemic stroke. [83] As cardiovascular disease is the main cause of death in patients with cerebral vascular disease it would seem appropriate to recommend bariatric surgery to the morbidly obese.

During the 2nd half of World War II severe food shortages occurred in West Germany, Finland, and Norway, but not in southern Germany or Switzerland. [84-87] People ate as little as 1,000-1,200 calories a day. In the countries with severe food shortages, this led to marked weight loss, their cholesterol levels fell from 230 to 140 mg/dL (5.95 to 3.62 mmol/L), and there were no deaths due to heart attacks or strokes. In western Germany, complicated atherosclerosis was absent at autopsy. Similarly, autopsies on prisoners of war who died of starvation had mainly smooth arteries with little atherosclerosis. [87] In Switzerland and Southern Germany, where there was no food shortage and obesity, heart attacks and strokes persisted throughout the war. Five years after the war, all these diseases reappeared in the countries where they had disappeared[7]. [86]

# Smoking

Smoking increases the risk of stroke 1.8-fold. There is a relative risk reduction of 50% within one year, and the risk is back to a baseline level five years after smoking cessation. [38]

# Antiplatelet Therapy & Primary Prevention

Three prospective trials of antiplatelet therapy for the primary prevention of stroke have not found convincing evidence of efficacy. [70-73] In 2021, the USPTF[8] issued the following draft recommendations. The decision to initiate low-dose aspirin use for the primary prevention of CVD in adults ages 40 to 59 years who have a 10% or greater 10-year CVD risk should be an individual one. Evidence indicates that the net benefit of aspirin use in this group is small. Persons who are not at increased risk for bleeding and are willing to take low-dose aspirin daily are more likely to benefit. The USPSTF recommends against initiating low-dose aspirin use for the primary prevention of CVD in adults age 60 years or older.

# References

1   Gunarathne A, et al. Secular trends in the cardiovascular risk profile and mortality of stroke admissions in an inner city, multiethnic population in the United Kingdom (1997–2005). *J Hum Hypertens* 2008;22(1):18–23.

2   Brown RD, et al. Stroke incidence, prevalence, and survival: Secular trends in Rochester, Minnesota, through 1989. *Stroke* 1996;27(3):373–380.

3   Kiely DK, et al. Familial aggregation of stroke. The Framingham Study. *Stroke* 1993;24(9):1366–1371.

4   Teunissen LL, et al. Risk factors for subarachnoid hemorrhage: A systematic review. *Stroke* 1996;27(3):544–549.

5   Ariesen MJ, et al. Risk factors for intracerebral hemorrhage in the general population: A systematic review. *Stroke* 2003;34(8):2060–2065.

6   Gage BF, et al. Validation of clinical classification schemes for predicting stroke: Results from the National Registry of Atrial Fibrillation. *JAMA* 2001;285(22):2864–2870.

7   I have informed patients of these facts. I have suggested that if they want to abolish their risk of stroke, they need to go on a starvation diet of 1200 calories/day!

8   https://www.uspreventiveservicestaskforce.org/uspstf/draft-recommendation/aspirin-use-to-prevent-cardiovascular-disease-preventive-medication#bootstrap-panel--6

7   Wang TJ, et al. A risk score for predicting stroke or death in individuals with new-onset atrial fibrillation in the community: The Framingham Heart Study. *JAMA* 2003;290(8):1049–1056.

8   Chobanian AV, et al. Seventh report of the Joint National Committee on Prevention, Detection, Evaluation, and Treatment of High Blood Pressure. *Hypertension* 2003;42(6):1206–1252.

9   Goldstein LB, et al. Primary prevention of ischemic stroke: A guideline from the American Heart Association/American Stroke Association Stroke Council: Cosponsored by the Atherosclerotic Peripheral Vascular Disease Interdisciplinary Working Group; Cardiovascular Nursing Council; Clinical Cardiology Council; Nutrition, Physical Activity, and Metabolism Council; and the Quality of Care and Outcomes Research Interdisciplinary Working Group: The American Academy of Neurology affirms the value of this guideline. *Stroke* 2006;37(6):1583–1633.

10  Metropolitan Life Insurance Company. *Blood pressure: Insurance experience and its implications*. New York: Metropolitan Life Insurance Company; 1961.

11  Veterans Administration Cooperative Study Group on Antihypertensive Agents. Effects of Treatment on morbidity in hypertension. Results in patients with diastolic blood pressures averaging 115 through 129 mm Hg. *JAMA* 1967;202(11):1028–1034.

12  Progress Study Group. Randomised trial of a perindopril-based blood-pressure-lowering regimen among 6,105 individuals with previous stroke or transient ischaemic attack. *Lancet* 2001;358(9287):1033–1041.

13  Singer DE, et al. Antithrombotic therapy in atrial fibrillation: American College of Chest Physicians Evidence-Based Clinical Practice Guidelines (8th edn). *Chest* 2008;133(6 Suppl):546S–592S.

14  Healey JS, et al. Risks and benefits of oral anticoagulation compared with clopidogrel plus aspirin in patients with atrial fibrillation according to stroke risk: The atrial fibrillation clopidogrel trial with irbesartan for prevention of vascular events (ACTIVE-W). *Stroke* 2008;39(5):1482–1486.

15  Go AS, et al. Anticoagulation therapy for stroke prevention in atrial fibrillation: How well do randomised trials translate into clinical practice?. *JAMA* 2003;290(20):2685–2692.

16  Man-Son-Hing M, Laupacis A. Anticoagulant-related bleeding in older persons with atrial fibrillation: Physicians' fears often unfounded. *Arch Intern Med* 2003;163(13):1580–1586.

17  Man-Son-Hing M, et al. Choosing antithrombotic therapy for elderly patients with atrial fibrillation who are at risk for falls. *Arch Intern Med* 1999;159(7):677–685.

18  Gage BF, et al. Incidence of intracranial hemorrhage in patients with atrial fibrillation who are prone to fall. *Am J Med* 2005;118(6):612–617.

19  Pirmohamed, M. (2006). "Warfarin: almost 60 years old and still causing problems." Br J Clin Pharmacol 62(5): 509-511. https://www.warf.org/event/the-warfarin-story-groundbreaking-ceremony-and-public-presentation/

20  Smith AG. Guidelines on oral anticoagulation: Second edition. *J Clin Pathol* 1991;44(1):86.

21  Saour JN, et al. Trial of different intensities of anticoagulation in patients with prosthetic heart valves. *N Engl J Med* 1990;322(7):428–432.

22  Pengo V, et al. A comparison of a moderate with moderate-high intensity oral anticoagulant treatment in patients with mechanical heart valve prostheses. *Thromb Haemost* 1997;77(5):839–844.

23  Acar J, et al. AREVA: Multicenter randomised comparison of low-dose versus standard-dose anticoagulation in patients with mechanical prosthetic heart valves. *Circulation* 1996;94(9):2107–2112.

24  Connolly SJ, et al. Dabigatran versus warfarin in patients with atrial fibrillation. *N Engl J Med* 2009;361(12):1139–1151.

25  Halliday A, et al. Prevention of disabling and fatal strokes by successful carotid endarterectomy in patients without recent neurological symptoms: Randomised controlled trial. *Lancet* 2004;363(9420):1491–1502.

26  Executive Committee for the Asymptomatic Carotid Atherosclerosis Study. Endarterectomy for asymptomatic carotid artery stenosis. *JAMA* 1995;273(18):1421–1428.

27  Rerkasem K, Rothwell PM. Temporal trends in the risks of stroke and death due to endarterectomy for symptomatic carotid stenosis: An updated systematic review. *Eur J Vasc Endovasc Surg* 2009;37(5):504–511.

28    Liapis CD, et al. ESVS guidelines. Invasive Treatment for carotid stenosis: Indications, techniques. *Eur J Vasc Endovasc Surg* 2009;37(4 Suppl):1–19.

29    Müller MD, Lyrer P, Brown MM, Bonati LH. Carotid artery stenting versus endarterectomy for treatment of carotid artery stenosis. *Cochrane Database of Systematic Reviews* 2020; (2).

30    National Institutes of Health ATP III. *Detection, evaluation, and Treatment of high blood cholesterol in adults*. Bethesda, Maryland: National Institutes of Health; 2002.

31    Amarenco P, et al. High-dose atorvastatin after stroke or transient ischemic attack. *N Engl J Med* 2006;355(6):549–559.

32    Contois JH, et al. Apolipoprotein B and cardiovascular disease risk: Position statement from the AACC Lipoproteins and Vascular Diseases Division Working Group on Best Practices. *Clin Chem* 2009;55(3):407–419.

33    Ridker PM, et al. Rosuvastatin to prevent vascular events in men and women with elevated C-reactive protein. *N Engl J Med* 2008;359(21):2195–2207.

34    Collins R, Reith C, Emberson J, et al. Interpretation of the evidence for the efficacy and safety of statin therapy. *The Lancet* 2016; 388(10059): 2532-61.

35    Force UPST. *Guide to clinical preventive services*. 2nd edn Baltimore: Williams & Wilkins; 1996.

36    Welin L, et al. Risk factors for coronary heart disease during 25 years of follow-up. The study of men born in 1913. *Cardiology* 1993;82(2–3):223–228.

37    Neter JE, et al. influence of weight reduction on blood pressure: A meta-analysis of randomised controlled trials. *Hypertension* 2003;42(5):878–884.

38    Wolf PA, et al. Cigarette smoking as a risk factor for stroke. The Framingham Study. *JAMA* 1988;259(7):1025–1029.

39    Flint AC, Conell C, Ren X, et al. Effect of Systolic and Diastolic Blood Pressure on Cardiovascular Outcomes. *N Engl J Med* 2019; 381(3): 243-51.

40    Douros A, Tölle M, Ebert N, et al. Control of blood pressure and risk of mortality in a cohort of older adults: the Berlin Initiative Study. *Eur Heart J* 2019; 40(25): 2021-8.

41    Chobanian AV, Bakris GL, Black HR, et al. Seventh report of the Joint National Committee on Prevention, Detection, Evaluation, and Treatment of High Blood Pressure. *Hypertension* 2003; 42(6): 1206-52.

42    Chen R, Suchard MA, Krumholz HM, et al. Comparative First-Line Effectiveness and Safety of ACE (Angiotensin-Converting Enzyme) Inhibitors and Angiotensin Receptor Blockers: A Multinational Cohort Study. *Hypertension* 2021; 78(3): 591-603.

43    Wright JT, Jr., Williamson JD, Whelton PK, et al. A Randomised Trial of Intensive versus Standard Blood-Pressure Control. *N Engl J Med* 2015; 373(22): 2103-16.

44    Gabb GM, Mangoni AA, Anderson CS, et al. Guideline for the diagnosis and management of hypertension in adults - 2016. *Med J Aust* 2016; 205(2): 85-9.

45    Whelton PK, Carey RM, Aronow WS, et al. 2017 ACC/AHA/AAPA/ABC/ACPM/ AGS/APhA/ASH/ ASPC/NMA/PCNA Guideline for the Prevention, Detection, Evaluation, and Management of High Blood Pressure in Adults: Executive Summary. *A Report of the American College of Cardiology/American Heart Association Task Force on Clinical Practice Guidelines* 2018; 71(19): 2199-269

46    Williams B, Mancia G, Spiering W, et al. 2018 ESC/ESH Guidelines for the management of arterial hypertension. *Eur Heart J* 2018; 39(33): 3021-104.

47    Neal B, Wu Y, Feng X, et al. Effect of Salt Substitution on Cardiovascular Events and Death. *New England Journal of Medicine* 2021.

48    Zhang W, Zhang S, Deng Y, et al. Trial of Intensive Blood-Pressure Control in Older Patients with Hypertension. *New England Journal of Medicine* 2021; 385(14): 1268-79.

49    Blumenthal JA, Hinderliter AL, Smith PJ, et al. Effects of Lifestyle Modification on Patients With Resistant Hypertension: Results of the TRIUMPH Randomized Clinical Trial. *Circulation*; 2021; 144(15):1212-1226.

50 January CT, Wann LS, Calkins H, et al. 2019 AHA/ACC/HRS Focused Update of the 2014 AHA/ACC/HRS Guideline for the Management of Patients with Atrial Fibrillation: A Report of the American College of Cardiology/American Heart Association Task Force on Clinical Practice Guidelines and the Heart Rhythm Society in Collaboration with the Society of Thoracic Surgeons. *Circulation* 2019; 140(2): e125-e51.

51 Turagam MK, Musikantow D, Whang W, et al. Assessment of Catheter Ablation or Antiarrhythmic Drugs for First-line Therapy of Atrial Fibrillation: A Meta-analysis of Randomised Clinical Trials. *JAMA Cardiology* 2021; 6(6): 697-705.

52 Hindricks G, Potpara T, Dagres N, et al. 2020 ESC Guidelines for the diagnosis and management of atrial fibrillation developed in collaboration with the European Association for Cardio-Thoracic Surgery (EACTS): The Task Force for the diagnosis and management of atrial fibrillation of the European Society of Cardiology (ESC) Developed with the special contribution of the European Heart Rhythm Association (EHRA) of the ESC. *European Heart Journal* 2020; 42(5): 373-498.

53 Martin DT, Bersohn MM, Waldo AL, et al. Randomised trial of atrial arrhythmia monitoring to guide anticoagulation in patients with implanted defibrillator and cardiac resynchronisation devices. *Eur Heart J* 2015; 36(26): 1660-8.

54 Bayés de Luna A, Baranchuk A, Martínez-Sellés M, Platonov PG. Anticoagulation in patients at high risk of stroke without documented atrial fibrillation. Time for a paradigm shift? *Ann Noninvasive Electrocardiol* 2017; 22(1).

55 Svennberg E, Friberg L, Frykman V, Al-Khalili F, Engdahl J, Rosenqvist M. Clinical outcomes in systematic screening for atrial fibrillation (STROKESTOP): a multicentre, parallel group, unmasked, randomised controlled trial. *The Lancet* 2021; 398(10310):1498-1506.

56 Svendsen JH, Diederichsen SZ, Højberg S, et al. Implantable loop recorder detection of atrial fibrillation to prevent stroke (The LOOP Study): a randomised controlled trial. *The Lancet* 2021; 398(10310):1507-1516

57 Seshadri DR, Bittel B, Browsky D, et al. Accuracy of Apple Watch for Detection of Atrial Fibrillation. *Circulation* 2020; 141(8): 702-3.

58 US Preventive Services Task Force. Screening for Asymptomatic Carotid Artery Stenosis: US Preventive Services Task Force Recommendation Statement. *JAMA* 2021; 325(5): 476-81.

59 AbuRahma AF, Avgerinos E, Chang RW, et al. Society for Vascular Surgery Clinical Practice Guidelines for Management of Extracranial Cerebrovascular Disease. *Journal of Vascular Surgery* 202; doi: 10.1016/j.jvs.2021.04.073. Online ahead of print.

60 Kleindorfer DO, Towfighi A, Chaturvedi S, et al. 2021 Guideline for the Prevention of Stroke in Patients with Stroke and Transient Ischemic Attack: A Guideline from the American Heart Association/American Stroke Association. *Stroke* 2021; 52(70): e364-e467.

61 Correction to: 2021 Guideline for the Prevention of Stroke in Patients with Stroke and Transient Ischemic Attack: A Guideline from the American Heart Association/American Stroke Association. *Stroke* 2021; 52(7): e483-e4.

62 Sett AK, Robinson TG, Mistri AK. Current status of statin therapy for stroke prevention. *Expert Review of Cardiovascular Therapy* 2011; 9(10): 1305-14.

63 Aradine E, Hou Y, Cronin CA, Chaturvedi S. Current Status of Dyslipidemia Treatment for Stroke Prevention. *Curr Neurol Neurosci Rep* 2020; 20(8): 31.

64 Poobalan A, Aucott L, Smith WCS, et al. Effects of weight loss in overweight/obese individuals and long-term lipid outcomes – a systematic review. *Obesity Reviews* 2004; **5**(1): 43-50.

65 Rosenthal RL. Effectiveness of altering serum cholesterol levels without drugs. *Proceedings (Baylor University Medical Center)* 2000; 13(4): 351-5.

66 Amarenco P, Bogousslavsky J, Callahan A, 3rd, et al. High-dose atorvastatin after stroke or transient ischemic attack. *N Engl J Med* 2006; 355(6): 549-59.

67 Grundy SM, Stone NJ. 2018 American Heart Association/American College of Cardiology Multisociety Guideline on the Management of Blood Cholesterol: Primary Prevention. *JAMA Cardiol* 2019; 4(5): 488-9.

68  Cannon CP, Blazing MA, Giugliano RP, et al. Ezetimibe Added to Statin Therapy after Acute Coronary Syndromes. *New England Journal of Medicine* 2015; 372(25): 2387-97.

69  Tomaszewski M, Stępień KM, Tomaszewska J, Czuczwar SJ. Statin-induced myopathies. *Pharmacol Rep* 2011; 63(4): 859-66.

70  Ridker PM, Cook NR, Lee IM, et al. A randomised trial of low-dose aspirin in the primary prevention of cardiovascular disease in women. *The New England journal of medicine* 2005; 352(13): 1293-304.

71   Bowman L, Mafham M, Wallendszus K, et al. Effects of Aspirin for Primary Prevention in Persons with Diabetes Mellitus. *The New England journal of medicine* 2018; 379(16): 1529-39.

72  Gaziano JM, Brotons C, Coppolecchia R, et al. Use of aspirin to reduce risk of initial vascular events in patients at moderate risk of cardiovascular disease (ARRIVE): a randomised, double-blind, placebo-controlled trial. *Lancet (London, England)* 2018; 392(10152): 1036-46.

73  McNeil JJ, Nelson MR, Woods RL, et al. Effect of Aspirin on All-Cause Mortality in the Healthy Elderly. *The New England journal of medicine* 2018; 379(16): 1519-28.

74  Chaturvedi S. To Screen or Not to Screen for Carotid Stenosis: Is That the Question? *JAMA Neurology* 2021.

75  Force USPST. Screening for Asymptomatic Carotid Artery Stenosis: US Preventive Services Task Force Recommendation Statement. *JAMA* 2021; 325(5): 476-81.

76  Goldstein LB. Screening for Asymptomatic Carotid Artery Stenosis: Lack of Clinical Benefit, Potential for Harm. *JAMA* 2021; 325(5): 443-4.

77  Keyhani S, Cheng EM. Screening for Asymptomatic Carotid Artery Stenosis in Adult Patients: Unclear Benefit but Downstream Risks. *JAMA Internal Medicine* 2021.

78  Smith-Bindman R, Bibbins-Domingo K. USPSTF Recommendations for Screening for Carotid Stenosis to Prevent Stroke—The Need for More Data. *JAMA Network Open* 2021; 4(2): e2036218-e.

79  Kernan WN, Ovbiagele B, Black HR, et al. Guidelines for the prevention of stroke in patients with stroke and transient ischemic attack: a guideline for healthcare professionals from the American Heart Association/American Stroke Association. *Stroke* 2014; 45(7): 2160-236.

80  Ingason AB, Hreinsson JP, Agustsson AS, et al. Rivaroxaban is associated with higher rates of gastrointestinal bleeding than other direct oral anticoagulants. *Annals of Internal Medicine* 2021; doi: 10.7326/M21-1474. Online ahead of print

81  Lachin JM, Orchard TJ, Nathan DM. Update on cardiovascular outcomes at 30 years of the diabetes control and complications trial/epidemiology of diabetes interventions and complications study. *Diabetes Care* 2014; 37(1): 39-43.

82  Singh G, Krauthamer M, Bjalme-Evans M. Wegovy (semaglutide): a new weight loss drug for chronic weight management. *J Investig Med* 2021; DOI: 10.1136/jim-2021-001952.

83  Moussa O, Ardissino M, Tang A, et al. Long-term cerebrovascular outcomes after bariatric surgery: A nationwide cohort study. *Clin Neurol Neurosurg* 2021; 203: 106560.

84  Vartiainen I. War-time and the mortality in certain diseases in Finland. *Ann Med Fenn* 1946;35: 234.

85  Strom A, Jensen RA. Mortality from circulatory diseases in Norway 1940-1945. *Lancet* 1951; 1(6647): 126-9.

86  Schornagel HE. The connection between nutrition and mortality from coronary sclerosis during and after World War II. *Documenta de medicina geographica et tropica* 1953; 5(2): 173-83.

87  Schettler G. Vorkrankheiten und Arteriosklerose. *Verh Dtsch Ges Inn Med* 1954; 60(60): 883-6.

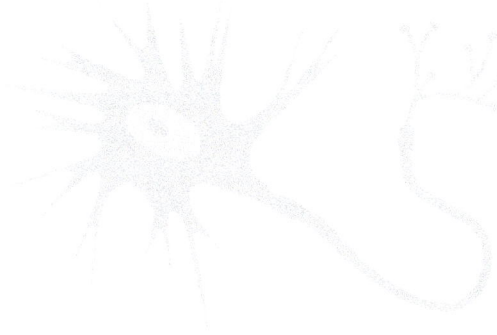

| Warning |
|---|
| The information in this appendix will be rapidly out of date. Always check the latest guidelines.[1] |

# Thrombolysis and Clot Retrieval for Ischaemic Stroke

## Abbreviations

**AHA/ASA**: American Heart Association/American Stroke Association, **ESO**: European Stroke Organisation,[1] **CT**: computerised tomography, **MRI**: magnetic resonance imaging, **mRS**: modified Rankin Score, **MT**: mechanical thrombectomy, **ICA**: internal carotid artery, **MCA**: middle cerebral artery, **t-PA**: tissue plasminogen activator or alteplase, **PT INR**: prothrombin time international normalisation ratio, **aPTT**: activated partial thromboplastin time. ⚷ = Key Point

There have been significant advances in acute stroke management since the first edition. One advance has been the role of imaging in determining the presence of an ischaemic penumbra, thus extending the therapeutic window beyond 3 hours. The second development has been clot-retrieval also referred to as mechanical thrombectomy (MT). Acute stroke is undergoing rapid changes and it is important to consult guidelines on a regular basis.

| ⚷ |
|---|
| Patients with acute stroke should be promptly referred to a centre that can administer thrombolysis and preferably mechanical thrombectomy. |

---

1  European Stroke organization: https://eso-stroke.org/guidelines/eso-guideline-directory/#acute-stroke
   AHA/ASA guidelines: https://professional.heart.org/en/guidelines-and-statements

# Thrombolytic therapy

At the 1995 AHA Stroke conference in San Antonia the NINDS funded t-PA (alteplase) trial results were presented[2]. We finally had a treatment that reduced acute stroke severity. IV alteplase within 3 hours of onset of stroke reduced severity as assessed by the mRS at 3 months.

The American Academy of Emergency Medicine and in particular Professor Jerome Hoffmann from UCLA criticised the trial. [3, 4] This criticism prompted a reanalysis that supported the original conclusions. [5, 6]

**Current guidelines** recommend intravenous thrombolysis with alteplase in patients with cerebral ischaemia within 3 (AHA/ASA) [7, 8] or up to 4.5 hours after onset (ESO). [9]. The dose is 0.9 mg/kg with a maximum dose of 90 mg administered over 60 minutes with 10% given as an initial bolus over one minute.

Although the time window for thrombolysis has been extended to 4.5 hours, [10-14] for the best results, t-PA should be administered as soon as possible after the onset of stroke, preferably within 60 minutes. As the benefit of therapy is time-dependent, thrombolysis should not be delayed for additional multimodal neuroimaging, such as CT and MRI perfusion imaging.

Alteplase improves the outcome for one in three patients treated between 1-3 hours from the onset and one in six patients treated in the 3-4.5-hour window. Beyond 4.5 hours, thrombolysis increases mortality. [11, 15]

Symptomatic intracerebral haemorrhage, including fatal bleeding, is the most dreaded complication of this therapy. It occurs in 1.7–7.3% of patients (depending on how symptomatic intracerebral haemorrhage is defined). [16, 17]

In 2022 the results of the Canadian Alteplase Compared to Tenecteplase (ACT) Randomized Controlled Trial was presented at the European Stroke Organisation conference in Lyon, France. [76] A single dose of 0.25mg/kg was found to be non-inferior to alteplase. Tenecteplase has distinct advantages including a single dose, more cost-effective and potentially faster.[3]

## Contraindications to thrombolysis

- Intracranial haemorrhage is the one absolute contraindication to thrombolysis.
- A platelet count of < 100,000 is a contraindication. As thrombocytopaenia is extremely rare, guidelines recommend proceeding with thrombolysis before the platelet count is known.
- Heparin within the preceding 24 hours.
- PT INR ≥ 1.7 or a PT ≥ 15 s.
- Severe uncontrolled hypertension (BP > 185mm Hg systolic or 110 mmHg diastolic.
- Severe head trauma or a stroke in the previous three months.
- Patients taking direct thrombin inhibitors or direct factor Xa inhibitors unless laboratory tests such as aPTT, INR, platelet count, ecarin clotting time, thrombin time, or appropriate direct factor Xa activity assays are normal or the patient has not received a dose of these agents for >48 h (assuming normal renal metabolising function).
- As hypoglycaemia may mimic stroke, the blood sugar should be normalised before considering thrombolysis.

---

2  I was present and the atmosphere was electric; Some neurologists made badges stating the dose they required based on their weight. There were many 90mg (maximum) doses!

3  I would urge caution and recommend waiting until the full paper has been peer reviewed and published before incorporating tenecteplase into clinical practice.

The elderly (>80 years of age), patients with severe stroke, diabetes with hyperglycaemia, rapidly improving deficit, or early ischaemic changes on CT scans are no longer considered contraindications to thrombolysis within three hours of onset. [7, 8, 18]

Three specific reversal agents for direct oral anticoagulants (DOACs) have been approved in the United States: idarucizumab for dabigatran reversal, andexanet alfa for apixaban and rivaroxaban (factor Xa inhibitors) reversal [19] and ciraparantag that reverses direct thrombin inhibitors, factor Xa inhibitors, and heparins. [20] Although there are isolated case reports of patients receiving t-PA after reversal of DOAC's [21-24] current the guidelines state that patients on DOAC's should not receive t-PA.

The latest **Japanese clinical guidelines** have taken a different view and recommend thrombolysis if the time of the last dose of direct oral anticoagulant exceeds 4 hours and if commonly available anticoagulation markers are normal or subnormal, i.e., international normalized ratio of prothrombin time <1.7 and activated partial thromboplastin time <1.5 times the baseline value (≤40 seconds only as a guide). [25]

## Wake-up Stroke

It is impossible to determine the exact onset time in the 15-20% of patients who awaken with a stroke. [26] Initially, these patients were denied thrombolysis. However, studies such as WAKE-UP [12] and DAWN [27] have defined a subgroup of these patients who can benefit (mRS 0-2 at 90 days 44-49% vs 13-16%) from thrombolysis. Perfusion-weighted imaging (PWI), diffusion-weighted imaging (DWI), and fluid-attenuated inversion recovery (FLAIR) image studies suggest the actual time of onset in patients with wake-up stroke may be close to the time of awakening. [28-30]

**Current guidelines** [7, 8, 31] recommend IV alteplase administration within 4.5 hours of stroke symptom recognition in patients with acute ischaemic stroke who awake with stroke symptoms or have unclear time of onset > 4.5 hours from last known well or at baseline state. MRI is used to identify diffusion-positive FLAIR-negative lesions in those who can benefit.

## Clot Retrieval-Mechanical Thrombectomy

In 2015, five published randomised trials EXTEND-IA [32],MR CLEAN [33],ESCAPE [34], REVASCAT [35], SWIFT PRIME [36] documented the benefits of mechanical thrombectomy (MT) in patients with occlusion of the distal intracranial internal carotid or proximal middle cerebral artery. MT requires the patient to be at an experienced stroke centre with rapid access to cerebral angiography, qualified neuro-interventionalists, and a comprehensive periprocedural care team. [8]

Acute assessment involves CT angiography with a CT perfusion study or MR angiography with diffusion-weighted magnetic resonance imaging with or without MR perfusion for certain patients. The CT perfusion can differentiate between the penumbra (potentially viable tissue) and the ischaemic core. (see figure F.1)

- **The core**
  - increased MTT/Tmax
  - markedly decreased CBF
  - markedly decreased CBV

- **The penumbra**
  - increased MTT/Tmax
  - moderately reduced CBF
  - near-normal or increased CBV

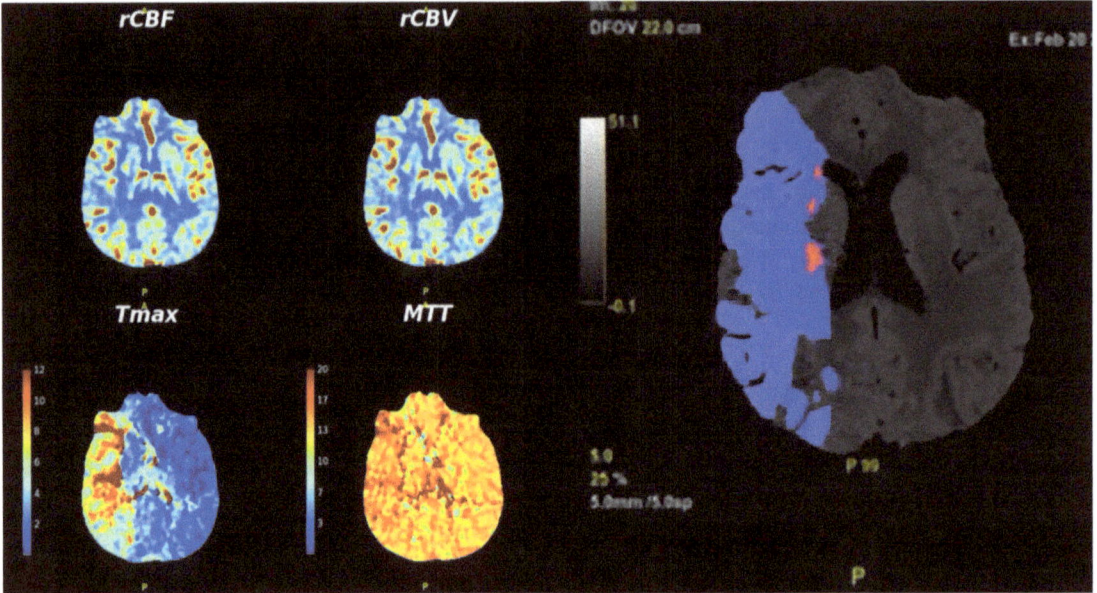

**Figure F.1** CT perfusion study. The Cerebral Blood Volume and Cerebral Blood Flow reduction look very similar indicating that there is very little dead brain (ischaemic core).The Tmax and MTT show delayed blood flow (reddened areas) indicating slow blood flow due to the blocked middle cerebral artery (MCA). The image on the right demonstrates the large area of reduced perfusion (decreased blood flow), ie., potentially salvageable brain. This was salvaged with clot retrieval as shown in figure F.2.

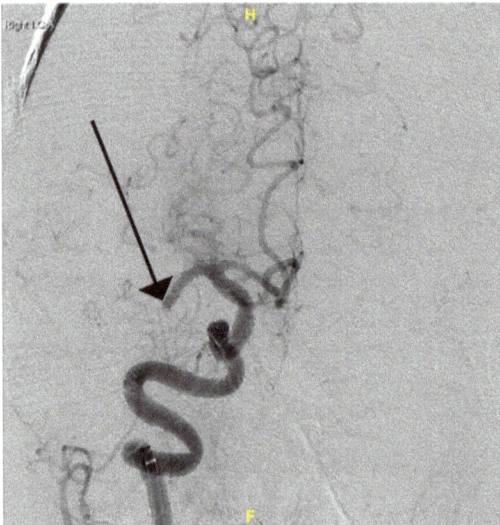

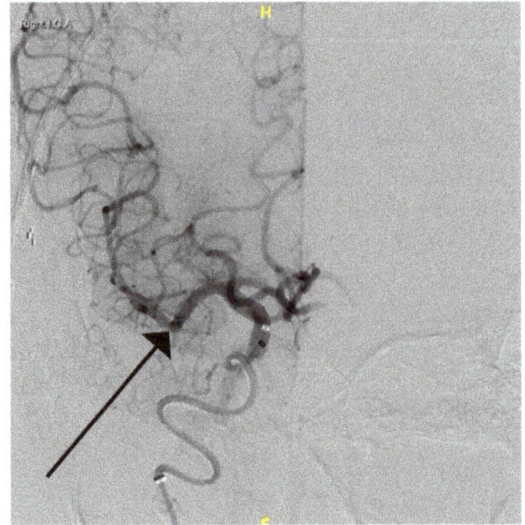

**Figure F.2** Cerebral angiography demonstrating clot retrieval. The image on the left shows occlusion of the middle cerebral artery (MCA) prior to clot retrieval and the image on the right shows successful re-opening of the MCA.

Mechanical thrombectomy (clot retrieval) [37-39] in acute stroke due to distal ICA/proximal MCA occlusion, is feasible and safe, high rates of recanalisation are achieved with favourable functional outcomes in some,[40, 41] but not all studies, particularly with severe stroke. [42] The odds of better disability outcomes at 90 days (mRS scale distribution) with the MT group declines with longer time from symptom onset to expected arterial puncture.

**The European Stroke Organisation guidelines** recommend MT ideally in < 6 hours but up to 24 hours after onset in patients with ischaemic stroke due to large vessel occlusion. [31]

**AHA/ASA guidelines** recommend MT for selected patients with acute ischaemic stroke within 6 to 16 hours of last known normal who have large vessel occlusion in the anterior circulation and meet other DAWN or DEFUSE3 (see below) [8]

# Extracranial Internal Carotid Artery Occlusion

In patients with extracranial internal carotid artery occlusion, the benefits of MT are less certain. There are no randomised trials. Complete recanalisation of the extracranial or intracranial ICA after t-PA was rare, occurring in only 10%. [43] Several small case studies have documented successful recanalisation. [42, 44-50] Often there is co-existent more distal occlusion of the ICA or proximal MCA that also required MT. In cases without intracranial large vessel occlusion, MT of acute ICA occlusion is associated with a risk of distal embolisation. [49]

**Current guidelines** state that although its benefits are uncertain, the use of MT with stent retrievers may be reasonable for patients with acute ischaemic stroke in whom MT treatment can be initiated within 6 hours of symptom onset. Inclusion criteria are a pre-stroke modified Rankin Score (mRS score) > 1, Alberta Stroke Program Early Computed Tomography Score (ASPECTS) > 6, or a National Institute of Health Stroke Scale (NIHSS) score < 6, and causative occlusion of the internal carotid artery (ICA). [8]

# Vertebral and Basilar Artery Occlusion

The benefits of MT are less clear with vertebral and basilar artery occlusion. The prognosis for basilar artery occlusion is poor but not uniformly fatal as once thought. [51, 52]

The BASICS study [52] failed to demonstrate any benefit from IV or intraarterial thrombolysis. Small studies of MT have achieved high recanalisation rates and a good outcome in about one-third with a mortality of approximately one-third. [53-56] in 2022 the ATTENTION trial demonstrated a significant benefit of clot retrieval in basilar artery occlusion performed within 12 hours after onset. [57, 58] A favourable functional outcome (mRS, 0 - 3) at 90 days — was achieved in 22.8% of the control group and in 46% of the endovascular group, giving an adjusted risk ratio of 2.1 ($P < .001$). The number needed to treat was just four.

**Current guidelines** stated that although the benefits are uncertain, the use of MT with stent retrievers may be reasonable for carefully selected patients with acute ischaemic stroke in whom treatment can be initiated (groin puncture) within 6 hours of symptom onset and who have causative occlusion of the vertebral or basilar artery. [8] In light of ATTENTION these guidelines will need to be updated. Once again emphasising the importance of constantly checking for the latest and up to date information.

# Extending the Thrombectomy Therapeutic Window

In patients with ICA or proximal MCA occlusion, either CT perfusion or MRI diffusion/perfusion analysed using automated software (RAPID) can determine the presence of an ischaemic penumbra (potentially salvageable ischaemic brain). Randomised trials of patients with an ischaemic penumbra and an ischaemic core of < 70ml on CT perfusion imaging [27, 59] confirmed the benefit (improved reperfusion and improved functional outcome) of MT in these patients and extended the therapeutic window up to 24 hours.

The Dawn [27], EXTEND-IA [32] and DEFUSE3 trials [59] were terminated early when interim analysis demonstrated the benefit of thrombectomy. The EXTEND-IA trial studied patients who had received IV t-PA < 4.5 hours after onset and randomised them to MT. DAWN and DEFUSE3 only studied MT in patients beyond 6 hours. EXTEND-IA and DEFUSE3 used a target mismatch profile on CT or MR perfusion imaging whilst DAWN used clinical-imaging mismatch (table F1).

Analysis of the AURORA (Analysis of Pooled Data from Randomized Studies of Thrombectomy More Than 6 Hours After Last Known Well) database [60] found no difference between clinical and target mismatch in terms of predicting outcome. On the other hand, analysis of the INSPIRE database [61] reported that target mismatch was superior to clinical mismatch. The question of whether a subset of patients with larger ischemic core volumes (>70 mL) could benefit from thrombectomy beyond 6 hours remains unanswered.[62, 63] Baron argues that the use of either mismatch profile could increase the currently small proportion of patients presenting more than six hours after stroke onset who could receive this beneficial and reasonably safe therapy.

# t-PA ± Mechanical Thrombectomy

Several trials (DIRECT MT, SKIP, DEVT, MR CLEAN NO IV, SWIFT DIRECT, THRACE) have compared t-PA and MT. As thrombolysis was the gold-standard treatment, most studies were designed to test noninferiority which they did. [64-69]

In most of these studies there was only a small difference in treatment outcome between bridging thrombolysis and direct thrombectomy approaches for the specific subset of patients who arrive at a major tertiary hospital and receive thrombectomy immediately.

In contrast, SWIFT-DIRECT[1] failed to demonstrate non-inferiority of MT alone compared to combined IV t-PA and MT. The preintervention reperfusion rate with intravenous thrombolysis was exceptionally low, the postintervention reperfusion rate was much higher in the IV t-PA arm. The authors concluded that in the current setting, there is no reason to skip intravenous thrombolysis in large vessel occlusions."

The 2021 **European Stroke Organisation guidelines** recommend mechanical thrombectomy and intravenous thrombolysis within six hours of onset for patients with large vessel occlusion in the anterior circulation. [70] MT and thrombolysis is recommended in the time window 6-24 hours for patients who fulfil the selection criteria in either the DEFUSE-3 [71] or DAWN study. [27]

---

4    Preliminary results presented at the 7th European Stroke Organisation Conference (ESOC 2021; 1–3 September, virtual) It is important to wait for the formal publication and detailed analysis of the study.

# t-PA after Mechanical Thrombectomy

The CHOICE trial [72] was published in 2022. It compared t-PA after not before MT. The hypothesis was that incomplete microcirculatory reperfusion might contribute to these suboptimal clinical benefits. In this trial, the proportion of participants with a modified Rankin Scale score of 0 or 1 at 90 days was 59.0% (36/61) with alteplase and 40.4% (21/52) with placebo (adjusted risk difference, 18.4%; 95% CI, 0.3%-36.4%; P = .047). The placebo group fared much better than studies of t-PA prior to MT where only 27% of patients are disability-free at 90 days. [73] The external applicability of this trial is uncertain. Of the 1825 patients who had received MT 748 (41%) fulfilled the angiographic criteria and yet only 121 (7%) patients were randomized of which 113 (6%) were treated as randomized. The dose of t-PA was smaller (0.225mg/kg, maximum dose 22.5mg). The study was terminated early due to difficulty enrolling patients during the COVID pandemic.

**The ACC/ASA guidelines** recommend eligible patients should receive thrombolysis and MT with a stent retriever if they meet all the following criteria:

1 prestroke mRS score of 0 to 1.
2 causative occlusion of the internal carotid artery or MCA segment 1 (M1).
3 age ≥18 years.
4 NIHSS score of ≥6.
5 ASPECTS of ≥6 and
6 MT can be initiated (groin puncture) within 6 hours of symptom onset.

**The Society of NeuroInterventional Surgery (SNIS) guidelines** [74] stated age greater than 80 is not a contraindication recommend MT for patients with NIHSS score ≥6 and

- Selected patients with anterior circulation acute ischaemic stroke (AIS) up to 24 hours after last seen well, stating that the best evidence is up to 16 hours.
- Patients with ICA occlusion (intracranial, cervical segment or tandem occlusion) and M1/M2 MCA occlusion
- Patients with anterior circulation AIS within the first six hours of symptom onset and either CT aspects ≥ 6, MRI DWI aspects ≥ 6, moderate-to-good collateral status on mCTA (>50% MCA territory), small (<50–70 mL) core infarct volumes, and/or significant penumbral to core mismatch on advanced perfusion imaging (CTP or MRI-DWI-PWI).
- MT may be reasonable within the first 6 hours of symptom onset in patients with a large core infarct volume such as CT ASPECTS of <6, MRI DWI or CTP-estimated core volume >70 mL.
- Patients with anterior circulation AIS due to intracranial ICA and/or M1 occlusion within 6–24 hours of symptom onset who meet the advanced MRI DWI-PWI or CTP imaging criteria for DAWN or DEFUSE 3.
- MT may be indicated in carefully selected patients with anterior circulation AIS within 6–24 hours of symptom onset who do not meet imaging criteria for DAWN and DEFUSE 3 but otherwise have a 'favourable' imaging profile such as CT ASPECTS of 6–10, MRI DWI ASPECTS of 6–10, moderate-to-good collateral status on mCTA, or small (<70 mL) core infarct on advanced MRI DWI-PWI or CTP imaging.

# ASPECTS

The ASPECTS (Alberta Stroke Program Early CT Score) is a method of assessing non-contrast CT scans for the area of ischaemia in the MCA territory. ASPECTS is calculated from two standard axial CT cuts. One is at the thalamus and basal ganglia level, and the other is just rostral to the ganglionic structures. The territory of the middle cerebral artery is allotted ten points. One point is subtracted for an area of early ischaemic change, such as focal swelling, or parenchymal hypoattenuation in each defined region. A normal CT scan has an ASPECTS value of 10 points. A score of 0 indicates diffuse ischaemia throughout the entire middle cerebral artery territory. [75] A score < 7 predicts a poor outcome as defined by an mRS > 0-2.

# Inclusion Criteria Defuse-3 and Dawn

| Inclusion Criteria | Defuse-3 [71] | Dawn[27] |
|---|---|---|
| Time Window | 6-16 hours since time last known well | 6-24 hours since time last known well |
| Age | 19-90 | ≥ 18 |
| mRS score before qualifying stroke | ≤ 2;life expectancy≥ 6 months | ≤ 1; life expectancy ≥ 6 months |
| NIHSS score | ≥ 6 | ≥ 10 (see below) |
| Arterial occlusion | ICA and/or M1* | ICA and/or M1 |
| Mismatch definition | Target mismatch profile on CT or MR perfusion imaging, as determined by an automated image postprocessing system: infarct call volume <70 mL † and mismatch volume >15 mL (Tmax greater than 6s‡) and mismatch ratio (penumbra/core) > 1.8 | Clinical-imaging mismatch age <80 years and NIHSS score ≥ 10 and infarct core 0-30 mL OR mismatch age <80 years and in IHS score ≥ 20 and infarct core 31-51 mL OR <80 years and NIHSS score ≥ 10 and infarct core 0-20 mL |

Table F1. * Carotid occlusions could be surgical or intracranial, with or without tandem MCA lesions in DEFUSE-3. † Based on CT perfusion or MRI diffusion. ‡ The size of the penumbra was estimated from the volume of tissue for which there was delayed arrival of an injected tracer agent (time to maximum of the residue function (Tmax) exceeding 6s. Abbreviations: ICA = internal cerebral artery; MCA = middle cerebral artery; mRS = modified Rankin Scale; NIHSS = National Institute of Health Stroke Scale.

# References

1.  Nogueira, R.G. and et.al., Endovascular treatment for acute basilar artery occlusion: A multicenter randomized controlled trial (ATTENTION), in *European Stroke Organisation Conference* (ESOC). 2022: Lyon, France.

2.  Tao, C., et al., Endovascular treatment for acute basilar artery occlusion: A multicenter randomized controlled trial (ATTENTION). *Int J Stroke*, 2022: p. 17474930221077164.

3.  Hoffman, J.R., Should physicians give tPA to patients with acute ischemic stroke? Against: and just what is the emperor of stroke wearing? *West J Med*, 2000. 173(3): p. 149-50.

4.  Goyal, D.G., et al. AAEM Position Statement on tPA: The Use of Intravenous Thrombolytic Therapy in the Treatment of Stroke. *AAEM Position Statements* 2007; Available from: https://www.aaem.org/resources/statements/position/aaem-position-statement-on-tpa-the-use-of-intravenous-thrombolytic-therapy-in-the-treatment-of-stroke.

5.  Ingall, T.J., et al., Findings from the reanalysis of the NINDS tissue plasminogen activator for acute ischemic stroke treatment trial. *Stroke*, 2004. 35(10): p. 2418-24.

6.  Saver, J.L., J. Gornbein, and S. Starkman, Graphic Reanalysis of the Two NINDS-tPA Trials Confirms Substantial Treatment Benefit. *Stroke*, 2010. 41(10): p. 2381-2390.

7.  Powers, W.J., et al., 2018 Guidelines for the Early Management of Patients With Acute Ischemic Stroke: A Guideline for Healthcare Professionals From the American Heart Association/American Stroke Association. *Stroke*, 2018. 49(3): p. e46-e110.

8.  Powers, W.J., et al., Guidelines for the Early Management of Patients With Acute Ischemic Stroke: 2019 Update to the 2018 Guidelines for the Early Management of Acute Ischemic Stroke: A Guideline for Healthcare Professionals From the American Heart Association/American Stroke Association. *Stroke*, 2019. 50(12): p. e344-e418.

9.  Berge, E., et al., European Stroke Organisation (ESO) guidelines on intravenous thrombolysis for acute ischaemic stroke. *European Stroke Journal*, 2021. 6(1): p. I-LXII.

10. Hacke, W., et al., Thrombolysis with alteplase 3 to 4.5 hours after acute ischemic stroke. N Engl J Med, 2008. 359(13): p. 1317-29.

11. Lees, K.R., et al., Time to treatment with intravenous alteplase and outcome in stroke: an updated pooled analysis of ECASS, ATLANTIS, NINDS, and EPITHET trials. *Lancet*, 2010. 375(9727): p. 1695-703.

12. Thomalla, G., et al., MRI-Guided Thrombolysis for Stroke with Unknown Time of Onset. *N Engl J Med*, 2018. 379(7): p. 611-622.

13. Ma, H., et al., Thrombolysis Guided by Perfusion Imaging up to 9 Hours after Onset of Stroke. *N Engl J Med*, 2019. 380(19): p. 1795-1803.

14. Koga, M., et al., Thrombolysis With Alteplase at 0.6 mg/kg for Stroke With Unknown Time of Onset: A Randomized Controlled Trial. *Stroke*, 2020. 51(5): p. 1530-1538.

15. Saver, J.L. and S.R. Levine, Alteplase for ischaemic stroke—much sooner is much better. *The Lancet*, 2010. 375(9727): p. 1667-1668.

16. Tissue plasminogen activator for acute ischemic stroke. The National Institute of Neurological Disorders and Stroke rt-PA Stroke Study Group. *N Engl J Med*, 1995. 333(24): p. 1581-7.

17. Wahlgren, N., et al., Thrombolysis with alteplase for acute ischaemic stroke in the Safe Implementation of Thrombolysis in Stroke-Monitoring Study (SITS-MOST): an observational study. *Lancet*, 2007. 369(9558): p. 275-82.

18. Demaerschalk, B.M., et al., Scientific Rationale for the Inclusion and Exclusion Criteria for Intravenous Alteplase in Acute Ischemic Stroke: A Statement for Healthcare Professionals From the American Heart Association/American Stroke Association. *Stroke*, 2016. 47(2): p. 581-641.

19. Cuker, A., et al., Reversal of direct oral anticoagulants: Guidance from the Anticoagulation Forum. *Am J Hematol*, 2019. 94(6): p. 697-709.

20. Hu, T.Y., V.R. Vaidya, and S.J. Asirvatham, Reversing anticoagulant effects of novel oral anticoagulants: role of ciraparantag, andexanet alfa, and idarucizumab. *Vasc Health Risk Manag*, 2016. 12: p. 35-44.

21. Pikija, S., et al., Idarucizumab in Dabigatran-Treated Patients with Acute Ischemic Stroke Receiving Alteplase: A Systematic Review of the Available Evidence. *CNS Drugs*, 2017. 31(9): p. 747-757.

22. Touzé, E., et al., Intravenous thrombolysis for acute ischaemic stroke in patients on direct oral anticoagulants. *Eur J Neurol*, 2018. 25(5): p. 747-e52.

23. Šaňák, D., et al., Intravenous Thrombolysis in Patients with Acute Ischemic Stroke after a Reversal of Dabigatran Anticoagulation with Idarucizumab: A Real-World Clinical Experience. *J Stroke Cerebrovasc Dis*, 2018. 27(9): p. 2479-2483.

24. Fang, C.W., et al., Intravenous Thrombolysis in Acute Ischemic Stroke After Idarucizumab Reversal of Dabigatran Effect: Analysis of the Cases From Taiwan. *J Stroke Cerebrovasc Dis*, 2019. 28(3): p. 815-820.

25. Toyoda, K., H. Yamagami, and M. Koga, Consensus Guides on Stroke Thrombolysis for Anticoagulated Patients from Japan: Application to Other Populations. *J Stroke*, 2018. 20(3): p. 321-331.

26. Roveri, L., et al., Wake-up stroke within 3 hours of symptom awareness: imaging and clinical features compared to standard recombinant tissue plasminogen activator treated stroke. J *Stroke Cerebrovasc Dis*, 2013. 22(6): p. 703-8.

27. Nogueira, R.G., et al., Thrombectomy 6 to 24 Hours after Stroke with a Mismatch between Deficit and Infarct. *N Engl J Med*, 2018. 378(1): p. 11-21.

28. Huisa, B.N., et al., Diffusion-weighted imaging-fluid attenuated inversion recovery mismatch in nocturnal stroke patients with unknown time of onset. *J Stroke Cerebrovasc Dis*, 2013. 22(7): p. 972-7.

29. Silva, G.S., et al., Wake-up stroke: clinical and neuroimaging characteristics. *Cerebrovasc Dis*, 2010. 29(4): p. 336-42.

30. Fink, J.N., et al., The stroke patient who woke up: clinical and radiological features, including diffusion and perfusion MRI. *Stroke*, 2002. 33(4): p. 988-93.

31. Turc, G., et al., European Stroke Organisation (ESO) European Society for Minimally Invasive Neurological Therapy (ESMINT) Guidelines on Mechanical Thrombectomy in Acute Ischemic Stroke. *Journal of NeuroInterventional Surgery*, 2019: p. neurintsurg-2018-014569.

32. Campbell, B.C., et al., Endovascular therapy for ischemic stroke with perfusion-imaging selection. *N Engl J Med*, 2015. 372(11): p. 1009-18.

33. Berkhemer, O.A., et al., A randomized trial of intraarterial treatment for acute ischemic stroke. *N Engl J Med*, 2015. 372(1): p. 11-20.

34. Goyal, M., et al., Randomized assessment of rapid endovascular treatment of ischemic stroke. *New England Journal of Medicine*, 2015. 372(11): p. 1019-1030.

35. Jovin, T.G., et al., Thrombectomy within 8 hours after symptom onset in ischemic stroke. *N Engl J Med*, 2015. 372(24): p. 2296-306.

36. Saver, J., M. Goyal, and A. Bonafe, Stent-retriever thrombectomy after intravenous t-PA vs. t-PA alone in stroke [published online April 17, 2015]. *N Engl J Med*. doi, 2015. 372(24): p. 2285-2295.

37. Coutinho, J.M., et al., Combined Intravenous Thrombolysis and Thrombectomy vs Thrombectomy Alone for Acute Ischemic Stroke: A Pooled Analysis of the SWIFT and STAR Studies. *JAMA Neurol*, 2017. 74(3): p. 268-274.

38. Pereira, V.M., et al., Prospective, multicenter, single-arm study of mechanical thrombectomy using Solitaire Flow Restoration in acute ischemic stroke. *Stroke*, 2013. 44(10): p. 2802-7.

39. Saver, J.L., et al., Solitaire flow restoration device versus the Merci Retriever in patients with acute ischaemic stroke (SWIFT): a randomised, parallel-group, non-inferiority trial. *Lancet*, 2012. 380(9849): p. 1241-9.

40. Ma, Y.D., et al., Mechanical thrombectomy with Solitaire stent for acute internal carotid artery occlusion without atherosclerotic stenosis: dissection or cardiogenic thromboembolism. *Eur Rev Med Pharmacol Sci*, 2014. 18(9): p. 1324-32.

41. Imai, K., et al., Clot removal therapy by aspiration and extraction for acute embolic carotid occlusion. *AJNR Am J Neuroradiol*, 2006. 27(7): p. 1521-7.

42. Díaz-Pérez, J., et al., Mechanical Thrombectomy in Acute Stroke Due to Carotid Occlusion: A Series of 153 Consecutive Patients. *Cerebrovasc Dis*, 2018. 46(3-4): p. 132-141.

43. Christou, I., et al., Intravenous tissue plasminogen activator and flow improvement in acute ischemic stroke patients with internal carotid artery occlusion. *J Neuroimaging*, 2002. 12(2): p. 119-23.

44. Hauck, E.F., et al., Emergent endovascular recanalization for cervical internal carotid artery occlusion in patients presenting with acute stroke. *Neurosurgery*, 2011. 69(4): p. 899-907; discussion 907.

45. Mishra, A., et al., Emergent extracranial internal carotid artery stenting and mechanical thrombectomy in acute ischaemic stroke. *Interv Neuroradiol*, 2015. 21(2): p. 205-14.

46. Bricout, N., et al., Day 1 Extracranial Internal Carotid Artery Patency Is Associated With Good Outcome After Mechanical Thrombectomy for Tandem Occlusion. *Stroke*, 2018. 49(10): p. 2520-2522.

47. Okumura, E., et al., Outcomes of Endovascular Thrombectomy Performed 6-24 h after Acute Stroke from Extracranial Internal Carotid Artery Occlusion. *Neurol Med Chir* (Tokyo), 2019. 59(9): p. 337-343.

48. de Castro-Afonso, L.H., et al., Endovascular Reperfusion for Acute Isolated Cervical Carotid Occlusions: The Concept of "Hemodynamic Thrombectomy". *Interventional Neurology*, 2019. 8(1): p. 27-37.

49. Mayer, L., et al., Management and prognosis of acute extracranial internal carotid artery occlusion. *Annals of Translational Medicine*, 2020. 8(19): p. 1268.

50. Cirillo, L., et al., Acute ischemic stroke with cervical internal carotid artery steno-occlusive lesion: multicenter analysis of endovascular approaches. *BMC Neurol*, 2021. 21(1): p. 362.

51. Kubik, C.S. and R.D. Adams, Occlusion of the basilar artery; a clinical and pathological study. *Brain*, 1946. 69(2): p. 73-121.

52. Mattle, H.P., et al., Basilar artery occlusion. *Lancet Neurol*, 2011. 10(11): p. 1002-14.

53. Wang, L., et al., Endovascular treatment of severe acute basilar artery occlusion. *Journal of Clinical Neuroscience*, 2015. 22(1): p. 195-198.

54. Meinel, T.R., et al., Mechanical thrombectomy for basilar artery occlusion: efficacy, outcomes, and futile recanalization in comparison with the anterior circulation. *Journal of NeuroInterventional Surgery*, 2019. 11(12): p. 1174.

55. Kwak, H.S. and J.S. Park, Mechanical Thrombectomy in Basilar Artery Occlusion. *Stroke*, 2020. 51(7): p. 2045-2050.

56. Schonewille, W.J., et al., Treatment and outcomes of acute basilar artery occlusion in the Basilar Artery International Cooperation Study (BASICS): a prospective registry study. *The Lancet Neurology*, 2009. 8(8): p. 724-730.

57. Liu, Z. and D.S. Liebeskind, Basilar Artery Occ Tao, C., et al. (2022). "Endovascular treatment for acute basilar artery occlusion: A multicenter randomized controlled trial (ATTENTION)." *Int J Stroke*: 17474930221077164.

58. Nogueira, R. G. and et.al. (2022). Endovascular treatment for acute basilar artery occlusion: A multicenter randomized controlled trial (ATTENTION). *European Stroke Organisation Conference* (ESOC). Lyon, France

59. Albers, G.W., et al., Thrombectomy for Stroke at 6 to 16 Hours with Selection by Perfusion Imaging. *N Engl J Med*, 2018. 378(8): p. 708-718.

60. Albers, G.W., et al., Assessment of Optimal Patient Selection for Endovascular Thrombectomy Beyond 6 Hours After Symptom Onset: A Pooled Analysis of the AURORA Database. *JAMA Neurol*, 2021. 78(9): p. 1064-1071.

61. Chen, C., et al., What Is the "Optimal" Target Mismatch Criteria for Acute Ischemic Stroke? *Frontiers in Neurology*, 2021. 11. 590766. eCollection 2020

62. Baron, J.-C., Selection of Patients for Thrombectomy in the Extended Time Window. *JAMA Neurology*, 2021. 78(9): p. 1051-1053.

63. Error in Figure. *JAMA Neurol*, 2021. 78(9): p. 1154.

64. Bracard, S., et al., Mechanical thrombectomy after intravenous alteplase versus alteplase alone after stroke (THRACE): a randomised controlled trial. *Lancet Neurol*, 2016. 15(11): p. 1138-47.

65. Yang, P., et al., Endovascular Thrombectomy with or without Intravenous Alteplase in Acute Stroke. *New England Journal of Medicine*, 2020. 382(21): p. 1981-1993.

66. Zi, W., et al., Effect of Endovascular Treatment Alone vs Intravenous Alteplase Plus Endovascular Treatment on Functional Independence in Patients With Acute Ischemic Stroke: The DEVT Randomized Clinical Trial. *JAMA*, 2021. 325(3): p. 234-243.

67. Suzuki, K., et al., Effect of Mechanical Thrombectomy Without vs With Intravenous Thrombolysis on Functional Outcome Among Patients With Acute Ischemic Stroke: The SKIP Randomized Clinical Trial. *JAMA*, 2021. 325(3): p. 244-253.

68. Treurniet, K.M., et al., MR CLEAN-NO IV: intravenous treatment followed by endovascular treatment versus direct endovascular treatment for acute ischemic stroke caused by a proximal intracranial occlusion—study protocol for a randomized clinical trial. *Trials*, 2021. 22(1): p. 141.

69. LeCouffe, N.E., et al., A Randomized Trial of Intravenous Alteplase before Endovascular Treatment for Stroke. *New England Journal of Medicine*, 2021. 385(20): p. 1833-1844.

70. Turc, G., et al., European Stroke Organisation (ESO) – European Society for Minimally Invasive Neurological Therapy (ESMINT) Guidelines on Mechanical Thrombectomy in Acute Ischaemic StrokeEndorsed by Stroke Alliance for Europe (SAFE). *European Stroke Journal*, 2019. 4(1): p. 6-12.

71. Albers, G.W., et al., A multicenter randomized controlled trial of endovascular therapy following imaging evaluation for ischemic stroke (DEFUSE 3). *Int J Stroke*, 2017. 12(8): p. 896-905.

72. Renú, A., et al., Effect of Intra-arterial Alteplase vs Placebo Following Successful Thrombectomy on Functional Outcomes in Patients With Large Vessel Occlusion Acute Ischemic Stroke: The CHOICE Randomized Clinical Trial. *JAMA*, 2022.

73. Goyal, M., et al., Endovascular thrombectomy after large-vessel ischaemic stroke: a meta-analysis of individual patient data from five randomised trials. *Lancet*, 2016. 387(10029): p. 1723-31.

74. Mokin, M., et al., Indications for thrombectomy in acute ischemic stroke from emergent large vessel occlusion (ELVO): report of the SNIS Standards and Guidelines Committee. *Journal of NeuroInterventional Surgery*, 2019. 11(3): p. 215.

75. Barber, P.A., et al., Validity and reliability of a quantitative computed tomography score in predicting outcome of hyperacute stroke before thrombolytic therapy. ASPECTS Study Group. Alberta Stroke Programme Early CT Score. *Lancet*, 2000. 355(9216): p. 1670-4.

76. Menon, B., et al. (2022). "Alteplase Compared to Tenecteplase (ACT) trial." *European Stroke Journal* 7(1_suppl): 546-588.

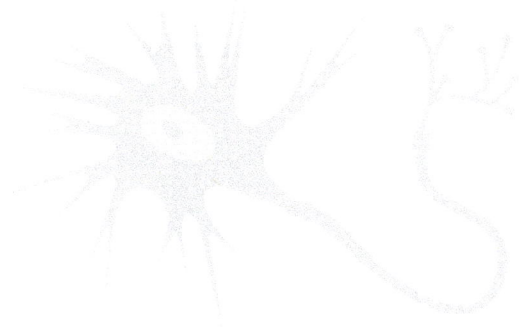

# Dysphagia Screen

All patients admitted with stroke or TIA symptoms must be screened for dysphagia before being given food or drink. Failure of the screen indicates dysphagia. The screen is completed by a speech pathologist, a doctor or a competency assessed nurse.

*Note:* A speech pathologist is available via pager 0800–1600 Mon/Fri and 0800–1030 Sat/Sun to review if the patient failed the screening test

- **Is the patient alert**
- **Speech sounds produced clearly**
- **Gag present**
- **Voice clear (say ah for several seconds)**
- **Cough strong**

If no to any of these questions:

- Make the patient nil by mouth.
- Position the patient in an upright position at 90º to sip some water ask the patient to take one, and then a second, then a third sip of water. If you can answer yes to the following questions, then ask the patient to drink one mouthful of water. If you can answer yes, then ask the patient to drink the rest of the cup.

  - Is the patient's voice clear after each swallow, after a sip, a mouthful, or the cup

- Is the patient breathing comfortably? After six, a mouthful and the cup
- If the answer to these two questions is no, the patient should be made Nil by mouth and referred to a speech therapist and dietician
- Take a baseline oxygen saturation level and then repeat two minutes after each sip, mouthful, or cup of water (record over page).
- If it falls by more than 2% the patient has failed the dysphagia screen.
- The patient should be nil by mouth, refer to speech therapist and dietician

**Screen pass** (all yes answers): patient can commence a full ward diet and thin fluids.

**Screen fail exception**: If oral drugs cannot be withheld or given by an alternative route (Pharmacy has a list of alternatives for dysphagic patients) then a Flexiflow NGT size 10 or 12 should be

# appendix G Dysphagia Screen

inserted primarily for drug administration, its position checked by chest X-ray and management orders written on admission

NGT inserted for medications: YES ☐    NO ☐

Continue to monitor for signs of dysphagia as described in the 'Dysphagia Screening After Stroke' learning package


Signature and designation _____


Date: _____ Time: _____


| Parameter | Baseline | 2 minutes post 1st sip water | 2 minutes post 2nd sip water | 2 minutes post 3rd sip water | 2 minutes post mouthful water | 2 minutes post cup water |
|---|---|---|---|---|---|---|
| Oxygen Saturation | | | | | | |

STROKE 121 DYSPHAGIA SCREEN

| Alert and responsive? | YES | NO |
|---|---|---|

| If patient | **1** |
|---|---|
| FAILS this: | |
| 1. Place NBM** without NGT (see exception below) | |
| 2. Refer to SP* | |
| 3. Refer to dietician | |

| Speech sounds produced clearly? | YES | NO |
|---|---|---|
| Gag present? | YES | NO<br>Absent, weak, unilateral |
| Voice clear?<br>(Say 'ah' for as long as you can) | YES | NO |
| Cough strong? | YES | NO |

| If patient | **2** |
|---|---|
| FAILS any: | |
| 1. Place NBM** without NGT (see exception below) | |
| 2. Refer to SP* | |
| 3. Refer to dietician | |

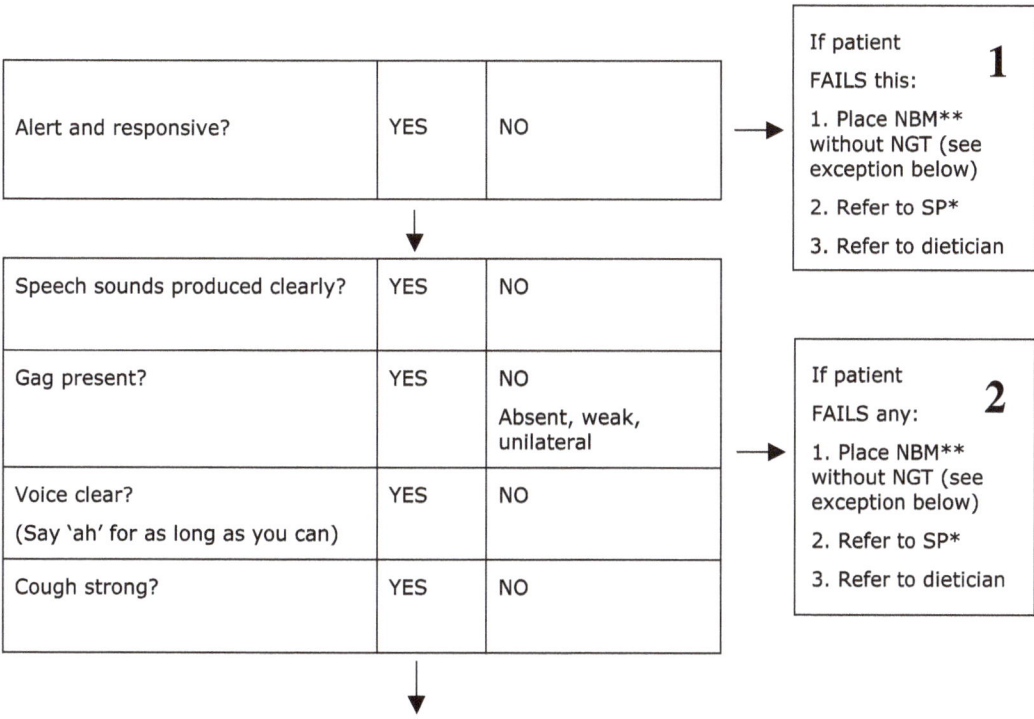

Position the patient in an upright position at 90° so that he/she can sip some water.

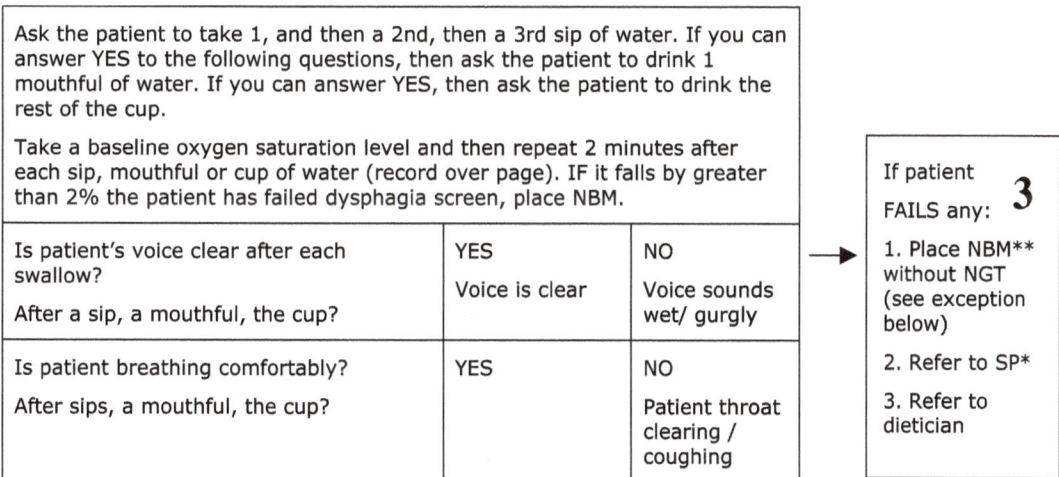

| Ask the patient to take 1, and then a 2nd, then a 3rd sip of water. If you can answer YES to the following questions, then ask the patient to drink 1 mouthful of water. If you can answer YES, then ask the patient to drink the rest of the cup. |
|---|
| Take a baseline oxygen saturation level and then repeat 2 minutes after each sip, mouthful or cup of water (record over page). IF it falls by greater than 2% the patient has failed dysphagia screen, place NBM. |

| | | |
|---|---|---|
| Is patient's voice clear after each swallow?<br><br>After a sip, a mouthful, the cup? | YES<br>Voice is clear | NO<br>Voice sounds wet/ gurgly |
| Is patient breathing comfortably?<br><br>After sips, a mouthful, the cup? | YES | NO<br>Patient throat clearing / coughing |

| If patient | **3** |
|---|---|
| FAILS any: | |
| 1. Place NBM** without NGT (see exception below) | |
| 2. Refer to SP* | |
| 3. Refer to dietician | |

* SP = speech pathologist

** NBM = nil by mouth

**Figure G1** Dysphagia Screen

479

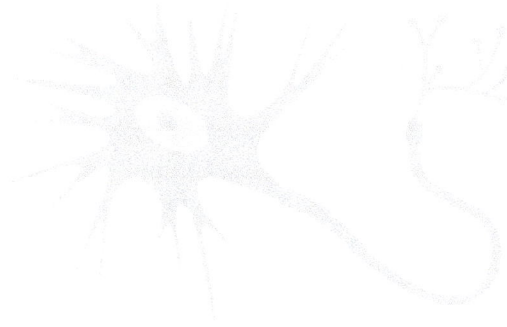

# Nerve Conduction Studies and Electromyography

Nerve conduction studies (NCS) are like any other test in that they have a sensitivity and specificity and positive and negative predictive values. NCS can help confirm a diagnosis and provide an objective measure of severity and can help in determining subsequent treatment and response to treatment.

## What to Tell the Patient to Expect

Many patients are very worried about NCS and electromyography (EMG), and it does not help if an explanation of what to expect is provided at the time of ordering the test. An explanation should always be, and usually is, provided at the time of the actual test. NCS are performed by taping a disc or a disposable recording electrode to the skin over the surface of the muscle and then applying a stimulating electrode and administering a small, safe, but at times uncomfortable, electrical impulse several times at different sites along course of various nerves. NOT all patients undergoing NCS will have a needle inserted into a muscle. A needle is inserted into muscle when performing EMG. Figures H.1 and H.2 can be used to show patients what to expect.

## How to Interpret NCS and EMG Reports

Most practitioners not familiar with NCS will simply read the conclusion. Neurophysiologists frequently use abbreviations that are confusing to the uninitiated. Table H.1 contains a list of the common terms and abbreviations used in NCS and EMG reports.

---

🔑

A Normal NCS do not exclude a diagnosis
when symptoms are intermittent in nature or of recent onset.

---

NCS reflect the degree of damage to the nerve and as such initially may be entirely normal or demonstrate minor and non-diagnostic abnormalities when the symptoms are either intermittent in nature or of recent onset. Repeat testing 3–6 months later will often demonstrate worsening

481

and be more conclusive. Patients with recent onset (a few weeks) symptoms of carpal tunnel syndrome often have normal NCS, as do patients in the first 1 or 2 weeks of acute inflammatory demyelinating peripheral neuropathy.

# When to Order NCS and EMG

The most useful application of electrophysiology is in carpal tunnel syndrome [1] where the sensitivity is high [2] and the response to surgery can be anticipated based on the severity of the findings [3]. In carpal tunnel syndrome if the degree of compression of the median nerve is mild the NCS can be normal. Table H.2 lists the findings on NCS with increasing severity of median nerve compression in the carpal tunnel. It is important to note that the NCS, even when positive, do NOT diagnose carpal tunnel syndrome; they simply localise the site of the problem to the region of the carpal tunnel in the wrist where carpal tunnel syndrome is the most probable cause. It is important to correlate the clinical symptoms with the NCS findings. In patients with persistent symptoms following surgery, a comparison between the pre- and postoperative studies allows assessment of whether the median nerve compression in the carpal tunnel has been decompressed or worse still the nerve has been damaged during surgery, a rare but recognised complication of surgery.

> Normal NCS do not exclude a mild carpal tunnel syndrome and abnormal NCS that are in keeping with carpal tunnel syndrome may not explain all the patient's symptoms.

- NCS are particularly useful at confirming and localising the exact site of compression in ulnar nerve lesions [7, 8]. Beware when the report shows slowing from above to below the elbow. Although this is a recognised technique the short distance means it can produce false positive results as a 0.5-1cm error in measuring the distance can represent a 10% difference. I prefer to compare the velocity and amplitude of the response from above the elbow to the wrist and below the elbow to the wrist. If there is change in either the amplitude or conduction velocity, I use Kimura's inching technique to determine the exact site of compression.[16]
- NCS ± EMG is also usually diagnostic in patients with suspected peripheral neuropathy – a normal study virtually excludes this diagnosis (except with recent onset symptoms or with small fibre neuropathy, see Chapter 12, 'Back pain and common leg problems with or without difficulty walking'). Occasionally NCS will detect subclinical neuropathy, particularly in diabetes [9].
- EMG is the test to order when looking for a disease of muscle such as polymyositis.
- NCS have a high sensitivity when a single nerve is damaged and in patients with a peripheral neuropathy. The exceptions to this are small fibre neuropathy, a common cause of burning feet syndrome where the NCS are normal and early in the course of AIDP where the initial NCS may be normal. Most protocols for electrophysiological examination of peripheral neuropathy require examination of motor and sensory nerves in at least two extremities [10].

- A condition where nerve conduction studies are often requested is impingement of the lateral cutaneous nerve of the thigh beneath the inguinal ligament, so-called meralgia paraesthetica (see Chapter 12, 'Back pain and common leg problems with or without difficulty walking'). It is important to warn the patient that the NCS are technically difficult, the test is very painful with electric stimuli to the groin and the sensitivity and specificity are poor.
- NCS and EMG for cervical and lumbar radiculopathy, even in competent hands, have a variable sensitivity [11, 12] in patients with suspected radiculopathy (29%) although results are a little better in patients with definite radiculopathy (72%) [11]. The most sensitive test is EMG [13].
- Similarly, nerve conduction studies in patients with shoulder and arm pain looking for brachial neuritis rarely if ever find any abnormality in patients who do not have objective signs of weakness or altered sensation. They involve very extensive and at time painful; testing with large amplitude prolonged stimuli required to stimulate the brachial plexus in the supraclavicular fossa.
- Repetitive stimulation studies to assess for myasthenia gravis or Lambert–Eaton Syndrome. [14]
- NCS for tarsal tunnel syndrome are technically difficult and of uncertain sensitivity and specificity. [15]

# What to Do When the Result is not what was Anticipated

- A normal study virtually excludes the suspected diagnosis when there are objective abnormal signs of a peripheral neuropathy or peripheral nerve lesion unless it was of recent onset (1–2 weeks). If NCS are normal in a patient with clinically suspected peripheral neuropathy, somatosensory evoked potentials may be abnormal. The other possibility is that the patient's symptoms, particularly those with burning feet are due to a small fibre neuropathy nit detected by NCS.
- In patients with intermittent symptoms a normal study does not exclude the diagnosis, particularly carpal tunnel syndrome. Approaches in this setting include wait-and-see with a repeat study in 3–6 months if symptoms persist. If symptoms are severe and classical for carpal tunnel syndrome in a patient who is unable to tolerate them it is not unreasonable to recommend a steroid injection or surgery in patients with classical carpal tunnel syndrome. However, as already alluded to, the results of surgery in the setting of normal NCS are less than optimal.
- In patients with atypical features of carpal tunnel syndrome and a normal NCS, the patient should be informed that there is no proof of the diagnosis, that their symptoms are not typical and may not resolve with surgery. The other alternative in this setting and the most useful is to seek a second opinion.

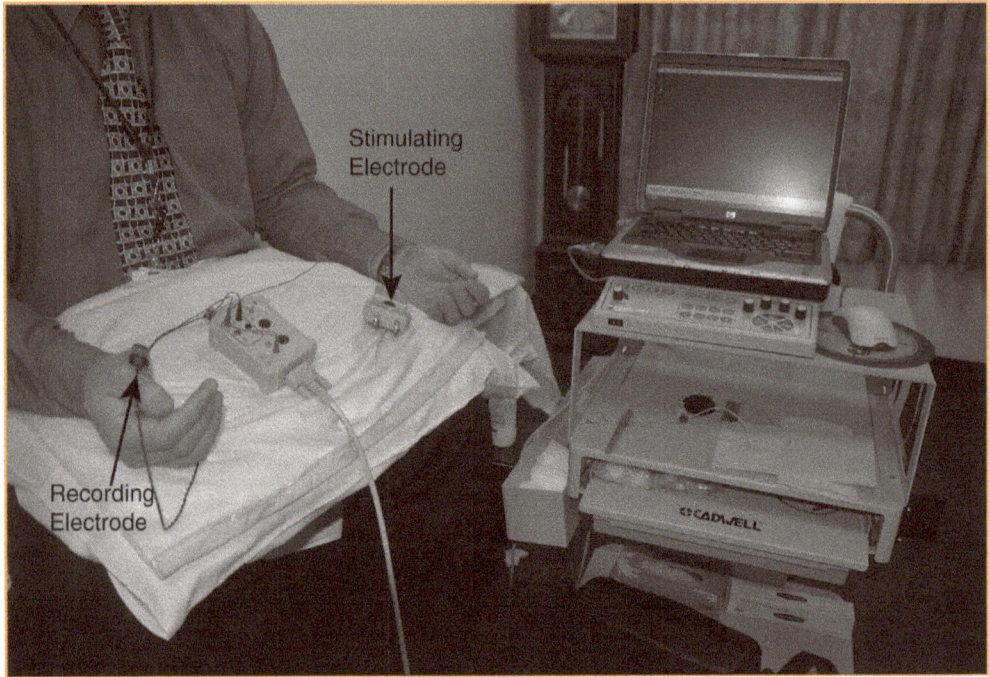

**Figure H.1** NCS set-up: The surface electrode is placed over the muscle (in this case the APB) and the stimulating electrode is placed over the nerve (not shown here) and a DC electrical impulse is applied to the nerve.

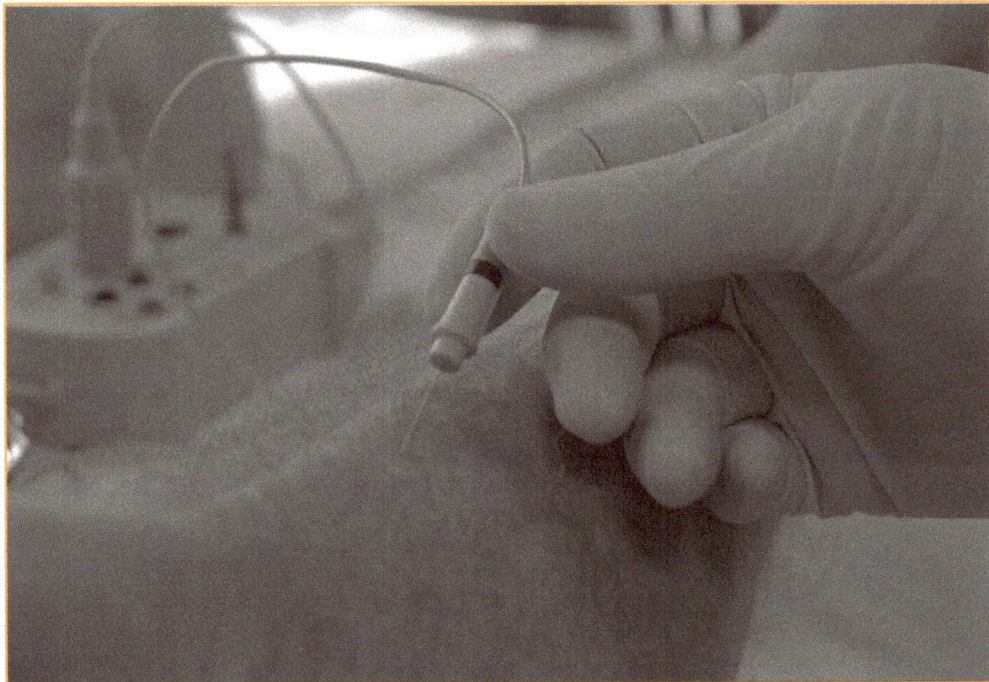

**Figure H.2** EMG set-up: The concentric needle electrode is shown in the muscle

| Term | Explanation |
|---|---|
| Distal motor latency (DML) | The latency between the distal point of stimulation of the nerve and the recording electrode on the surface of the muscle |
| Motor nerve conduction velocity (MNCV) | The conduction velocity between two points of stimulation along the motor nerve |
| Sensory nerve conduction velocity (SNCV) | The conduction velocity along the sensory nerve |
| Sensory nerve action potential (SNAP) | The response on stimulating the sensory nerve |
| Compound motor action potential (CMAP) | The response recorded over the muscle when stimulating the motor nerve |
| Single fibre electromyography (SFEMG) | Using a fine needle to record the response in a single muscle fibre, particularly useful in myasthenia gravis |
| F-wave latency (F-Wave) | The time taken for the impulse to spread from the point of stimulation distally in the limb in a retrograde manner back to the anterior horn cell in the spinal cord and then back down to the recording electrodes; this latency is very dependent on the length of the limb |
| Insertional activity* | Refers to the initial potentials recorded on insertion of the needle into the muscle |
| Spontaneous activity* | Refers to abnormal muscle fibre activity such as fibrillation potentials, positive sharp waves and fasciculations seen in enervated muscle or the inflammatory myopathies |
| Recruitment* | Refers to the number of motor units fire (recruit) with active muscle contraction |

**Table H.1** Common terms used in electromyography (*) and nerve conduction studies

| Severity of carpal tunnel syndrome | Increasing severity of NCS findings* |
|---|---|
| Very mild or recent onset | Normal |
| Mild | Prolonged sensory latency, either palm to wrist or finger to wrist (with or without a reduction in the amplitude of the response) but only in comparison with the corresponding ulnar SNAP (> 0.3 ms difference) |
| Mild–moderate | Prolonged absolute sensory latency (palm to wrist) |
| Moderate | As above + prolonged median 2nd lumbrical to ulnar 4th interosseous latency (> 0.4 ms difference) [6] |
| Moderate–severe | Prolonged median distal motor latency (DML) compared to corresponding ulnar DML (> 0.5 ms) ± absent median SNAP. Prolonged absolute median distal motor latency (> 4.7 ms) |
| Severe | Absent median motor and sensory responses but retained lumbrical response. |
| Very Severe | No response in the motor, sensory or lumbrical studies |

**Table H.2** NCS findings in carpal tunnel syndrome with increasing severity of median nerve compression
* *Note:* This is like the severity rating scale proposed by Bland [4], except he does not refer to the absent responses or the median lumbrical studies. These latter studies are particularly useful and may help to confirm carpal tunnel syndrome in patients with coexistent peripheral neuropathy. [5]

# References

1    American Association of Electrodiagnostic Medicine. American Academy of Neurology and American Academy of Physical Medicine and Rehabilitation. Practice parameter for electrodiagnostic studies in carpal tunnel syndrome: Summary statement. *Muscle Nerve* 2002;25(6):918–922.

2    American Association of Electrodiagnostic Medicine. Guidelines in electrodiagnostic medicine. Practice parameter for electrodiagnostic studies in carpal tunnel syndrome. *Muscle Nerve Suppl* 1999;8:S141–S167.

3    Schrijver HM, et al. Correlating nerve conduction studies and clinical outcome measures on carpal tunnel syndrome: Lessons from a randomized controlled trial. *J Clin Neurophysiol* 2005;22(3):216–221.

4    Bland JD. A neurophysiological grading scale for carpal tunnel syndrome. *Muscle Nerve* 2000;23(8):1280–1283.

5    Preston DC, Logigian EL. Lumbrical and interossei recording in carpal tunnel syndrome. *Muscle Nerve* 1992;15(11):1253–1257.

6    Boonyapisit K, et al. Lumbrical and interossei recording in severe carpal tunnel syndrome. *Muscle Nerve* 2002;25(1):102–105.

7    Kern RZ. The electrodiagnosis of ulnar nerve entrapment at the elbow. *Can J Neurol Sci* 2003;30(4):314–319.

8    American Association of Electrodiagnostic Medicine. American Academy of Neurology, and American Academy of Physical Medicine and Rehabilitation. Practice parameter: Electrodiagnostic studies in ulnar neuropathy at the elbow. *Neurology* 1999;52(4):688–690.

9    Liu MS, et al. [Clinical and neurophysiological features of 700 patients with diabetic peripheral neuropathy]. *Zhonghua Nei Ke Za Zhi* 2005;44(3):173–176.

10   American Association of Electrodiagnostic Medicine. Guidelines in electrodiagnostic medicine. *Muscle Nerve* 1992;15:229–253.

11   Nardin RA, et al. Electromyography and magnetic resonance imaging in the evaluation of radiculopathy. *Muscle Nerve* 1999;22(2):151–155.

12   Robinson LR. Electromyography, magnetic resonance imaging, and radiculopathy: It's time to focus on specificity. *Muscle Nerve* 1999;22(2):149–150.

13   American Association of Electrodiagnostic Medicine and American Academy of Physical Medicine and Rehabilitation. Practice parameters for needle electromyographic evaluation of patients with suspected cervical radiculopathy: Summary Statement. *Muscle Nerve Supplement* 1999;22(8):S211–S322.

14   American Association of Electrodiagnostic Medicine Quality Assurance Committee. Practice parameter for repetitive nerve stimulation and single fiber EMG evaluation of adults with suspected myasthenia gravis or Lambert–Eaton myasthenic syndrome: Summary statement. *Muscle Nerve* 2001;24(9):1236–1238.

15   Patel AT, et al. Usefulness of electrodiagnostic techniques in the evaluation of suspected tarsal tunnel syndrome: An evidence-based review. *Muscle Nerve* 2005;32(2):236–240.

16   Machida M, Kimura J. [Nerve conduction study using inching technique]. *No To Shinkei* 1987; 39(9): 825-35.

# Diagnostic Criteria for Multiple Sclerosis

| Warning |
| --- |
| The information in this appendix will be rapidly out of date. Always check the latest guidelines. |

| McDonald Criteria for Diagnosis of MS | |
| --- | --- |
| **Number of lesions with objective clinical evidence** | **Additional data needed for a diagnosis of multiple sclerosis** |
| ≥2 clinical attacks ≥2 None* | None |
| ≥2 clinical attacks 1 (as well as clear-cut historical evidence of a previous | None |
| ≥2 clinical attacks 1 | Dissemination in space demonstrated by an additional clinical attack implicating a different CNS site or by MRI‡ |
| 1 clinical attack ≥2 | Dissemination in time demonstrated by an additional clinical attack or by MRI§ OR demonstration of CSF-specific oligoclonal bands¶ |
| 1 clinical attack 1 | Dissemination in space demonstrated by an additional clinical attack implicating a different CNS site or by MRI‡ AND Dissemination in time demonstrated by an additional clinical attack or by MRI§ OR demonstration of CSF-specific oligoclonal bands |

**Table I.1** 2017 revisions to the McDonald diagnostic criteria for multiple sclerosis [1]

| McDonald Criteria Dissemination in Space and Time |
|---|
| **Primary progressive multiple sclerosis can be diagnosed in patients with:**<br>• 1 year of disability progression (retrospectively or prospectively determined) independent of clinical relapse<br>**Plus, two of the following criteria:**<br>• One or more T2-hyperintense lesions* characteristic of multiple sclerosis in one or more of the following brain regions: periventricular, cortical or juxtacortical, or infratentorial<br>• Two or more T2-hyperintense lesions* in the spinal cord<br>• Presence of CSF-specific oligoclonal bands |
| Dissemination in space can be demonstrated by one or more T2-hyperintense lesions* that are characteristic of multiple sclerosis in two or more of four areas of the CNS: periventricular, † cortical or juxtacortical, and infratentorial brain regions, and the spinal cord |
| • Dissemination in time can be demonstrated by the simultaneous presence of gadolinium-enhancing and non-enhancing lesions* at any time or by a new T2-hyperintense or gadolinium-enhancing lesion on follow-up MRI, with reference to a baseline scan, irrespective of the timing of the baseline MRI |

**Table I.2** 2017 McDonald criteria for demonstration of dissemination in space and time by MRI in a patient with a clinically isolated syndrome. *Unlike the 2010 McDonald criteria, no distinction between symptomatic and asymptomatic MRI lesions is required. †In some patients—e.g., individuals older than 50 years or those with vascular risk factors—it might be prudent for the clinician to seek a higher number of periventricular lesions.

| McDonald Criteria Primary Progressive MS |
|---|
| **Primary progressive multiple sclerosis can be diagnosed in patients with:**<br>• 1 year of disability progression (retrospectively or prospectively determined) independent of clinical relapse<br>**Plus, two of the following criteria:**<br>• One or more T2-hyperintense lesions* characteristic of multiple sclerosis in one or more of the following brain regions: periventricular, cortical or juxtacortical, or infratentorial<br>• Two or more T2-hyperintense lesions* in the spinal cord<br>• Presence of CSF-specific oligoclonal bands |

**Table I.3** 2017 McDonald criteria for diagnosis of primary progressive multiple sclerosis. *Unlike the 2010 McDonald criteria, no distinction between symptomatic and asymptomatic MRI lesions is required.

# References

1    Thompson AJ, Banwell BL, Barkhof F, et al. Diagnosis of multiple sclerosis: 2017 revisions of the McDonald criteria. *The Lancet Neurology* 2018; 17(2): 162-73.

# Treatment of Parkinson's Disease

| Warning |
|---|
| The information in this appendix will be rapidly out of date. Always check the latest guidelines. |

## Introduction

There is no effective treatment to arrest the progression of the disease.

Management is primarily the alleviation of symptoms whilst minimizing the side effects of medications. Initial treatment options include levodopa1 combined with a decarboxylase inhibitor, a dopamine agonist, or a monoamine oxidase type B inhibitor. Treatment should commence early as delayed treatment results in a more inferior quality of life. [1]

As a general principle, starting with the smallest possible dose is advisable and gradually increasing to the minimum effective or maximum tolerated amount when starting treatment. In the initial stages, patients respond well to 1-2 tablets of levodopa with each meal. As the disease worsens, the benefit duration diminishes in patients, and patients require more frequent levodopa, or the addition of other drugs discussed below. In the late stages of Parkinson's, it is often necessary to reduce therapy to alleviate troublesome and involuntary movements referred to as dyskinesia.

## Levodopa – The Drug of First Choice

Levodopa forms the mainstay of treating the motor symptoms in Parkinson's as it replaces the dwindling dopamine. Levodopa was first investigated in 1967 by George Cotzias and colleagues. [2] Levodopa results in more symptomatic benefit and is better tolerated than the dopamine agonists. [3] However, levodopa has a higher risk of developing dyskinesia. [4, 5] Levodopa is combined with a peripheral decarboxylase inhibitor, either carbidopa or benserazide. These reduce the peripheral side effects seen with large doses of pure levodopa. The decarboxylase inhibitor also inhibits the peripheral degradation of levodopa, thus boosting the amount of levodopa reaching the central nervous system. The plasma half-life of levodopa in

---

1 The word levodopa in this document implies a combination of levodopa and a decarboxylase inhibitor.

the immediate-release formulation is approximately 90 minutes with a duration of action of about 3-4 hours.

Parkinson's disease is a life-long problem. Thus, there is no need to rapidly increase the dose of any of the recommended drugs. One approach is to commence Levodopa with the lowest possible dose, half a 100/25mg tablet per day. The dose is increased by half a tablet per day each week. The patient is reviewed at eight weeks when they have been on one tablet three times per day for two weeks, allowing enough time to assess the benefit. If the benefit is suboptimal, the dose is slowly increased by half a tablet per day each week up to two tablets three times per day.

In Parkinson's disease, the initial response to levodopa is very gratifying. Some patients benefit more than others. A small number of patients are drug-resistant. [6] *A lack of improvement should prompt a review of the diagnosis*. The levodopa unresponsive patients had rigidity, bradykinesia, and gait disturbance without tremor. Without a diagnostic test, it is unclear whether such patients have Parkinson's disease with loss of dopamine neurons.

The maximum dose very much depends on the development of side effects. Most patients will require 400-2000 mg per day divided into 2-8 hourly doses. However, the German [7] guidelines recommend a much lower maximum dose of only 400 mg per day. In the initial stages, the dose-limiting side effects include nausea and postural hypotension, whilst dyskinesia, hallucinations, and confusion influence the dose in the latter stages of the disease.

Levodopa improves bradykinesia and rigidity. In some, but not all patients, it alleviates the severity of the tremor. Levodopa does not benefit the non-motor symptoms such as autonomic dysfunction, gastrointestinal symptoms, disturbances of sleep and mood, or dementia.

# End of Dose Failure vs the On-Off Phenomena

Initially, the benefit duration from a single dose may last several (5-6) hours, and thus levodopa is prescribed with each meal. After a few years, the duration of the benefit progressively shortens. A phenomenon referred to as end-of-dose failure or motor fluctuations.

Significant motor fluctuations, referred to as the on-off phenomenon, develop in patients with more Parkinson's. The on-off phenomenon is when dyskinesia alternates with severe symptoms of Parkinson's, <u>unrelated to the timing of medication</u>. Patients experience potentially disabling "off" periods that do not respond to increased levodopa.

To differentiate between motor fluctuations with dyskinesia and the on-off phenomenon, it is essential to clarify the exact time patients take each drug, how long the benefit persists and the time when dyskinesia develops. Patients can complete a daily chart if there is some uncertainty, as shown in figure one. Patients need a careful explanation to assist them in differentiating between the involuntary movement of dyskinesia with the tremor of Parkinson's. There are three types of levodopa-induced dyskinesia. Peak-dose dyskinesia (when levodopa level is at its maximum), the wearing off or off period dyskinesia (when the levodopa level is low) and diphasic dyskinesia.

| Time of Day | 0600 | 0700 | 0800 | 0900 | 1000 | 1100 | 1200 | 1300 | 1400 | 1500 |
|---|---|---|---|---|---|---|---|---|---|---|
| Good control | | | | | | | | | | |
| Off | | | | | | | | | | |
| Dyskinesia | | | | | | | | | | |
| Time of medication | | | | | | | | | | |

| Time of Day | 1600 | 1700 | 1800 | 1900 | 2000 | 2100 | 2200 | 2300 | 2400 | |
|---|---|---|---|---|---|---|---|---|---|---|
| Good control | | | | | | | | | | |
| Off | | | | | | | | | | |
| Dyskinesia | | | | | | | | | | |
| Time of medication | | | | | | | | | | |

**Figure 1.** A chart for patients with significant motor fluctuations to document their symptoms. The patient places a mark in the relevant box depending upon whether they are experiencing a significant off period, feel they are well controlled or experiencing the involuntary movements of dyskinesia.

The dyskinesia is typically choreiform but may be dystonic, myoclonic, or ballistic. Peak-dose dyskinesia usually commences about 30 minutes after each dose of levodopa and may last up to 3 hours. Peak-dose dyskinesia is managed by reducing the individual doses of the levodopa, discontinuing, or reducing COMT and MAO-B inhibitors, switching to immediate-release preparations and considering adding amantadine. A different approach is needed with off-period dyskinesia, diphasic dyskinesia and the dyskinesia seen with the on-off phenomenon. [8]Nocturnal off-period dystonia is treated with long-acting levodopa formulations at bedtime. COMT inhibitors, Mayo-B inhibitors and dopamine agonists treat daytime off-period dystonia. Diphasic dyskinesia is difficult to treat. Currently, subcutaneous infusions of apomorphine, Levodopa/carbidopa intestinal gel, and deep brain stimulation are recommended.

Many patients prefer to have dyskinesia rather than be immobile from Parkinson's.[2] Dyskinesia and the on-off phenomenon were once thought to result of toxicity from long time use of levodopa. This led to the recommendation that levodopa therapy should be deferred for as long as possible. The LEAP study [1, 9] and the neurotoxin MPTP [10, 11] (1-methyl-4-phenyl-1,2,3,6-tetrahydropyridine) induced Parkinsonism have shown this to be incorrect. [3]Levodopa should be introduced early on when symptoms interfere with the patient's quality of life.

There are several different approaches to managing patients with motor fluctuations that result in significant off periods. [8] One method is to reduce the interval between doses. It is not uncommon for patients with long-standing Parkinson's to be taking half a tablet every 2-3 hours or swallowing 30 mL of liquid levodopa. They need to have an alarm to remind them that a dose is due. Other options include slow and rapid release forms of levodopa, either as individual drugs or combined into a single drug, liquid levodopa, dopamine agonists, catechol-O-methyltransferase (COMT) inhibitors, monoamine oxidase type B (MAO-B) inhibitors, apomorphine and duo-dopa. Not all these medications are available in every country. There is little comparative data to help in selecting one from the other.

Managing the on-off phenomenon is far more complex. The aim is to minimize the fluctuations in the serum levels of medications. Continuous or slow-release levodopa should be discontinued as it makes controlling levodopa levels difficult. Options include liquid levodopa, dopamine agonists (including rotigotine transdermal patches), continuous subcutaneous apomorphine, COMT inhibitors and adenosine A2A antagonists.

Rescue therapy is used in patients with frequent off periods. Rescue medications act more rapidly and include madopar rapid, liquid levodopa administered either orally or sublingually and apomorphine subcutaneous or sublingual [12, 13] are appropriate.

---

2 Personal observation

3 These so-called "side-effects" may simply reflect the severity of the underlying disease and the paucity of dopamine receptors. Individuals with MPTP poisoning destroyed virtually all their dopamine receptors and developed the "long-term side-effects" within months of commencing levodopa.

# Extended or Controlled-Release Levodopa

Extended or controlled release levodopa combines immediate and slow-release forms of levodopa with a decarboxylase inhibitor. Controlled-release levodopa reduces the bioavailability (71vs 99%) but prolongs the serum half-life of levodopa. In theory, this eliminates the fluctuations in the levodopa level. The time to peak levodopa concentrations is twice that of the standard levodopa-decarboxylase formulation.[14]

# Liquid Levodopa

If patients can tolerate the increased fluid (not all patients can), oral liquid levodopa is a viable option. The total daily dose of the levodopa-decarboxylase combination is dissolved either in a bottle of dry ginger ale or 1 L of water containing 500 mg of vitamin C. Both have the necessary pH for the levodopa to survive in the liquid. Liquid levodopa must be made up every day. Patients drink 60 mL every hour. In this way, they are drip-feeding a continuous supply of levodopa into the circulation, avoiding large surges in levodopa levels that occur when taking tablets or capsules. Continuous intravenous dopaminergic delivery reduces motor fluctuations. [15] A continuous subcutaneous infusion of liquid levodopa results in significantly less off-time and increased on-time without troublesome dyskinesia. [16, 17] Co-administration of entacapone results in higher serum levels of levodopa during continuous subcutaneous infusion. [17]

# Continuous Dopaminergic Stimulation

Continuous dopaminergic stimulation is recommended in patients with advanced Parkinson's who take levodopa 4-5 times per day because of end of dose failure. Continuous dopamine stimulation is one of the device-aided treatments (DATs). Device-aided treatment of Parkinson's refers to deep brain stimulation (DBS), levodopa-carbidopa intestinal gel infusion (LCIG), and subcutaneous infusion of the dopamine agonist apomorphine.

Jejunal levodopa-carbidopa intestinal gel infusion is as equally effective as deep brain stimulation. [18]

# Duo-Dopa

Duo-dopa is a solution (20mg/ml) of dopamine combined with a decarboxylase inhibitor administered via a permanent percutaneous endoscopic gastrostomy (PEG) tube containing a smaller intestinal tube terminating in the duodenum. The solution is 20mg/ml, and 100ml is administered slowly throughout the day resulting in smoother intestinal drug uptake. It is recommended for patients who are not suitable for deep-brain stimulation or cannot manage subcutaneous apomorphine. [19] Duo-dopa is resource-consuming and expensive. It requires a multidisciplinary team to ensure optimal patient care. Duo-dopa is used in patients with advanced Parkinson's to alleviate motor fluctuations.

# Dopamine Agonists

Dopamine agonists are either ergoline and non-ergoline agonists. The ergoline agonists include bromocriptine, pergolide, lisuride, and cabergoline, whereas ropinirole (2-24 mg per day, once per day) and pramipexole are non-ergoline agonists. The dopamine agonists have a serum half-life of six or more hours and act directly on dopamine receptors mimicking the endogenous neurotransmitter. The ergoline dopamine agonists have been discontinued because they cause retroperitoneal fibrosis and cardiac valve abnormalities. Dopamine agonists can be used alone but are more frequently added to levodopa, allowing a 20-30% reduction in the dose of levodopa[4]. In advanced Parkinson's, dopamine agonists decrease "off" time. The decrease in the levodopa dosage results in less dyskinesia. Nausea, postural hypotension, and dyskinesia occur with higher doses.

Apomorphine is a non-ergoline dopamine agonist. [12, 13, 20] Before initiating apomorphine, all antiparkinsonian medications should be temporarily withheld. Pre-treatment with domperidone 20 mg TDS is required to prevent significant nausea that can occur. Apomorphine is administered either by subcutaneous injections (10-30mg) or continuous subcutaneous infusion (30-180 mg per day). However, long term use of continuous subcutaneous infusion runs the risk of crystallization of apomorphine in the catheter, leading to the formation of thrombi. [21]

One very disturbing side-effect of dopamine agonists is sudden sleep attacks whilst driving! [22, 23] These are exceedingly rare, occurring in less than 2% of patients. Patients who experience these episodes should stop driving until the dose of their dopamine agonist is reduced. Patients should be warned of the possibility of developing impulse control disorders, such as gambling, compulsive sexual behaviour, and binge-eating disorder that are other potential side effects of dopamine agonists. [24]

# COMT Inhibitors

Catechol-O-methyltransferase (COMT) inhibitors block the enzyme COMT that breaks down dopamine. The COMT inhibitors include entacapone (200mg), tolcapone (100-200mg) and opicapone(50mg). Tolcapone can cause fatal level failure and is rarely used. The main side-effects include nausea, abdominal discomfort, constipation, or diarrhoea. It is important to warn patients that their urine may change colour. Each dose of levodopa is combined with a dose of entacapone, whilst opicapone is once-a-day therapy.

# MAO-B Inhibitors

At one stage, thought to be monoamine oxidase type B (MAO-B) inhibitors such as selegiline and rasagiline were neuroprotective. This is no longer the case. Both drugs provide a small symptomatic benefit, less than levodopa but fewer side effects. [25]

Safinamide inhibits MAO-B and reduces dopamine reuptake. It is associated with significant improvement in motor function with reduced off time and less dyskinesia. [26, 27] The half-life is 20-30 hours; thus, it can be taken once daily. The commencing dose is 50 mg per day, and the maximum amount is 100 mg per day.

---

4   personal observation, previously untreated patients do not notice the same significant improvement with the dopamine agonists as they do with levodopa preparations.

# Adenosine A2A antagonists

Istradefylline has a different mechanism of action than all other Parkinson's drugs. It blocks the chemical and no zine in the brain, boosting the signalling of dopamine. It significantly decreases off time. [28, 29]

# Glutamate Antagonists- Amantadine

Amantadine is a complex drug with glutaminergic, dopaminergic, anticholinergic, and serotoninergic activity. It is helpful for levodopa-induced dyskinesia and for treating motor fluctuations. [30]

# Rescue Therapy

Rescue therapy refers to rapidly acting drugs in patients with significant motor fluctuations and significant off-periods.

# Madopar Rapid

Madopar rapid (50/12.5 or 100/25 mg dispersible tablets) is dissolved in 25-50 mL of water. It provides a short-term boost and is easier to swallow for patients with dysphagia. [31]

# Sinemet Fizz

Take one 250ml bottle of ginger ale. Drop-in one 250/25 Sinemet or three and a half Sinemet 100/10 tablets. The ginger ale will have approximately 1 mg per ml of Sinemet. Keep cool, and it will remain stable for 24 hours. The patient carries the bottle and takes one mouthful every 5-10 minutes until improvement.

# Inhaled Levodopa

Inhaled levodopa, as with all forms of levodopa, is associated with motor fluctuations and dose-limiting dyskinesias. It is a dry powder that is inhaled, delivering levodopa to the alveolar membrane, where it is rapidly absorbed within minutes. Improvement was noticed within ten minutes and sustained for one hour.[31] The USFDA approved Inbrija (levodopa inhalation powder) in 2018.

# Apomorphine

Apomorphine as a subcutaneous bolus (7-10 mg per bolus, up to 75 mg per day) has been available as rescue therapy for some time. [12] Recently, a sublingual form has been developed. [13] The initial dose is 10 mg but can be increased by 5 mg each day to a maximum of 35 mg.

# Levodopa Resistant Tremor
## Drug Therapy

In patients with levodopa unresponsive tremor, the dopamine agonists (bromocriptine, pramipexole, ropinirole, rotigotine and injectable apomorphine), anticholinergics (benztropine and trihexyphenidyl) [32] and the MAO-B inhibitor safinamide [33]are recommended. Neurosurgery is an option if medical therapy fails. [34, 35]

# Neurosurgery

There are several neurosurgical interventions directed to various parts of the basal ganglia. The invasive techniques are ablative surgery to the pallidum, thalamus, subthalamus, and deep brain stimulation. The non-invasive methods include focused high-frequency ultrasound and transcranial magnetic stimulation.

# Lesion Therapy

Ablative lesions of the basal ganglia include pallidotomy, thalamotomy and subthalamotomy. They are not applied bilaterally due to the risk of speech, swallowing, and cognitive deficits. Lesions to the ventral intermediate nucleus were highly effective in alleviating tremor. Thalamotomy has been replaced by pallidotomy and deep brain stimulation with fewer side effects.

Unilateral pallidotomy results in significant bilateral improvement of contralateral rigidity, bradykinesia, tremor and drug-induced dyskinesia, and a significant short-term improvement in ipsilateral rigidity bradykinesia and drug-induced dyskinesia as well as gait and "off"-period freezing.

Subthalamotomy, either unilateral and bilateral, has not been studied in randomized controlled trials. Case series suggests improvement in UPDRS[5] motor scores but with the risk of developing chorea. [36]

## High-Frequency Focused Ultrasound

Unilateral focused ultrasound delivered at high frequencies to the thalamus, first used in the 1950s, is a newer FDA-approved lesion technique. [37]

# Deep Brain Stimulation

Deep brain stimulation to the ventral intermediate nucleus of the thalamus is highly effective for tremor, in some instances, leading to complete resolution of contralateral tremor. [38-41]

Deep brain stimulation of the internal globus pallidus improves the "off-medicine" UPDRS motor sub score, bradykinesia, rigidity, tremor, and gait. The benefit gradually declines over the ensuing years, although the reduction in dyskinesia persists.

Deep brain stimulation to the subthalamic nucleus improves all the cardinal motor symptoms.

Deep brain stimulation enables a reduction in the dose of antiparkinsonian drugs, and side effects that occur with stimulation can be modified by altering the frequency of stimulation.

---

5 Unified Parkinson's Disease Rating Scale.

Patients with deep brain stimulators require frequent monitoring and adjustment of the settings. This implies regular visits to the clinic, although this can be done remotely with a local health care provider. [42]

Deep brain stimulation is indicated in patients with motor fluctuations, end of dose (also referred to as wearing off) dyskinesia and patients with medication unresponsive tremor. It does not benefit gait, balance, freezing, speech or swallowing difficulties, or cognitive changes. Deep brain stimulation is unhelpful in patients who no longer respond to levodopa at all. It can be done bilaterally. The procedure is contraindicated in patients with significant cognitive impairment, severe depression, psychosis, and it is not recommended for patients who have had Parkinson's for less than four years. The Congress of Neurological Surgeons has published guidelines. [40] They regard bilateral DBS to the subthalamic nucleus and globus pallidus internus as equally effective. If the goal is to reduce the dose of levodopa, they recommend DBS to the subthalamic nucleus.

## Transcranial Magnetic Stimulation

Transcranial magnetic stimulation studies have provided insights into the central role of the primary motor cortex in the movement disorder of Parkinson's disease; at this point, its effectiveness in treating Parkinson's remains unproven. [43]

## Unproven

Embryonic stem cell transplants, gene therapy and growth factors are under investigation.

## Physical Activity

Physical therapy has a vital role in patients with Parkinson's disease, particularly in the more advanced stages. Patients must not overexert themselves to the point of exhaustion. Cueing strategies to improve gait; cognitive movement strategies to improve transfers; exercises to improve balance; and training of joint mobility and muscle power to improve physical capacity. [44] The optimal mix of interventions for everyone varies according to the stage of disease progression and the patient's preferred form of exercise, capacity for learning, and age. [45]

## Non-Motor Symptoms of Parkinson's

Non-motor manifestations of Parkinson's have a significant impact on patients' quality of life and do not respond to levodopa or other drugs used to treat the motor manifestations of Parkinson's. Depression, constipation, and postural hypotension are the more troublesome non-motor symptoms of Parkinson's. [46-50]

### Excessive Drooling

Excessive drooling[6] (sialorrhea) is a common symptom of Parkinson's and can cause awkwardness in social situations. It ranges from mild wetting of the pillow during sleep to embarrassing outpourings of saliva during unguarded moments.

---

6   https://www.parkinson.org/Understanding-Parkinsons/Symptoms/Movement-Symptoms/Drooling

Drooling, along with speech and swallowing issues, is included among non-movement symptoms even though the root cause is motor: decreased coordination, slowness of movement (bradykinesia) and rigidity of the muscles of the mouth and throat.

Parkinson's causes a reduction in automatic actions, including swallowing, creating an inability to manage the flow of saliva in and around the mouth. In Parkinson's disease, the amount of saliva produced is normal, but <u>swallowing difficulties</u> with swallowing less often or not completely – lead to saliva pooling in the mouth.

When severe, drooling is an indicator of more severe difficulty with swallowing (also known as dysphagia), which can cause the person to choke on food and liquids and develop aspiration pneumonia.

## Managing Drooling

A speech pathologist can assess patients with excess drooling. They can perform a swallow test (dysphagia screen) and recommend strategies to help with drooling. Sucking on hard candy or chewing gum activates the jaw and the automatic swallowing reflex, which can help clear saliva, providing temporary relief from drooling. Another tactic is wearing a sweatband to wipe the mouth as needed discretely.

If these lifestyle strategies are ineffective, adjusting antiparkinsonian medications may make it easier to swallow. Prescription medication to dry up saliva production include:

**Oral anticholinergic medications,** as a class, decrease the production of saliva. Side effects include drowsiness, confusion, vomiting, dizziness, blurred vision, constipation, flushing, headache, and urinary retention.

**Glycopyrrolate and other oral anticholinergic medications** (trihexyphenidyl, benztropine, hyoscine):

**Scopolamine patch**:

**One percent atropine eye drops** given as 1-2 drops under the tongue per day to dry the mouth. Systemic side effects are much less likely with this local treatment.

**Botulinum toxin A** (Botox) injections into the salivary glands can decrease saliva production. Saliva production is reduced without side effects, except for the thickening of oral mucus secretion. Botox is not always effective, but when it works, the benefit can last for several months before re-injection is necessary. Botulinum toxin should be avoided when oral secretions are already deep and thick.

**Tricyclic antidepressants** such as amitriptyline or nortriptyline commonly cause a dry mouth and can be used to treat excess saliva. Older patients do not always tolerate them.

## Constipation

Constipation occurs in up to two-thirds of Parkinson's disease patients, reducing their quality of life. There is little evidence for a specific intervention in patients with Parkinson's disease, and general principles apply. Increasing dietary fibre, water consumption and physical activity are appropriate. Probiotics and prebiotics may reduce symptom burden with minor risk of side effects. If possible, cease drugs that cause constipation, such as analgesics, anticholinergics, iron supplements, calcium channel blockers and antacids containing aluminium. Hydrophilic organic polymers (including psyllium and bran) are an appropriate next step. When constipation is severe, it may be necessary to use medications such as osmotic agents (lactulose, glycerin, polyethylene glycol), stool softeners (docusate) and short-term use of stimulant laxatives (bisacodyl, coloxyl with senna). [51, 52]

# Excessive Daytime Somnolence

Modafinil should be considered for patients who subjectively experience excessive daytime somnolence.

# Impotence

Sildenafil citrate (Viagra) may be considered to treat erectile dysfunction

# Depression

Depression is common and significantly impacts the quality of life. The tricyclic antidepressants nortriptyline in doses up to 150 mg resulted in substantial improvement in one randomized placebo-controlled trial. It is likely amitriptyline would show a similar benefit. Selective serotonin reuptake inhibitors (SSRIs) have not been subjected to randomized trials, but they have demonstrated efficacy in two large uncontrolled studies. [53, 54]

# Psychosis

medication-induced visual hallucinations are common in patients with advanced Parkinson's disease, necessitating a reduction in the dose. In some patients, atypical antipsychotics such as clozapine or prototyping are required to control psychosis. Olanzapine and risperidone are not recommended. Typical antipsychotics such as largactil, haloperidol, thioridazine and fluphenazine should be avoided as they will exacerbate the symptoms of Parkinson's disease. [54]

| Drug | Daily Dose | Doses/day |
|---|---|---|
| Levodopa/Decarboxylase inhibitor | 150-2,000 mg | Variable 4-12 |
| **Dopamine Agonists** | | |
| Bromocriptine | 1.25-40 mg | 3-4 |
| Cabergoline | 0.5-3 mg | 1 |
| Pramipexole | 0.75-4 mg | 3 |
| Ropinerole | 0.25-4 mg | 1 |
| Rotigotine transdermal patch | 2-16 mg | 1 |
| **Glutamate Antagonist** | | |
| Amantadine | 100-400 mg | 1-4 |
| **Anticholinergics** | | |
| Artane | 1-10 mg | 4 |
| Orphenadrine | 50-300 mg | 2 |
| **COMT Inhibitors*** | | |
| Entacapone | 2000-1600 mg | variable |
| Tolcapone | 100-200 mg | variable |
| Opicapone | 50 mg | variable |

| Drug | Daily Dose | Doses/day |
|---|---|---|
| **MAO-B Inhibitors** | | |
| Selegiline | 5-10 mg | 2 |
| Rasagiline | 1 mg | 1 |
| Safinamide | 50-100 mg | 1 |
| **Adenosine A2A Receptor Antagonist** | | |
| Istradefylline | 20-40 mg | 1 |

**Table J1:** Current drugs used in Parkinson's and their dose. * One tablet of a COMT inhibitor with each dose of levodopa

# References

1.  Verschuur, C.V.M., et al., Randomized Delayed-Start Trial of Levodopa in Parkinson's Disease. *New England Journal of Medicine, 2019. 380(4): p. 315-324.*

2.  Cotzias, G.C., M.H. Van Woert, and L.M. Schiffer, Aromatic amino acids and modification of parkinsonism. *N Engl J Med*, 1967. 276(7): p. 374-9.

3.  Gray, R., et al., Long-term effectiveness of dopamine agonists and monoamine oxidase B inhibitors compared with levodopa as initial treatment for Parkinson's disease (PD MED): a large, open-label, pragmatic randomised trial. *Lancet*, 2014. 384(9949): p. 1196-205.

4.  Del Sorbo, F. and A. Albanese, Levodopa-induced dyskinesias and their management. *J Neurol*, 2008. 255 Suppl 4: p. 32-41.

5.  Pandey, S. and P. Srivanitchapoom, Levodopa-induced Dyskinesia: Clinical Features, Pathophysiology, and Medical Management. *Ann Indian Acad Neurol*, 2017. 20(3): p. 190-198.

6.  Mones, R.J., Absence of Response to Levodopa in Parkinson's Disease. *JAMA*, 1971. 217(9): p. 1245-1245.

7.  Bhatia, K., et al., Guidelines for the management of Parkinson's disease. The Parkinson's Disease Consensus Working Group. *Hosp Med*, 1998. 59(6): p. 469-80.

8.  Pahwa, R., et al., Practice Parameter: treatment of Parkinson disease with motor fluctuations and dyskinesia (an evidence-based review): report of the Quality Standards Subcommittee of the American Academy of Neurology. *Neurology,* 2006. 66(7): p. 983-95.

9.  Verschuur, C.V.M., et al., Randomized Delayed-Start Trial of Levodopa in Parkinson's Disease. *N Engl J Med*, 2019. 380(4): p. 315-324.

10. Davis, G.C., et al., Chronic Parkinsonism secondary to intravenous injection of meperidine analogues. *Psychiatry Res*, 1979. 1(3): p. 249-54.

11. Langston, J.W., et al., Chronic Parkinsonism in humans due to a product of meperidine-analog synthesis. *Science*, 1983. 219(4587): p. 979-80.

12. Hughes, A.J., et al., Subcutaneous apomorphine in parkinson's disease: Response to chronic administration for up to five years. *Movement Disorders*, 1993. 8(2): p. 165-170.

13. Olanow, C.W., et al., Apomorphine sublingual film for off episodes in Parkinson's disease: a randomised, double-blind, placebo-controlled phase 3 study. *Lancet Neurol*, 2020. 19(2): p. 135-144.

14. Margolesky, J. and C. Singer, Extended-release oral capsule of carbidopa-levodopa in Parkinson disease. *Ther Adv Neurol Disord*, 2018. 11: p. 1756285617737728.

15. Wright, B.A. and C.H. Waters, Continuous dopaminergic delivery to minimize motor complications in Parkinson's disease. *Expert Rev Neurother*, 2013. 13(6): p. 719-29.

16. Olanow, C.W., et al., Continuous Subcutaneous Levodopa Delivery for Parkinson's Disease: A Randomized Study. *J Parkinsons Dis*, 2021. 11(1): p. 177-186.

17. Giladi, N., et al., ND0612 (levodopa/carbidopa for subcutaneous infusion) in patients with Parkinson's disease and motor response fluctuations: A randomized, placebo-controlled phase 2 study. *Parkinsonism Relat Disord*, 2021. 91: p. 139-145.

18. Liu, X.D., Y. Bao, and G.J. Liu, Comparison Between Levodopa-Carbidopa Intestinal Gel Infusion and Subthalamic Nucleus Deep-Brain Stimulation for Advanced Parkinson's Disease: A Systematic Review and Meta-Analysis. *Front Neurol*, 2019. 10: p. 934.

19. Karlsborg, M., et al., Duodopa pump treatment in patients with advanced Parkinson's disease. *Dan Med Bull*, 2010. 57(6): p. A4155.

20. Stocchi, F., Use of apomorphine in Parkinson's disease. *Neurol Sci*, 2008. 29 Suppl 5: p. S383-6.

21. Manson, A.J., et al., Intravenous apomorphine therapy in Parkinson's disease: clinical and pharmacokinetic observations. *Brain*, 2001. 124(Pt 2): p. 331-40.

22. Frucht, S., et al., Falling asleep at the wheel: motor vehicle mishaps in persons taking pramipexole and ropinirole. *Neurology*, 1999. 52(9): p. 1908-10.

23. Homann, C.N., et al., Sleep attacks in patients taking dopamine agonists: review. *Bmj,* 2002. 324(7352): p. 1483-7.

24. Weintraub, D., et al., Impulse control disorders in Parkinson disease: a cross-sectional study of 3090 patients. *Arch Neurol*, 2010. 67(5): p. 589-95.

25. Dezsi, L. and L. Vecsei, Monoamine Oxidase B Inhibitors in Parkinson's Disease. *CNS Neurol Disord Drug Targets*, 2017. 16(4): p. 425-439.

26. Borgohain, R., et al., Randomized trial of safinamide add-on to levodopa in Parkinson's disease with motor fluctuations. *Movement Disorders*, 2014. 29(2): p. 229-237.

27. Stocchi, F., et al., A randomized, double-blind, placebo-controlled trial of safinamide as add-on therapy in early Parkinson's disease patients. *Movement Disorders*, 2012. 27(1): p. 106-112.

28. LeWitt, P.A., et al., Adenosine A2A receptor antagonist istradefylline (KW-6002) reduces "off" time in Parkinson's disease: A double-blind, randomized, multicenter clinical trial (6002-US-005). *Annals of Neurology*, 2008. 63(3): p. 295-302.

29. Sako, W., et al., The effect of istradefylline for Parkinson's disease: A meta-analysis. *Sci Rep*, 2017. 7(1): p. 18018.

30. Rascol, O., M. Fabbri, and W. Poewe, Amantadine in the treatment of Parkinson's disease and other movement disorders. *The Lancet Neurology*.

31. Steiger, M.J., et al., The clinical efficacy of oral levodopa methyl ester solution in reversing afternoon "off" periods in Parkinson's disease. *Clin Neuropharmacol*, 1991. 14(3): p. 241-4.

32. Fox, S.H., et al., International Parkinson and movement disorder society evidence-based medicine review: Update on treatments for the motor symptoms of Parkinson's disease. *Mov Disord*, 2018. 33(8): p. 1248-1266.

33. Blair, H.A. and S. Dhillon, Safinamide: A Review in Parkinson's Disease. *CNS Drug*s, 2017. 31(2): p. 169-176.

34. Lyons, K.E. and R. Pahwa, Deep brain stimulation and tremor. *Neurotherapeutic*s, 2008. 5(2): p. 331-8.

35. Marjama-Lyons, J. and W. Koller, Tremor-predominant Parkinson's disease. Approaches to treatment. *Drugs Aging*, 2000. 16(4): p. 273-8.

36. Bond, A.E., et al., Safety and Efficacy of Focused Ultrasound Thalamotomy for Patients With Medication-Refractory, Tremor-Dominant Parkinson Disease: A Randomized Clinical Trial. *JAMA Neurol*, 2017. 74(12): p. 1412-1418.

37. Xu, Y., et al., Safety and efficacy of magnetic resonance imaging-guided focused ultrasound neurosurgery for Parkinson's disease: a systematic review. *Neurosurgical Review*, 2021. 44(1): p. 115-127.

38. Obeso, J.A., et al., Deep-brain stimulation of the subthalamic nucleus or the pars interna of the globus pallidus in Parkinson's disease. *N Engl J Med*, 2001. 345(13): p. 956-63.

39. Lee, D.J., et al., Current surgical treatments for Parkinson's disease and potential therapeutic targets. *Neural Regen Res*, 2018. 13(8): p. 1342-1345.

40. Rughani, A., et al., Congress of Neurological Surgeons Systematic Review and Evidence-Based Guideline on Subthalamic Nucleus and Globus Pallidus Internus Deep Brain Stimulation for the Treatment of Patients With Parkinson's Disease: Executive Summary. *Neurosurgery*, 2018. 82(6): p. 753-756.

41. Deuschl, G., et al., A Randomized Trial of Deep-Brain Stimulation for Parkinson's Disease. *New England Journal of Medicine*, 2006. 355(9): p. 896-908.

42. Li, D., et al., Remotely Programmed Deep Brain Stimulation of the Bilateral Subthalamic Nucleus for the Treatment of Primary Parkinson Disease: A Randomized Controlled Trial Investigating the Safety and Efficacy of a Novel Deep Brain Stimulation System. *Stereotactic and Functional Neurosurgery,* 2017. 95(3): p. 174-182.

43. Cantello, R., R. Tarletti, and C. Civardi, Transcranial magnetic stimulation and Parkinson's disease. *Brain Res Brain Res Rev*, 2002. 38(3): p. 309-27.

44. Keus, S.H., et al., Evidence-based analysis of physical therapy in Parkinson's disease with recommendations for practice and research. *Mov Disord*, 2007. 22(4): p. 451-60; quiz 600.

45. Morris, M.E., C.L. Martin, and M.L. Schenkman, Striding out with Parkinson disease: evidence-based physical therapy for gait disorders. *Phys Ther*, 2010. 90(2): p. 280-8.

46. Antonini, A. and P. Barone, Dopamine agonist-based strategies in the treatment of Parkinson's disease. *Neurol Sci*, 2008. 29 Suppl 5: p. S371-4.

47. Bloem, B.R., M.S. Okun, and C. Klein, Parkinson's disease. *The Lancet*, 2021. 397(10291): p. 2284-2303.

48. Seppi, K., et al., The Movement Disorder Society Evidence-Based Medicine Review Update: Treatments for the non-motor symptoms of Parkinson's disease. *Mov Disord,* 2011. 26 Suppl 3(0 3): p. S42-80.

49. Sethi, K., Levodopa unresponsive symptoms in Parkinson disease. *Movement disorders: official journal of the Movement Disorder Society*, 2008. 23 Suppl 3: p. S521-33.

50. Zesiewicz, T.A., et al., Practice parameter: therapies for essential tremor: report of the Quality Standards Subcommittee of the American Academy of Neurology. *Neurology*, 2005. 64(12): p. 2008-20.

51. Pedrosa Carrasco, A.J., L. Timmermann, and D.J. Pedrosa, Management of constipation in patients with Parkinson's disease. *NPJ Parkinsons Dis*, 2018. 4: p. 6.

52. Selby, W. and C. Corte, Managing constipation in adults. Australian Prescriber, 2010. 33: p. 116-119.

53. Andersen, J., et al., Anti-depressive treatment in Parkinson's disease. A controlled trial of the effect of nortriptyline in patients with Parkinson's disease treated with L-DOPA. *Acta Neurol Scand,* 1980. 62(4): p. 210-9.

54. Miyasaki, J.M., et al., Practice parameter: initiation of treatment for Parkinson's disease: an evidence-based review: report of the Quality Standards Subcommittee of the American Academy of Neurology. *Neurology*, 2002. 58(1): p. 11-7.

# Hypertension is Secondary to, not the cause of Arteriosclerosis

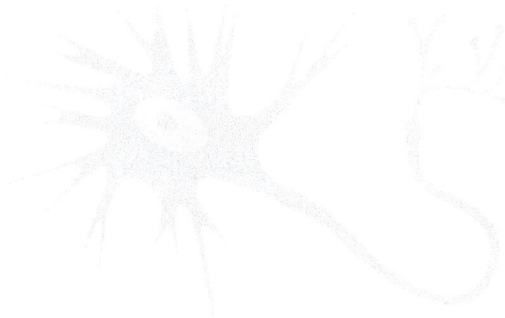

The views expressed here are not, at this point, universally accepted.

This appendix reprints my hypothesis that essential hypertension is the consequence of and not the cause of arteriosclerosis with superimposed atherosclerosis. It is published in Medical Hypotheses 2020:144;110236. The last sentence was not in the original publication.

This hypothesis is based on extensive reading of the literature related to arteriosclerosis and superimposed atherosclerosis.

# Abstract

The arterial system is a closed loop and the pressure within this loop reflects cardiac output, resistance to outflow, volume of fluid within the circulation and stiffness of the arterial wall. Increased resistance to outflow or Bayliss's phenomena cannot be the cause as it reverses with treatment of hypertension. There is no evidence for increased cardiac output in essential hypertension. Increased blood volume contributes to hypertension in obesity just as it does in hypertension due to renal failure. The principal cause of essential hypertension is increasing stiffness of the arterial wall. This is a consequence of arteriosclerosis that commences in utero and that progressively increases in severity with increasing age. Arteriosclerotic arterial wall stiffening antedates the onset of essential hypertension by decades. It not only explains the increasing incidence of essential hypertension with increasing age, but it is the only thing that fulfils Koch's first postulate and that is it is present in 100% of individuals with essential hypertension.

# Introduction

It is almost 400 years since William Harvey[1] inserted a pipe into the carotid artery of a horse and observed the pulsatile nature of blood pressure (BP). Despite centuries of research there is no consensus regarding the aetiology of essential hypertension (EH). Any theory must explain the increasing incidence of EH with increasing age and fulfill Koch's first postulate, it must be present in 100% of cases.

This review details the evidence that stiffening of the arterial wall due to arteriosclerosis antedates the onset of essential hypertension by decades and argues that arteriosclerosis with superimposed atherosclerosis together with a contribution from increased intravascular blood volume in the setting of obesity is the aetiology not the consequence of essential hypertension.

# The Hypothesis

That arteriosclerotic stiffening of the arterial wall with superimposed atherosclerosis is the principal cause, not the consequence of essential hypertension.

# Empirical data

This section examines the evidence for arteriosclerosis being the cause of arterial wall stiffness and then discusses how arterial wall stiffness contributes to increased arterial pressure.

Although symptoms from atherosclerotic vascular disease usually develop years after the onset of hypertension the reason why essential hypertension cannot be the primary cause of arteriosclerosis is because it <u>develops decades before the onset of essential hypertension</u>.

The terms arteriosclerosis and atherosclerosis have often been used interchangeably but they are distinct entities. Arteriosclerosis is thickening of the intima and media together with rupture of the internal elastic lamina without the presence of lipid deposits. Almost certainly the consequence of the physical damage exerted by the pulsatile flow of blood at high pressure in the arteries. Arteriosclerosis is the cause of increased arterial wall stiffness; is present in 100% of individuals to a varying degree and the severity increases with increasing age. Arteriosclerosis can occur in the absence of atherosclerosis, atherosclerosis with the accumulation of lipid deposits in the arterial wall is <u>always</u> superimposed on arteriosclerosis.

The stiffness of the arterial wall is in part due to the failure of the elastic fibres to recoil after being stretched and in part related to thickening of the intima and media. There is overwhelming autopsy evidence that arteriosclerosis, the cause of arterial wall stiffening precedes the onset of essential hypertension by decades. The earliest changes have been documented in stillborn foetuses.[2-4] Changes in the internal elastic lamina are present in the coronary arteries of children at birth.[5] Lesions identical with the early phases of arteriosclerosis in adults occur in the coronary arteries in children and adolescents.[6] Gross evidence of coronary artery arteriosclerosis with superimposed atherosclerosis was detected in 77% of Korean War Veterans with an average age of only 22.1 years.[7] Three percent had completely occluded coronary arteries. Reduced elasticity of the aorta due to the failure of the elastic fibres to recoil and thickening of the intima increases in severity with increasing age. [8] Arteriosclerosis, to a varying degree is present in every individual, [9] Significant atherosclerosis was found in 60-80% of 3,000 subjects aged 15-34 in the Pathobiological Determinants of Atherosclerosis in Youth (PDAY) study and yet only

15.5% had hypertension.[10] Furthermore, other risk factors such as smoking, elevated cholesterol, obesity and impaired glucose tolerance were present in a minority of these individuals.

In addition to post-mortem findings ultrasound has documented increased arterial wall stiffness and endothelial dysfunction in severely obese children aged 4-17 years of age in the absence of hypertension.[11] Increased common carotid artery intima-media thickness and reduced elasticity is present in pre-hypertension.[12]

Having established that worsening arterial wall stiffness precedes the onset of essential hypertension by decades the next question is how does it cause arterial hypertension?

The arterial system is a closed loop. Logically increased pressure within a closed loop <u>can only result</u> from one or more of the following four mechanisms:
- Increased pump pressure (in this case cardiac output)
- Increased volume of fluid within the loop (only possible with non-rigid walls)
- Increased stiffness of the arterial wall and
- Increased resistance to outflow

# Evaluation of the hypothesis

Increased cardiac output cannot be the cause of EH as left ventricular hypertrophy only develops after prolonged and poorly controlled hypertension. It is however, the mechanism in the secondary hypertension of hyperthyroidism,[13] chronic renal failure[14] and Cushing's.[15]

Neither is increased resistance to outflow the explanation. The small arteries and arterioles are the site of altered vascular resistance. This is influenced by several mechanisms; the length of the vessel, sympathetic nerve innervation, increased blood viscosity and the contraction of arterioles as a reflex response to distension, the so-called Bayliss effect.[16] The Bayliss effect essentially controls tissue perfusion and diminishes transmission of high pressures into more fragile blood vessels. Long-standing hypertension precedes the hypertrophy of the vascular smooth muscle. Peripheral resistance diminishes with treatment of hypertension[17,18] implying that resistance to outflow is secondary to and not the cause of hypertension. Peripheral resistance is increased in Cushing's[15], noradrenaline secreting pheochromocytoma[19] and with elevated low-density lipoproteins (LDL) secondary to increased blood viscosity.[20] Drugs such as Phenylephrine hydrochloride, Phenylpropanolamine, Pseudoephedrine hydrochloride and Caffeine all increase peripheral resistance.[21]

This leaves increased blood volume and/or stiffness of the arterial wall as the only plausible explanations for the aetiology of EH.

Increased volume of fluid within the circulatory system contributes to hypertension in obese individuals but cannot be the primary cause as it is not present in 100% of individuals. The blood volume in males and females with a BMI of 25 kg/m² is approximately 4.8 L and 4.7 L respectively. This increases to 6.6 and 6.4 L in morbid obesity (BMI of 45 kg/m²).[22] This increased blood volume exacerbates the hypertension and can resolve with weight loss. The prevalence of hypertension is approximately 20-25% in underweight or normal; 34-38% overweight and 55-65% in obese (class 2 and 3) individuals.[23] Aortic dilation is related to increasing age and obesity as measured by body surface area. This would provide a larger reservoir to accommodate the increased blood volume and why hypertension may not occur in obesity. Obesity influences blood pressure via other mechanisms[24,25] that are not relevant to the current discussion. Increased blood volume contributes to the hypertension seen in chronic renal failure. Typically, pre-dialysis systolic blood pressure is often greater than 160 mm Hg falling by 20-30 mm Hg with the removal of as much as 2 litres of excess fluid during dialysis.[26] Increased intravascular blood volume is also a characteristic of hypertension secondary to drugs such as NSAIDS, Corticosteroids, Danazol, Oral Contraceptives containing oestrogen and progestogen,[21] Cushing's,[15] primary (Conn's syndrome)[27] and secondary hyperaldosteronism[28]

Once established hypertension will create a vicious cycle of worsening arteriosclerosis and increasingly severe hypertension.

Other theories such as sympathetic overactivity, alterations in the renin-angiotensin system, vasoconstriction of the small arteries and arterioles as suggested by Pickering and excess salt consumption do not stand up to scrutiny as none of them fulfil Koch's first postulate nor can they account for the increased incidence of EH with increasing age. Increasing age is associated with reduced salt consumption[29], reduced sympathetic activity[30] and a 50% reduction of plasma renin activity and the aldosterone secretion.[31] Although a recent study suggested that primary hyperaldosteronism may be common on the basis of a lowering of the threshold for the diagnosis it cannot explain the increased incidence with age nor does it fulfil Koch's first postulate.[32]

A further argument against the renin-aldosterone hypothesis is that renin and aldosterone levels are not raised in prehypertension.[33] Against the hypothesis that sympathetic nerve activity is causative is that resting muscle sympathetic nerve activity and plasma noradrenaline levels are similar in both borderline hypertensive and normotensive individuals and do not correlate with blood pressure measurements.[34] Finally there is no evidence that vasoconstriction increases with age.

The evidence and logic presented in this paper justifies the conclusion that essential hypertension is primarily the result of increased stiffness of the arterial wall due to arteriosclerosis and not the reverse. Arteriosclerotic stiffening of the arterial wall both fulfils Koch's first postulate and more importantly is the only mechanism that can explain the increasing incidence of essential hypertension with increased age.

# Consequences of the hypothesis

If this theory is correct, that essential hypertension is the consequence of age-related physical damage to arteries then the only way we can reduce its devastating consequences is through the avoidance of excessive weight gain and excess salt consumption.

The other conclusion is that clinically undetectable atherosclerosis is almost certainly the cause of most if not all cryptogenic strokes.

## References

1.  W. H. Exercitationes de generatione animalium. London: O. Pulleyn; 1651.

2.  Napoli C, D'Armiento FP, Mancini FP, *et al.* Fatty streak formation occurs in human fetal aortas and is greatly enhanced by maternal hypercholesterolemia. Intimal accumulation of low density lipoprotein and its oxidation precede monocyte recruitment into early atherosclerotic lesions. *The Journal of clinical investigation* 1997; 100(11): 2680-90.

3.  Matturri L, Lavezzi AM, Ottaviani G, *et al.* Intimal preatherosclerotic thickening of the coronary arteries in human fetuses of smoker mothers. *J Thromb Haemost* 2003; 1(10): 2234-8.

4.  Milei J, Ottaviani G, Lavezzi AM, *et al.* Perinatal and infant early atherosclerotic coronary lesions. *The Canadian journal of cardiology* 2008; 24(2): 137-41.

5.  Levene CI. Atherosclerosis--disease of old age or infancy? *J Clin Pathol Suppl (R Coll Pathol)* 1978; 12: 165-73.

6.  Moon HD. Coronary arteries in fetuses, infants, and juveniles. *Circulation* 1957; 16(2): 263-7.

7.  Enos WF, Holmes RH, Beyer J. Landmark article, July 18, 1953: Coronary disease among United States soldiers killed in action in Korea. Preliminary report. By William F. Enos, Robert H. Holmes and James Beyer. *Jama* 1986; 256(20): 2859-62.

8.  Wilens SL. The Postmortem Elasticity of the Adult Human Aorta. Its Relation to Age and to the Distribution of Intimal Atheromas. *The American journal of pathology* 1937; 13(5): 811-34.3.

9.  Geiringer E. The Gerontological Aspects of Atheroma: An Approach to a Pathology of Senescence. *British Journal of Social Medicine* 1948; 2: 132-8.

10. Zieske AW, Malcom GT, Strong JP. Natural history and risk factors of atherosclerosis in children and youth: the PDAY study. *Pediatric Pathology & Molecular Medicine* 2002; 21(2): 213-37.

11. Tounian P, Aggoun Y, Dubern B, *et al.* Presence of increased stiffness of the common carotid artery and endothelial dysfunction in severely obese children: a prospective study. *Lancet (London, England)* 2001; 358(9291): 1400-4.

12. Femia R, Kozakova M, Nannipieri M, *et al.* Carotid intima-media thickness in confirmed prehypertensive subjects: predictors and progression. *Arteriosclerosis, thrombosis, and vascular biology* 2007; 27(10): 2244-9.

13. Prisant LM, Gujral JS, Mulloy AL. Hyperthyroidism: a secondary cause of isolated systolic hypertension. *Journal of clinical hypertension (Greenwich, Conn)* 2006; 8(8): 596-9.

14. Kim KE, Onesti G, Schwartz AB, *et al.* Hemodynamics of hypertension in chronic end-stage renal disease. *Circulation* 1972; 46(3): 456-64.

15. Cicala MV, Mantero F. Hypertension in Cushing's syndrome: from pathogenesis to treatment. *Neuroendocrinology* 2010; 92 Suppl 1: 44-9.

16. Bayliss WM. On the local reactions of the arterial wall to changes of internal pressure. *The Journal of physiology* 1902; 28(3): 220-31.

17. Sivertsson R, Hansson L. Effects of blood pressure reduction on the structural vascular abnormality in skin and muscle vascular beds in human essential hypertension. *Clinical science and molecular medicine Supplement* 1976; 3: 77s-9s.

18. Hansson L, Sivertsson R. Regression of structural cardiovascular changes by antihypertensive therapy. *Hypertension (Dallas, Tex : 1979)* 1984; 6(6 Pt 2): III147-9.

19. Zuber SM, Kantorovich V, Pacak K. Hypertension in pheochromocytoma: characteristics and treatment. *Endocrinology and metabolism clinics of North America* 2011; 40(2): 295-311, vii.

20. Sloop GD, Garber DW. The effects of low-density lipoprotein and high-density lipoprotein on blood viscosity correlate with their association with risk of atherosclerosis in humans. *Clinical science (London, England : 1979)* 1997; 92(5): 473-9.

21. Grossman E, Messerli FH. Drug-induced hypertension: an unappreciated cause of secondary hypertension. *The American journal of medicine* 2012; 125(1): 14-22.

22. Nadler SB, Hidalgo JH, Bloch T. Prediction of blood volume in normal human adults. *Surgery* 1962; 51(2): 224-32.

23. Must A, Spadano J, Coakley EH, *et al.* The Disease Burden Associated With Overweight and Obesity. *Jama* 1999; 282(16): 1523-9.

24. Frohlich ED, Messerli FH, Reisin E, *et al.* The problem of obesity and hypertension. *Hypertension (Dallas, Tex : 1979)* 1983; 5(5 Pt 2): Iii71-8.

25. Orr JS, Gentile CL, Davy BM, *et al.* Large Artery Stiffening With Weight Gain in Humans. *Hypertension (Dallas, Tex : 1979)* 2008; 51(6): 1519-24.

26. Passauer J, Petrov H, Schleser A, *et al.* Evaluation of clinical dry weight assessment in haemodialysis patients using bioimpedance spectroscopy: a cross-sectional study. *Nephrol Dial Transplant* 2010; 25(2): 545-51.

27. Conn JW, Cohen EL, Rovner DR. Landmark article Oct 19, 1964: Suppression of plasma renin activity in primary aldosteronism. Distinguishing primary from secondary aldosteronism in hypertensive disease. By Jerome W. Conn, Edwin L. Cohen and David R. Rovner. *Jama* 1985; 253(4): 558-66.

28. Gottam N, Nanjundappa A, Dieter RS. Renal artery stenosis: pathophysiology and treatment. *Expert review of cardiovascular therapy* 2009; 7(11): 1413-20.

29. Loria CM, Obarzanek E, Ernst ND. Choose and prepare foods with less salt: dietary advice for all Americans. *The Journal of nutrition* 2001; 131(2s-1): 536s-51s.

30. Novak V, Lipsitz LA. Aging and the Autonomic Nervous System. In: Robertson D, ed. Primer on the autonomic nervous system 2nd ed; 2004: 191-3.

31. Noth RH, Lassman MN, Tan SY, *et al.* Age and the renin-aldosterone system. *Arch Intern Med* 1977; 137(10): 1414-7.

32. Brown JM, Siddiqui M, Calhoun DA, *et al.* The Unrecognized Prevalence of Primary Aldosteronism. *Annals of internal medicine* 2020.

33. Kotchen TA, Guthrie GP, Jr., Cottrill CM, *et al.* Low renin-aldosterone in "prehypertensive" young adults. *The Journal of clinical endocrinology and metabolism* 1982; 54(4): 808-14.

34. Schobel HP, Heusser K, Schmieder RE, *et al.* Evidence against elevated sympathetic vasoconstrictor activity in borderline hypertension. *Journal of the American Society of Nephrology : JASN* 1998; 9(9): 1581-7.

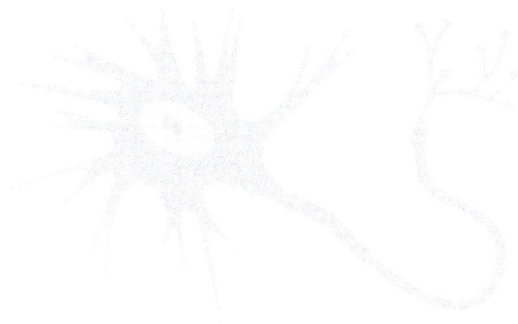

# Hypothesis:
# Could Meniere's be a Channelopathy?

> The views expressed here are not, at this point, universally accepted.

## Abstract

Meniere's disease is a clinical syndrome of uncertain aetiology. Meniere's is believed to be related to endolymphatic hydrops. Clinically, it is a paroxysmal disorder with vertigo and subsequent deafness after repeated attacks. It is sensitive to sodium in the diet and responds to acetazolamide. These are the features of channelopathies. The present paper explores the possibility that Meniere's may be a channelopathy. (Intern Med J 2005; 35: 488–489)

**Key words**: Meniere's, channelopathy, vertigo, acetazolamide, deafness.

Reproduced and modified from: *Internal Medicine Journal* 2005; 35: 488–489

## The Hypothesis

I attended a talk on channelopathies discussing episodic ataxias, hemiplegic migraine and migrainous vertigo. It occurred to me that Meniere's disease has the features of a channelopathy. Like many channelopathies, it is a paroxysmal disorder with attacks precipitated by an ion (in this case sodium) in the diet. Attack frequency is reduced by acetazolamide. After repeated attacks, it results in a permanent deficit, namely deafness.

Meniere's disease is a disease of the inner ear characterized by a triad of symptoms: vestibular and auditory symptoms with a feeling of pressure in the ear. Meniere's disease was initially described by Prosper Meniere in 1861.[1] The course of the disease may be progressive or non-progressive. The age of onset is usually 20–60 years of age, [2] but can occur in childhood.[3]

# appendix L Aetiology of Meneire's

The exact histopathological findings in Meniere's disease are unclear.[4] Damage to the hair cells and the supporting cells within the sensory region of the membranous labyrinth are one of the earliest pathological changes of Meniere's disease and precede neuronal loss. In advanced disease, there is dilatation of the membranous labyrinth with an increase in the endolymph volume relative to the perilymph, termed endolymphatic hydrops. A blinded study comparing histological sections of the sacs from the temporal bones of patients with Meniere's disease with those from controls did not significantly differ in endolymphatic sac fibrosis.[5] Endolymphatic hydrops is not present in all patients with advanced Meniere's disease. Endolymphatic hydrops occurs in the absence of any clinical symptoms.[6] Kiang has suggested that the central dogma of endolymphatic hydrops as the final common pathway is unproven, and that hydrops may be an epiphenomenon.[7]

Inner hair cells have at least two distinct potassium (K+) channels in their basolateral membrane. They also express calcium channels. Outer hair cells have at least three types of K+ channels. In the cochlear, the hair cell channel is KCNQ4. This is a voltage-gated potassium channel expressed prominently in outer hair cells. Mutations result in non-syndromic autosomal dominant, progressive hearing loss.[8] Mutations in two other genes encoding K+ channel subunits, KCNQ1 and KCNE1, have been detected in syndromic hereditary deafness.[8] Deafness is one of the hallmarks of advanced Meniere's disease. Linkage studies in autosomal dominant non-syndromic progressive sensorineural hearing loss have mapped the disease to the DFNA9 locus (DFNA refers to autosomal dominant) on chromosome 14, the COCH gene.[9] Autosomal dominant non-syndromic progressive sensorineural hearing loss is associated with vestibular dysfunction, symptoms consistent with the criteria for Meniere's disease,

Anticipation in familial Meniere's disease (with successive generations there is an earlier age of onset and a tendency to more severe manifestations) has been described and suggests that there may be a trinucleotide expansion as the possible genetic lesion.[10] Trinucleotide repeats have been described with spinocerebellar atrophy [6] and myotonic dystrophy, both channelopathies.[11,12]

Although missense and truncating mutations have been found in familial hemiplegic migraine and episodic ataxia type 2, a unique mutation in the CACNA1A gene, a G-to-A substitution has been identified, resulting in an arginine-to-glutamine change at codon 583 of this calcium channel alpha 1A-subunit. This results in several different phenotypes, including spinocerebellar ataxia (SCA) 6 and familial hemiplegic migraine.[13] Cerebral autosomal dominant arteriopathy with subcortical infarcts and leukoencephalopathy (CADASIL) (where patients experience a high incidence of migraine with aura and prolonged neurological dysfunction) has recently been linked to mutations in the human homolog of the notch3 gene locus that lies in close proximity to the CACNA1A4 Ca2+ channel gene that carries the causative mutation in familial hemiplegic migraine and familial episodic ataxia type-2.[14]

Sensitivity to a dietary ion is seen in channelopathies. Hypokalaemic periodic paralysis is sensitive to sodium and hyperkalaemic periodic paralysis is sensitive to potassium.[15]

Patients with channelopathies are responsive to acetazolamide. [16–19] Acetazolamide reduces the number of attacks of vertigo but does not influence the hearing loss in Meniere's disease. [20] Weller *et al.* have described a patient with CADASIL who had a dramatic reduction in migraine attacks with acetazolamide.[14]

# Conclusion

None of the above discussions proves that Meniere's disease is a channelopathy. I simply raise the concept as a possibility. On the other hand, if this hypothesis is correct, then it may lead to a more effective treatment for a rare but disabling disease. If it *is* a channelopathy, the fact that K+ channel mutations affecting the hair cells have been linked to deafness suggests it may be a K+ channelopathy.

# References

1   Baloh RW. Prosper Meniere and his disease. *Arch Neurol* 2001; 58: 1151–6.

2   da Costa SS, de Sousa LC, Piza MR. Meniere's disease: overview, epidemiology, and natural history. *Otolaryngol Clin North Am* 2002; 35: 455–95.

3   Akagi H, Yuen K, Maeda Y, Fukushima K, Kariya S, Orita Y *et al.* Meniere's disease in childhood. *Int J Pediatr Otorhinolaryngol* 2001; 61: 259–64.

4   Sando I, Orita Y, Hirsch BE. Pathology and pathophysiology of Meniere's disease. *Otolaryngol Clin North Am* 2002; 35: 517–28.

5   Wackym PA, Schuknecht HF, Ward PH, Linthicum FH, Aframian D, Bell T. Blinded controlled study of endolymphatic sac fibrosis in Meniere's disease. In: Filipo R, Barbara M (eds) *Meniere's Disease: Perspectives in the '90s. Proceedings of the* Third International Symposium. Amsterdam: Kugler; 1994: 209–15.

6   Rauch SD, Merchant SN, Thedinger BA. Meniere's syndrome and endolymphatic hydrops. Double-blind temporal bone study. *Ann Otol Rhinol Laryngol* 1989; 98: 873–83.

7   Kiang NYS. *An auditorium physiologist's view of Meniere's syndrome.* In: Nadol JB Jr (ed.) Second International Symposium on Meniere's Disease. Amsterdam: Kugler and Ghedini; 1989: 13–24.

8   Kubisch C, Schroeder BC, Friedrich T, Lutjohann B, El-Amraoui A, Marlin S *et al.* KCNQ4, a novel potassium channel expressed in sensory outer hair cells, is mutated in dominant deafness. *Cell* 1999; 96: 437–46.

9   Fransen E, Verstreken M, Verhagen WI, Wuyts FL, Huygen PL, D'Haese P *et al.* High prevalence of symptoms of Meniere's disease in three families with a mutation in the COCH gene. *Hum Mol Genet* 1999; 8: 1425–9.

10  Fung K, Xie Y, Hall SF, Lillicrap DP, Taylor SA. Genetic basis of familial Meniere's disease. *J Otolaryngol* 2002; 31: 1–4.

11  Frontali M. Spinocerebellar ataxia type 6: channelopathy or glutamine repeat disorder? *Brain Res Bull* 2001; 56: 227–31.

12  Mankodi A, Takahashi MP, Jiang H, Beck CL, Bowers WJ, Moxley RT *et al.* Expanded CUG repeats trigger aberrant splicing of CIC-1 chloride channel pre-mRNA and hyperexcitability of skeletal muscle in myotonic dystrophy. *Mol Cell* 2002; 10: 35–44.

13  Alonso I, Barros J, Tuna A, Coelho J, Sequeiros J, Silveira I *et al.* Phenotypes of spinocerebellar ataxia type 6 and familial hemiplegic migraine caused by a unique CACNA1A missense mutation in patients from a large family. *Arch Neurol* 2003;60: 610–14.

14  Weller M, Dichgans J, Klockgether T. Acetazolamide-responsive migraine in CADASIL. *Neurology* 1998; 50: 1505.

15  Miller TM, Dias da Silva MR, Miller HA, Kwiecinski H, Mendell JR, Tawil R *et al.* Correlating phenotype and genotype in the periodic paralyses. *Neurology* 2004; 63: 1647–55.

16  Lubbers WJ, Brunt ER, Scheffer H, Litt M, Stulp R, Browne DL *et al.* Hereditary myokymia and paroxysmal ataxia linked to chromosome 12 is responsive to acetazolamide. *J Neurol Neurosurg Psychiatry* 1995; 59: 400–5.

17   Zasorin NL, Baloh RW, Myers LB. Acetazolamide–responsive episodic ataxia syndrome. *Neurology* 1983; 33: 1212–14.

18   Pulkes T. Episodic ataxia type 2: an uncommon inherited CNS channelopathies. *J Med Assoc Thai* 2003; 86: 376–80.

19   Jen J. Familial episodic ataxias and related ion channel disorders. *Curr Treat Options Neurol* 2000; 2: 429–31.

20   Corvera J, Corvera G. Long-term effect of acetazolamide and chlorthalidone on the hearing loss of Meniere's disease. *Am J Otolaryngol* 1989; 10: 142–5.

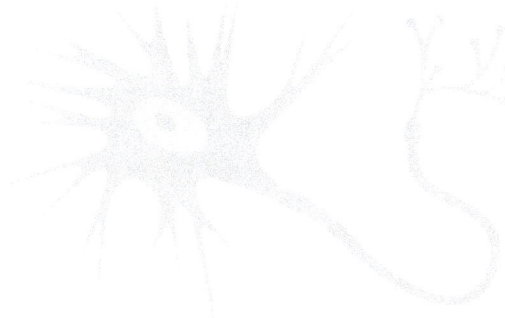

# Insights into the Management of Idiopathic Intracranial Hypertension

The views expressed here are not, at this point, universally accepted.

Idiopathic Intracranial Hypertension (IIH) is a syndrome of raised intracranial pressure (>25cmH$_2$O) with normal CSF and no alternative cause detected by imaging. [1] What triggers the initial rise in CSF pressure is unknown.

The aetiology is unknown. IIH is predominantly but not exclusively seen in pre-menopausal overweight females. The 2015 Cochrane review concluded that there is no current consensus on the best management strategy for IIH. [2]

## The known facts:

1. In IIH, there is a shift of CSF into the cerebral hemispheres resulting in intracellular and extracellular oedema as shown by MRI [3, 4] and brain biopsy. [5]
2. Transverse venous sinus narrowing is secondary to the raised intracranial pressure [6, 7] and thus cannot be the primary cause.
3. Venous sinus stenting [8], regarded as unproven in the current guidelines [9] results in improvement or resolution of the IIH. [10]. This implies that the secondary transverse sinus compression must play a role in perpetuating the problem. A view shared by others. [11, 12]
4. Although the exact mechanism has not been established, a lumbar puncture can lead to a resolution of IIH. [13] In some patients, this occurs when they develop a low-pressure headache, in most resolution occurs in the absence of low-pressure headache.
5. Resolution of IIH occurs in the setting of low-pressure headaches. [14, 15]
6. Lumboperitoneal and ventriculoperitoneal shunts alleviate symptoms when the shunt pressure is set at 15cm H$_2$O.
7. If the shunt is dislodged or blocked, recurrence is almost invariable[16], indicating that shunts do not reverse the pathology.

8. Reversal of transverse sinus compression occurs with an LP-induced CSF pressure reduction. [7, 17, 18] The level of reduction has varied from as low as 8cm $H_2O$ [18] up to 23 cm $H_2O$. [7]

9. Transient opening of the transverse sinuses with a reduced CSF pressure to low levels does not lead to a resolution of IIH. [7, 18]

10. High dose acetazolamide is the recommended treatment in patients who do not respond to an initial lumbar puncture. [19] However, in the NORDIC Idiopathic Intracranial Hypertension Study, although visual function improved, there was no improvement in headache in the treating group compared to the placebo group.

11. One of our patients developed a low-pressure headache in the setting of a malfunctioning shunt necessitating occlusion of the shunt. This patient remained free of symptoms of IIH for ten years when recurrence occurred with significant weight gain.

12. Overnight resolution of IIH is not observed with carbonic anhydrase inhibitors.

# Interpretation of these Facts

Resolution of IIH is possible with either a non-pencil point LP needle induced CSF leak or the insertion of a temporary external lumbar drain.

Patients with IIH who develop a low-pressure headache following a lumbar puncture experience immediate resolution of their IIH symptoms. It is as if a switch has been thrown. A low-pressure headache reflects prolonged drainage of CSF at a rate greater than it is produced, reducing the CSF pressure. This fall in the CSF pressure would eliminate the transverse sinus narrowing (similar to stenting), breaking the vicious cycle and allowing for egress of the CSF from the cerebrum. This mechanism could also explain the resolution of IIH following a lumbar puncture in the absence of a low-pressure headache, where the transverse sinus constriction is relieved at a pressure not low enough to produce a low-pressure headache.

Although lumboperitoneal and ventriculoperitoneal shunts reduce intracranial pressure, relieve the headache, and improve papilloedema, recurrence of symptoms is almost invariable if the shunt is dislodged or blocked. The likely explanation is that the shunts decrease the CSF pressure to approximately 15cm H2O, sufficiently low enough level to relieve symptoms but not low enough to reverse the transverse sinus constriction and break the vicious cycle of raised intracranial pressure.

Resolution of idiopathic intracranial hypertension could be achieved by lowering the CSF pressure to relieve the transverse sinus compression, thus breaking the vicious cycle. The CSF pressure needs to be reduced for long enough to enable egress of CSF out of the cerebrum into the subarachnoid space. This can be achieved with either an LP induced CSF leak using a non-pencil point lumbar puncture needle or insertion of a temporary external lumbar drain. The rate of CSF drainage with a lumbar drain needs to exceed the rate of production in order to reflect what occurs with an LP induced CSF leak causing a low pressure headache.

We have observed immediate (within 72 hours) and sustained resolution of IIH in several patients with the insertion of a temporary lumbar drain. [20-25] Although not subjected to a randomised trial immediate resolution is not a feature of medically treated IIH. One could argue that when a therapy alters the "natural history" of an illness that a randomised trial may not be required.

# References

1. Friedman, D.I., G.T. Liu, and K.B. Digre, *Revised diagnostic criteria for the pseudotumor cerebri syndrome in adults and children. Neurology*, 2013. 81(13): p. 1159-65.

2. Piper, R.J., et al., Interventions for idiopathic intracranial hypertension. *Cochrane Database Syst Rev,* 2015. 2015(8): p. Cd003434.

3. Gideon, P., et al., Increased brain water self-diffusion in patients with idiopathic intracranial hypertension. *American Journal of Neuroradiology*, 1995. 16(2): p. 381.

4. Moser, F.G., et al., MR imaging of pseudotumor cerebri. *AJR Am J Roentgenol*, 1988. 150(4): p. 903-9.

5. Sahs, A.L. and R.J. Joynt, Brain Swelling of Unknown Cause. *Neurology*, 1956. 6(11): p. 791.

6. King, J.O., et al., Manometry combined with cervical puncture in idiopathic intracranial hypertension. *Neurology*, 2002. 58(1): p. 26-30.

7. Buell, T., et al., Transient resolution of venous sinus stenosis after high-volume lumbar puncture in a patient with idiopathic intracranial hypertension. *Journal of Neurosurgery*, 2017. 129: p. 1-4.

8. Higgins, J.N., et al., Venous sinus stenting for refractory benign intracranial hypertension. *Lancet,* 2002. 359(9302): p. 228-30.

9. Mollan, S.P., et al., Evaluation and management of adult idiopathic intracranial hypertension. *Pract Neurol*, 2018. 18(6): p. 485-488.

10. Dinkin, M.J. and A. Patsalides, Venous Sinus Stenting in Idiopathic Intracranial Hypertension: Results of a Prospective Trial. *J Neuroophthalmol*, 2017. 37(2): p. 113-121.

11. De Simone, R., et al., The role of dural sinus stenosis in idiopathic intracranial hypertension pathogenesis: the self-limiting venous collapse feedback-loop model. *Panminerva Med*, 2014. 56(3): p. 201-9.

12. Buell, T., et al., Resolution of venous pressure gradient in a patient with idiopathic intracranial hypertension after ventriculoperitoneal shunt placement: A proof of secondary cerebral sinovenous stenosis. *Surg Neurol Int,* 2021. 12: p. 14.

13. Johnston, I., A. Paterson, and M. Besser, The treatment of benign intracranial hypertension: A review of 134 cases *Surg Neurol,* 1981. 16(3): p. 218-224.

14. Loh, Y., R.J. Labutta, and E.S. Urban, Idiopathic intracranial hypertension and postlumbar puncture headache. *Headache*, 2004. 44(2): p. 170-3.

15. McGonigal, A., I. Bone, and E. Teasdale, Resolution of transverse sinus stenosis in idiopathic intracranial hypertension after L-P shunt. *Neurology*, 2004. 62(3): p. 514-5.

16. Wang, V.Y., et al., Complications of lumboperitoneal shunts. *Neurosurgery,* 2007. 60(6): p. 1045-8; discussion 1049.

17. De Simone, R., et al., Sudden re-opening of collapsed transverse sinuses and longstanding clinical remission after a single lumbar puncture in a case of idiopathic intracranial hypertension. Pathogenetic implications. *Neurol Sci,* 2005. 25(6): p. 342-4.

18. Lee, S.W., et al., Idiopathic intracranial hypertension; immediate resolution of venous sinus "obstruction" after reducing cerebrospinal fluid pressure to<10cmH(2)O. *J Clin Neurosci,* 2009. 16(12): p. 1690-1692.

19. Wall, M., et al., Effect of acetazolamide on visual function in patients with idiopathic intracranial hypertension and mild visual loss: the idiopathic intracranial hypertension treatment trial. *JAMA*, 2014. 311(16): p. 1641-51.

20. Gates, P., P. McNeill, and N. Shuey, Indication to use a non-pencil-point lumbar puncture needle. P*ract Neurol*, 2019. 19(2): p. 176-177.

21. Gates, P. and P. McNeill, A Possible Role for Temporary Lumbar Drainage in the Management of Idiopathic Intracranial Hypertension. *Neuroophthalmology*, 2016. 40(6): p. 277-280.

22. Gates, P.C., et al. Resolution of idiopathic intracranial hypertension with low pressure headache. *Australian New Zealand Association of Neurology*. 2011. Hobart.

515

23. Gates, P.C. Immediate resolution of idiopathic intracranial hypertension with prolonged drainage of CSF at low pressure. in *65th Annual American Academy of Neurology*. March 16-23 2013. San Diego.

24. Gates, P.C., Resolution of idiopathic intracranial hypertension after sustained lowering of cerebrospinal fluid pressure. *World Journal of Neurology*, 2015. 5(1): p. 47-51.

25. Gates, P.C., et al., Low pressure headache not low CSF pressure appears to predict immediate resolution of idiopathic intracranial hypertension (IIH). in *ANZAN Annual Meeting*. 2010: Melbourne.

# List of Videos

To access these videos go to:

www.understandingneurology.com

Click on the heading book and then textbook videos

The above videos and access to a section on common neurological problems not seen in hospitals are free with purchase of the book. A subscription to the website will gain access to further lectures on common neurological problems and intermittent disturbances, over 60 videos of patients with neurological problems covering history taking, the cerebral hemispheres, the brainstem, the upper and lower limbs and over 35 multiple choice questions based on cases seen by Professor Gates in clinical practice (more will be added over time).

# Proof Readers of First Edition

Charles Austin-Woods, BSc(Hons), MBBS
Registrar, Wollongong Hospital, Wollongong, NSW

Cheyne Bester, BSc(Hons)
Benjamin C Cheah, BSc(Hons), BA
Prince of Wales Medical Research Institute, Prince of Wales Clinical School, University of New South Wales, Sydney, NSW

Hsu En Chung, BMedSc, MBBS
Junior Medical Officer, Austin Health, Melbourne, Vic

Richard P Gerraty, MD, FRACP
Neurologist, The Alfred Hospital, Melbourne, Vic, Associate Professor, Department of Medicine, Monash University

Matthew Kiernan, DSc, FRACP
Professor of Medicine – Neurology, University of New South Wales, Consultant Neurologist, Prince of Wales Hospital, Sydney, NSW

Shane Wei Lee, MBBS(Hons), PostGradDip (surgical anatomy)
Resident, Royal Melbourne Hospital, Melbourne, Vic

Michelle Leech, MBBS(Hons), FRACP, PhD
Consultant Rheumatologist, Monash Medical Centre, Associate Professor and Director of Clinical Teaching Programs, Southern Clinical School, Monash University, Melbourne, Vic

Sarah Jensen, BMSc, MBBS
Junior Medical Officer, The Canberra Hospital, ACT

James Padley, PhD, BMedSc(Hons)
4th year medical student, University of Sydney, Sydney, NSW

Claire Seiffert, BPhysio(Hons), MBBS
Junior Medical Officer, Wagga Wagga Base Hospital, Wagga Wagga, NSW

Selina Watchorn, BA, BNurs, MBBS
Junior Medical Officer, The Canberra Hospital, ACT

John Waterston, MD, FRACP
Consultant Neurologist, The Alfred Hospital, Melbourne, Vic, Honorary Senior Lecturer, Department of Medicine, Monash University

# Reviewers of First Edition

**Charles Austin-Woods,** BSc(Hons), MBBS
Registrar, Wollongong Hospital, Wollongong, NSW

**Cheyne Bester,** BSc(Hons)
**Benjamin C Cheah**, BSc(Hons), BA
Prince of Wales Medical Research Institute, Prince of Wales Clinical School, University of New South Wales, Sydney, NSW

**Hsu En Chung**, BMedSc, MBBS
Junior Medical Officer, Austin Health, Melbourne, Vic

**Richard P Gerraty**, MD, FRACP
Neurologist, The Alfred Hospital, Melbourne, Vic, Associate Professor, Department of Medicine, Monash University

**Matthew Kiernan**, DSc, FRACP
Professor of Medicine – Neurology, University of New South Wales, Consultant Neurologist, Prince of Wales Hospital, Sydney, NSW

**Shane Wei Lee**, MBBS(Hons), PostGradDip (surgical anatomy)
Resident, Royal Melbourne Hospital, Melbourne, Vic

**Michelle Leech**, MBBS(Hons), FRACP, PhD
Consultant Rheumatologist, Monash Medical Centre, Associate Professor and Director of Clinical Teaching Programs, Southern Clinical School, Monash University, Melbourne, Vic

**Sarah Jensen**, BMSc, MBBS
Junior Medical Officer, The Canberra Hospital, ACT

**James Padley**, PhD, BMedSc(Hons)
4th year medical student, University of Sydney, Sydney, NSW

**Claire Seiffert**, BPhysio(Hons), MBBS
Junior Medical Officer, Wagga Wagga Base Hospital, Wagga Wagga, NSW

**Selina Watchorn**, BA, BNurs, MBBS
Junior Medical Officer, The Canberra Hospital, ACT

**John Waterston**, MD, FRACP
Consultant Neurologist, The Alfred Hospital, Melbourne, Vic, Honorary Senior Lecturer, Department of Medicine, Monash University

# Extracts Book Reviews First Edition

**Professor Neil Scolding**
Burden Professor of Clinical Neurosciences,
University of Bristol Institute of Clinical Neurosciences, Department of Neurology, Frenchay
Hospital, Bristol BS16 1LE, UK, Pract Neurol 2011; 11: 178–179.

*"…I hesitantly suggest we may be seeing the birth of a new classic educational and training neurology textbook. I recommend it highly.*

*…The next chapter is really quite unusual, entitled 'After the history and examination, what next?' This is not a prosaic list of investigations and when to use them but rather a thoughtful, much broader and to my mind potentially very helpful discussion of strategies and options, depending on the degree of certainty of the doctor and the degree of 'illness' of the patient. Perhaps I should get out more but I have not seen such an account before, and I strongly suspect it would have made a great difference to my own early years in neurology, and could do so for current and future generations."*

---

**Professor Tissa Wijeratne**
Neurologist and Head, Stroke Unit and Research Unit Western Hospital, Melbourne, VIC
*A cure for neurophobia*
MJA 2011 Vol. 194 Issue 4 Pages 193, Demystifying Neurology for Students and Teachers.

*"…this book will help many medical students and young residents come to enjoy neurology as the fascinating subject that it is."*
World Federation of Neurology June 2011

---

**Professor Richard Gerraty**
Epworth HealthCare,Department of Medicine,
Monash University, Richmond, Vic 3121, Australia
Journal of Clinical Neuroscience 2011 Vol. 18 Issue 12 Pages 1749

*"Medical students, hospital medical officers and neurology registrars will benefit from having their own copy of this book and consulting it often and soon reading the whole of it. They will take to this book as it is clear and understandable and so obviously relevant to what they need. For anyone teaching students and resident staff there are many lessons in this book for how to approach the task. Some of the material will date, requiring subsequent editions, but the most important chapters will remain relevant for years and this is a book that will last".*

---

**Professor Michelle. Leech, Rheumatologist**
Monash University, Melbourne, Victoria, Australia
Internal Medicine Journal **40** (2010) 869

*"The result is a text of enormous utility to medical students, postgraduate students and importantly teachers of those students. Non-neurology clinicians would also find this text illuminating. It makes neurology highly accessible and allows any reader to integrate clinically relevant neuroanatomy with clinical neurological presentations in order to make diagnoses confidently."*

# Glossary

**Allodynia**: Hypersensitivity reaction to touch and gentle palpation (allopathia is sometimes used if the hypersensitivity is such as to lead to feelings of burning, electric shocks and excessive pins and needles)

**Amaurosis fugax**: A fleeting loss of vision; if it occurs in one eye it is referred to as monocular amaurosis fugax (carotid territory); if it is bilateral it is vertebrobasilar territory (amaurosis is the Greek word for darkening, dark or obscure; fugax is related to fugitive/fleeing, fleeting or short-lived)

**Amyotrophy**: Progressive wasting of muscle

**Apraxia**: Total or partial loss of the ability to perform coordinated movements or manipulate objects in the absence of motor or sensory impairment

**Aura**: The brief warning that may precede an actual seizure or headache; a peculiar sensation (visual, auditory, somatic or gustatory disturbance) forerunning the appearance of more definite symptoms [1]

**Cerebral infarction**: Loss of brain tissue subsequent to the transient or permanent loss of circulation and/or oxygen delivery to that region of the brain

**Chiari malformation**: Congenital malformation where the cerebellar tonsils protrude through the foramen magnum into the cervical spinal canal

**Circumstantial evidence**: Information in the past, family and social history, that only increases the likelihood of a particular illness, it does not indicate the presence of that diagnosis

**Clonus**: Upper motor neuron sign with repetitive contractions of muscles induced by a sudden movement

**Déjà vu**: The experience of feeling sure that one has witnessed or experienced a new situation previously

**Dermatome**: Area of the skin supplied by a specific spinal nerve root

**Dysaesthesia**: Unpleasant sensation evoked by lightly stroking or touching the skin

**Dysarthria**: Speech disorder in which the pronunciation is unclear although the meaning of what is said is normal

**Dysphagia**: Difficulty swallowing

**Dystonia**: Impairment of the ability to understand and use the symbols of language, both spoken and written

**Epilepsy**: A condition characterised by recurrent seizures

**Erb's point**: A site at the lateral root of the brachial plexus located 2–3 cm above the clavicle

# Glossary

**Foramen magnum**: The opening in the occipital bone at the base of the skull, where the lower aspect of the brainstem becomes the upper aspect of the spinal cord

**Herniation**: Brain tissue, cerebrospinal fluid and blood vessels are moved or pressed away from their usual position in the head, typically down through the tentorium

**Ictus**: Strictly defined as a blow or sudden attack, it is another term used to describe a seizure

**Intracerebral haemorrhage**: Haemorrhage inside the brain

**Jamais vu**: A feeling of unfamiliarity, a sense of seeing the situation for the first time, despite rationally knowing that he or she has been in the situation before

**Lacunar infarction**: Small area of cerebral infarction (diameter 0.2–1.5 cm) related to the occlusion of small arteries (30–300 um)

**Lewy body**: An eosinophilic intracytoplasmic neuronal inclusion

**Ligamentum flavum**: Ligament that connects the lamina of adjacent vertebra, from the axis bone to the first segment of the sacrum

**Likely pathology**: Established by eliciting the exact mode of onset and progression of symptoms

**Lower motor neuron (LMN)**: Signs that indicate involvement of the peripheral nervous system

**Meridians of longitude**: The descending motor pathway and the two ascending sensory pathways. Could also refer to the visual pathway from the eye to the occipital lobe and the vestibular pathway that arises in the inner ear and ends in the brainstem and cerebellum as these are long pathways with different abnormalities along those pathways that indicate the site of the problem

**Myelopathy**: A disorder in which the tissue of the spinal cord is diseased or damaged; a disturbance or disease of the spinal cord

**Myopathy**: Any of several diseases of muscle that are not caused by a disorder of the nerves

**Myositis**: Inflammation of muscle

**Myotome**: The muscles supplied by a particular spinal nerve root

**Myotonia**: Tonic spasm of a muscle, typically seen in myotonic dystrophy where the patient has difficulty relaxing the muscle (e.g. after gripping an object the fingers are peeled slowly off the object)

**Negative predictive value**: Concerned only with negative test results. For any diagnostic test, the positive predictive value will fall as the prevalence of the disease falls while the negative predictive value will rise

**Paraesthesia**: Any subjective sensation, experienced as numbness, tingling or a 'pins-and-needles' feeling

**Parallels of latitude**: The dermatomes, myotomes and reflexes in the limbs, the dermatomes on the trunk, the cranial nerves in the brainstem, the cerebellum and the cortical symptoms and signs in the cerebral hemispheres

**Paraparesis**: Partial weakness affecting the lower limbs

**Paraplegia**: Total weakness of the lower limbs

**Pathognomonic**: A sign or symptom that is so characteristic of a disease that it makes the diagnosis

**Periodic paralysis**: Intermittent episodes of muscle weakness, typically used to refer to the genetic muscle disorders hypokalaemic and hyperkalaemic periodic paralysis, also seen in hyperthyroidism

**Phonophobia**: Increased sensitivity to noise

**Photophobia**: Increased sensitivity to light

**Photopsia**: Perceived flashes of light

**Positive predictive value**: The chance that a positive test result will be correct. For any diagnostic test, the positive predictive value will fall as the prevalence of the disease falls, while the negative predictive value will rise. In practice, since most diseases have a low prevalence, even when the tests we use have apparently good sensitivity and specificity, the positive predictive value may be very low

**Post-ictal**: Period of time immediately after the seizure

**Primary prevention**: Measures taken to reduce the incidence of subsequent cerebral vascular disease before the first symptomatic event

**Quadriparesis**: Partial weakness of all four limbs

**Quadriplegia**: Total weakness of all four limbs, also referred to as tetraparesis

**Radiculopathy**: Dysfunction of a nerve root that can cause weakness or sensory symptoms in a specific pattern corresponding to that nerve root. C, T, L and S are the abbreviations used to refer to the cervical, thoracic, lumbar and sacral regions, respectively. The number of the nerve root is placed after the letter, e.g. C6

**Rhabdomyolysis**: Rapid disintegration of striated muscle tissue accompanied by the excretion of myoglobin in the urine

**Secondary prevention**: Measures taken to reduce the incidence of subsequent cerebral vascular disease after the development of symptoms of cerebral vascular disease

## Glossary

**Seizure**: Sudden change in behaviour due to an abnormal firing of nerve cells in the brain or symptoms of cerebral dysfunction resulting from paroxysmal discharges of neurons involving the cerebral cortex

**Sensitivity**: Indication of how good a test is at correctly identifying people who have the disease

**Specificity**: Indication of how good a test is at correctly excluding people who do not have the condition

**Spondylolisthesis**: Forward dislocation of one vertebra over the one beneath

**Spondylosis**: Degenerative arthritis, osteoarthritis of the spinal vertebrae in which osteophytes (abnormal bone outgrowths) cause a narrowing of the spinal canal and produce compression of the spinal cord and nerve roots

**Subarachnoid haemorrhage (SAH)**: Bleeding within the head into the space between two membranes that surround the brain; the bleeding is beneath the arachnoid membrane and just above the pia mater (the arachnoid is the middle of three membranes around the brain while the pia mater is the innermost one)

**Subdural haemorrhage**: Bleeding within the inner meningeal layer of the dura (the outer protective covering of the brain)

**Subhyaloid haemorrhages**: Dark red, globular swellings around the optic disc that are thought to be caused by rapid venous engorgement secondary to the rapid increase in intracranial pressure that results from the initial subarachnoid haemorrhage

**Tentorium**: Flap of the meninges separating the cerebral hemispheres from the brainstem and cerebellum in the posterior fossa

**Tone**: Resistance to passive movement, increased with upper motor neuron problems and normal or decreased with lower motor neuron problems

**Transient ischaemic attack (TIA)**: Sudden, focal neurological deficit that lasts for less than 24 hours, presumed to be of vascular origin, and confined to an area of the brain or eye

**Upper motor neuron (UMN)**: Signs that indicate involvement of the central nervous system

**Valsalva**: Forced expiration against a closed glottis, increasing intrathoracic pressure

**Visual obscurations**: Inability to see in a particular part of the visual field for a period of time

**Whiplash**: Injury to the neck (the cervical vertebrae) resulting from rapid acceleration or deceleration

## References

1: *Dorland's medical dictionary*, 31st edn Philadelphia. Elsevier; 2007.
2: *Mosby's Dictionary of Medicine, Nursing & Health Professions*, 2nd Australian and New Zealand Edition. Elsevier; 2009.

# Index

# Index

# Index

# Index

# Index

# Index

# Index

# Index

# Index

# Index

# Index

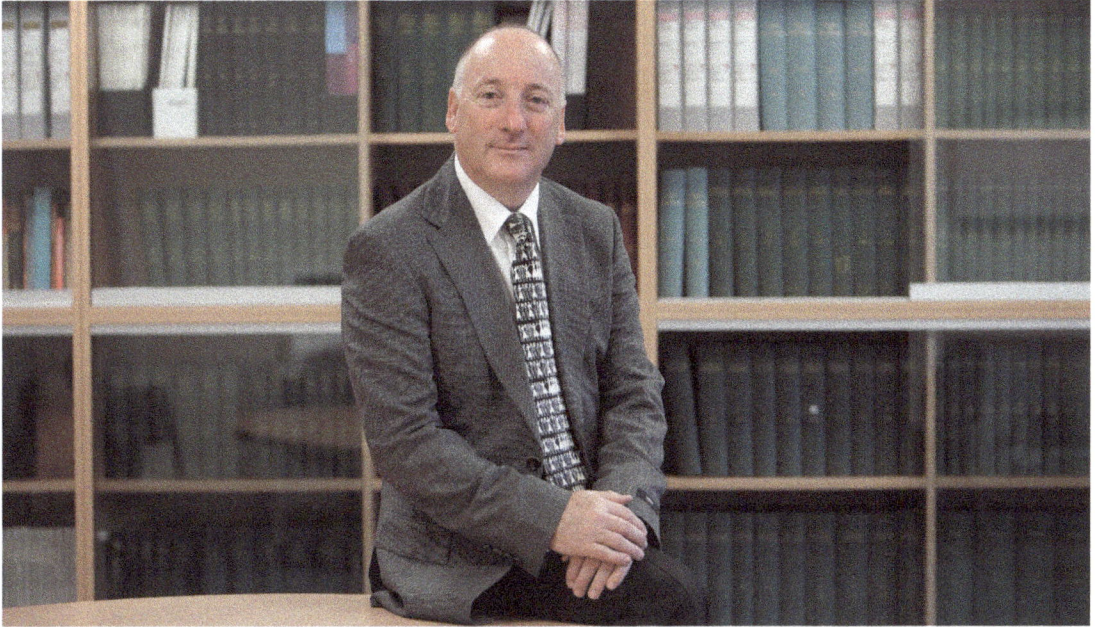

**Peter Gates – Affiliate Professor Deakin University Waurn Ponds and Associate Professor Melbourne University Parkville, Australia Email: prof.petergates@gmail.com**

**1986**

The inaugural most innovative and effective teaching award

Medical Students St Vincent's Hospital Clinical School Melbourne Victoria Australia

**2005 & 2006**

Richard Hallowes Teaching Award Hospital Medical Officers

Barwon Health, Geelong Victoria Geelong Victoria Australia

**2021:** Order of Australia (OAM)

**Website:** http://www.understandingneurology.com/

**10 Formal Powerpoint Presentations**

- History Taking
- Understanding the Brainstem and the Rule of 4
- Cerebral Hemispheres
- Upper Limb (5*3*5 rule)
- Lower Limb (2*2*4 rule)
- Intermittent Disturbances of Neurological Function
- Headache
- Dizziness
- Carpal Tunnel Syndrome
- Ulnar Nerve Lesions

**Plus**

60+ videos of clinical neurology cases, some illustrate the method of history taking, others demonstrate cases involving every single nerve and nerve root lesion in the upper and lower limbs as well as hemisphere and brainstem problems plus 40 multiple choice questions.

A Life-time subscription A$100.00

www.ingramcontent.com/pod-product-compliance
Lightning Source LLC
Chambersburg PA
CBHW052336210326
41597CB00031B/5277